APPLETON & LANGE'S REVIEW FOR THE

PHYSICIAN ASSISTANT

APPLETON & LANGE'S REVIEW FOR THE

PHYSICIAN ASSISTANT

Editors
Patrick J. Cafferty, PA-C
Neurosurgical Associates of Western Kentucky
Paducah, Kentucky

Linford J. Stillson, PA-C
New England College of Osteopathic Medicine
Biddeford, Maine

APPLETON & LANGE
Norwalk, Connecticut/San Mateo, California

Copyright © 1991 by Appleton & Lange
A Publishing Division of Prentice Hall

91 92 93 94 95 / 10 9 8 7 6 5 4 3 2

Prentice Hall International (UK) Limited, *London*
Prentice Hall of Australia Pty. Limited, *Sydney*
Prentice Hall Canada, Inc., *Toronto*
Prentice Hall Hispanoamericana, S.A., *Mexico*
Prentice Hall of India Private Limited, *New Delhi*
Prentice Hall of Japan, Inc., *Tokyo*
Simon & Schuster Asia Pte. Ltd., *Singapore*
Editor Prentice Hall do Brasil Ltda., *Rio de Janeiro*
Prentice Hall, *Englewood Cliffs, New Jersey*

Library of Congress Catologing-in-Publication Data

Appleton & Lange's review for the physician assistant / editors,
    Patrick J. Cafferty. Linford J. Stillson.
        p. cm.
    Includes bibliographical references.
    ISBN 0-8385-0121-4
    1. Physicans' assistants--Examinations, questions, etc.
I. Cafferty, Patrick J. II. Stillson, Linford J. III. Title:
Appleton and Lange's review for the physician assistant
    [DNLM: 1. Physicians' Assistants--examination questions.   W 18
A64943]
R697.P45A67 1991
610.69'53'076--dc20
DNLM/DLC
for Library of Congress   90-14440
                                                                    CIP

Acquisitions Editor: Jamie Mount Sokol

Production Editor: Susan Meiman

PRINTED IN THE UNITED STATES OF AMERICA

Contributors

Joan Alfiero, PA-C
Clinical Coordinator, AIDS Program
Yale New Haven Hospital
New Haven, Connecticut

Mary S. Andresen, MS, PA
Instructor in Pediatrics
Child Health Associate Program
University of Colorado
Denver, Colorado

Deborah Geltman Aragon, MS, PA-C
Instructor in Pediatrics
Child Health Associate Program
University of Colorado
Denver, Colorado

Lynne P. Boldstad, PA-C
Private Practice, Internal Medicine
Oneonta, New York

Patrick J. Cafferty, PA-C
Neurosurgical Associates of Western Kentucky
Paducah, Kentucky

William K. Chapman, PA-C
Private Practice, Internal Medicine
Stockton, California

Mark A. Colloton, MS, PA-C
Instructor in Pediatrics
Child Health Associate Program
University of Colorado
Denver, Colorado

Kevin T. Fitzpatrick, PA-C
Trauma and Surgical Intensive Care Research
Duke University Medical Center
Durham, North Carolina

Robert Howell, PA-C
Private Practice, Nephrology
Bridgeport, Connecticut

Robert Jarski, PhD, PA-C
Associate Professor
Director of Clinical Research Program
School of Health Sciences
Oakland University
Rochester, Michigan

Peter Juergensen, PA-C
Lecturer in Internal Medicine
Yale University School of Medicine
New Haven, Connecticut

Janet Stayer Kozel, PA-C
Private Practice, Psychiatry
Lexington, Kentucky

Lecturer in Psychiatry
University of Kentucky Physician Assistant Program
Lexington, Kentucky

Deborah H. Lawrason, PA-C
Associated Internists of Danbury
Danbury, Connecticut

Janet Rigberg Mayes, PA-C
Department of Surgery
University Hospitals of Cleveland
Cleveland, Ohio

Denyse Mahoney, PA-C
Department of Obstetrics and Gynecology
Booth Memorial Medical Center
Flushing, New York

Mary McClure, PA-C
Newington Childrens Hospital
Newington, Connecticut

Ricky D. Miller, PA-C
Sand Lake Emergency Department
Orlando, Florida

Doris Rapp, PharmD, PA-C
Private Practice, Internal Medicine
Lexington, Kentucky

Associate Professor
University of Kentucky Physician Assistant Program
        and College of Pharmacy
Lexington, Kentucky

William Reynolds, PA-C
Lake Buena Vista Urgent Care
Orlando Regional Medical Center
Orlando, Florida

Linford J. Stillson, PA-C
New England College of Osteopathic Medicine
Biddeford, Maine

Heidemarie Watts, PA-C
Department of Dermatology
Kaiser Permanente HMO
Tucker, Georgia

Patricia Connor Young, MS, PA-C
Instructor in Pediatrics
Child Health Associate Program
University of Colorado
Denver, Colorado

Contents

Preface

The Physician Assistant profession has grown dramatically since its inception at Duke University in 1965, from a handful of Physician Assistants to over 20,000, with an additional 1,200 graduates per year. With growth came the need for standardization and a method of ensuring high quality Physician Assistants for placement. With this goal in mind the National Commission on the Certification of Physician Assistants (NCCPA) was formed with the responsibility of providing a means by which to assess the competence of Physician Assistants and certifying them by the means of a national, standardized test. In addition, the NCCPA offers periodic recertification examinations to ensure Physician Assistants maintain competency.

The first review book for the National Certification Examination was published by ARCO Publishing and came out in 1980. Although the book met with great success, over the past ten years there have been changes in both the content and format of the examination, and the book is now outdated. Presented herein, in an effort to meet the current needs of both the new student and the recertification applicant, is not simply an updated version of the previous edition, but a new book entirely.

The text has been compiled by Physician Assistants from all over the country who are specialists in particular subject areas. We have made every effort to research the appropriate level of material for examination preparation, and have had extensive input from survey information of program directors, new students who have just taken the examination, and recertification applicants. By reviewing old examinations, and applying data from our current survey efforts, we have compiled what we feel is a thorough review book.

The text is organized into three sections. The first section (Chapters 1 and 2) is a discussion of the examination and strategies with which the student may improve performance. We have also included a discussion on the clinical skills problems and provided suggestions for improving performance on this segment of the examination.

The second section of the book (Chapters 3 through 9) contains questions, answers, and explanations divided into subject areas, with information presented in the exact format currently used on the National Certification Examination. The questions have been generated by Physician Assistants who specialize in these fields in an effort to offer both the basic information as well as some of the more advanced materials that might be encountered on the examination. We have organized this section by subject so that the student can concentrate on particular areas of weakness. Answers and detailed explanations are provided, with primary references cited for further study

The third and final section of the text (Chapter 10) is a Practice Examination consisting of 200 questions. This section offers integrated materials similar in format to the current examination. We believe that through careful use of this final section, the student will significantly improve test results by becoming familiar with the examination format.

We wish you the best of luck with the examination. We are confident that this book will prove a useful study tool for you.

Patrick J. Cafferty, PA-C
Linford J. Stillson, PA-C

Acknowledgments

The editors would like to express their sincere appreciation to a number of people, particularly Malcolm Beinfield, MD and Elaine Grant, PA-C for their encouragement in proceeding with this endeavor. In addition, we would like to thank Marilyn Fitzgerald and Vince Grande of the American Academy of Physician Assistants for their help in locating Physician Assistants in various fields of specialty. We would also like to thank the number of Physician Assistant graduates and educators who have provided us with the insight with which we have created this text. We would also like to express our appreciation to the contributing authors for their efforts and particularly Jamie Mount Sokol for her never-ending support throughout this project.

CHAPTER 1

Introduction

This book has been designed as a study aid to review for the Physician Assistant National Certification and Recertification Examination. Here, in one package, is a comprehensive review resource with more than 1000 questions presented in the same format as those seen in the national examinations. Each of these questions is answered with referenced, paragraph-length answers. In addition, the final section of the book is a 200-question practice test for self-assessment purposes. The entire book has been organized by specialty area to help evaluate your areas of relative strength and weakness and further direct your study effort with the available references.

ORGANIZATION

This books is divided into 11 chapters; the first 9 review the major areas of medicine. Chapter 6, Internal Medicine, is subdivided into 10 sections covering its subspecialties. The final chapters are the practice test and master bibliography.

This introduction provides information on question types, methods for using this book, and specific information on the National Certifying and Recertifying Examinations.

QUESTIONS

The National Certifying Examinations contain four different types of questions. In general, about 40% of these are "one best answer—single item" questions; 45% are "multiple true–false or K type", 10% are "one best answer—matching set"; and 5% are "comparison-matching set" questions. In some cases, a group of two or three questions may be related to a situational theme. In addition, some questions have illustrative material (graphs, x-rays, tables) that require understanding and interpretation on your part. Finally, some of the items are stated in the negative. In such instances, we have printed the negative word in capital letters (e.g., "All of the following are correct **EXCEPT**;" "Which of the following choices is **NOT** correct;" and "Which of the following is **LEAST** correct").

One Best Answer—Single Item Question

This type of question presents a problem or asks a question and is followed by five choices, only **one** of which is entirely correct. The directions preceding this type of question will generally appear as below:

DIRECTIONS: Each of the numbered items or incomplete statements in this section is followed by answers or by completions of the statement. Select the <u>ONE</u> lettered answer or completion that is <u>BEST</u> in each case.

An example for this item type follows:

1. An obese 21-year-old woman complains of increased growth of coarse hair on her lip, chin, chest, and abdomen. She also notes menstrual irregularity with periods of amenorrhea. The most likely cause is

   (A) polycystic ovary disease
   (B) an ovarian tumor
   (C) an adrenal tumor
   (D) Cushing's disease
   (E) familial hirsutism

   In this type of question, choices other than the correct answer may be partially correct, but there can only be one *best* answer. In the question above, the key work is "most." Although ovarian tumors, adrenal tumors, and Cushing's disease are causes of hirsutism (described in the stem of the question), polycystic ovary disease is a much more common cause. Familial hirsutism is not associated with the menstrual irregularities mentioned. Thus, the *most* likely cause of the manifestations described can only be "(A)-polycystic ovary disease."

One Best Answer—Matching Sets

These questions are essentially matching questions that are usually accompanied by the following general directions:

DIRECTIONS (Questions 2 through 4): Each group of items in this section consists of lettered headings followed by a set of numbered words or phrases. For each numbered word or phrase, select the ONE lettered heading that is most closely associated with it. Each lettered heading may be selected once, more than once, or not at all.

Any number of questions (usually two to six) may follow the five headings:

Questions 2 through 4

For each adverse drug reaction listed below, select the antibiotic with which it is most closely associated.

 (A) Tetracycline
 (B) Chloramphenicol
 (C) Clindamycin
 (D) Cefotaxime
 (E) Gentamicin

2. Bone marrow suppression
3. Pseudomembranous enterocolitis
4. Acute fatty necrosis of liver

Note that, unlike the single-item questions, the choices in the matching sets questions *precede* the actual questions. As with the single-item questions, however, only **one** choice can be correct for a given question.

DIRECTIONS (Questions 5 and 6): Each group of items in this section consists of lettered headings followed by a set of numbered words or phrases. For each numbered word or phrase, select

 A if the item is associated with (A) only,
 B if the item is associated with (B) only,
 C if the item is associated with both (A) and (B),
 D if the item is associated with neither (A) nor (B).

Any number of questions (usually two to six) may follow the four headings:

Questions 5 and 6

 (A) polymyositis
 (B) polymyalgia rheumatica
 (C) both
 (D) neither

5. Pain is a prominent syndrome
6. Associated with internal malignancy in adults

Note that, as with the other matching-set questions, the choices precede the actual questions. Once again, only **one** choice can be correct for a given question.

Multiple True–False or K-Type Questions
These questions are considered the most difficult (or tricky), and you should be certain that you understand and follow the directions that always accompany these questions:

DIRECTIONS: For each of the items in this section, ONE or MORE of the numbered options is correct. Choose the answer

 (A) if only 1, 2, and 3 are correct.
 (B) if only 1 and 3 are correct.
 (C) if only 2 and 4 are correct.
 (D) if only 4 is correct.
 (E) if all are correct.

This code is always the same (i.e., (D) would never say "if 3 is correct"), and it is repeated throughout this book in a summary box (see below) at the top of any page on which multiple true–false item questions appear.

SUMMARY OF DIRECTIONS				
(A)	**(B)**	**(C)**	**(D)**	**(E)**
1, 2, 3 only	1, 3 only	2, 4 only	4 only	All are correct

A sample question follows:

7. The superficial perineal space contains which of the following?

 (1) crura of the clitoris
 (2) the deep transverse perineal muscle
 (3) the ischiocavernosus muscle
 (4) the anal sphincter

You first need to determine which choices are right and wrong, and then which code corresponds to the correct numbers. In the example above, (A) and (C) are both structures contained in this space, and therefore (B) is the correct answer to this question.

Answers, Explanations, and References
In each of the sections of this book, the question sections are followed by a section containing the answers, explanations, and references for the questions. This section (1) tells you the answer to each question; (2) gives you an explanation and reviews the reason the answer is correct, background information on the subject matter, and the reason the other answers are incorrect; and (3) tells you where you can find more in-depth information on the subject matter in other books and journals. We encourage you to use this section as a basis for further study and understanding.

If you choose the correct answer to a question, you can then read the explanation (1) for reinforcement and (2) to add to your knowledge of the subject matter (remember that the explanations usually tell not only why the answer is correct, but often also why the other choices are incorrect). If you choose the wrong answer to a question, you can read the explanation for an instructional review of the material in the question. Furthermore, you can note the reference cited (e.g., Pritchard, p. 250), look up the complete source in the references at the end of the chapter (e.g., Pritchard, JA: Williams Obstetrics, 19th ed. Norwalk, CT., Appleton & Lange, 1987), and refer to the pages cited for a more in-depth discussion.

Practice Test

The 200-question Practice Test at the end of the book covers and reviews all the topics covered in Chapters 1 through 9. The questions are grouped according to question type (one best answer—single item, one best answer—matching sets, comparison matching sets, then multiple true–false items or type K questions), with the subject areas integrated. Specific instructions for how to take the Practice Test are given later.

The Practice Test is followed by a subspecialty list that will enable you to analyze your areas of strength and weakness and thereby focus your review. For example, by checking off your incorrect answers, you may find that a pattern develops in that you are incorrect on most or all of the pediatric questions. In this case, you could note the references (in the Answers and Explanations section) for your incorrect answers and read those sources. You might also want to purchase a pediatric text or review book to do a much more thorough review. We think you will find this subspecialty list very helpful and we urge you to use it.

HOW TO USE THIS BOOK

There are two logical ways to get the most value from this book. We will call them Plan A and Plan B.

In **Plan A**, you go straight to the Practice Test and complete it according to the instructions given. Using the subspecialty list, analyze your areas of strength and weakness. This will be a good indicator of your initial knowledge of the subject and will help to identify specific areas for preparation and review. You can now use the first nine chapters of the book to help you improve your relatively weak points.

In **Plan B**, you go through Chapters 1 through 9 checking off your answers, and then comparing your choices with the answers and discussions in the book. Once you have completed this process, you can take the Practice Test and see how well prepared you are. If you still have a major weakness, it should be apparent in time for you to take remedial action.

In Plan A, by taking the Practice Test first, you get quick feedback regarding your initial areas of strength and weakness. You may find that you have a good command of the material, indicating that perhaps only a cursory review of the first nine chapters is necessary. This, of course, would be good to know early in your exam preparation. On the other hand, you may find that you have many areas of weakness. In this case, you could then focus on these areas in your review—not just with this book, but also with textbooks.

It is, however, unlikely that you will not study prior to taking the National Boards (especially since you have this book). Therefore, it may be more realistic to take the Practice Test after you have reviewed the first nine chapters (as in Plan B). This will probably give you a more realistic type of testing situation, as very few of us merely sit down to a test without studying. In this case, you will have done some reviewing (from superficial to in-depth), and your Practice Test will reflect this study time. If, after reviewing the first nine chapters and taking the Practice Test, you still have some weaknesses, you can then go back to the first of these chapters and supplement your review with your texts.

SPECIFIC INFORMATION ON THE EXAMINATIONS

The official source for all information on the Certification or Recertification process is the National Commission on Certification of Physician Assistants, Inc. (NCCPA), 2845 Henderson Mill Road, N.E., Atlanta, Georgia 30341. This organization is comprised of representatives from the major organizations of medicine including the American Academy of Physician Assistants and the Association of Physician Assistant Programs. Their function is to formulate and administer the annual certification examination and to provide the means for recertification.

Eligibility requires completion or near completion of a Physician Assistant or Surgeon's Assistant program that is accredited by the American Medical Association's Committee on Allied Health and Accreditation. Details regarding registration are available from the NCCPA.

The examination consists of several portions, the first is the general examination. This is a 200-question examination addressing all aspects of Physician Assistant education including anatomy, physiology, history taking, physical examination, laboratory and radiographic interpretation, as well as treatment modalities. The extended-core written examinations include surgery and primary care. Each of these are 150 questions in length and focus on that specialty. The examinee must choose one of these extended-core exams; however, for an additional fee you may take both extended-core exams. The score of the examination is a composite of your performance on the general and clinical skills portions. Tips for improving your score on the written exam are provided in the next chapter.

CLINICAL SKILLS PROBLEMS

The final component of the National Board Examination is a series of clinical scenarios in which the physician assistant examinee is asked to demonstrate his or her ability to correctly perform a problem-oriented physical examination. The examinee will be provided with three problems. Two of these will be examinations limited to 10-minutes, whereas one will be a 20-minute exam and invariably will involve a neurologic assessment. The examinee is expected to interpret the organ system or systems involved in the scenario and correctly perform a series of physical examination maneuvers related to the potential problems presented in this scenario. There is no requirement of obtaining historical information and there is limited communication between the examinee and the simulated patient. The patient can respond to simple commands, for example, "Does this hurt?" and directions to perform various physical examination maneuvers. The method used for scoring the clinical skills problems is a simple check sheet for the completion both accurately and in appropriate sequence of physical examination maneuvers related to the presenting problem. There are no penalties or point deductions for performing excessive or unwarranted physical examination maneuvers during the allotted time. Hence, the examinee would be best advised to perform all appropriate maneuvers within their allotted time. It is the responsibility of the examinee to provide all equipment appropriate to the examination and this should be assembled far in advance of the examination date. Please see Table 1–1 for a checklist of suggested equipment. A sample clinical scenario would be the following. *A 47-year-old-white female with a history of hypertension develops complaints of lightheadedness and it is noted that she fell to the ground striking her head with a resultant brief loss of consciousness.*

It is clear that this is a complicated presentation involving syncope as well as a closed head injury. The patient would need to be evaluated for her level of consciousness and associated neurologic deficits. In addition, one would need to evaluate the underlying cause of her syncopal episode. This would include evaluation of the carotid vessels for bruits, careful auscultation of the heart for evidence of murmurs or clicks as well as other evidence of cardiac pathology. Care must be taken to also include in your assessment the acquisition of vital signs, a frequently overlooked portion of the physical examination. In this particular patient scenario, one would wish to include checking the orthostatic blood pressure and/or

TABLE 1–1. RECOMMENDED EQUIPMENT

1. Otoscope and opthalmoscope
2. Flashlight or penlight
3. Tongue depressors
4. Ruler and flexible tape measure
5. Thermometer
6. Watch with a second hand
7. Sphygmomanometer
8. Stethoscope
9. Reflex hammer
10. Tuning fork
11. Safety pins
12. Test tubes containing scents and tastes for selected neurologic examination
13. Cotton
14. Paper and pen or pencil

blood pressure in both arms. While conducting the examination, there are occasionally points when you will be observing certain findings, and it would be prudent to talk through the examination both as a reminder to yourself and to help point out to the examiner exactly for what you are looking or listening. This will avoid any misconceptions as to what you might have been observing.

We hope that through careful use of this book whether through plan A or plan B, you find this text a useful and beneficial study guide.

CHAPTER 2

Test-Taking Skills—Tips and Techniques

Robert Jarski

Machine-scorable written exams measure not only medical knowledge but also test-taking skills. Through examples, practice, and explanations, this chapter is designed to help the physician assistant student or graduate use appropriate methods for answering the types of written questions found on standardized board exams. Information on preparing for board exams will also be included.

To pass written board exams, three conditions are generally necessary: (1) knowing about or recognizing the medical information contained in the questions; (2) using appropriate test-taking skills; and (3) avoiding situations that are likely to cause mistakes or impede performance. Test anxiety is an example.

Standardized exams can be intimidating and result in test anxiety. However, remembering that most test questions were created by well-intentioned clinicians can help keep the exam's purpose in perspective. In addition, multiple-choice questions are limited in what they can evaluate; they generally assess only fundamental cognitive knowledge. Test-wise individuals use strategies that enable them to perform their best in responding to questions on fundamental knowledge.

The fact is, written tests—even at their "state-of-the art" best—are crude evaluation devices (Snelbecker, 1985; Maatsch, 1983). Multiple-choice questions cannot reflect a clinician's total fund of medical skills. For example, patient rapport and the mechanics of examining patients are not accurately measured through multiple-choice questions. Multiple-choice questions can, however, successfully measure certain cognitive or knowledge skills. Machine-scored exams have limited assessment capabilities. Test taking is a discrete skill that is different from clinical skills, and expert clinicians are not necessarily expert test takers.

Test takers should master the skill of test taking the same way he or she has mastered the skill of physical examination. This may be accomplished by practicing the methods suggested in this chapter while answering the questions that follow in this text.

This chapter primarily presents information based on objective studies and sound psychological theories of test taking, perception, and recall (Snelbecker, 1985; U.S. Department of Education, 1986; DeCecuo and Crawford, 1974; Carman, 1984; Phipps, 1983). The chapter is organized in four sections: (1) what to do when preparing for the exam; (2) what to do during the exam; (3) illustrative questions; and (4) do's and don'ts that bring together the strategies explained in the previous three sections.

Objectives

In this chapter the student or graduate physician assistant will

1. identify proven techniques from the psychology of learning and educational measurement that will enhance test performance;
2. identify information from testing theory that will help avoid "careless" errors; and
3. practice using clues to help identify correct and incorrect responses to exam questions.

WHAT TO DO WHEN PREPARING FOR THE EXAM

Getting into Practice

To develop test-taking skills, you must actively practice what you will be doing on the test, that is, answering multiple-choice questions. Reading and reviewing texts is rarely enough. To become proficient in suturing wounds, you not only read about suturing, but you practice suturing. Some physician assistants have not taken a written exam in weeks, months, or years. Do not attempt to sit for board exams without practicing answering multiple-choice questions any sooner than you would suture a facial laceration without having sutured skin in weeks, months, or years. Responding to questions similar to those encountered on the boards is invaluable for exam preparation. The present text is designed for this purpose.

Areas to Emphasize

Direct your studying to the primary care areas with which you are least familiar. Although you may enjoy studying the areas relating directly to your practice, the task at hand is to pass the boards. This is best accomplished by achieving a fundamental knowledge of each medical discipline appearing on the exam.

Write several of your own test questions—those who do so frequently comment that their questions were surprisingly similar to those on the boards. This is probably so because only a limited amount of knowledge is amenable to the written exam format. In addition to identifying clinical information that is likely to be tested, you will gain valuable insight into the logic of test item construction that in turn helps in selecting correct answers.

Scheduling Preparation Time

Using a calendar, schedule specific periods for test preparation, setting aside specific times for reviewing and answering multiple-choice questions. Regular preparation over several months is preferred to cramming; studying just before the exam is usually nonproductive.

For the recertification exam, the amount of preparation needed depends largely upon your practice setting. If your knowledge in primary care family medicine is current, you probably need less preparation than a physician assistant in a subspecialty practice. Although an attempt is made to compare a physician assistant's practice profile to board scores by discipline, primary care knowledge will enhance test performance. A certain knowledge level in primary care is assumed. In addition, preparation in speciality disciplines is encouraged for graduates sitting for speciality board exams.

The usual learning aids, such as the use of mnemonics, are highly recommended. The reader is referred to appropriate references (Carman, 1984; Phipps, 1983) for general information about study skills. The remainder of this chapter will address specific information about the board exams.

WHAT TO DO DURING THE EXAM

Physical Needs

Find a seat with few or no distractions, avoiding places near doorways and thoroughfares. Repeated interference can hinder your test performance. Take your watch in case a clock is not easily visible. Nonsmokers should ascertain through the proctor that they will have a smoke-free environment.

Speak with the proctor about any reasonable and specific needs you may have. Consider the proctor your advocate. He or she is there (usually voluntarily and with pay) to provide a favorable testing environment. It is the proctor's responsibility to provide it.

Consider nutritional and other personal needs. It is recommended that a heavy meal not be eaten within 2 hours prior to the exam. You may wish to bring with you a complex carbohydrate snack, packaged drinks, and other supplies, such as tissues and cough drops. Keep food and drinks handy for breaks if consuming them during the exam is restricted. Get adequate sleep and rest before the exam.

Time Allowance

Before beginning each section of the exam, calculate the amount of time you can spend on each question. Never go over the calculated time limit on your first attempt at each question. If you do not know an answer, come back to it at the end. When calculating your time allotment, allow for a few extra minutes at the end so you can return to skipped items. Your subconscious will process those items while you work on the other questions. Also, hints often appear in other test items.

Time is usually not an obstacle in the board exam; you probably will have more time than needed.

Attitude

During the test, maintain a positive, confident attitude. Remind yourself that you prepared as best you could, and use some other effective techniques such as those described below.

Do not become discouraged by questions you cannot answer. Many test items are, by design, those having been answered incorrectly by a large number of test takers. Test questions having a predetermined discrimination level are retained for use in future exams. If too many test takers answer a particular test item correctly, it is not used again. Therefore, most of the items you will be answering are those that many test takers have failed. So keep in mind that there will be a number of questions you are not expected to answer correctly.

Also be aware that numerous experimental questions are found on most standardized exams. Experimental questions are those being field tested, and they are not counted in your score. Because you do not know which items these are, assume that any absurd question is experimental. Try not to become irate or unnecessarily concerned about any question.

Self-coaching and imaging techniques (Greenberg, 1987; Pelletier, 1977; Hiebert et al, 1983) may be helpful for all test takers. Stress management methods (Greenberg; Benson, 1975; Hiebert et al, 1983) may be especially useful for anxious test takers. Most professional athletes and stage performers master and routinely use these techniques to avoid situations likely to interfere with optimal performance.

These techniques will not bring to mind medical knowledge never encountered, but they may help in retrieving learned information and in avoiding exam errors due to extreme stress. Managing stress generally results in improved concentration and the ability to reason logically. The suggested techniques may be learned through special courses and by consulting appropriate references (Greenberg, 1987; Pelletier, 1977; Benson, 1975; Hiebert et al, 1985). Techniques should be learned and practiced several weeks before the exam and used the day of the exam; certain brief imaging procedures may be used for relaxing and improving concentration during the exam.

Concentration

During the exam, think of nothing except the questions in front of you. When working in the operating room, you concentrate on the operative field. Similarly, give the exam your full, serious, and undivided attention. Problems at work or home should be left at the exam room doorstep; your one and only task during the exam period is to answer questions to the best of your ability.

Test Mechanics

Before beginning each section of the exam, read the directions. Formats could change. Never find yourself having answered an entire section incorrectly because you failed to read the instructions.

You are allowed to mark on the test booklet unless instructed otherwise. It has been found that errors can be minimized by marking your answers in the test booklet, and then marking the machine scorable answer sheet after every 20 to 30 questions. This process varies the task, allows some psychological rest and forces you to periodically check for accuracy in marking the correct item number on the answer sheet.

If you do not know the answer to a question, skip it and continue answering the questions you know. Frequently, you will find clues in other questions that will help you answer those you left blank. In addition, your subconscious will have processed the questions you skipped. It has been found that a great deal of information is stored in memory, but information retrieval is often faulty. Methods such as rest and varying mental tasks enhance retrieval. Come back later to the questions you left blank.

Changing Your Answer

Contrary to some popular misconceptions, if you doubt an answer selection and want to change it, it is suggested that you do so. In numerous studies across disciplines examining thousands of changed responses, answers were changed approximately twice as often from incorrect responses to correct ones (Welch and Leichner, 1988; Fabrey and Case, 1985; Shababudin, 1983). If you really have no idea which response is correct and you find yourself purely guessing, perhaps your first instinct is accurate. However, if you have a reason to change your answer, you will probably change from an incorrect to a correct response.

Answering by Elimination

Selecting your answer by the process of elimination increases the probability of choosing the correct response. Using the stem of the question, form a sentence with each choice provided. Be cautioned against selecting the first answer you think is correct; consider all possibilities before making a final selection.

Most test questions have in common the following anatomic features: (1) one choice is easily recognized as an outlyer and incorrect; (2) two choices appear plausible as either slightly off the topic or the opposite of the correct answer (e.g., artery versus arteriole, left versus right hemithorax); (3) two choices are correct, but one is better than the other.

The test taker's job is to (1) eliminate the outlyer; (2) identify the two plausible choices and reject them after weighing them against the two that are more likely to be correct; and then (3) select the better answer of the remaining two. Similar to a differential diagnosis, this job is accomplished effectively through the process of elimination.

By using the process of elimination, almost anyone can eliminate the outlyer. In doing so, the probability of selecting the wrong answer by guessing alone is decreased by 20%. If the two plausible but incorrect choices are identified, the test taker then has two remaining items and a 50–50 chance of guessing the correct answer.

Always Triage First

On some exams, points for selecting unnecessarily dangerous, invasive, expensive, or potentially harmful choices are tallied separately. On the exam, as in real life, you are allowed very few such errors. Screen each and every question for potentially harmful or invasive choices. Just as patients are triaged, you should similarly triage each test item encountered. There are three question categories that should be identified.

The first is the "friendly" question—the one that assesses your medical knowledge simply by asking for information. The second category includes those questions designed to trap. Unlike the "friendly" question, the item designed to trap has a preconceived attracter or distracter that may catch the test taker off guard. The third type of question is the one containing a potentially harmful choice. It may refer to a treatment, procedure, finding, or diagnosis.

The third category might not be necessarily tricky, but the test item writer had in mind a possible pitfall that must not be selected. This pitfall should be identified in your triaging. As you read each test item, place it into one of the three categories before selecting your answer.

Detailed examples of each question type are presented under the section, "Illustrative Questions."

About Type K Questions

Type K questions are multiple combination, multiple-choice questions. Memorize the following combination schemes before the exam:

Mark A if only 1, 2, and 3 are correct.
Mark B if only 1 and 3 are correct.
Mark C if only 2 and 4 are correct.
Mark D if only 4 is correct.
Mark E if all are correct.

This will avoid confusion and loss of time you could put to better use.

When answering questions, form a sentence using the stem with each foil, as you would with single-answer multiple-choice questions. Mark only those you are *sure* are true or false. Then rule out among answers A through E those that are not possibilities. For example, if you are sure that foil 3 is false, eliminate A, B, and E. By guessing alone, you now have a 50–50 chance of selecting (C) or (D) as the correct answer.

It is especially important to practice using the Type K scheme before the actual exam. In addition, writing several of your own test questions is highly recommended. Valuable insights will be gained by doing so.

Type Ks require that you consider more chance probabilities and answer combinations than single-answer multiple-choice questions. Test takers who learn to play and enjoy the game of answering Type Ks tend to report success. The opposite appears true of those who are hostile toward the format.

Some General Hints

Certain "hints" of test taking apply to most multiple-choice tests. These hints are not, however, as likely to work on standardized exams as on other tests, but they may be useful as a last resort for answering some test items.

The choices "all of the above" or "none of the above" have an increased probability of being correct. If in a single answer multiple-choice question two alternatives mean exactly the same thing, they probably are both incorrect.

Finally, if you must make a pure guess, (C) is most likely the correct choice. The next most likely choice is (B). Board exam test writers try to guard against these probabilities, but the odds might prove useful to you if all else fails.

ILLUSTRATIVE QUESTIONS

You will encounter the following types of questions on board exams. Each example presented illustrates a strategy to help identify correct choices. As always, first triage each question and identify its category.

The Oversimplification

Some questions appear tricky because you think "no question could be this simple!" If you really know the answer to a question, answer it without belaboring or looking for booby traps that are not there. The following is an example.

A 22-year-old woman presents with abdominal pain and fever of 2 days duration. During the digital pelvic exam, she experiences exquisite pain when the cervix is moved. This suggests a diagnosis of

(A) uterine fibroids
(B) vaginitis
(C) peritonitis
(D) cystitis
(E) cervical carcinoma

The foil least likely to cause pain, E, is eliminated. Any of the remaining four are possibilities, but peritonitis of some etiology is usually a safe diagnostic consideration. Do not get bogged down considering the unlikely diagnostic possibilities when an obvious choice is present. The oversimplification in this case was the correct answer, (C).

The Oversimplification That Is Dangerous by Omission.

As always, triage questions for traps. In the following question, the correct choice is an oversimplification that is dangerous by omission.

A painless testicular mass is found in an otherwise normal 38-year-old. Which of the following diagnoses should be pursued?

(A) varicocele
(B) carcinoma
(C) furuncle
(D) torsion
(E) strangulation

Choices C, D, and E are ruled out because they usually are painful. A and B, however, usually are painless. Because of its prognosis if left untreated, a testicular mass should be considered cancer until proven otherwise. Not to do so would be considered a life-threatening omission. Although a simple and obvious component of the self-exam and the primary care exam, the correct choice was (B).

Always screen questions for dangerous or critical choices whether harmful by omission or commission. A potentially harmful choice may present as an oversimplification.

Clues from Logic

Sometimes a logical (and correct) answer is contained in the stem, as shown in the following example.

The diagnosis of congenital hip dislocation is made

(A) in utero
(B) at birth
(C) at 6 weeks of age
(D) at 6 months of age
(E) fluoroscopically

The term "congenital" means "present at birth." This is when the diagnosis of congenital hip dislocation is made. The correct choice was (B).

Clues from Related Areas

Similarly to "Clues from Logic," knowledge about related disciplines can provide additional hints.

An obese 45-year-old woman presents with acute genital pain. Upon examination you find a 2 × 3 cm soft mass in the right labia majora. This is most likely

(A) an inguinal hernia
(B) a femoral hernia
(C) a femoral aneurysm
(D) marked lymphadenopathy
(E) neurofibroma

If the mass were located in the scrotum of an obese man, you would probably not miss the common diagnosis of inguinal hernia. Remembering from developmental anatomy that the labia majora and scrotum are corresponding tissues, (A) would be selected as the correct response, even if the test taker had minimal knowledge about surgical emergencies.

The "Odd" Choice
This test-taking clue is demonstrated by way of two examples. The first example comes from psychiatry.

Which of the following is <u>not</u> a sign of transsexualism?

(A) rejecting one's anatomic sex
(B) sex identity problems during childhood
(C) dressing in clothing of the opposite sex
(D) aversion toward one's own genitalia
(E) sex identity problems during adolescence

Transsexualism is considered pathological because the patient considers a mutilating procedure preferable to living as his/her designated sex. Each choice except (C) implies pathology—rejecting one's own anatomy, sex identity problems, and aversion. The odd choice, (C), has, however, no associated pathology and was the correct response.

The second example follows.

A 65-year-old man complains of burning pain of the distal extremities especially upon exposure to heat. Upon examination, the hands and feet are warm and erythematous. The findings are most consistent with

(A) diabetes mellitus
(B) arteriosclerosis
(C) Raynaud's phenomenon
(D) thromboembolism
(E) erythromelalgia

With the limited amount of information provided in the stem, it is unlikely that you can differentiate precisely among the choices provided. Your only clue is the odd choice. Even if you are unfamiliar with the infrequently seen problem of erythromelalgia, notice that choices A through D are associated with problems causing impaired circulation and cold extremities. "Erythro" or "red" implies increased circulation and warmth. (E), the odd choice among the options provided, was the correct answer.

Qualifying Words
Test-item stems containing qualifying words such as most, more, usually, often, less seldom, few, etc., will sometimes lead you to the correct answer.

You see in the outpatient clinic a 32-year-old man whom you suspect is suffering from alcohol withdrawal. The most likely finding would be

(A) visual hallucinations
(B) auditory hallucinations
(C) fine motor tremors
(D) major motor seizures
(E) autonomic hyperactivity

Any of the above may be seen with alcohol withdrawal. However, fine motor tremors are the most common by far. The stem contains a qualifying word suggesting (C) as the correct choice.

If a qualifying word appears among the choices presented, it deserves special attention. Words such as best,

entirely, completely, always, and all imply that something is always true; words such as worst, never, no, and none imply that something is never true. In clinical practice, always and never are rarely correct.

The Overqualified Choice
To make an answer acceptable, test-item writers sometimes must qualify a choice to the point at which the test taker recognizes the ploy. The following example illustrates the overqualified choice.

In a 66-year-old emphysematous man with a 100 pack-year smoking history, clubbing is most appropriately described as

(A) discoloration
(B) a flattened angle between the dorsal surface of the distal phalanx and the proximal nail
(C) an abnormal inwardly curved nail
(D) a pack-year history
(E) a measurably increased eponychium

The overqualified (lengthy) choice, (B), is likely to be correct, as in this example.

However, remember the "Odd Choice" described above! Sometimes the very short "Odd Choice" is correct. You will recognize this variation because it will be attractively precise and succinct. Having at least some knowledge of the item, you will identify it as accurate.

Strange Terms
Choices containing completely unfamiliar words are likely to be distracters. Do not assume that you somehow missed an important chapter of Harrison's or that there was a gap in your education. If the choice appears completely bizarre, the test-item writer was probably scraping the barrel for a distracter.

On a routine peripheral blood smear from a 13-year-old boy, you see a nucleated cell that is filled with bright red granules and is approximately three times the diameter of a typical red blood cell. This should be recognized as a (an)

(A) Franz–Kulig cell
(B) myelocyte
(C) eosinophil
(D) Olson cell
(E) Kuppler cell

Choices A, D, and E are completely fictitious—the test-item writer obviously did not lack imagination. B is familiar—remember basic anatomy or hematology? However, identifying a myelocyte on the peripherial smear is not basic primary care, which the board exam covers. Hence, physician assistants should recognize the morphology and significance of an eosinophil. The correct response was (C).

"Apple Pie" Choices
There are some responses to which no one would object. Consider the following test question.

When evaluating a 23-year-old woman with vaginal bleeding, the most important clinical information is gained from the

(A) prothrombin time
(B) partial thromboplastin time
(C) CBC and iron studies
(D) physical exam
(E) detailed history

A patient's history provides a clinician's best information and is almost never incorrect. (E) is an "apple pie" choice.

The "apple pie" choice, however, can also be used by test-item writers to set traps.

The most important physical exam component(s) in the emergency evaluation of an unconscious patient is (are)

(A) body symmetry
(B) a carefully performed and prompt neurological exam
(C) the cardiopulmonary exam
(D) vital signs
(E) blood gasses

The initial triage of this question would identify it as a "trap" question because of the critical nature of the scenario combined with an incorrect "apple pie" choice. Blood gasses are promptly dismissed because they are not physical exam components, for which the stem asks. B appears attractive because of its "apple pie" component. Nevertheless, remember your ABCs of emergency care! The correct response was (D).

Hints from Inconsistencies in Terminology

Grammar inconsistencies between the stem and a choice (e.g., tense, number, gender) are usually recognized by expert educational evaluators who screen board exam test questions. You will, therefore, seldom encounter this type of "hint" on board exams, although it will be found more frequently in classroom situations. Hints due to inconsistencies in terminology are more frequent than other types of hints because expert test-item reviewers frequently lack a medical background. Therefore, you may benefit from recognizing inconsistencies in terminology.

A 19-year-old unconscious motorcycle accident victim with suspected multiple trauma is brought to the emergency room. The most significant physical findings usually will result from

(A) undressing the patient
(B) a prompt neurological exam
(C) interviewing the family
(D) interviewing a witness to the accident
(E) all the above

Choices C and D can be excluded because they refer to historical, not physical findings. This also excludes foil E. Because critical, life-saving information across organ systems may be gained from observing the patient, choice (A)

was correct. Similarly, choice E, blood gasses, in the previous example was eliminated because it was inconsistent with the information asked for in the stem.

Rank Orders

When given a list of numbers or other rank orders, the correct response most often occurs somewhere between the extremes, as shown in these examples.

A 17-year-old woman presents with a history of pelvic discomfort during menses. Through questioning, you determine that the amount of blood lost during each cycle is normal. The amount of her blood loss would be approximately

(A) 25 mL
(B) 35 mL
(C) 70 mL
(D) 100 mL
(E) 125 mL

Here is the second example.

In reviewing the chart of a 45-year-old man, you notice a past diagnosis of chronic schizophrenia. To be termed *chronic*, this disorder was present for at least

(A) 3 months
(B) 1 year
(C) 2 years
(D) 3 years
(E) 4 years

Most test-item writers try to bury the correct answer somewhere in the middle. (C) was the correct answer in each example.

As with "Hints from Inconsistencies in Terminology," this clue does not work as often on board exams as it does on classroom tests. Educational evaluators try to randomize the position of correct responses as much as possible. However, when in doubt, it is better to avoid the extremes when presented with rank ordered options.

DO'S AND DON'TS

The following "do's and don'ts" summarize some of the important points made earlier in this chapter.

DO practice what you will be doing during the exam, that is, answering multiple-choice questions. Answering these questions is a skill different from knowing clinical information. Get into practice for answering multiple-choice questions by actually answering them. This is imperative for the clinician who has not taken a multiple-choice exam recently.

DO direct your studying to the primary care areas with which you are least familiar. Passing the boards is best accomplished by achieving a fundamental knowledge level in each medical discipline assessed on the exam.

DO write your own multiple-choice questions (including Type K). Not only will you gain insights into the mechanics of test-item writing and correctly answering questions, but it is likely that the content of many of your items will resemble those of actual board exam questions.

DO get adequate sleep and rest before the exam.

DO relate test questions to your own practice and experience. Test-item writers are people who have derived many test questions from their own clinical experience. What would *you* expect a primary care physician assistant to know? Use this mind set to understand the goal of a question and to keep a positive attitude throughout the exam.

DO change your answer if you have a good reason to do so. You are twice as likely to change from an incorrect response to a correct one. However, if you are only playing a hunch with no information about the topic at all, your first "gut" reaction might be correct.

DO triage each and every question before selecting your answer. Evaluate it as a question designed to (1) test knowledge in a "friendly" way; (2) trap by including common pitfalls; or (3) trap by including potentially dangerous choices. In the first case, the apparent oversimplification is probably the correct choice. In questions designed to trap, beware of the "apple pie" choice—ommission or commission. On the test, as in real clinical life, you cannot afford to make many dangerous errors.

DO use the process of elimination. Your job is to find the single best answer. As with a patient's differential diagnosis, this usually is done by *elimination*. Avoid choosing an answer until after you have considered each choice.

DO read the question stem and combine it with each foil to form a sentence. After doing this, use the process of elimination to arrive at the final answer.

DO mark your answers in the test booklet and transfer them to the machine scorable answer sheet after every 20 to 30 questions. This procedure tends to minimize errors and provide psychological rest.

DO consider the proctor your colleague. He or she is there to support you and to facilitate your best performance on the exam. Expect and demand this kind of treatment.

DO leave items blank if you are not sure of the answer. Return to these items when you finish the rest of the exam or at a time when you gain information from other questions.

DO pace yourself, allowing a calculated amount of time per question. In your time allocation, allow for some extra minutes at the end for returning to items left blank.

DO make educated guesses, if you must guess. Use the information provided in this chapter to help in your decision. By also using your medical knowledge and judgment, your chances will be much improved.

DO be alert for qualifying words such as most, more, usually, often, less seldom, few, etc., which will sometimes lead you to the correct answer.

DO consider choices containing completely unfamiliar words distractors. If the choice appears completely unfamiliar, the answer is probably incorrect.

DO consider "apple pie" choices as probably correct. However, beware that they may also be used to trap.

DO consider choices that are different from the others—the "odd choice." This may involve the choice having the "odd" meaning or the "odd" length—long or short. The overqualified choice is often correct.

DO select item (C) when purely guessing—it is most frequently the correct response on many one-choice only multiple-choice questions. If you can somehow eliminate C as a possibility, (B) is the next most likely choice. This is a "last ditch" strategy that works more often on classroom tests than on board exams.

DO select "all the above" or "none of the above" as a last ditch strategy. When appearing as choices, they are likely to be correct.

DO read all instructions for each section of the exam. Be aware of any change in format.

DO use the hints in this chapter pertaining to single-answer multiple-choice questions for answering Type K questions. As with other formats on the board exam, triage each item and beware of dangerous or potentially harmful responses—choosing even a few incorrectly may result in failing the exam.

DO avoid situations that might put you in an unfavorable mindset before the exam. For example, if you anticipate heavy highway traffic, arrive at the exam site a day early. If disturbances bother you during an exam, come early and select a seat in a far corner of the testing room. Let nothing interfere with your best possible performance on the day of the exam.

DO consider taking the exam a positive experience. Keep your motivation high through self-coaching and imaging techniques. Use recommended stress management techniques, especially if you are anxious when taking tests.

DO plan to reward yourself for a good performance after the exam. This facilitates a positive attitude.

DON'T cram at the last minute. This kind of preparation will not be adequate for an exam that covers mostly primary care breadth rather than depth.

DON'T eat a large meal within 2 hours of the beginning of the exam. Be well nourished, but not full.

DON'T think of anything except the exam in front of you. Think of it as your "operative field." Concentrate on giving your best possible performance.

DON'T become irate over seemingly absurd questions. Answer them to the best of your ability, realizing that they probably are experimental questions that will not affect your score. Other test takers probably will also consider them absurd.

DON'T guess randomly. Even if you are completely unsure of the answer to a question, use the hints suggested in this chapter to increase the probability of "guessing" the correct response. Make educated, not random guesses.

DON'T leave any item blank at the end of the exam. Unanswered items generally will be counted wrong. However, it is better to leave an item blank than to choose an incorrect response involving an incorrect dangerous, invasive, or otherwise potentially harmful item.

REFERENCES

Benson H. *The Relaxation Response*. New York: Avon Books; 1975.

Carman RA. *Study Skills: A Student's Guide for Survival*, 2nd ed. John Wiley: New York; 1984.

DeCecco JP., Crawford WR. *The Psychology of Learning and Instruction*, 2nd ed. Englewood Cliffs, NJ: Prentice-Hall; 1974.

Fabrey L, Case SM. Further support for changing multiple-choice answers. *J Med Educ*. June 1985: 488–490.

Greenberg JS. *Comprehensive Stress Management*, 2nd ed. Dubuque, IA: Wm. C. Brown Company Publishers; 1987.

Hiebert B, Cardinal J, Dumka L, Marx RW. Self-instructed relaxation: A therapeutic alternative. *Biofeedback Self-Regul*. December 1983: 601–617.

Maatsch, JL. *The Predictive Value of Medical Speciality Examinations: Final Report*. Washington, D.C.: National Center for Health Services Research, Contract No. HS-02-038-04; 1983.

Pelletier KR. *Mind as Healer, Mind as Slayer*. New York: Dell; 1977.

Phipps R. *The Successful Student's Handbook: A Step-by-Step Guide to Study, Reading and Thinking Skills*. Seattle, WA: University of Washington Press; 1983.

Shababudin SH. Pattern of answer changes to multiple-choice questions in physiology. *Med Educ*. March 1983: 316–318.

Snelbecker GE. *Learning Theory, Instructional Theory and Psychoeducational Design*. Lanham, MD: University Printers of America; 1985.

U.S. Department of Education. *What Works: Research About Teaching and Learning*. Washington, D.C.: U.S. Department of Education; 1986.

Welch J, Leichner P. Analysis of changing answers on multiple-choice examination for nationwide sample of Canadian psychiatry residents. *J Med Educ*. February 1988: 133–135.

CHAPTER 3

Surgery

Patrick J. Cafferty, Linford J. Stillson, Janet Rigberg Mayes

Questions

DIRECTIONS (Questions 1 through 7): Each of the numbered items or incomplete statements in this section is followed by answers or by completions of the statement. Select the ONE lettered answer or completion that is BEST in each case.

1. Which of the following disorders of hemostasis is most commonly seen in the bleeding surgical patient?

   (A) Thrombocytopenia
   (B) Disseminated intravascular coagulopathy (DIC)
   (C) Von Willebrand's disease (Factor VIII)
   (D) Christmas disease (Factor IX)
   (E) Classical hemophilia (Factor VIII)

Questions 2 through 5

Match the following symptoms or signs with the most likely diagnosis

2. lower extremity paresthesias

3. muffled heart sounds

4. fracture of the femur

5. tachycardia and warm skin

   (A) neurogenic shock
   (B) septic shock
   (C) insulin shock
   (D) hypovolemic shock
   (E) cardiogenic shock

6. Which of the following symptoms are **LEAST** likely to be associated with carcinoma of the breast?

   (A) nipple retraction
   (B) erythema or skin discoloration
   (C) skin dimpling
   (D) breast pain
   (E) axillary lymphadenopathy

7. Mammography is indicated

   (A) annually in all women of child-bearing age
   (B) annually in women more than 35 years of age
   (C) at 40 years of age and then annually after the age of 50
   (D) to evaluate a palpable breast mass
   (E) none of the above

DIRECTIONS (Question 8): For each of the items in this section, ONE or MORE of the numbered options is correct. Choose the answer

   A if only 1, 2, and 3 are correct,
   B if only 1 and 3 are correct,
   C if only 2 and 4 are correct,
   D if only 4 is correct,
   E if all are correct.

8. Which of the following is/are of historical importance in evaluating the patient with a breast mass?

   (A) use of oral contraceptives
   (B) age of the first childbirth
   (C) family history of breast cancer
   (D) history of benign breast mass

DIRECTIONS (Questions 9 through 13): Each of the numbered items or incomplete statements in this section is followed by answers or by completions of the statement. Select the ONE lettered answer or completion that is BEST in each case.

9. Diffuse abdominal pain that is "wave-like" and associated with vomiting is most likely

   (A) pancreatitis
   (B) peptic ulcer disease
   (C) appendicitis
   (D) bowel obstruction
   (E) cholelithiasis

10. Abdominal pain that is sudden in onset and severe is **NOT** associated with

    (A) perforated peptic ulcer
    (B) ureteral colic
    (C) biliary colic
    (D) ruptured abdominal aneurysm
    (E) pancreatitis

11. If intestinal obstruction is suspected, then which radiologic procedure is indicated initially?

    (A) barium enema
    (B) abdominal ultrasound
    (C) abdominal CAT scan
    (D) flat and upright abdomen
    (E) upper GI series with small bowel follow through

12. "Pain out of proportion" with physical findings is associated with which diagnosis?

    (A) perforated peptic ulcer
    (B) peritonitis
    (C) mesenteric occlusion
    (D) Crohn's disease
    (E) cecal volvulus

13. Which nervous structure is at greater risk during thyroidectomy?

    (A) cervical sympathetic chain
    (B) recurrent laryngeal nerve
    (C) vagus nerve
    (D) superior laryngeal nerve
    (E) inferior laryngeal nerve

DIRECTIONS (Questions 14 and 15): For each of the items in this section, ONE or MORE of the numbered options is correct. Choose the answer

    A if only 1, 2, and 3 are correct,
    B if only 1 and 3 are correct,
    C if only 2 and 4 are correct,
    D if only 4 is correct,
    E if all are correct.

14. Which of the following might be associated with thyroid carcinoma?

    (1) hoarseness
    (2) dysphagia
    (3) palpable mass
    (4) Delphian node

15. Which factor is most significant as a precursor to thyroid carcinoma?

    (1) family history of medullary thyroid cancer
    (2) history of hyperthyroidism
    (3) irradiation of the neck
    (4) history of goiter

DIRECTIONS (Questions 16 and 17): Each of the numbered items or incomplete statements in this section is followed by answers or by completions of the statement. Select the ONE lettered answer or completion that is BEST in each case.

16. The most useful diagnostic test in the preoperative evaluation of a solid thyroid mass is

    (A) ultrasound
    (B) thyroid function test
    (C) needle aspiration
    (D) radioactive scan
    (E) needle biopsy

17. Which thyroid malignancy has the best prognosis following surgical excision?

    (A) follicular carcinoma
    (B) papillary carcinoma
    (C) medullary carcinoma
    (D) anaplastic carcinoma
    (E) lymphoma

DIRECTIONS (Questions 18 through 21): For each of the items in this section, ONE or MORE of the numbered options is correct. Choose the answer

    A if only 1, 2, and 3 are correct,
    B if only 1 and 3 are correct,
    C if only 2 and 4 are correct,
    D if only 4 is correct,
    E if all are correct.

18. Primary hyperparathyroidism **IS NOT** caused by

    (1) parathyroid adenoma
    (2) hyperplasia of the parathyroid
    (3) carcinoma of the parathyroid
    (4) vitamin D deficiency

19. The most common cause(s) of hypoparathyroidism is/are

    (1) idiopathic
    (2) metastatic carcinoma
    (3) renal failure
    (4) surgery

20. Which of the following is/are branches of the superior mesenteric artery?

    (1) right colic artery
    (2) left colic artery
    (3) middle colic artery
    (4) sigmoid artery

21. Characteristic features of the colon include

    (1) taenia coli
    (2) valvulae conniventes
    (3) haustra
    (4) ligament of Treitz

DIRECTIONS (Questions 22 through 26): Each group of items in this section consists of lettered headings followed by a set of numbered words or phrases. For each numbered word or phrase, select

   A if the item is associated with (A) only,
   B if the item is associated with (B) only,
   C if the item is associated with both (A) and (B),
   D if the item is associated with neither (A) nor (B).

Match the following sign/symptom with the most commonly associated form of colitis

   (A) Crohn's colitis
   (B) ulcerative colitis

22. discontinuous involvement

23. transmural involvement

24. bleeding

25. anal fissures

26. abdominal mass

DIRECTIONS (Questions 27 and 28): Each of the numbered items or incomplete statements in this section is followed by answers or by completions of the statement. Select the ONE lettered answer or completion that is BEST in each case.

27. Antibiotic induced colitis results from overgrowth of

    (A) *Bacteroides fragilis*
    (B) *Escherichia coli*
    (C) *Clostridium tetani*
    (D) *Clostridium dificile*
    (E) *Bacteroides vulgatus*

28. Treatment of pseudomembranous colitis consists of

    (A) steroids
    (B) sulfasalizine
    (C) ampicillin 500 mg PO qid
    (D) vancomycin 500 mg PO qid
    (E) colectomy

DIRECTIONS (Questions 29 through 32): For each of the items in this section, ONE or MORE of the numbered options is correct. Choose the answer

   A if only 1, 2, and 3 are correct,
   B if only 1 and 3 are correct,
   C if only 2 and 4 are correct,
   D if only 4 is correct,
   E if all are correct.

29. Radiographic finding in Crohn's colitis include

    (1) cobblestoning
    (2) fistulization
    (3) stenosis
    (4) calcium deposits

30. Complications of ulcerative colitis include

    (1) toxic megacolon
    (2) hemorrhage
    (3) perforation
    (4) carcinoma

31. Initial treatment of colitis includes

    (1) azulfidine
    (2) ACTH
    (3) prednisone
    (4) surgical resection

32. Surgical management of ulcerative colitis includes

    (1) ileostomy
    (2) abdominoperineal resection
    (3) total colectomy
    (4) regional resection

DIRECTIONS (Questions 33 and 34): Each of the numbered items or incomplete statements in this section is followed by answers or by completions of the statement. Select the ONE lettered answer or completion that is BEST in each case.

33. Bleeding from diverticulosis is

    (A) rare
    (B) indolent
    (C) often the only symptom
    (D) associated with abdominal pain
    (E) never life threatening

34. The diagnostic procedure of choice for massive lower GI bleeding is

    (A) CT scan
    (B) colonoscopy
    (C) barium enema
    (D) Arteriography
    (E) radionucleotide imaging

DIRECTIONS (Question 35): For each of the items in this section, ONE or MORE of the numbered options is correct. Choose the answer

    A if only 1, 2, and 3 are correct,
    B if only 1 and 3 are correct,
    C if only 2 and 4 are correct,
    D if only 4 is correct,
    E if all are correct.

35. Diverticulitis frequently presents as

    (1) pain
    (2) fever
    (3) anorexia
    (4) vomiting

DIRECTIONS (Questions 36 and 37): Each of the numbered items or incomplete statements in this section is followed by answers or by completions of the statement. Select the ONE lettered answer or completion that is BEST in each case.

36. Which is NOT a complication of diverticulitis?

    (A) obstruction
    (B) perforation
    (C) fistula
    (D) carcinoma
    (E) bleeding

37. Which of the following have NO malignant potential?

    (A) Polyposes coli
    (B) tubular adenoma
    (C) villous adenoma
    (D) familial polyposis
    (E) juvenile polyposis

DIRECTIONS (Question 38): For each of the items in this section, ONE or MORE of the numbered options is correct. Choose the answer

    A if only 1, 2, and 3 are correct,
    B if only 1 and 3 are correct,
    C if only 2 and 4 are correct,
    D if only 4 is correct,
    E if all are correct.

38. Indications for hemorrhoidectomy include

    (1) pain
    (2) bleeding
    (3) prolapse
    (4) thrombosis

DIRECTIONS (Question 39): Each of the numbered items or incomplete statements in this section is followed by answers or by completions of the statement. Select the ONE lettered answer or completion that is BEST in each case.

39. Anal fissure is NOT associated with

    (A) Crohn's disease
    (B) tuberculosis
    (C) trauma
    (D) diabetes
    (E) syphilis

DIRECTIONS (Questions 40 through 42): For each of the items in this section, ONE or MORE of the numbered options is correct. Choose the answer

    A if only 1, 2, and 3 are correct,
    B if only 1 and 3 are correct,
    C if only 2 and 4 are correct,
    D if only 4 is correct,
    E if all are correct.

40. Screening for carcinoma of the colon should include

    (1) hemoccult
    (2) barium enema
    (3) colonoscopy
    (4) carcinoembryonic antigen (CEA) titers

41. Esophageal achalasia consists of

    (1) relaxation of lower esophageal sphincter
    (2) absence of esophageal peristalsis
    (3) gastroesophageal reflux
    (4) contraction of lower esophageal sphincter

42. Therapy for esophageal achalasia consists of

    (1) esophagomyotomy
    (2) vagal denervation
    (3) esophageal dilation
    (4) Nissan fundoplication (antireflux procedure)

DIRECTIONS (Question 43): Each of the numbered items or incomplete statements in this section is followed by answers or by completions of the statement. Select the ONE lettered answer or completion that is BEST in each case.

43. The complications of gastroesophageal reflux include all the following EXCEPT

(A) bleeding
(B) Barretts esophagus
(C) esophageal contractures
(D) esophageal ulceration
(E) Mallory Weiss syndrome

DIRECTIONS (Questions 44 and 45): For each of the items in this section, ONE or MORE of the numbered options is correct. Choose the answer

A if only 1, 2, and 3 are correct,
B if only 1 and 3 are correct,
C if only 2 and 4 are correct,
D if only 4 is correct,
E if all are correct.

44. Which of the following are important in the diagnosis of esophageal motility disorders?

(1) manometry
(2) endoscopy
(3) contrast radiography
(4) CT scanning

45. Complications associated with diaphragmatic hernias include

(1) volvulus
(2) obstruction
(3) ischemia
(4) carcinoma

DIRECTIONS (Questions 46 and 47): Each of the numbered items or incomplete statements in this section is followed by answers or by completions of the statement. Select the ONE lettered answer or completion that is BEST in each case.

46. The earliest feature of esophageal carcinoma is

(A) dyspnea
(B) hematemesis
(C) pain
(D) dysphagia
(E) weight loss

47. The main duct emptying the pancreas is

(A) ampulla of Vater
(B) duct of Sylvius
(C) duct of Wirsung
(D) duct of Santorini
(E) ampulla of Laffaye

DIRECTIONS (Questions 48 and 49): For each of the items in this section, ONE or MORE of the numbered options is correct. Choose the answer

A if only 1, 2, and 3 are correct,
B if only 1 and 3 are correct,
C if only 2 and 4 are correct,
D if only 4 is correct,
E if all are correct.

48. The diagnosis of acute pancreatitis is based on

(1) elevated amylase
(2) elevated calcium
(3) history and physical
(4) abdominal radiographs

49. Treatment of pancreatitis consists of

(1) IV fluids
(2) NG suction
(3) Analgesics
(4) exploratory laparotomy

DIRECTIONS (Questions 50 and 51): Each of the numbered items or incomplete statements in this section is followed by answers or by completions of the statement. Select the ONE lettered answer or completion that is BEST in each case.

50. The most common complications of acute pancreatitis is

(A) pseudocyst
(B) abscess
(C) diabetes
(D) steatorrhea
(E) chronic pancreatitis

51. Diagnosis of chronic pancreatitis has been easier with the advent of

(A) CT scan
(B) ultrasound
(C) MRI—magnetic resonance imaging
(D) ERCP—endoscopic retrograde cholecystpancreatography
(E) radionucleotide imaging

DIRECTIONS (Question 52): For each of the items in this section, ONE or MORE of the numbered options is correct. Choose the answer

A if only 1, 2, and 3 are correct,
B if only 1 and 3 are correct,
C if only 2 and 4 are correct,
D if only 4 is correct,
E if all are correct.

52. Classic findings in a patient with chronic pancreatitis might include

(1) diabetes
(2) steatorrhea
(3) weight loss
(4) fever

DIRECTIONS (Question 53): Each of the numbered items or incomplete statements in this section is followed by answers or by completions of the statement. Select the ONE lettered answer or completion that is BEST in each case.

53. Treatment of a pancreatic pseudocyst consists of

(A) observation
(B) total pancreatectomy
(C) endoscopic cannulation and drainage
(D) internal drainage
(E) percutaneous drainage under CT scan

DIRECTIONS (Questions 54 through 56): For each of the items in this section, ONE or MORE of the numbered options is correct. Choose the answer

A if only 1, 2, and 3 are correct,
B if only 1 and 3 are correct,
C if only 2 and 4 are correct,
D if only 4 is correct,
E if all are correct.

54. Symptoms of carcinoma of the pancreas may include

(1) pruritis
(2) epigastric pain
(3) weight loss
(4) jaundice

55. In the Whipple procedure (pancreaticoduodenectomy), which of the following is/are removed?

(1) head of the pancreas
(2) gallbladder
(3) duodenum
(4) spleen

56. Normal splenic function consists of

(1) hematopoiesis
(2) production of tissue thromboplastin
(3) vitamin K synthesis
(4) erythrocyte sequestration

DIRECTIONS (Questions 57 through 61): Each group of items in this section consists of lettered headings followed by a set of numbered words or phrases. For each numbered word or phrase, select the ONE lettered heading that is most closely associated with it. Each lettered heading may be selected once, more than once, or not at all.

Match the following hernias to their definitions

57. strangulated hernia

58. incarcerated hernia

59. direct hernia

60. indirect hernia

61. sliding hernia

(A) an organ is involved in the hernia
(B) unreducible
(C) ischemia
(D) patent tunica vaginalis
(E) Hesselbach's triangle

DIRECTIONS (Question 62): Each of the numbered items or incomplete statements in this section is followed by answers or by completions of the statement. Select the ONE lettered answer or completion that is BEST in each case.

62. The most common type of hernia in females is

(A) indirect hernia
(B) direct hernia
(C) femoral hernia
(D) ventral hernia
(E) spigelian hernia

DIRECTIONS (Question 63): For each of the items in this section, <u>ONE</u> or <u>MORE</u> of the numbered options is correct. Choose the answer

    A if only <u>1, 2, and 3</u> are correct,
    B if only <u>1 and 3</u> are correct,
    C if only <u>2 and 4</u> are correct,
    D if only <u>4</u> is correct,
    E if <u>all</u> are correct.

63. Complications of hernia repair include

    (1) testicular edema
    (2) recurrence
    (3) bleeding
    (4) ilioinguinal nerve damage

DIRECTIONS (Question 64): Each of the numbered items or incomplete statements in this section is followed by answers or by completions of the statement. Select the <u>ONE</u> lettered answer or completion that is <u>BEST</u> in each case.

64. Which of the following is the most common tumor of the brain?

    (A) glioblastoma
    (B) meningioma
    (C) astrocytoma
    (D) metastases
    (E) acoustic neuroma

DIRECTIONS (Question 65): For each of the items in this section, <u>ONE</u> or <u>MORE</u> of the numbered options is correct. Choose the answer

    A if only <u>1, 2, and 3</u> are correct,
    B if only <u>1 and 3</u> are correct,
    C if only <u>2 and 4</u> are correct,
    D if only <u>4</u> is correct,
    E if <u>all</u> are correct.

65. Which is/are symptom(s) of a brain tumor?

    (1) headache
    (2) loss of vision
    (3) seizure
    (4) hemiparesis

DIRECTIONS (Question 66): Each of the numbered items or incomplete statements in this section is followed by answers or by completions of the statement. Select the <u>ONE</u> lettered answer or completion that is <u>BEST</u> in each case.

66. A 29-year-old male presents with complaints of severe low back and leg pain following a sneeze. His pain extends from the buttocks posteriorly to the sole of the foot. On examination you note an absent ankle jerk and weakness of plantar flexion. The most likely diagnosis is

    (A) spinal cord tumor
    (B) S1 radiculopathy
    (C) L5 radiculopathy
    (D) pulled hamstring
    (E) spondylolysis

DIRECTIONS (Questions 67 through 73): For each of the items in this section, <u>ONE</u> or <u>MORE</u> of the numbered options is correct. Choose the answer

    A if only <u>1, 2, and 3</u> are correct,
    B if only <u>1 and 3</u> are correct,
    C if only <u>2 and 4</u> are correct,
    D if only <u>4</u> is correct,
    E if <u>all</u> are correct.

67. Gastric acid secretion is

    (1) increased by vaguely released acetylcholine
    (2) inhibited by secretin (cholecystokinin)
    (3) stimulated by gastrin released from the duodenal mucosa
    (4) inhibited by calcium ions

68. Which of the following enhance, or enhances, the secretion of gastrin?

    (1) the presence of acid in the antrum
    (2) the presence of acid in the duodenum
    (3) sympathetic neural stimulation
    (4) antral distention

69. Which of the following is/are true regarding the digestive functioning of the stomach?

    (1) the antrum plays no role in digestion
    (2) lipase in gastric acid secretions aids in early fat digestion
    (3) salivary amylase activity is enhanced by gastric acid
    (4) pepsin is a pH-dependent enzyme

SUMMARY OF DIRECTIONS				
A	**B**	**C**	**D**	**E**
1, 2, 3 only	1, 3 only	2, 4 only	4 only	All are correct

70. Atrophic gastritis is associated with

    (1) achlorhydria or hypochlorhydria
    (2) pernicious anemia due to chronic gastrointestinal blood loss
    (3) a greater incidence of gastric cancer
    (4) bloody vomitus

71. Which of the following statements about melena are true?

    (1) melena usually indicates upper gastrointestinal tract bleeding
    (2) the tarry color is a result of the production of the acid hematin by the action of gastric acid on hemoglobin
    (3) as little as 50 mL of blood may produce melena
    (4) only blood is capable of producing black stools

72. Which of the following are true regarding proximal gastric ulceration?

    (1) stress is often a precipitating factor
    (2) incidence increases with age
    (3) acid hypersecretion is an associated factor
    (4) in the United States gastric ulcers are much less common than duodenal ulcers.

73. Which of the following would be most likely to decrease gastric acid production?

    (1) parietal cell vagotomy
    (2) antrectomy
    (3) proximal Gastrectomy
    (4) pyloroplasty

DIRECTIONS (Questions 74 through 77): Each of the numbered items or incomplete statements in this section is followed by answers or by completions of the statement. Select the ONE lettered answer or completion that is BEST in each case.

74. The most common abnormal physiologic mechanism of duodenal ulcer formation is

    (A) increased secretion of gastric acid
    (B) rapid gastric emptying
    (C) fasting hypergastrinemia
    (D) hyperpepsinogenemia
    (E) deficient duodenal buffers

75. A 70-year-old female presents with massive melena and associated hypotension which is corrected with IV fluid and blood. Which of the following should be done first to determine the source of gastrointestinal bleeding?

    (A) a lower gastrointestinal barium enema
    (B) Sigmoidoscopy
    (C) colonoscopy
    (D) radionuclide imaging
    (E) selective arteriography

76. A 60-year-old diabetic male presents with a bleeding duodenal ulcer. He is treated with nasogastric suctioning, saline lavage, and blood transfusions as needed. However, he continues to bleed actively and requires more than 12 U of blood in the first 24 hours. Prior to this he was otherwise healthy. The treatment of choice is

    (A) systemic infusion of vasopressin (pitressin)
    (B) angiographic catheterization of the gastroduodenal artery and gel foam embolization
    (C) proximal gastric vagotomy
    (D) oversewing the ulcer, bilateral truncal vagotomy and pyloroplasty
    (E) bilateral truncal vagotomy, antrectomy and Billroth II gastrojejunostomy

77. The treatment of choice for a 50-year-old male with biopsy-documented gastric lymphoma would be

    (A) wide local excision
    (B) chemotherapy
    (C) subtotal gastrectomy and radiotherapy
    (D) subtotal gastrectomy
    (E) radiotherapy

DIRECTIONS (Questions 78 through 82): Each group of items in this section consists of lettered headings followed by a set of numbered words or phrases. For each numbered word or phrase, select the ONE lettered heading that is most closely associated with it. Each lettered heading may be selected once, more than once, or not at all.

For each characteristic below select the disorder with which it is most likely to be associated.

    (A) Gastric ulcer
    (B) Duodenal ulcer
    (C) Stress ulceration
    (D) Chronic gastritis
    (E) Prepyloric ulcer

78. parietal cell antibodies

79. blood group O

80. brought on by ischemia

81. increased risk of cancer

82. cause of gastric outlet obstruction

DIRECTIONS (Questions 83 through 86): For each of the items in this section, ONE or MORE of the numbered options is correct. Choose the answer

A if only 1, 2, and 3 are correct,
B if only 1 and 3 are correct,
C if only 2 and 4 are correct,
D if only 4 is correct,
E if all are correct.

83. Most gall stones contain

   (1) cholesterol
   (2) calcium
   (3) bile pigments
   (4) oxalates

84. Gall stone formation has been associated with

   (1) hemolytic disease
   (2) aortic valve replacement
   (3) use of birth control pills
   (4) Ileal resection

85. Which of the following statements regarding the use of HIDA isotope scans to define gall bladder functions are correct?

   (1) they can be used to define obstruction of the extrahepatic ducts.
   (2) they are seldom effective when the patient's serum bilirubin level is higher than 3.5 mg per 100 mL.
   (3) they are the diagnostic tools of choice for defining acute cholecystitis secondary to cystic duct obstruction
   (4) their toxicity is approximately the same as that of IV cholangiography

86. Which of the following statements regarding sclerosing cholangitis are true?

   (1) it produces a clinical and laboratory picture of extrahepatic jaundice
   (2) it occurs more frequently in males than females
   (3) it has been seen in association with ulcerative colitis
   (4) it is thought to result from trauma during the passage of gall stones

DIRECTIONS (Questions 87 through 92): Each of the numbered items or incomplete statements in this section is followed by answers or by completions of the statement. Select the ONE lettered answer or completion that is BEST in each case.

87. Lithogenic bile is characterized by a low ratio of concentration of

   (A) cholesterol to bile salts
   (B) cholesterol to lecithin and bile salts
   (C) cholesterol to lecithin
   (D) bilirubinate to cholesterol
   (E) lecithin and bile salts to cholesterol

88. The major stimulus for gall bladder emptying is mediated by

   (A) stimulation of the sympathetic system
   (B) release of cholecystokinin
   (C) stimulation of the parasympathetic (vagal) system
   (D) release of secretin
   (E) secretion of hydrochloric acid

89. The treatment of radiolucent gall stones with chenodeoxycholic acid for 2 years results in a complete dissolution in what percentage of patients?

   (A) less than 5%
   (B) 15%
   (C) 25%
   (D) 35%
   (E) greater than 40%

90. In patients with asymptomatic gall stones who were treated without surgery, symptoms developed in

   (A) less than 10%
   (B) 20%
   (C) 30%
   (D) 40%
   (E) 50%

91. A 40-year-old female complains of recurrent postprandial attacks of colicky right upper quadrant pain. Ultrasonography does not demonstrate gall stones. She presently is pain free. The next diagnostic test should be

   (A) flat plate of the abdomen
   (B) oral cholecystography
   (C) HIDA scan
   (D) CT scan of the gall bladder
   (E) percutaneous transhepatic cholangiography (PCT)

92. A 65-year-old male who has previously undergone cholecystectomy presents in the Emergency Room with jaundice, fever, and right upper quadrant abdominal pain. Initial treatment should be

    (A) antibiotics
    (B) endoscopic sphincterotomy
    (C) percutaneous transhepatic drainage
    (D) T-tube decompression of the common bile duct
    (E) emergency exploratory laparotomy

DIRECTIONS (Questions 93 through 96): Each group of items in this section consists of lettered headings followed by a set of numbered words or phrases. For each numbered word or phrase, select the ONE lettered heading that is most closely associated with it. Each lettered heading may be selected once, more than once, or not at all.

    (A) acute cholecystitis
    (B) chronic cholecystitis
    (C) both
    (D) neither

93. cystic duct obstruction

94. empyema

95. requires immediate operation

96. HIDA scan is the specific diagnostic test

DIRECTIONS (Questions 97 through 101): For each of the items in this section, ONE or MORE of the numbered options is correct. Choose the answer

    A if only 1, 2, and 3 are correct,
    B if only 1 and 3 are correct,
    C if only 2 and 4 are correct,
    D if only 4 is correct,
    E if all are correct.

97. Which of the following statements about liver anatomy is/are true?

    (1) the caudate lobe involves both the anatomic right and anatomic left lobes
    (2) the quadrate lobe is within the medial segment of the left lobe
    (3) the left lobe extends to the right of the falciform ligament
    (4) the right lobe is divided into the inferior and superior segments

98. Physiologic functions of the liver include which of the following?

    (1) it is the only site of albumen synthesis
    (2) during fasting it supplies glucose by glycogenolysis and glyconeogenesis

    (3) it is the primary site of cholesterol synthesis
    (4) it actively secretes secondary bile acids

99. Which of the following statements is/are true about the hepatic arterial supply?

    (1) normal arterial anatomy is present in only 50% of persons
    (2) it provides 75% of blood flow to the liver
    (3) it parallels the portal venous system within the liver
    (4) the most common variant is right hepatic artery arising from the gastroduodenal artery

100. Which form or forms of viral hepatitis is/are usually transmitted parenterally?

    (1) hepatitis B
    (2) non-A non-B hepatitis
    (3) delta-associated hepatitis
    (4) hepatitis A

101. Which of the following statements are true regarding non-A non-B hepatitis?

    (1) it rarely leads to cirrhosis even in chronic cases
    (2) it is the most common cause of posttransfusion hepatitis
    (3) previous exposure hepatitis B protects against non-A non-B hepatitis infection
    (4) it results in chronic hepatitis more frequently than hepatitis B

DIRECTIONS (Questions 102 through 107): Each of the numbered items or incomplete statements in this section is followed by answers or by completions of the statement. Select the ONE lettered answer or completion that is BEST in each case.

102. The most common primary tumor site associated with hepatic metastases is

    (A) pancreas
    (B) stomach
    (C) colon
    (D) breast
    (E) lung

103. Which of the following is/are true regarding the treatment of primary hepatocellular carcinoma

    (A) most lesions are amenable to resection with a resulting 5-year survival rate of approximately 30%
    (B) most lesions are NOT amenable to partial resection and are best treated with radiation
    (C) orthotopic liver transplanation has become the treatment of choice

(D) mean survival of untreated patients is 3–4 months from the time of onset of the symptoms

(E) both systemic chemotherapy and hepatic arterial chemotherapy produce a response rate of approximately 60%

104. The demonstration of an elevated level of alpha fetoprotein in the serum of an adult suggests the diagnosis of

(A) metastatic cancer of the liver
(B) primary cancer of the liver
(C) focal nodular hyperplasia of the liver
(D) pyogenic liver abscess
(E) biliary cirrhosis

105. The most common cause of portal hypertension is related to

(A) extrahepatic venous outflow obstruction
(B) intrahepatic portal venous obstruction (presinusoidal)
(C) increased hepatopetal blood flow
(D) extrahepatic portal venous obstruction
(E) intrahepatic–hepatic venous obstruction (postsinusoidal)

106. Which of the following best determines long-term survival following a shunting procedure of an alcoholic patient with cirrhosis of the liver?

(A) control of ascites
(B) a low-protein diet
(C) a low-salt intake
(D) use of lactulose
(E) abstinence from alcohol

107. Which of the following criteria in a patient with alcoholic cirrhosis provides the most acceptable indication for portal systemic shunting with the best chance of survival?

(A) documented varices that have never bled but are large
(B) documented varices that have bled several times in the recent past and have not responded to endoscopic variceal sclerosis
(C) documented acutely bleeding varices that have not stopped after 10 U of transfused blood
(D) large esophageal varices and mild encephalopathy
(E) very high portal pressure discovered during abdominal surgery

DIRECTIONS (Questions 108 through 112): Each group of items in this section consists of lettered headings followed by a set of numbered words or phrases. For each numbered word or phrase, select the ONE lettered heading that is most closely associated with it. Each lettered heading may be selected once, more than once, or not at all.

Select the type of hepatic abscess described best by the following statements

(A) amebic liver abscess
(B) pyogenic liver abscess
(C) both
(D) neither

108. usually single

109. predominately involves the right lobe of the liver

110. the cultures are usually sterile

111. treatment is primarily medical

112. treatment is primarily surgical

DIRECTIONS (Questions 113 through 121): For each of the items in this section, ONE or MORE of the numbered options is correct. Choose the answer

A if only 1, 2, and 3 are correct,
B if only 1 and 3 are correct,
C if only 2 and 4 are correct,
D if only 4 is correct,
E if all are correct.

113. True statements regarding benign tumors of the small bowel include

(1) they are most often found in the ileum
(2) they often produce no symptoms and are difficult to diagnose by either clinical or radiological examination
(3) they most commonly present with bleeding and obstruction
(4) they obstruct the bowel either by encroachment on the lumen or by causing intussusception

SUMMARY OF DIRECTIONS

A	B	C	D	E
1, 2, 3 only	1, 3 only	2, 4 only	4 only	All are correct

114. True statements regarding malignant small bowel tumors include

 (1) carcinoid is the most common malignancy of the small intestine
 (2) they account for 2% of all gastrointestinal malignancies
 (3) 5-year survival is highest with adenocarcinoma followed by lymphoma, and still lower with leiomyosarcoma
 (4) wide resection with regional lymphadenectomy is the preferred operation

115. True statements regarding carcinoid tumors include

 (1) there is a tendency toward multicentricity
 (2) the cell of origin is the Kupffer cell
 (3) prognosis is related to tumor size, location, and histologic pattern
 (4) the rectum is the most common site of origin

116. True statements regarding Meckel's diverticulum include

 (1) they occur in 50% of the population in one form or another
 (2) they are true diverticula
 (3) diverticulitis is the most common complication
 (4) some can be visualized with technetium pertechnetate scans

117. Considering the function of the appendix, which of the following is/are true?

 (1) it is a vestigial organ with no known function
 (2) its immunological function protects against development of colon cancer
 (3) the infantile appendix is the sole source of maturation for the thymus independent lymphocytes.
 (4) it is part of the secretory immune system

118. Which of the following are true in acute appendicitis?

 (1) anorexia is usually present
 (2) pain often begins in the periumbilical area
 (3) obstipation or diarrhea often occur
 (4) vomiting usually precedes pain

119. Which of the following is/are true regarding acute appendicitis in the elderly?

 (1) symptoms and physical findings may be minimal
 (2) it is associated with a high rate of perforation
 (3) perforation often results in diffuse peritonitis
 (4) perforation is associated with a 50% mortality rate

120. Which of the following are true regarding the pathogenesis of acute appendicitis?

 (1) fecaliths are identified in most patients with uncomplicated appendicitis
 (2) fecaliths are more often found with gangrenous appendicitis than with simple appendicitis
 (3) when examined carefully, a congenital narrowing of the appendiceal–cecal junction can frequently be identified.
 (4) luminal obstruction is the most important factor in the development of appendicitis

121. Which of the following regarding the anatomy of the appendix is/are true?

 (1) in the adult the base of the appendix is located in the posteromedial aspect of the cecum below the ileal cecal valve.
 (2) the position of the tip in acute appendicitis is a function of the source of infection
 (3) the Tinea coli form the outer longitudinal muscle layer
 (4) the position of the tip is relatively constant and is approximately under McBurney's point

DIRECTIONS (Questions 122 through 125): Each of the numbered items or incomplete statements in this section is followed by answers or by completions of the statement. Select the ONE lettered answer or completion that is BEST in each case.

122. In the evaluation of a female patient with right lower quadrant pain which of the following should be included in the differential diagnosis?

 (A) twisted ovarian cyst or tumor
 (B) diverticulitis of the sigmoid colon
 (C) ruptured ectopic pregnancy
 (D) epiploic appendagitis
 (E) all of the above

123. Which of the following regarding appendicitis during pregnancy is true?

 (A) may present with right upper quadrant or right flank pain

(B) should initially be treated with antibiotics in an attempt to avoid operation

(C) occurs more frequently than in nonpregnant women

(D) when perforated it is associated with a fetal mortality of 80% and a maternal mortality of 10%

(E) all of the above

124. Which of the following radiological findings are associated with acute appendicitis?

(A) distended loop of small bowel in the right lower quadrant

(B) partial filling of the appendix on barium enema

(C) a gas-filled appendix

(D) a mass effect in the cecum on barium enema

(E) all of the above

125. For which of the following patients would nonoperative treatment of appendicitis be appropriate?

(A) a pregnant woman during her first trimester

(B) a 35-year-old patient with subsiding symptoms and a right lower quadrant mass

(C) an elderly patient with coexisting cardiac disease

(D) a 20-year-old woman with Crohn's disease

(E) none of the above

DIRECTIONS (Questions 126 through 129): For each of the items in this section, ONE or MORE of the numbered options is correct. Choose the answer

A if only 1, 2, and 3 are correct,
B if only 1 and 3 are correct,
C if only 2 and 4 are correct,
D if only 4 is correct,
E if all are correct.

126. Which of the following statements are true regarding serum acid phosphatase in prostatic disease?

(1) acid phosphatase has been useful as a tumor marker in assessing treatment results for prostatic cancer

(2) acid phosphatase may be elevated after rectal examination of a normal prostate.

(3) acid phosphatase that is elevated in a patient with prostatic cancer usually precludes a surgical cure.

(4) acid phosphatase elevations are specific to prostatic cancer

127. A male patient in good health presents with an asymptomatic prostate nodule. Biopsy reveals adenocarcinoma. The metastatic work-up is negative. Which one or more of the following therapies may be appropriate?

(1) transurethral prostate resection (TURP)

(2) radical prostatectomy

(3) orchiectomy

(4) local radiotherapy alone

128. A 30-year-old male presents with a nontender hard testicular lump. Appropriate treatment includes which one or more of the following

(1) determination of serum alpha fetoprotein and human chorionic gonadotropin levels

(2) incisional biopsy via a scrotal incision

(3) orchiectomy via an inquinal incision

(4) incisional biopsy via an inquinal incision

129. An adolescent male presents with a 3-hour history of severe scrotal pain. The examination reveals scrotal swelling and tenderness that does not permit discrete palpation of the epididymis. The best treatment at this point is

(1) heat, scrotal elevation, and antibiotics

(2) manual attempt at detorsion

(3) analgesics and reexamination

(4) surgical exploration

DIRECTIONS (Questions 130 and 131): Each of the numbered items or incomplete statements in this section is followed by answers or by completions of the statement. Select the ONE lettered answer or completion that is BEST in each case.

130. A testicular mass in a 25-year-old would most likely be which of the following

(A) benign tumor

(B) seminoma

(C) teratocarcinoma

(D) choriocarcinoma

(E) embryonal cell carcinoma

131. Urinary tract calculi are most commonly composed of

(A) uric acid

(B) cystine

(C) calcium oxalate

(D) ammonium magnesium phosphate

(E) pure calcium phosphate

DIRECTIONS (Questions 132 through 138): Each group of items in this section consists of lettered headings followed by a set of numbered words or phrases. For each numbered word or phrase, select the ONE lettered heading that is most closely associated with it. Each lettered heading may be selected once, more than once, or not at all.

Questions 132 through 138

Match the type of joint with its appropriate example

(A) elbow
(B) skull sutures
(C) public symphysis

B **132.** fibrous joint

c **133.** fibrocartilaginous joint

A **134.** diarthrodial joint

Questions 135 through 138

Match the following primary shoulder disorders with their appropriate clinical characteristic

(A) pain extending along the proximal humeral groove
(B) unrelenting pain not relieved by change in position
(C) limitation of internal rotation and full abduction
(D) surgical repair may be required

B **135.** subacrominal bursitis

A **136.** bicipital tendonitis

C **137.** supraspinatus tendonitis

D **138.** rotator cuff tear

DIRECTIONS (Questions 139 through 142): Each of the numbered items or incomplete statements in this section is followed by answers or by completions of the statement. Select the ONE lettered answer or completion that is BEST in each case.

139. Physiologic interruption of nerve conduction caused by a transient incomplete or complete paralysis of a peripheral nerve is referred to as

(A) axonopraxia
(B) neuropraxia
(C) axonotmesis
(D) Wallerian degeneration
(E) neurotmesis

140. A tear of the lateral meniscus is best diagnosed by a means of

(A) an accurate history
(B) physical examination
(C) arthroscopy
(D) arthrotomy
(E) arthrography

141. Regarding chondromalacia of the patella, which of the following statements is true?

(A) radiographs show characteristic changes early in the course of the disease
(B) The pain is aggravated by knee flexion, kneeling, and descending stairs
(C) the progressive nature of the disease warrants early surgical intervention
(D) the initial changes usually occur on the lateral aspect of the patella
(E) patellectomy is the only proven form of successful surgical therapy

142. Which of the following is most sensitive to anoxia?

(A) peripheral nerves
(B) striated muscle
(C) skin
(D) tendon
(E) bone

DIRECTIONS (Questions 143 through 148): Each group of items in this section consists of lettered headings followed by a set of numbered words or phrases. For each numbered word or phrase, select

A if the item is associated with (A) only,
B if the item is associated with (B) only,
C if the item is associated with both (A) and (B),
D if the item is associated with neither (A) nor (B).

DIRECTIONS (Questions 143 and 144

(A) pain in the calf
(B) pain in the buttock
(C) both
(D) neither

B **143.** aortic occlusion

A **144.** superficial femoral artery occlusion

Questions 145 and 146

(A) deep venous thrombosis
(B) congestion, loss of sensory and motor function, danger of limb loss from cessation of arterial flow
(C) both
(D) neither

145. phlegmasia alba dolens

146. phlegmasia cerulea dolens

Questions 147 and 148

    (A) gangrenous digits
    (B) tropic ulcers
    (C) both
    (D) neither

147. diabetes mellitus

148. Buerger's disease

DIRECTIONS (Questions 149 through 152): For each of the items in this section, <u>ONE</u> or <u>MORE</u> of the numbered options is correct. Choose the answer

    A if only <u>1, 2, and 3</u> are correct,
    B if only <u>1 and 3</u> are correct,
    C if only <u>2 and 4</u> are correct,
    D if only <u>4</u> is correct,
    E if <u>all</u> are correct.

149. Patients complaining of leg pain and cold feet may show signs of chronic tissue ischemia including

    (1) loss of hair from digits
    (2) atrophy of skin
    (3) brittle nails
    (4) rubor on dependency

150. Which of the following abnormal finding(s) produced by an arterial injury is (are) most important?

    (1) paralysis
    (2) pain
    (3) paresthesia
    (4) pallor

151. Congenital arteriovenous fistula

    (1) port wine stain
    (2) massively hypertrophied extremity
    (3) may produce a thrill or bruit
    (4) should be treated aggressively

152. Following arterial repair for trauma of the femoral artery, postoperative pulses are now absent. What is the recommended course of action?

    (1) conservative therapy—wait and see if pulses return
    (2) arteriogram
    (3) anticoagulant therapy
    (4) reexploration and thrombectomy

DIRECTIONS (Questions 153 through 156): Each of the numbered items or incomplete statements in this section is followed by answers or by completions of the statement. Select the <u>ONE</u> lettered answer or completion that is <u>BEST</u> in each case.

153. Which of the following is/are the best method(s) for the control of bleeding?

    (A) tourniquet
    (B) tourniquet and direct digital pressure
    (C) direct digital pressure
    (D) tourniquet and packing the wound with gauze and applying a pressure dressing
    (E) direct digital pressure and packing the wound with gauze and applying a pressure dressing

154. The following statements about anterior compartment syndrome are true **EXCEPT**

    (A) it results from the compromise of the outflow of fluid from a closed space
    (B) the elevated intracompartmental pressure affects the tibial artery, the anterior tibial nerve, and the anterior tibial, extensor digitorium longus, peroneus tertius and extensor hallicus longus muscles
    (C) is best treated by decompression fasciotomy following disappearance of pedal pulses
    (D) must be differentiated from shin splits
    (E) early treatment may result in complete return of function

155. Which of the following ankle brachial indices reflects that of a diabetic with complaints of stocking neuropathy?

    (A) 0.25
    (B) 0.50
    (C) 0.75
    (D) 1.00
    (E) 1.25

156. The most important laboratory examination in arterial occlusive disease is

    (A) arteriography
    (B) B-mode ultrasonography
    (C) Doppler ultrasound
    (D) plethysmography
    (E) magnetic resonance

DIRECTIONS (Questions 157 and 158): Each group of items in this section consists of lettered headings followed by a set of numbered words or phrases. For each numbered word or phrase, select

A if the item is associated with (A) only,
B if the item is associated with (B) only,
C if the item is associated with both (A) and (B),
D if the item is associated with neither (A) nor (B).

(A) the first sign of unrecognized heart disease
(B) cardioarterial embolization
(C) both
(D) neither

157. thrombi

158 emboli

DIRECTIONS (Question 159): Each of the numbered items or incomplete statements in this section is followed by answers or by completions of the statement. Select the ONE lettered answer or completion that is BEST in each case.

159. A patient presents to you with complaints of swollen legs that have become increasingly brown in color. The patient is likely to have

(A) chronic venous insuffiency
(B) venous thrombosis
(C) varicose veins
(D) lymphedema
(E) atherosclerotic occlusive disease

DIRECTIONS (Question 160): For each of the items in this section, ONE or MORE of the numbered options is correct. Choose the answer

A if only 1, 2, and 3 are correct,
B if only 1 and 3 are correct,
C if only 2 and 4 are correct,
D if only 4 is correct,
E if all are correct.

160. What treatment course should be taken for patients with an embolic event to their lower extremity?

(1) prompt administration of IV heparin
(2) under local anesthesia, removal of emboli with fogarty balloon catheter through short incisions
(3) fasciotomy
(4) operative angiography

DIRECTIONS (Question 161): Each of the numbered items or incomplete statements in this section is followed by answers or by completions of the statement. Select the ONE lettered answer or completion that is BEST in each case.

161. Which arterioscleortic aneurysm is most common?

(A) abdominal aortic aneurysm
(B) carotid artery aneurysm
(C) popliteal aneurysm
(D) femoral aneurysm
(E) subclavian artery aneurysm

DIRECTIONS (Questions 162 through 173): Each group of items in this section consists of lettered headings followed by a set of numbered words or phrases. For each numbered word or phrase, select

A if the item is associated with (A) only,
B if the item is associated with (B) only,
C if the item is associated with both (A) and (B),
D if the item is associated with neither (A) nor (B).

Questions 162 and 163

(A) proliferative reaction in the media causing narrowing of the arterial lumen
(B) degenerative changes in the media
(C) both
(D) neither

162. Abdominal aortic aneurysm

163. Atherosclerotic occlusive disease

Questions 164 and 165

(A) impotence
(B) claudication
(C) both
(D) neither

164. abdominal aortic aneursym

165. aortoiliac occlusive disease

Questions 166 through 168

For each set of symptoms, select the associated disorder

(A) painless, cold cyanosis of the hands and feet
(B) red, warm painful extremities
(C) persistant mottled reddish-blue discoloration of the skin of the extremities

166. livedo reticularis

167. erythromegalia

168. acrocyanosis

Questions 169 through 171

(A) recurrent episodes of vasoconstriction in the upper extremities initiated by exposure to cold or emotional stress
(B) secondary manifestation of a more serious disorder of the vascular system
(C) both
(D) neither

169. Raynaud's phenomenon

170. Raynaud's disease

171. Buerger's disease

Questions 172 and 173

(A) edema and redness of the affected part without necrosis of the skin
(B) formation of blisters
(C) both
(D) neither

172. first-degree frostbite injury

173. second-degree frostbite injury

DIRECTIONS (Questions 174 and 175): Each of the numbered items or incomplete statements in this section is followed by answers or by completions of the statement. Select the ONE lettered answer or completion that is BEST in each case.

174. The best temperature range for rewarming cold exposed tissue should be

(A) 25°–30° C
(B) 32°–36° C
(C) 40°–44° C
(D) 48°–52° C
(E) 55°–60° C

175. The following statements about Buerger's disease are correct **EXCEPT** for

(A) the distribution of arterial involvement is the same as that of atherosclerosis

(B) the distribution of disease in the lower extremity is similar to the typical arterial involvement in the diabetic
(C) early in the course of the disease, the superficial veins undergo recurrent superficial thrombophlebitis
(D) it is most often seen in men who are between the ages of 20 and 40
(E) a history of at least 20 cigarettes per day habit is present

DIRECTIONS (Questions 176 through 180): For each of the items in this section, ONE or MORE of the numbered options is correct. Choose the answer

    A if only 1, 2, and 3 are correct,
    B if only 1 and 3 are correct,
    C if only 2 and 4 are correct,
    D if only 4 is correct,
    E if all are correct.

176. Diminution or absence of femoral pulses combined with absence of popliteal and pedal pulses is most likely to occur in patients with

(1) abdominal aortic aneurysm
(2) diabetes mellitus as well as aortoiliac occlusion
(3) Buerger's disease
(4) aortoiliac occlusive disease

177. The rationale behind education of diabetics to the importance of proper foot care includes the following

(1) it is likely that diabetics will develop atherosclerosis in their lower extremities
(2) diabetics may not notice minor trauma
(3) diabetics have a propensity for developing infections
(4) the foot of the diabetic has distinct characteristics that can quickly progress to threaten life and limb

178. Patients with aortoiliac occlusive disease may also have

(1) coronary artery atherosclerosis
(2) aneurysmal disease
(3) cerebral atherosclerosis
(4) hypercoagulability

SUMMARY OF DIRECTIONS				
A	**B**	**C**	**D**	**E**
1, 2, 3 only	1, 3 only	2, 4 only	4 only	All are correct

179. What is usually responsible for the development of venous stasis ulcers at the ankle?

     (1) greater saphenous vein
     (2) perforator or communicating vein
     (3) lesser saphenous vein
     (4) venous valvular incompetance

180. Ischemic stroke

     (1) refers to cerebral infarction occurring as a result of impairment of regional blood flow
     (2) is secondary to cerebral embolization of thrombi that originate in the heart
     (3) is due to fibromuscular hyperplasia
     (4) is associated with obliterative arteritis of the great vessels

DIRECTIONS (Questions 181 through 183): Each group of items in this section consists of lettered headings followed by a set of numbered words or phrases. For each numbered word or phrase, select the ONE lettered heading that is most closely associated with it. Each lettered heading may be selected once, more than once, or not at all.

Select the study that will be helpful in establishing the diagnosis of the following diseases.

     (A) Adson's maneuver
     (B) Allen's test
     (C) submersion test
     (D) exercise stress test
     (E) valsalva maneuver

181. Raynaud's disease

182. thoracic outlet syndrome

183. femoropopliteal disease

DIRECTIONS (Question 184): Each of the numbered items or incomplete statements in this section is followed by answers or by completions of the statement. Select the ONE lettered answer or completion that is BEST in each case.

184. The statements below are true EXCEPT for

     (A) venous valves assure proximal flow and prevent distal reflux
     (B) the number of venous valves increase the greater the distance from the heart
     (C) venous valves have little if any role in venous disease
     (D) venous valves may be weakened in patients with varicose veins
     (E) venous valves are absent from the vena cava and the common iliac veins

DIRECTIONS (Questions 185 through 187): For each of the items in this section, ONE or MORE of the numbered options is correct. Choose the answer

     A if only 1, 2, and 3 are correct,
     B if only 1 and 3 are correct,
     C if only 2 and 4 are correct,
     D if only 4 is correct,
     E if all are correct.

185. The lymphedema associated with radiation following mastectomy may be

     (1) primary lymphedema
     (2) secondary lymphedema
     (3) unavoidable and treated with a compression stocking
     (4) due to infection caused by staphylococcus or beta hemolytic streptococcus

186. Which disease(s) has (have) been known to cause heart disease in children?

     (1) varicella or chickenpox
     (2) rubella
     (3) diphtheria
     (4) rheumatic fever

187. The main physiologic disturbances resulting from congenital heart disease are

     (1) obstructive lesions
     (2) pulmonary congestion
     (3) left-to-right shunts
     (4) right-to-left shunts

DIRECTIONS (Question 188): Each of the numbered items or incomplete statements in this section is followed by answers or by completions of the statement. Select the ONE lettered answer or completion that is BEST in each case.

188. The following statements about congenital heart disease are true EXCEPT

     (A) congenital heart disease occurs as an isolated malformation resulting from defective embryonic development without known cause
     (B) atrial or ventricular septal defects result from incomplete formation of the respective septa
     (C) transposition and other abnormalities of the aorta result from abnormalities in the spiral division of the primitive bulbus cordis

(D) although a large number of congenital heart defects have been recognized, in a large pediatric cardiac clinic three malformations will comprise the majority of abnormalities seen

(E) cardiac development occurs early in uterine life, for virtually all fetal heart structures are formed between the third and eighth week of pregnancy.

DIRECTIONS (Questions 189 through 192): Each group of items in this section consists of lettered headings followed by a set of numbered words or phrases. For each numbered word or phrase, select

A if the item is associated with (A) <u>only,</u>
B if the item is associated with (B) <u>only,</u>
C if the item is associated with <u>both</u> (A) <u>and</u> (B),
D if the item is associated with <u>neither</u> (A) <u>nor</u> (B).

(A) acyanotic
(B) cyanotic
(C) both
(D) neither

189. tetralogy of Fallot

190. ventricular septal defect

191. atrial septal defect

192. transposition of the great vessels

DIRECTIONS (Questions 193 and 194): For each of the items in this section, <u>ONE</u> or <u>MORE</u> of the numbered options is correct. Choose the answer

A if only <u>1, 2, and 3</u> are correct,
B if only <u>1 and 3</u> are correct,
C if only <u>2 and 4</u> are correct,
D if only <u>4</u> is correct,
E if <u>all</u> are correct.

193. What are the most common forms of congenital heart disease?

(1) atrial septal defects
(2) ventricular septal defects
(3) patent ductus arteriosus
(4) tetralogy of Fallot

194. In obtaining the history of a 3-year-old patient who presents with signs and symptoms of recurrent pneumonia, what other questions should be asked of the mother?

(1) did the mother have rubella in the first trimester?
(2) does anyone in the family have congenital heart disease?

(3) has she noticed the child's lips, finger tips, or lobes of the ears turning blue?
(4) does the child squat frequently while walking or during outdoor play?

DIRECTIONS (Question 195): Each of the numbered items or incomplete statements in this section is followed by answers or by completions of the statement. Select the <u>ONE</u> lettered answer or completion that is <u>BEST</u> in each case.

195. All the following physical findings point to a severe congenital cardiac malformation **EXCEPT**

(A) hepatic enlargement
(B) clubbing of the fingers and toes
(C) delayed growth and development
(D) normal growth and development
(E) cyanotic lips

DIRECTIONS (Questions 196 and 197): Each group of items in this section consists of lettered headings followed by a set of numbered words or phrases. For each numbered word or phrase, select

A if the item is associated with (A) <u>only,</u>
B if the item is associated with (B) <u>only,</u>
C if the item is associated with <u>both</u> (A) <u>and</u> (B),
D if the item is associated with <u>neither</u> (A) <u>nor</u> (B).

(A) hypertension, headaches, epistaxis, leg fatigue
(B) fatigue, dyspnea, angina, syncope
(C) both
(D) neither

196. congenital aortic stenosis

197. coarctation of the aorta

DIRECTIONS (Questions 198 through 201): Each group of items in this section consists of lettered headings followed by a set of numbered words or phrases. For each numbered word or phrase, select the <u>ONE</u> lettered heading that is most closely associated with it. Each lettered heading may be selected once, more than once, or not at all.

(A) loud harsh systolic murmur heard best at the second left interspace
(B) continuous machinery murmur
(C) pansystolic murmur along the left sternal border in the 3rd or 4th intercostal spaces
(D) soft systolic murmur audible in the 2nd or 3rd left intercostal spaces
(E) systolic murmur heard over the left hemithorax

198. pulmonic stenosis

199. atrial septal defect

200. ventricular septal defect

201. patent ductus arteriosus

DIRECTIONS (Questions 202 through 206): For each of the items in this section, ONE or MORE of the numbered options is correct. Choose the answer

A if only 1, 2, and 3 are correct,
B if only 1 and 3 are correct,
C if only 2 and 4 are correct,
D if only 4 is correct,
E if all are correct.

202. Which of the following is(are) (a) late sign(s) of advanced cardiac disease?

(1) dysnpea
(2) edema
(3) syncope
(4) angina

203. Which symptom(s) is(are) the hallmark(s) of coronary artery disease?

(1) dyspnea
(2) syncope
(3) arrhythmia
(4) angina

204. Extracorporeal circulation includes

(1) a roller pump to provide practically nonpulsatile flow of blood
(2) a disposable membrane or bubble oxygenator
(3) heparinization
(4) the use of protamine

205. Problems from perfusion include

(1) derangement of normal clotting mechanisms
(2) renal insufficiency
(3) transient neurological abnormalities
(4) multiple organ injury

206. Myocardial preservation may be accomplished by

(1) topical hyperthermia
(2) arresting the heart with cold blood potassium technique
(3) blood cardioplegia
(4) crystalloid cardioplegia

DIRECTIONS (Questions 207 and 208): Each of the numbered items or incomplete statements in this section is followed by answers or by completions of the statement. Select the ONE lettered answer or completion that is BEST in each case.

207. The most serious complication following extracorporeal circulation is

(A) postoperative bleeding
(B) cardiac arrhythmias
(C) stroke
(D) renal failure
(E) respiratory insufficiency

208. The cerebral anoxia following circulatory arrest produces brain damage within

(A) 30 to 60 seconds
(B) 1 to 2 minutes
(C) 3 to 4 minutes
(D) 5 to 7 minutes
(E) 6 to 8 minutes

DIRECTIONS (Questions 209 and 210): Each group of items in this section consists of lettered headings followed by a set of numbered words or phrases. For each numbered word or phrase, select

A if the item is associated with (A) only,
B if the item is associated with (B) only,
C if the item is associated with both (A) and (B),
D if the item is associated with neither (A) nor (B).

(A) syncope
(B) dyspnea
(C) both
(D) neither

209. mitral stenosis

210. aortic stenosis

DIRECTIONS (Question 211): Each of the numbered items or incomplete statements in this section is followed by answers or by completions of the statement. Select the ONE lettered answer or completion that is BEST in each case.

211. Which is the most common clinical cardiac problem?

(A) stable angina of varying severity
(B) asymptomatic: angiographically significant

coronary artery disease with little or no angina
(C) unstable angina
(D) acute infarction
(E) postinfarction angina

DIRECTIONS (Questions 212 through 217): For each of the items in this section, <u>ONE</u> or <u>MORE</u> of the numbered options is correct. Choose the answer

A if only <u>1, 2, and 3</u> are correct,
B if only <u>1 and 3</u> are correct,
C if only <u>2 and 4</u> are correct,
D if only <u>4</u> is correct,
E if <u>all</u> are correct.

212. The myocardial ischemia produced by coronary artery disease can cause one or more of the following events

  (1) angina pectorus
  (2) sudden death
  (3) myocardial infarction
  (4) congestive heart failure

213. The best therapy for acute myocardial infarction includes

  (1) angioplasty
  (2) IV administration of a thrombolytic agent
  (3) intracoronary administration of a thrombolytic agent
  (4) immediate bypass preceded by intraaortic balloon support

214. Occlusion of a vein graft within the first 5 years following coronary artery bypass grafting may be due to

  (1) anastomotic technique
  (2) trauma to the vein graft at the time of operation
  (3) postoperative adhesions
  (4) the use of dipyridamole and aspirin

215. Which is/are the best bypass grafting material(s)?

  (1) brachial vein
  (2) greater saphenous vein
  (3) lesser saphenous vein
  (4) internal mammary artery

216. Chronic constrictive pericarditis may be due to

  (1) viral pericarditis
  (2) *Haemophilus influenzae*
  (3) intensive radiation
  (4) *Staphylococcus*

217. Which pacemaker(s) has (have) the ability to cause ventricular fibrillation?

  (1) demand pacemaker
  (2) atrioventricular pacemaker
  (3) programmable pacemaker
  (4) fixed-rate asynchronous pacemaker

DIRECTIONS (Questions 218 and 218): Each of the numbered items or incomplete statements in this section is followed by answers or by completions of the statement. Select the <u>ONE</u> lettered answer or completion that is <u>BEST</u> in each case.

218. The findings listed below are typical of a mild pericardiotomy syndrome **EXCEPT**

  (A) fever
  (B) pericardial friction rub
  (C) pleural effusion
  (D) elevated white blood cell count
  (E) normal white blood cell count

219. The statements about left ventricular aneurysms are true **EXCEPT** for

  (A) the aneurysm usually enlarges a moderate degree and then becomes stationary
  (B) they are due to a severe transmural myocardial infarction
  (C) the aneurysm undergoes progressive enlargement and rupture
  (D) more than 80% of aneurysms are in the anterolateral portion of the left ventricle
  (E) lateral or posterior aneurysms are uncommon

DIRECTIONS (Questions 220 through 222): Each group of items in this section consists of lettered headings followed by a set of numbered words or phrases. For each numbered word or phrase, select

A if the item is associated with (A) <u>only</u>,
B if the item is associated with (B) <u>only</u>,
C if the item is associated with <u>both (A) and (B)</u>,
D if the item is associated with <u>neither (A) nor (B)</u>.

  (A) penetrating cardiac trauma
  (B) blunt cardiac trauma
  (C) both
  (D) neither

220. steering wheel injury

221. tamponade and hemorrhage

222. pericardial effusion and chest pain

Answers
and Explanations

1. **(A)** Thrombocytopenia is by far the most common bleeding disorder seen in the postoperative patient. This results from platelet consumption in the control of bleeding or may be the result of drug interaction or in cases of massive blood transfusion. The most common cause of bleeding in a surgical patient is poor local control. This should be suspected in patients who are bleeding from a single site, not multiple sites. *(Schwartz. pp. 115–120)*

Shock is a clinical entity in which the cardiovascular system cannot adequately perfuse the vital organs and can be caused by trauma, metabolic derangement, infection, or cardiac injury

2. **(A)** Lower extremity paresthesis is most commonly associated with neurogenic shock, as the symptom of paresthesias is associated with a neurologic injury. This causes interruption of the sympathetic innervation responsible for vasoconstriction and results in hypotension.

3. **(E)** Cardiogenic shock. Muffled heart sounds, especially in the hypotensive patient with distended neck, veins should suggest the presence of cardiac tamponade.

4. **(D)** Hypovolemic shock. The fracture of a femur is associated with a large loss of blood into the surrounding tissue and depletes the intravascular space. This in turn causes the reduction in the volume which the heart can pump and decreases the systemic blood pressure.

5. **(B)** Septic shock. The individual with an overwhelming infection becomes hyperdynamic, meaning his/her heart is working very hard; however, the toxins produced by the bacteria, notably gram-negative, will cause a vasodilation. This vasodilation is responsible for the decrease in blood pressure and also the warmth of skin, because there is more blood flowing there. *(Shires et al, pp. 139–140)*

6. **(D)** Pain is not a symptom associated with carcinoma of the breast. This is more commonly seen in mastitis, pregnancy, or in fat necrosis following trauma. The remainder of the symptoms are all suspicious of carcinoma and should be thoroughly evaluated. *(Rush, pp. 556–559)*

7. **(C)** Mammography is indicated initially at the age of 40. All women should be encouraged to have annual or biannual examinations up to the age of 50 at which point the indication is an annual examination. This examination should consist of a physician or physician's assistant breast examination as well as mammography. Studies have documented that the early findings on mammogram have led to earlier detection of malignant lesions. *(American Cancer Society Guidelines; Rush, p. 556)*

8. **(E)** All these are important historical points ascertained in the evaluation of the patient with a breast mass. There are associated risks of breast carcinoma in females who had had no children or their first child after the age of 30. In addition, there is an increased risk of breast cancer in those patients with family history of carcinoma and in those people with benign breast lesions. *(Rush, p. 556–558; Wilson, p. 533)*

9. **(D)** Diffuse abdominal pain that is "wave-like" and associated with vomiting is most likely the result of a luminal-type obstruction. Generally, this is a bowel obstruction either small or large. Pancreatitis, which is also associated with diffuse abdominal pain, is generally a constant pain that often radiates into the back. The remaining choices are occasionally colicky or "wave-like" although they are generally not diffuse in nature. *(Schwartz, pp. 1065, 1074–1079; Cope, pp. 20–27)*

10. **(C)** Biliary colic is often an insidious pain that is postprandial in its onset. Perforation of viscus, ureteral colic, the rupturing of an abdominal aneu-

rysm, or severe pancreatitis can be severe in onset and, in fact, can cause a patient to collapse. (Schwartz, p. 1065; Cope, pp. 21–23)

11. (D) When evaluating a patient with abdominal pain that you suspect to be an intestinal obstruction, a flat and upright of the abdomen will provide you with sufficient information to determine a simple obstruction or a dynamic ileus from a perforation of a viscus by the demonstration of free air. Further radiographic investigation would involve the use of a barium enema that would outline the inferior margins of an obstructing lesion. (Schwartz, pp. 1078–1079)

12. (C) Pain out of proportion to physical findings is a clue to an underlying vascular etiology. The ischemic pain resulting from either a venous or arterial occlusion process is significant with minimal signs, that is peritonitis or localized tenderness. This unfortunately is often a diagnosis of exclusion that is only made via arteriography. (Adams, pp. 1504–1505)

13. (B) The recurrent laryngeal nerve lies in the tracheoesophageal groove bilaterally and is responsible for innervation of the vocal cord on the ipsilateral side. It must be identified during thyroidectomy to avoid iatrogenic injury. The cervical sympathetic chain and vagus nerve lie along the path of the carotid artery and jugular vein and are not usually encountered during thyroid surgery. The laryngeal nerves lie adjacent to the superior and inferior thyroid arteries and are identified during ligation of those vessels. (Kaplan, p. 1614; Zollinger et al, pp. 346–347)

14. (E) Findings associated with thyroid carcinoma include those of pressure within the neck such as dysphagia, which may be the result of pressure on the esophagus. In addition, tumor invasion may result in injury to the recurrent laryngeal nerve with resultant vocal cord paralysis and hoarseness. Palpable mass is associated with both benign and malignant processes within the thyroid but should certainly be suspect for a malignant process. A Delphian node is usually palpable on the trachea just above the thyroid isthmus and is usually associated with malignant disease or thyroiditis. (Kaplan, pp. 1633–1638)

15. (B) The historical information that places an individual at high risk for cancer involves previous irradiation to the head and neck. In addition, there have been increased instances of carcinoma of the thyroid demonstrated in individuals who have family members with histories of medullary thyroid carcinoma. This is most likely a result of the famil-

ial medullary carcinoma syndrome that is a genetic inheritance in 50% of their offspring. Changes in thyroid function, either hyperfunctioning or hypofunctioning glands, have not been proven to increase the risks of carcinoma. (Kaplan, p. 1631)

16. (E) The most useful diagnostic test in the preoperative evaluation of a solid thyroid mass is a needle biopsy. Ultrasound and needle aspiration are useful in the determination of cystic lesions. The radioactive scan is important in the differentiation of a cold or nonfunctioning nodule; however, the majority of benign lesions are also cold and this is not in any way diagnostic of carcinoma. In addition, thyroid function tests have no role, because the majority of patients with thyroid carcinoma are found to be euthyroid. (Kaplan, p. 1632)

17. (B) Papillary carcinoma of the thyroid has an excellent prognosis following surgical excision. In recent studies, 10-year survival rates were approximately 89%. Follicular carcinoma has a propensity for a mulicentric focus of carcinoma. Studies have shown this to have a 10-year survival of between 44%–86% based upon the apparent invasiveness of the original tumor. (Kaplan, pp. 1634–1635)

18. (D) Vitamin D deficiency is not a cause of primary hyperparathyroidism. Parathyroid adenomas, hyperplasia of the parathyroid gland, as well as carcinoma of the parathyroid gland are all cited in the etiology of primary hyperparathyroidism. In addition, nonparathyroid tumors can secrete a parathormone-like substance that can mimic primary hyperparathyroidism. (Kaplan, pp. 1649–1654)

19. (D) The most common causes of hypoparathyroidism are related to surgery. This is the result of either surgical removal, trauma, or devascularization during thyroid surgery. Metastatic carcinoma and renal failure are generally associated with elevation of the serum calcium level. Idiopathic hypoparathyroidism is an exceedingly rare condition and would present prior to the age of 16. (Kaplan, p. 1677)

20. (B) The superior mesenteric artery gives rise to the right colic, middle colic, and ileocolic vessels. The inferior mesenteric artery gives rise to the left colic, sigmoid, and hemorrhoidal vessels. Collateral circulation is provided by the marginal artery of Drummond which traverses the mesenteric border of the colon. (Zollinger et al, p. 13; Cohn and Nance, p. 983)

21. (B) The taenia coli, which are longitudinal muscles of the colon, and the haustra, which are outpouchings between the taenia, give the colon its classic appearance. Valvulae conniventes are semicircular valves seen in the small intestine. The ligament of Treitz is a landmark denoting the end of the duodenum and start of jejunum. *(Cohn and Nance, p. 983)*

22. (A); 23. (A); 24. (B); 25. (A); 26. (A) Crohn's colitis is associated with a number of anorectal complications including anal fistulae and fissures. It is a disease of the entire alimentary tract that can be seen in different sections with normal tissue between the involved areas. Crohn's is almost always a full-thickness disease in contrast to ulcerative colitis, which generally involves the mucosa and submucosa only. Because of Crohn's transmural involvement, it can cause localized perforation and inflammatory masses in the abdomen. *(Goldberg et al, pp. 1246–1247)*

27. (D) Overgrowth of *Clostridium dificile* and the increased production of exotoxin are responsible for the colitis seen after antibiotic use. This can result from the use of most antibiotics. However, ampicillin and clindamycin are most frequently associated. *(Goldberg et al, pp. 1251–1252)*

28. (D) Treatment of pseudomembranous colitis involves the cessation of all present antibiotics, the replacement of fluid and electrolytes, and the use of vancomycin 500 mg PO qid. Steroids, sulfasalizine, and colectomy are not used for treatment of this type of colitis. *(Goldberg et al, p. 1252)*

29. (A) Cobblestoning results from the changes in mucosal pattern and loss of haustra seen in colitis. In addition, Crohn's frequently causes perforation and fistulazation with adjacent structures, that is, bladder and rectum. Stenosis and stricture result from long-standing inflammatory reaction. *(Schwartz et al, p. 1246)*

30. (E) There are a number of complications associated with ulcerative colitis including all those listed. Each of them is, in and of itself, serious, and justify surgical intervention. The prognosis for cancer in patients with colitis is poor. A 20% 5-year survival is seen in this group compared to 40% in the general population. *(Goldberg, et al, pp. 1239–1242)*

31. (A) An initial management of colitis includes the use of sulfasalizine (azulfidine), ACTH, corticosteroids, and occasionally azathioprine. Surgery is indicated for the management of specific complications, that is, perforation or hemorrhage. *(Glickman and Robert, p. 128)*

32. (B) Surgical management of ulcerative colitis involves total colectomy and creation of an ileostomy, as the disease is confined to the colon. This is often a curative approach. A number of procedures have been devised to provide continence of the fecal stream via ileal pouches or anastomosis of the ileum to the rectal musculature. *(Goldberg et al, pp. 1242–1243)*

33. (C) Bleeding from diverticulosis represents about two thirds of all massive lower gastrointestinal bleeds. It is usually the only symptom and can be sudden in onset and profuse, requiring emergent surgical repair. *(Goldberg et al, pp. 1255–1259)*

34. (D) Angiography is the most beneficial study in massive lower GI bleeding that is greater than 2.0 mL/min. It accurately localizes the bleeding site and allows the use of selective intraarterial vasoconstrictive agents. Technetium-labeled RBC is helpful in bleeding as slow as 0.5 mL/min. The remaining studies have limited value in brisk bleeding. *(Schwartz p. 1091)*

35. (A) Diverticulitis results from inflammation of a diverticulum and presents with pain, fever, anorexia, and change in bowel habits. Nausea is frequent; however, vomiting is infrequent unless there is obstruction. *(Goldberg et al, p. 1256)*

36. (D) Carcinoma is not a complication of diverticulitis although they may present with similar symptoms. The remaining are all associated with diverticulitis and can necessitate surgical resection. *(Goldberg et al, pp. 1257–1260)*

37. (E) Juvenile polyposis has no malignant potential and the usual symptoms includes bleeding. Polyposes coli is seen in Gardner's syndrome and along with villous adenoma and familial polyposis all have significant malignant potential. Tubular adenomas generally remain carcinoma in situ, since they rarely extend beyond the muscularis. *(Goldberg et al, pp. 1264–1270)*

38. (E) All these are indications for surgical relief of hemorrhoidal symptoms. Failure of dietary manipulation, topical medications and/or rubber band ligation often lead to surgery. *(Goldberg et al, pp. 1302–1303)*

39. (D) Diabetes is not associated with anal fissure although the inability to heal wounds is associated with diabetes. Conservative management to include anal hygiene, laxatives, and lubricants should precede surgery unless the fissure is associated with perirectal abscess, which should be incised and drained. *(Goldberg et al, p. 1303)*

40. (B) Screening for colon carcinoma involves hemoccult study and colonoscopy. The hemoccult study or stool for blood is a very sensitive and inexpensive test that can be done by the patient at home. Colonoscopy should be done once in the fourth or fifth decade and then biannually. CEA is a useful blood test for determining recurrence of tumor. *(American Cancer Society Guidelines; Goldberg et al, pp. 1277–1278)*

41. (C) Characteristically, esophageal achalasia has unsynchronized contractions of the esophagus that gives it the absence of peristalsis. Failure of the lower esophageal sphincter to relax makes it impossible for food to pass into the stomach. Gastroesophageal reflux is not seen in this condition unless it results from mechanical dilation of the lower esophageal sphincter. *(Pairolero, et al, pp. 1109–1111)*

42. (B) There is at present no cure for esophageal achalasia. A number of procedures have been proposed with regard to therapy for this condition. Of late, esophagomyotomy has proven to be the most successful in relieving the diffuse esophageal spasm. This procedure involves dissection of the muscular layer of the esophagus through a thoracic approach down onto the gastric wall. This is offered to all but the worse of surgical risk patients, in which case esophageal dilation would be performed. Vagal denervation is avoided in these patients, as this would relax the lower esophageal sphincter but is associated with a high incidence of esophageal reflux. The Nissan fundoplication, which is an antireflux procedure, is of no benefit in esophageal achalasia. *(Pairolero et al, pp. 1112–1113)*

43. (E) Mallory Weiss syndrome is not a complication of gastroesophageal reflux. This is a condition seen after repeated forceful vomiting and is associated with bleeding and pain. The remainder are all associated complications of gastroesophageal reflux. As a result of the distal esophagus being persistently exposed to the low PHs from the stomach, esophageal ulceration with bleeding occurs and, following prolonged exposure, muscle contractures and mucosal changes such as Barrett's esophagus. *(Pairolero et al, p. 1151)*

44. (B) The evaluation of esophageal motility is most often done through manometric means. There are several devices that through the use of balloon-covered transformers, will measure the upper and lower esophageal sphincters as well as the pressures generated within the esophageal mucosa. In addition, the use of contrast radiography, specifically Cine radiography or the barium swallow, is also an important adjunct in the diagnosis of motility disorders. Endoscopy, although critical for the evaluation of esophageal disease per se, is not of significant value in the evaluation of esophageal function. *(Pairolero et al, pp. 1106–1110)*

45. (A) Complications associated with herniation of the abdominal viscera through the diaphragm are volvulus and obstruction. Should this condition persist, an ischemic injury will occur to the abdominal viscera. There is, however, no increased incidence of carcinoma either within the hernia itself or within the abdominal viscera. This condition is usually amenable to simple reduction and surgical repair. *(Pairolero et al, pp. 1118–1123)*

46. (D) The earliest and almost constant feature associated with carcinoma of the esophagus is dysphagia. This is initially seen with the swallowing of solid foods, but if undetected, will eventually progress to involve liquids and even saliva. Advanced stage malignancies will be associated with painful swallowing and, to some extent, bleeding, although massive bleeding is not associated with esophageal malignancies. *(Pairolero et al, pp. 1138–1139)*

47. (C) The main duct emptying the pancreas is the duct of Wirsung. The minor duct is the duct of Santorini. These enter into the second part of the duodenum at the ampulla of Vater. *(Silen and Steer, pp. 1413–1414)*

48. (B) Acute pancreatitis is often a clinical diagnosis, although elevation of the serum amylase is helpful. A more reliable indicator is total urinary amylase in 2 hours. Care must be taken not to ascribe an elevated serum amylase alone to pancreatitis, as this can occur with cholecystitis, perforated ulcer, infarcted bowel, renal failure, and mumps. *(Silen and Steer, pp. 1420–1421)*

49. (A) The mainstay of therapy for acute and chronic pancreatitis is supportive; repletion of fluids and electrolytes is paramount, because these patients are frequently dehydrated secondary to nausea, vomiting, and thirdspacing of fluid. In addition, the GI tract is put at rest with nasogastric suctioning to avoid stimulus of the exocrine function; and, last, analgesics are used for the pain. Surgery is not indicated unless a complication ensues such as pseudocyst, abscess, necrosis, or hemorrhage. *(Silen and Steer, pp. 1421–1422)*

50. **(A)** The development of a pancreatic pseudocyst is the most common complication of pancreatitis. It should be suspected in those patients with anorexia, weight loss, and upper abdominal pain after an episode of pancreatitis. *(Silen and Steer, p. 1421)*

51. **(D)** The advent of ERCP has made it possible to document the status of the pancreatitic ducts and the presence of intraductal calcification. In the patient with chronic pancreatitis, such repeated episodes lead to deposition of calcium and eventual ductal obstruction. This is frequently the cause of the pain in these patients. CT and ultrasound are helpful in evaluating the pancreas for pseudocyst or abscess. *(Silen and Steer, pp. 1427–1428; Bradley and Zeppa, p. 1186)*

52. **(A)** The classic triad of weight loss, diabetes, and steatorrhea should indicate severe pancreatic disease. The presence of fever would be associated with complications such as an infected pseudocyst. *(Bradley and Zeppa, p. 1189)*

53. **(D)** Drainage of a pancreatic pseudocyst is recommended to avoid the complications of infection or hemorrhage into the cyst. This would ideally involve total excision of the cyst; however, this is rarely possible. Hence, these are incised and internally drained by anastomosis to the stomach or duodenum. *(Silen and Steer, pp. 1428–1429)*

54. **(E)** All these symptoms may be seen in a patient with carcinoma of the pancreas. Pruritis is related to increasing bilirubin and often precedes the onset of jaundice. It is often thought that pain is not associated with carcinoma of the pancreas; however, retrospectively, about 75% of patients complain of dull epigastric aching that radiates to the back or lower quadrants. *(Silen and Steer, p. 1430)*

55. **(A)** The Whipple procedure consists of a resection involving the distal stomach, pylorus, duodenum, proximal pancreas and gallbladder. The remaining jejunum is anastamosed to the biliary and pancreatic duct as well as to the stomach. The spleen is not involved in this resection. *(Zollinger et al, p. 212; Silen and Steer, pp. 1432–1433)*

56. **(D)** The primary function of the spleen is the sequestration of aging erythrocytes. It is not involved in the production of erythrocytes nor in the formation of products for the clotting cascade. *(Schwartz, pp. 1442–1443)*

57. **(C)** An unreducible hernia in which the content of the hernia develops ischemia is said to be strangulated. *(Morton, p. 1525)*

58. **(B)** A hernia through which bowel or omentum extend and then becomes edematous, usually secondary to venous congestion, is unreducible. The contents are then incarcerated. *(Morton, p. 1525)*

59. **(E)** A direct hernia occurs as the result of weakened muscles in the floor of the inguinal canal. This occurs in Hesselbach's Triangle, the boundaries of which are medial to the inferior epigastric artery, lateral to the rectus sheath, and superior to the inguinal ligament. *(Morton, pp. 1526–1527)*

60. **(D)** The indirect hernia in males extends through the internal ring and is found within the spermatic cord and cremasteric fibers. The path of herniation is along the tunica vaginalis. This has not completely closed since descent of the testicle. These are also referred to as congenital hernias. *(Gray's Anatomy, p. 1051; Morton, pp. 1527–1528)*

61. **(A)** A sliding hernia is the situation in which one wall of the hernia sac is composed of an intraperitoneal organ such as cecum or sigmoid colon. This may coexist with other forms of hernia, that is, indirect hernia. Care must be taken in resection of the hernia sac to rule out this possibility. *(Morton, p. 1525)*

62. **(C)** The most common type of hernia in a female is the femoral hernia. This starts off with a defect in the transversalis fascia; however, it extends under the inguinal ligament and can often grow quite large prior to its diagnosis. *(Morton, p. 1528)*

63. **(E)** All these are complications associated with herniorrhaphy. Hemorrhage, severing of the vas deferens, ilioinguinal, iliohypogastric, or genitofemoral nerves are potential complications. Testicular swelling may result from a tight closure of the inguinal ring. Recurrence is a complication that may occur in 20% to 30% of patients according to varying sources. Underlying problems such as diabetes, obesity, and infection all increase the risk of recurrence. *(Morton, pp. 1543–1544; SCNA [1983], pp. 1363–1371)*

64. **(A)** Brain tumors occur in five patients per 100,000 in the United States and account for about 2.7% of all cancer deaths. Glioblastomas comprise about 40% of the brain tumors. Meningiomas occur in about 15% to 20% and metastatic lesions represent 5% to 10% of intracranial lesions *(Youman's pp. 2682–2685; Spencer et al, pp. 1847–1848)*

65. (E) All these can be seen with brain tumors. Signs and symptoms will vary according to the location of the tumor. Increased intracranial pressure will generally cause headache and, because of its long course, the 6th cranial nerve is also sensitive to pressure, which can cause double vision. Seizures, weakness, and visual change arise according to tumor location. Any of these symptoms should raise suspicion of brain tumor. *(Youman's, pp. 2874–2875; Spencer et al, pp. 1848–1849)*

66. (B) This patient most likely has a ruptured disc between the L5 and S1 vertebrae, which has caused weakness in the gastrocnemius muscles and elimination of the ankle jerk, which are both controlled by the 1st sacral nerve root. This can also involve hypalgesia of the lateral aspect of the foot. The L5 nerve root classically causes pain along the posterolateral leg to the dorsum of the foot along with dorsiflexion weakness. *(Youman's, pp. 2540–2543; Spencer et al, pp. 1871–1872)*

67. (A [1,2,3]) Release of acid from parietal cells is a direct result of vagal stimulation. Gastrin is also released from the antrum under vagal control. Although the antrum is the primary source of gastrin, the duodenal mucosa also secretes gastrin. Secretin inhibits gastric acid secretion, and is released when the duodenum detects the presence of acid. Calcium is a stimulator of gastric acid secretion. *(Moody et al, pp. 1162–1163)*

68. (D [4]) The release of gastrin is a result of antral distension, the presence of protein in the antrum, and vagal stimulation. As the gastric pH decreases, a feedback mechanism inhibits the secretion of gastrin and, therefore, gastric acid. Gastrin release ceases when the gastric pH is 1.5 or less. *(Moody et al, p. 1163)*

69. (C [2,4]) The stomach digests food both by chemical and mechanical means. The antrum functions by grinding food particles into smaller particles and then returning the particles to the proximal stomach. Fat, protein, and carbohydrates are enzymatically digested in the stomach. Salivary amylase is rendered inactive by gastric acid. Pepsinogen, however, requires a low pH in order to be converted to its active form. *(Moody et al, p. 1161)*

70. (B [1,3]) Atrophic gastritis is associated with achlorhydria as a result of a loss of parietal cells (the primary acid-producing cells). Pernicious anemia results from the loss of the production of intrinsic factor (from the parietal cell) and not from chronic blood loss. Patients with atrophic gastritis are at a higher risk for developing gastric cancer. Atrophic gastritis itself does not produce any symptoms. *(Moody et al, p. 1181)*

71. (A [1,2,3]) Melena is generally produced from upper gastrointestinal tract bleeding. Red or currant-jelly stools, however, may be produced if the bleeding is massive. The stimulatory effect of intraluminal blood increases gastrointestinal motility and will produce a rapid transit time. Melena results from the interaction of gastric acid and hemoglobin, and as little as 50 mL of blood may be enough to produce melena. Other substances, especially iron have been known to cause black stools. Black stools can persist for up to 5 days after a significant upper gastrointestinal hemorrhage. *(Schwartz, p. 1085)*

72. (C) The incidence of gastric ulcer increases with age. In Western countries, duodenal ulcers are much more prevalent than are gastric ulcers. Increased acid production and stress are associated with duodenal, **NOT** gastric, ulcers. *(Moody, et al, pp. 1168–1175)*

73. (A) There are several surgical procedures designed to decrease gastric acid production. Parietal cell vagotomy would denervate parietal cells, or the acid-producing cells of the stomach. Antrectomy would lead to decreased gastrin production, and proximal gastrectomy removes the acid-producing cells. A procedure such as pyloroplasty will increase gastric emptying but should not significantly affect gastric acid secretion. *(Moody et al, pp. 1172–1173)*

74. (A) The pathophysiology of duodenal ulcer formation has a multifaceted etiology. Forty percent of patients have gastric acid hypersecretion secondary to an increase in the parietal cell mass. Fasting gastrin levels are usually normal. Increased pepsinogen production, rapid gastric emptying, and an absence of sufficient duodenal buffers have all been implicated in the role of duodenal ulcers, but as yet the role has not been proven. *(Moody et al, pp. 1168–1169)*

75. (D) Radionuclide imaging is emerging as an effective, minimally invasive, and safe method for determining gastrointestinal bleeding. Because most gastrointestinal bleeding is not a continuous process and radionuclide imaging can be continued for up to 24 hours, it is a useful method for determining the source of such bleeding. The accuracy and sensitivity of this imaging is as good as selective angiography, although the imaging cannot pinpoint the site of bleeding as well as does angiography. Colonoscopy is of little use in detecting the cause of massive gastrointestinal bleeding because the amount of bleeding obscures the bleeding site. Barium enema should not be performed as an early procedure because the contrast material involved will obscure subsequent angiograms. *(Schwartz, pp. 1088–1089)*

76. **(D)** For those patients in whom medical therapy has not been successful, surgical treatment of bleeding peptic ulcer is necessary. All the options listed in this question are capable of controlling upper gastrointestinal hemorrhage caused by peptic ulcer. However, the procedure that offers the lowest mortality and morbidity rates, reasonable long-term protection from recurrence, and control of the bleeding is oversewing the ulcer bilateral truncal vagotomy and a pyloroplasty. *(Moody et al, pp. 1174–1175)*

77. **(E)** Of all the gastric malignancies, lymphoma accounts for approximately 2%. The treatment of choice for those with gastric lymphoma is radiotherapy. This accounts for a 5-year survival rate of approximately 40%. If outlet obstruction is present, the treatment of choice would be subtotal gastrectomy with postoperative radiotherapy. *(Moody et al, p. 1178)*

78–82 **78 (D); 79 (B); 80 (C); 81 (D); 82 (E)** Severe stresses such as trauma, sepsis, or burns can cause ischemia of the gastric mucosa and subsequent ulceration (so called stress ulcers). In chronic (atrophic) gastritis, gastric atrophy occurs and increases the risk of gastric cancer. Prepyloric ulcers can obstruct the gastric outlet causing gastric distention, cramps, pain, and nausea. Several factors are known to increase the instance of duodenal ulcers. One of these is blood type O. Parietal cell antibodies have been associated with the less common of two types of chronic gastritis, the type associated with vitamin B type absorption. *(Moody et al, pp. 1166–1182)*

83. **(A)** Gallstones are usually composed of a combination of calcium, bile pigments, and cholesterol. Cholesterol stones, which are the most predominate type of gallstone in the United States, are formed when the proportion of bile salts and lecithin in the bile are inadequate to form micelles to dissolve cholesterol. It is possible to have pure cholesterol stones; however, this is rare. Approximately 30% of patients diagnosed with gallstones in the United States will have pigmented stones. Pigmented stones are of two types: black pigmented stones are associated with hemolysis, cirrhosis, and old age; brown pigmented stones (or earthy stones) are usually associated with infection. *(Schwartz, pp. 1390–1391)*

84. **(E)** Cholelithiasis may be present whenever conditions occur that alter the concentrations of the major elements involved in gallstone formation. Pigmented stones may occur in patients who have hematological diseases associated with increased hemolysis. Also, hemolysis caused by mechanical trauma such as that found in a patient with aortic valve replacement results in the formation of pigmented stones. Increases in the concentration of cholesterol in the blood and bile and suppression of gall bladder emptying may be found with prolonged administration of estrogen, such as that found in the use of birth control pills. People who have undergone ileal resection of the distal third of their small intestine have an interruption in their enterohepatic circulation and a decrease of the secretion of bile salts and phospholipids, both necessary for the solubility of cholesterol. It is likely that such patients will develop cholelithiasis. *(Schwartz, pp. 1390–1391)*

85. **(B)** The HIDA scan or technetium 99-labeled N substituted imino diacetic acid scan uses a gamma emitting isotope with a 6-hour half life. These isotopes are selectively extracted by the liver and secreted into the bile. In patients with acute cholecystitis secondary to cystic duct obstruction, the isotope will fail to enter the gall bladder. This makes it the diagnostic choice for such a condition. This technique can also define obstruction of extrahepatic bile ducts, in which case the radionuclides fail to enter the intestine. These scans are associated with less toxicity than the contrast media involved in IV cholangiography. They provide adequate visualization even when bilirubin levels are as high as 10 to 20 mg per 100 mL. *(Schwartz, p. 1388)*

86. **(A)** Sclerosing cholangitis appears to occur more frequently in males than in females, which is in contrast to acute cholecystitis. There have been a significant number of sclerosing cholangitis cases found to be associated with ulcerative colitis. Because it has been found that most individuals who have sclerosing cholangitis do not have stones in their gall bladder or common bile duct, this disease does not appear to be caused by irritation of the common duct due to the passage of gallstones. The cause of the disease is unknown, although it has been suggested that it may be related to viral infection. The entire extrahepatic and intrahepatic bile duct system may be involved, or the hepatic duct may be spared and the disease restricted to the common duct. The gall bladder is usually not involved. The clinical and laboratory presentation is usually that of extrahepatic jaundice. It is usually noted that the serum alkaline phosphatase level is elevated out of proportion to that of the serum bilirubin level. *(Schwartz, pp. 1400–1401)*

87. **(E)** The solubility of cholesterol depends on the relative concentrations of conjugated bile salts, cholesterol, and phospholipids (lecithin being predominant). Cholesterol is insoluble in aqueous solution,

but becomes soluble when incorporated into lecithin bile salt micelles. The ratio of the sum of the molar concentrations of bile salts plus lecithin to the molar concentration of cholesterol is termed the lithogenous ratio. A lowering of this ratio by either a decrease in the concentration of bile salts or lecithin, or an increase in the concentration of cholesterol, makes the cholesterol less soluble and results in a more lithogenic bile. Bilirubinate, a major constituent of pigmented stones, has no effect on the solubility on other bile constituents. *(Schwartz, pp. 1390–1391)*

88. **(B)** Cholecystokinin, which is released from the intestinal mucosa in response to food (particularly fat) and enters into the duodenum, is the primary stimulus for gall bladder emptying. Cholecystokinin also relaxes the terminal bile duct, the sphincter of Oddi, and the duodenal musculature. Vagal stimulation causes the gall bladder to contract, but the rate of gall bladder emptying is unchanged following the vagotomy. Sympathetic stimulation is inhibitory to the motor activity of the gall bladder, whereas secretin and hydrochloric acid have little effect on motor activity. *(Schwartz, p. 1385)*

89. **(B)** Chenodeoxycholic acid replenishes the bile acid pool and so tends to return super-saturated bile to a more normal composition. It has also been found to decrease hepatic cholesterol synthesis. Chenodeoxycholic acid is less effective in dissolving large (1.5 cm) than small stones, and radiopaque rather than radiolucent stones. When treatment is terminated, cholelithiasis is likely to return. Side effects of this type of treatment include clinically significant hepatotoxicity. *(Schwartz et al, p. 1391)*

90. **(E)** In several large series of asymptomatic patients with gallstones who were followed and who did not receive surgical treatment, symptoms developed in 50% and serious complications developed in 20%. An operative mortality of 0.7% has been reported for asymptomatic patients in contrast to a 5% mortality rate for patients with acute cholecystitis. Based on a high incidence of ultimate development of symptoms or complications and the small risk of operative mortality, it is generally felt that, unless there is a strong contraindication, the presence of cholelithiasis with or without symptoms is an indication for a cholecystectomy. *(Schwartz, p. 1391)*

91. **(B)** In patients with chronic cholecystitis, ultrasonography is approximately 95% accurate for the detection of gallstones and has, for the most part, replaced oral cholecystography as the initial method of diagnosis. Oral cholecystography is still useful, however, in the evaluation of patients with typical symptoms of chronic cholecystitis who have equivocal and negative ultrasounds. HIDA scanning is most useful in the diagnosis of acute cholecystitis. CT scans can demonstrate gallstones, but this method is not appropriate for initial screening evaluations. Direct visualization of the bile duct by percutaneous transhepatic cholangiography is important in the evaluation of common duct obstruction. *(Schwartz, pp. 1386–1388, 1398)*

92. **(A)** Charcot's Triad consisting of fever, jaundice, and abdominal pain, is the clinical hallmark of acute cholangitis. Initial treatment consists of fluid resuscitation and antibiotics to cover gram-negative organisms, aerobes, and enterococci. If the patient improves with these measures, cholangiographic assessment of the biliary tract is carried out in order to plan definitive therapy. Most cases of acute cholangitis are caused by calculous disease, although benign strictures and malignancies must be excluded. If the patient does not respond to initial nonoperative therapy, decompression of the biliary tract must be carried out. This may be done either surgically, or through percutaneous techniques. *(Schwartz, p. 1399)*

93–96. **93 (C); 94 (A); 95 (D); 96 (A))** Cholecystitis is considered to be acute or chronic dependent on the clinical presentation. The pathophysiology of both implies that the cystic duct is obstructed, usually by gallstones. In acute cholecystitis, persistent obstruction of the cystic duct leads to a chemical and bacterial inflammation of the gall bladder wall itself and potential complications of empyema, gangrene, perforation, and fistula formation. HIDA scan is considered a specific test for acute cholecystitis because of the low rate of false-positive studies. Acute cholecystitis require cholecystectomy but the timing of the operation is controversial. Early cholecystectomy prevents complications and recurrent symptoms and has shown to be as safe in terms of morbidity and mortality as the delayed operation when symptoms resolve. Proponents of the delayed cholecystectomy have suggested that because most episodes of acute cholecystitis resolve, and because the operation may be more difficult in the case of acute inflammatory process, the operation is more appropriately carried out later. In chronic cholecystitis, intermittent cystic duct obstruction produces biliary colic. The diagnosis is usually made on the basis of symptoms, and an ultrasound demonstrating cholelithiases. Chronic cholecystitis is treated by elective cholecystectomy. *(Schwartz, pp. 1395–1398)*

97. (A [1, 2, and 3]) Anatomically, the liver is divided into right and left lobes by a plane between the gall bladder fossa and inferior vena cava. The left lobe is divided into medial and lateral segments by the falciform ligament. The right lobe is divided into the anterior and posterior segments that do not have external landmarks. (Meyers, p. 1054)

98. (A [1, 2, and 3]) The liver performs a wide range of synthetic and metabolic functions and is an important component of the reticuloendothelial systems. Albumin and other plasma proteins such as urea, fibrinogen, and most coagulation factors are principally synthesized in the liver. The liver also has a central role in lipid and glucose metabolism. In the well-fed state, the liver is a site of glycogen synthesis and during periods of fasting it provides energy substrate by glycogenolysis and gluconeogenesis as well as by the formation of ketone bodies. In addition, the liver is also the primary site of cholesterol synthesis and it has a controlling function in the entero-hepatic circulation. Primary bile acids are synthesized, conjugated, actively secreted and then effectively retrieved during this process. Furthermore, the liver is critical in the role of metabolism of fat and water-soluble vitamins, and is the site of the initial 25 hydroxylation of vitamin D. The liver is responsible for the metabolism of many drugs and toxins by the oxidative reactions of the cytochrome P 450 system. (Meyers, p. 1063)

99. (B [1 and 3]) The hepatic arterial supply is normally derived from the celiac axis by way of the proper hepatic artery, which becomes the common hepatic artery after giving off the gastroduodenal branch. The common hepatic artery subsequently bifurcates into the right and left hepatic branches. In approximately 15%-20% of persons, the right hepatic artery can arise from the superior mesenteric artery. The left hepatic artery may originate from the left gastric artery in 15% of persons. These variations must be kept in mind when considering surgical approaches. The hepatic arterial blood supply accounts for approximately 25% of the hepatic blood flow with the remainder supplied by the portal vein. (Schwartz, pp. 1327–1328)

100. (A [1, 2, and 3]) Four types of viral hepatitis are currently recognized. Each of these is caused by a distinct and different etiologic agent. Hepatitis A virus is usually transmitted by a fecal–oral route and does not constitute a particular risk to those involved in surgery. Hepatitis B virus, non-A, non-B hepatitis, and delta-associated hepatitis (which requires the presence of hepatitis B virus) are usually transmitted by the parenteral route, although nonparenteral transmission can occur. Blood transfusion is the classic method of parenteral transmission. Blood products do not all carry an equal risk of hepatitis. Most whole blood and its derivatives have a relatively small risk when compared with products prepared with pooled plasma for the administration of clotting factors. (Hamilton, p. 1123)

101. (C [2 and 4]) Approximately 20% of all cases of hepatitis are of a non-A, non-B variety. The specific virus or antigen responsible for this has not yet been identified. Because there are no screening tests available to eliminate non-A, non-B hepatic virus from blood products, it therefore represents the most common cause of posttransfusion hepatitis. Previous exposure of one type of hepatitis does not protect against subsequent infection with other types. It is thought that non-A, non-B infection develops into chronic hepatitis more frequently than does hepatitis B and that as many as 30% of patients with chronic active hepatitis may become cirrhotic. A vaccine is available for active immunization against hepatitis B, but not for non-A, non-B hepatitis. (Hamilton, p. 1123)

102. (E) The most common primary tumor associated with metastases to the liver is bronchogenic carcinoma. However, considering patients with primary cancers, those with gastrointestinal primaries will develop liver metastases in a greater percentage than those with lung cancers. When colorectal cancers metastasize, they do so commonly to the liver. The diagnosis of hepatic metastases is confirmed by CT scan, ultrasound, or biopsy. (Meyers, p. 1083)

103. (D) Surgical excision is the only definitive treatment for primary hepatocellular carcinoma. Three criteria should be met before attempts are made for surgical resection. (1) The cancer should be solitary. (2) There should be no involvement of the lymph nodes, vasculature, or bile ducts. (3) There should be no distant metastases. Even with the advances of improved surgical techniques, anesthesia, and blood replacement, hepatic resection has only reached an acceptable level of less than 5%. Overall, only 20% to 30% of patients can undergo resection, and 5-year survival rates approach 30%. In the face of extensive cirrhosis, and with its associated morbidity and mortality, resection is contraindicated. Orthotopic liver transplantation results have not been encouraging. Radiation and/or chemotherapy have not been shown to prolong survival. (Schwartz, pp. 1347–1349)

104. (B) The protein alpha fetoprotein (AFP) is normally present in the fetus at birth, but disappears after a few weeks. In patients in the United States

with primary hepatic neoplasms, 30% will be found to have AFP in their serum. If present, AFP may be used as a marker because resection of the tumor converts the test to negative. Recurrence of the same tumor would be evident by a return of AFP to the serum. The AFP may also be elevated in embryonic tumors of the ovary and testes, giving a false-positive test result. In metastatic tumors of the liver, the AFP is usually negative. *(Schwartz, p. 1348)*

105. **(E)** The etiology of portal hypertension arises from four categories of pathology: (1) increased hepatopetal flow without obstruction, such as that seen with hepatic arterial–portal venous fistulas; this is an infrequent cause; (2) extrahepatic outflow obstruction, as in Budd–Chiari syndrome or endophlebitis of the hepatic veins; (3) obstruction of the extrahepatic portal venous system, as in cavernomatous transformation of the portal vein. The most common etiologic factor in this category in childhood is some form of infection carried by a patent umbilical vein (neonatal omphalitis); (4) the overwhelming majority of cases of portal hypertension are caused by intrahepatic obstruction. This category accounts for 90% of all cases. Cirrhosis (nutritional, postnecrotic, or biliary) is the most common reason for this type of postsinusoidal obstruction to portal blood flow. *(Schwartz, pp. 1352–1355)*

106. **(E)** In a patient with alcoholic cirrhosis, abstinence from alcohol is the most important factor in determining survival postshunting. A low-salt diet, control of ascites, a low-protein diet, and the use of lactulose are various therapies that are used depending on the severity of the disease. *(Langer and Grieg, p. 1116)*

107. **(B)** Bleeding from varices that have not responded to endoscopic sclorosis in an alcoholic cirrhotic patient is the most accepted indication for surgery. Because only 30% of cirrhotic patients with varices, regardless of size, will ever bleed, choice *A* is incorrect. Emergency shunting results in an operative survival of 50% to 71% and a 7-year survival in 42% of patients. If possible, emergency shunting should be avoided. Prophylactic shunts, such as for choice *E* do not increase survival, and may produce encephalopathy. If at all possible, patients with encephalopathy should not be shunted. *(Schwartz, pp. 1362–1374)*

108–112. **108 (A); 109 (C); 110 (A); 111 (A); 112 (B)** Hepatic abcesses are related to two distinct types of pathogens: *Entamoeba histolytica,* and pyogenic bacteria. With pyogenic abcesses, *Escherichia coli* or other gram-negative bacteria are the most commonly isolated organism. The most common source of these bacteria is a contiguous infection in the biliary system. Amebic abscesses are caused by *histolytica* and no bacteria are typically isolated from these abscesses. However, in 22% of patients, secondary infection is a complication. Pyogenic abscesses may be solitary, multiple, and multilocular. Amebic abscesses are usually single. The right lobe of the liver is commonly involved in any abscesses of the liver because of the so-called streaming effect in the portal vein. Treatment of pyogenic abscesses consists of appropriate antibiotics plus surgical drainage. The mortality rate with a solitary pyogenic abscess is 24%, whereas multiple abscesses carry a 70% mortality. Undrained pyogenic abscesses have a mortality rate approaching 100%. With amebic abscesses, the treatment is conservative, consisting of the use of amebicidal drugs. Aspiration is indicated if the patient fails to respond to medication or if signs of secondary infection develop. With amebic abscesses, the mortality rate is only 7% in uncomplicated cases and 43% in cases where complications such as secondary infection develop. *(Schwartz et al, pp. 1334–1340)*

113. **(E)** Approximately 60% of benign tumors of the small bowel occur in the ileum. 25% occur in the jejunum, and 15% in the duodenum. Often, these tumors are discovered at autopsy and are asymptomatic during life. Unless obstruction is present, the physical diagnosis is rarely helpful and radiologic examination may fail to show an existing tumor, even if suspected clinically. The two most common clinical manifestations are bleeding and obstruction. Bleeding occurs in roughly 30% of patients and is rarely gross hemorrhage. The bleeding is usually occult. Obstruction is either from encroachment, in which case the obstruction is chronic and partial, or by intussusception. *(Townsend and Thompson, pp. 1205–1206)*

114. **(C)** Malignant tumors of the small bowel are relatively infrequent, accounting for about 2% of all gastrointestinal malignancies. Histologically, adenocarcinoma is the most frequent, followed by carcinoid, lymphoma, and leiomyosarcoma. Survival is lowest with adencarcinoma (20%) and higher with the other cell types (40%). Treatment of malignant small bowel tumors is wide resection including regional lymph nodes. This requires pancreaticoduodenectomy in duodenal lesions. With lymphomas, postoperative radiation and/or chemotherapy is indicated but has no effect with the other cell types. *(Townsend and Thompson, pp. 1207–1209)*

115. **(B)** Carcinoid tumors were histologically first described in 1808, although their potential for malignancy was not recognized until 1911. The cells of origin are the Kultschitzsky cell, and carcinoid tumors may arise anywhere in the gastrointestinal tract that these cells occur, that is, from stomach to anus. The appendix is however, the most frequently involved, followed by the ileum, and rectum. Carcinoid tumors may also be found outside the gastrointestinal tract including the bronchus and ovary. Carcinoid tumor has a tendency for multicentricity that exceeds any other neoplasm of the gastrointestinal tract. The prognosis is a function of tumor size and its site of origin, along with its histological type. *(Townsend and Thompson, pp. 1208–1209)*

116. **(C)** Meckel's diverticulum is the most frequently encountered diverticulum of the small intestine. It occurs in 2% of the population. It is a true diverticulum and is found on the antimesenteric border of the ileum about 2 feet from the ileocecal valve. Complications of Meckel's diverticulum include intestinal obstruction, which is the most common, followed by bleeding and, finally, Meckel's diverticulitis. Occasionally, Meckel's diverticulum contains ectopic gastric mucosa and can be seen with a technetium pertechnetate scan. *(Townsend and Thompson, p. 1212)*

117. **(D)** The appendix is usually referred to as a vestigal organ. This is however, not the case. Current evidence suggests that the appendix is a highly specialized part of the gastrointestinal tract. The appendix participates in the secretory immune system in the gut as part of the gut-associated lymphoid tissues (GALT). It is not, however, indispensable. The immunoglobulin system shows no detectable defect upon removal of the appendix. The appendix also plays a role in the maturation of the B lymphocytes, along with the tonsils and Peyer's patches. In the 1960s it was felt that patients who had had their appendix removed had a higher risk of developing cancer of the colon. Most recent studies have not shown this relationship to be true. *(Schwartz, p. 1315)*

118. **(A)** Abdominal pain is the prime symptom of appendicitis. Classically, the pain is initially diffuse, but centered in the periumbilical region. The pain is characterized as a steady, moderately severe, occasionally crampy, type of pain. Usually within 4 to 6 hours, the pain localizes in the right lower quadrant. There is, however, a high degree of variability to this classic sequence. Anorexia is so closely associated with acute appendicitis that the diagnosis should be questioned if the patient is not anorectic. Vomiting occurs in about 75% of patients, but is not prolonged. Changes in bowel function, in particular obstipation or constipation, frequently occur but are of little diagnostic value. In more than 95% of patients with acute appendicitis, anorexia is the first symptom, followed by abdominal pain and then vomiting, if vomiting occurs. The diagnosis should be questioned if vomiting precedes the onset of abdominal pain. *(Schwartz, p. 1317)*

119. **(A)** Acute appendicitis in the elderly is a very serious disease. Less than 10% of patients operated on for appendicitis are more than 60, but greater than 50% of all deaths from appendicitis are in this age group. Classic symptoms and physical findings may be present but are generally much milder or difficult to elicit. Fever and/or leukocytosis are less than expected and in some patients, normal. Because of these conditions, 67% to 90% of elderly patients will have a ruptured appendix at the time of operation. This often results in a diffuse peritonitis. Mortality rates of ruptured appendicitis in the elderly is about 15%, a fivefold increase from the overall rate. *(Schwartz, p. 1321)*

120. **(C)** Obstruction of the lumen of the appendix is the principle factor in the pathogenesis of acute appendicitis. Fecaliths are the most common cause of appendiceal obstruction. Other less common causes of appendiceal obstruction are vegetable and fruit seeds, intestinal worms, and inspissated barium from x-ray studies. Fecaliths are found in simple appendicitis in about 40% of cases. In gangrenous appendicitis without rupture, they are found in approximately 65%; if the appendix is gangrenous and ruptured, a fecalith is found approximately 90% of the time. *(Schwartz, pp. 1316–1317)*

121. **(B)** At birth, the appendix arises from the inferior tip of the cecum. Through growth and differentiation, the appendix in the adult comes to lie on the posteriormedial aspect of the cecum, below the ileocecal valve. The base of the appendix and its relationship to the cecum is relatively constant. The distal end may, however, be found in a variety of places, such as the pelvis, retrocecal, or even on the left side. The three taeniae coli are a useful surgical landmark in that they converge at the junction of the cecum and the appendix. Here, they form the outer longitudinal muscle layer of the appendix. *(Schwartz, p. 1315)*

122. **(E)** With acute appendicitis, the differential diagnosis is essentially that of the acute abdomen. A diverse number of pathologies can present with a seemingly identical picture of appendicitis. In general, about 85% of the cases diagnosed preoperatively as appendicitis are positive, accounting for an acceptable 15% false-negative rate. The most common inaccurate preoperative diagnoses include,

mesenteric lymphadenitis, no pathology found; acute pelvic inflammatory disease; twisted ovarian cyst; and epiploic appendagitis. Diverticulitis of the sigmoid colon, particularly that portion that lies on the right side, is also included in the differential. The diagnosis of appendicitis depends on three factors: (1) the location of the inflamed appendix, (2) the sex and age of the patient, and (3) the type of appendicitis, that is, ruptured or simple. *(Schwartz, pp. 1319–1321)*

123. **(A)** The diagnosis of acute appendicitis in a pregnant patient is a difficult one. Abdominal pain and nausea are common in pregnancy as well as in appendicitis. Because of the ever-expanding uterus, the appendix is displaced so that the location of the point of maximal tenderness is shifted to a higher and more lateral position. There is no difference in the rate of occurrence of appendicitis between pregnant and nonpregnant females. Maternal mortality is about 0.2% and is almost always associated with generalized peritonitis. Fetal mortality is 8.5% in simple appendicitis, but rises to 35% with perforation. There is only one treatment for acute appendicitis and that is surgery. To attempt to treat appendicitis with antibiotics alone ignores the obstructive pathogenesis of the disease and is not a acceptable therapy. *(Schwartz, pp. 1321–1322)*

124. **(E)** Although acute appendicitis is a diagnosis of clinical findings, radiography may be used to narrow the list of the differential diagnosis or to demonstrate complications of appendicitis. Radiographic findings consistent with, but not diagnostic, of appendicitis include distended loop(s) of small bowel in the right lower quadrant, visualization of a gas-filled appendix, and a partially filled appendix on barium enema examination. Some studies show that, with barium enema examination, the findings of a partially filled appendix, a mass effect on the medial and inferior borders of the cecum, and a mass effect or mucosal changes of terminal ileum, are pathognomonic for acute appendicitis. *(Schwartz, p. 1318)*

125. **(B)** Acute appendicitis is a surgical disease. Delaying surgery places the patient at greater risk for increased morbidity and mortality. In pregnancy, there is a fourfold increase in fetal mortality associated with appendiceal rupture. In the elderly, nonoperative treatment increases the chance of rupture and death. In patients with periappendiceal abscess formation, the treatment is controversial. Nonoperative treatment initially, in combination with antibiotic therapy, and close monitoring of the patient's clinical and laboratory course is an acceptable option in a patient with subsiding symptoms and a palpable right lower quadrant mass. An elec-

tive appendectomy should be performed in 6 weeks to 3 months later, if the patient remains stable. The interval appendectomy is needed because of the high rate of recurrence. *(Schwartz p. 1322)*

126. **(A)** Carcinoma of the prostate is the most frequent malignant tumor in males over the age of 65. It should be noted, however, that many men die with carcinoma of the prostate and not because of it. Elevations in the serum acid phosphatase occurs from many sources, including multiple myeloma, bony tumors, benign prostatic disease, and acute urinary retention. The portion of the total serum acid phosphatase that comes from the prostate may be detected by the addition of tartate to the serum, making it a more specific test. An elevation of the prostatic serum acid phosphatase is not specific for carcinoma. The normal prostate contains acid phosphatase and minor serum elevations may be seen following rectal examinations. These elevations may persist for up to 36 hours. The presence of an elevated serum acid phosphatase in cases of prostatic cancer usually indicates metastatic disease or extensive local disease, precluding surgical cure. It is useful as a tumor marker to gauge effectiveness of treatment. It is not generally elevated in early disease and so it is not useful as a screening method. Digital examination of the rectum and prostate is the most important method of detecting asymptomatic prostate cancer. *(Weinerth, p. 1686)*

127. **(C)** Detection of the asymptomatic prostate nodule is essential in order to find prostate cancer in its potentially curable form. The vast majority are found on routine physical examination. Greater than 50% of prostatic nodules palpated on rectal examination are found to be positive for carcinoma on biopsy. The objective of treatment for asymptomatic prostate cancers should be to cure. Only surgical excision, namely, radical prostatectomy, or radical radiation therapy can offer a cure for this disease. The 5-year survival rate in selected cases can be greater than 50%. *(Frank, p. 1766)*

128. **(B)** Benign tumors of the testis are very rare. Whenever a testicular mass is found it should be considered malignant until proven otherwise. Testicular malignancies account for 1% of all cancers in the male. The average age at diagnosis is 32 years. Patients typically present with a nonpainful lump in the testis, which is hard, nontender, and solid. The mass does not transilluminate. If a testicular tumor is suspected, surgical exploration is indicated. Serum alpha fetoprotein and human chorionic gonadotropin should be obtained, as these are useful tumor markers in many testicular tumors. Exploration via an inguinal incision, so as to control the spermatic vessel at the inguinal ring, is the

preferred method. Palpation of induration of the testis is the indication for orchiectomy. In that these tumors are heterogeneous, incisional biopsy has no role. *(Frank, pp. 1768–1770)*

129. (D) The differential in this patient is that of acute epididymitis verses testicular torsion. Because prompt treatment of testicular torsion is necessary to prevent testicular infarction, it may occasionally be required that the patient with acute epididymitis be explored in order to prevent the loss of a testis from torsion. Four hours appears to be the maximal amount of time that a testis can undergo torsion, after which irreversible damage is done. If time allows, isotopic scanning of the testis may show the characteristic absence of testicular blood flow. However, time should not be wasted in order to confirm the diagnosis. *(Frank, p. 1735)*

130. (B) Testicular masses are malignant until proven otherwise. Testicular masses are most often found in the 20 to 35-year-old age group. Benign tumors, usually fibromas of the tunica vaginalis, are in the differential diagnosis but are rare. Of malignant tumors, germinal cell tumors are the most common. This cell type includes seminoma (40%), embryonal cell carcinoma (25%), teratocarcinoma (25%), and choriocarcinoma (1%). *(Frank, pp. 1768–1769)*

131. (C) The composition of urinary calculi is significant, in that therapy aimed at prevention of recurrence and the etiological abnormality may both be determined by knowing the make-up of the calculi. Calcium oxalate stones are the most common urinary calculi. They account for approximately 75% of all urinary stones. Ammonium-magnesium phosphate stones makeup 15% of stones and are typically found in infected urine. Uric acid stones constitute about 8% of all calculi. Finally, cystine stones represent only 1% of urinary calculi. *(Frank, p. 1748)*

132–134.   132 (B); 133 (C); 134 (A) Joints are either fibrous or cartilaginous based on the nature of the tissue joining the bones together. A fibrous joint, such as the sutures of the skull, is made up of bones united by fibrous tissue. When bones are joined by either hyline cartilage or fibrocartilage, they are called cartilaginous joints. The pubic symphysis and the intervertebral discs are examples of this type of joint. Synovial joints also known as diarthrodial joints are movable joints united by a capsule. This capsule is lined with synovium. Most joints of the extremities are synovial joints. *(Duthie and Hoaglund, p. 1981)*

135–138.   135 (B); 136 (A); 137 (C); 138 (D) After the age of 35, pain after minor strains of the shoulder or spontaneous pain is common. Before attaching the

diagnosis to a local condition of the shoulder, one must be certain to rule out diseases that may cause referred pain to the shoulder. Cardiac, pulmonary, and gastrointestinal pathologies may all cause referred pain to the shoulder. Pathology in the neck including cervical arthritis and brachial plexus irritation, Pancoast's tumors, and central nervous system disease need to be considered. Once the pathology has been located at the shoulder, knowledge of the anatomy of the shoulder makes the diagnosis easier. Disorders of the rotator cuff, bicipital tendonitis, and subacromial bursitis are the three most common causes of primary painful shoulder disorders. The rotator cuff is made up of the common tendonous insertions of the supraspinatus, infraspinatus, teres minor, and the subscapularis muscle tendons (SITS). The rotator cuff is intimately adherent to the shoulder capsule that lies just beneath it. The rotator cuff comes in contact with the undersurface of the coracoacromial ligament when the arm is abducted past 90° or is fully elevated. This may lead to mechanical irritation and subsequent degeneration. The subacromal bursa lies between the coracoacromial ligament, the acromion, and the rotator cuff. Inflammation may occur here as a result of the mechanical irritation, causing bursitis. This typically causes unrelenting pain that is unaffected by position changes. With supraspinatous tendonitis, the patient usually complains of low-grade shoulder pain with sudden motion or with full internal rotation and the extremes of abduction. Bicipital tendonitis presents with similar symptoms but differentiation may be made on the basis of the anatomical location of the biceps tendon. Pain and tenderness are found over the bicipital groove. A rotator cuff tear is a physical disruption of the rotator cuff and is usually partial. Partial tears can be treated with shoulder immobilization in a sling. Complete tears may be treated conservatively but surgical repair is often required. *(Duthie and Hoaglund, pp. 2001–2002)*

139. (B) Injury to the peripheral nerves may accompany soft tissue injuries with or without fractures. The clinical manifestations of these injuries are dependent on the severity of the injury. Neurapraxia is the least severe type of nerve injury and is characterized by a transient loss of nerve conduction. With more severe injuries, Wallerian degeneration of the axon may take place. The Schwann sheath may remain intact. The combination is termed *axonotmesis*. If the nerve is completely divided, the term used is *neurotmesis*. *(Spencer et al, p. 1845)*

140. (C) As with any pathology, the history and physical examination are important. In internal derangements of the knee, however, the practitioner is rarely able to make an accurate diagnosis. Arthroscopy, especially of the lateral compartment, is more accurate than arthrography, and permits visualization of portions of the knee that are not viewed at arthrotomy. *(Duthie and Hoaglund, pp. 1966–1967)*

141. **(B)** Chondromalacia of the patella represents degeneration of the cartilage surface of the patella and the earliest changes occur on its medial facet. X-rays are negative early in the disease but are used to rule out other forms of pathology. The cause of chondromalcia is unknown, but repetitive trauma may play a role. The patient will typically complain of discomfort in the knee with acute flexion or when kneeling or walking down stairs. Most patients may be treated conservatively with good results. In those patients who do not respond to conservative management, surgical treatment is needed. Realignment of the quadriceps patellar mechanism, or patellectomy are the surgical treatments of choice. *(Duthie and Hoaglund, pp. 1995–1996)*

142. **(A)** Peripheral nerves are most sensitive to anoxia. Paralysis and anesthesia quickly develop when arterial blood flow is severely decreased. Striated muscle is almost equally sensitive and will usually become necrotic if arterial blood flow is decreased to such a degree that anesthesia and paralysis are present. Skin, bone, and tendon may survive an ischemic injury that produces irreversible extensive muscle necrosis. *(Imparato and Riles, p. 936)*

143. **(B)**

144. **(A)** In acute arterial occlusion, the level of arterial obstruction may be diagnosed from the history because the exertional muscle pain occurs one joint distal to the site of occlusion. Superficial femoral artery occlusion results in calf pain. An occlusion in the external iliac artery can produce thigh pain and aortic occlusion may be diagnosed by buttock pain. The level of occlusion can often be estimated from the color and temperature level as well as the pulse findings. The arterial pulse is absent at the site of occlusion, frequently with accentuation of the pulse immediately proximal to this point. Sensory impairment varies from hypesthesia to anesthesia, and motor disturbances from weakness to paralysis. *(Imparato and Riles, p. 951)*

145. **(A)**

146. **(C)** The clinical manifestations of major venous thrombosis involving the deep venous system of the thigh and pelvis produces pain, pitting edema, and blanching, termed *phlegmasia alba dolens*. It can occur in pregnancy secondary to compression of the left iliac vein, relaxation of the vessel wall, or from hormonal effects on the blood. Mechanical factors can also decrease left iliac vein drainage, such as compression of the right iliac artery, overdistended

bladder, and congenital webs within the vein. As venous thrombosis progresses, the venous return slows from the extremity. The buildup of venous blood can cause cessation of arterial flow and endanger the limb. The congested limb with both sensory and motor loss is referred to as *phelgmasia cerulea dolens*. Unless venous flow is restored, venous gangrene is likely to develop. *(Schwartz et al, p. 1014)*

147. **(C)**

148. **(A)** The gangrenous digits represent occlusion of a critical digital artery. Diabetics may have a type of arterial occlusive disease that typically involves the popliteal artery and its branches down to the pedal arches. Minor trauma, unnoticed by diabetics because of their diabetic neuropathy, may progress to gangrene of the toes. Trophic ulcers, which are usually sharply demarcated, punched-out areas on the sole of the foot overlying a pressure point, are frequently found in diabetics. Palpable pedal pulses may be present. Buerger's disease, a form of chronic arterial insuffiency in which tobacco plays a major role in its progression, superficial ulceration, and gangrene will develop if arterial circulation is not improved. *(Imparato and Riles, pp. 971–972, 995)*

149. **(E)** Signs of chronic tissue ischemia include loss of hair from the digits, atrophy of the skin, brittle opaque nails, and rubor on dependency. Muscle atrophy in the feet with increasing prominence of the interosseous spaces may be present. The importance of the examination of the foot is emphasized by the fact that gangrene seldom appears in an extremity with chronic vascular disease until these stigmata of chronic ischemia are present. *(Imparato and Riles, p. 949)*

150. **(B)** The classic five abnormal findings associated with acute ischemia are pain, paralysis, paresthesia or anesthesia, absent pulses, and pallor. Paralysis and paresthesia are most important because loss of neurologic function indicates a degree of tissue ischemia that will progress to gangrene unless arterial blood flow is improved. *(Imparato and Riles, pp. 936–939)*

151. **(A)** Congenital arteriovenous fistulas constitute one manifestation of a number of more commonly related abnormalities of the vascular system. The appearance may vary from a simple port wine stain to the massively hypertrophied extremity that has multiple arteries, capillaries, and veins dilated and visible in and through the skin with or without abnormal arteriovenous communications. The hallmark of the complex congenital arteriovenous fistula is the palpation of a thrill and the auscultation of a bruit. The key note to treatment is conservativ-

ism. The decision to treat malformations on the surface of the body need only to be based upon whether a lesion threatens to ulcerate or bleed, whether the hemihypertrophy of the extremity may lead to serious orthopedic problems, or whether the deformity is so cosmetically repulsive that the patient must have help. (Imparato and Riles, p. 934)

152. (C) The most important consideration following operation is to detect peripheral pulses, which indicate satisfactory restoration of arterial flow. If pulses cannot be detected or if previously palpable pulses disappear, an arteriogram should be performed or the site of anastomosis should be reexplored. The important principle to emphasize is that, with modern vascular techniques, traumatic injury of a normal artery can almost always be successfully repaired. Anticoagulant therapy is not recommended routinely after arterial repair, for it provides little protection from thrombus but does increase the risk of bleeding into the wound. (Imparato and Riles, p. 938)

153. (E) Control of bleeding is the most urgent immediate problem and can usually be accomplished by direct digital pressure on the bleeding site or by tightly packing the wound with gauze and applying a pressure dressing. Tourniquets are best avoided for most injuries. If they are used, they must be carefully padded to avoid the risk of permanent injury to peripheral nerves. (Imparato and Riles, p. 937)

154. (C) Anterior compartment syndrome should be treated by decompression fasciotomy early to avoid anoxic necrosis of the muscle mass. The dorsalis pedis pulse may be normal, diminished, or absent. Its absence is a late sign and occasionally follows the loss of motor power of the muscles of the anterior compartment. (Imparato and Riles, p. 940)

155. (E) Diabetics may have high ankle brachial indices due to calcification of the arterial wall. Claudicators range from 0.50 to 1.00. Patients with more advanced degrees of ischemia will generally have an index less than 0.50. The ankle brachial index is a ratio between the pressure of the affected extremity and the normal systolic blood pressure. (Imparato and Riles, p. 949)

156. (A) Noninvasive studies using ultrasound, plethysmography, x-ray, and magnetic resonance have been useful in confirming the diagnosis and differentiating arterial diseases from other syndromes. Arteriography continues to be the most important laboratory technique. A high-quality study is essential in planning the surgical approach to reconstruction. (Imparato and Riles, p. 949)

157. (D)

158. (C) Emboli arising from the heart, constituting the majority of emboli seen, are referred to as cardioarterial embolization. In about 90% of patients with lower extremity emboli, the embolus originates in the heart from one of three causes: mitral stenosis, atrial fibrillation, or myocardial infarction. In some patients, it is the first sign of unrecognized heart disease. Emboli and thrombi are terms that are not interchangeable. A thrombus is a blood clot obstructing a blood vessel. A thrombosis is inferred when there are signs of diffuse vascular disease. An embolism may occur during atrial fibrillation when there is a dislodgement of a thrombus from the left ventricle. (Imparato and Riles, p. 950; DeGowin and De-Gowin, p. 427; Taber, T-26)

159. (A) Incompetent valves of the deep veins enable a long column of blood to transmit pressures of over 100 mm Hg to venules. This promotes fluid and protein loss into tissues. The perivascular fibrinous deposits interfere with normal oxygenation and metabolism of tissues. This causes the thickening and liposclerosis of the subcutaneous tissues to produce the characteristic nonpitting edema. In patients with long-standing chronic venous insufficiency, hemosiderin deposits from the red cells are responsible for the brown pigment. (Greenfield, p. 1029)

160. (E) The prompt IV administration of heparin to inhibit the development of thrombi distal to the embolus is the most important therapeutic measure in the treatment of an arterial embolus. For operations on the lower extremity, local anesthesia may be used. The emboli can be removed by the insertion of a Fogarty balloon catheter through a short incision placed directly over the uppermost level of the arterial occlusion. If the embolus is localized to the incision site, the balloon catheter should be used to clear out the entire artery. An operative arteriogram should be performed to confirm the patency of the artery. A fasciotomy may help preserve limb viability if embolectomy has been delayed beyond 4 to 6 hours and increased muscle turgor was palpated before operation. (Imparato and Riles, p. 954)

161. (A) Abdominal aortic aneurysms are the most common of the atherosclerotic aneurysms. Men are affected more frequently than women in a ratio approximating 10:1. Except for traumatic and congenital malformations, almost all peripheral aneurysms result from arteriosclerosis. The majority of the peripheral aneurysms are in the popliteal artery. Infrequent sites include the femoral, carotid, and subclavian arteries. (Schwartz, p. 988)

162. (B)

163. (A) The majority of abdominal aneurysms are arteriosclerotic in nature and their pathogenesis is probably different from occlusive disease. Aneurysms result from degenerative changes in the media. Atherosclerotic occlusion results from a proliferative reaction in the media causing narrowing of the lumen. The distribution of the two processes is also different. The atherosclerotic occlusive process involves the aorta at sites of bifurcations, attachments, tapers, and curvatures. Aneurysmal disease occurs at the abdominal aorta, popliteal, carotid, femoral, iliac, and subclavian arteries. *(Imparato and Riles, p. 981)*

164. (D)

165. (C) In the 1940s, Leriche described the clinical characteristics of occlusion of the abdominal aorta. These are claudication, sexual impotence in the male, and absence of gangrene. The lumen narrowing may be due to fibrointimal thickening, ulceration of atherosclerotic plaques, and superimposed thrombus or embolization of portions of atherosclerotic plaques. The progress of aortoiliac occlusive disease is slow. Symptoms of claudication appear with exercise. Sexual impotence is frequent because of decreased blood flow through the hypogastric arteries. Patients with abdominal aortic aneurysms are usually asymptomatic. They may have associated lesions but for the most part do not complain of claudication or impotence. Occasionally, low back pain caused by tension on retroperitoneum by the aneurysm may be a patient's complaint. *(Imparato and Riles, pp. 957, 982)*

166. (C)

167. (B)

168. (A) Livedo reticularis, an unusual vasomotor condition, is characterized by a persistent mottled reddish blue discoloration of the skin of the extremities. It is most prominent in the legs and although it never disappears, it does worsen on exposure to the cold. The pathologic feature apparently is a stenosis of the arterioles that pierce the cutis at right angles and arborize into peripheral capillaries of the skin, which accounts for the nature of the discolorization. Peripheral pulses are normal. Acrocyanosis is a disorder characterized by persistent but painless cold and cyanosis of the hands and feet. The basic pathologic condition is a slow rate of blood flow through the skin, the result of chronic arteriolar constriction, that results in a high percentage of reduced hemoglobin in the blood in the capillaries and production of the cyanotic color. This disorder is usu-ally found in young women who note persistent coldness and blueness of the fingers or hands for many years, worsening on exposure to the cold. Peripheral pulses are normal. In erythromelalgia, the basic abnormality is an unusual sensitivity to warmth. Skin temperatures of 32° to 36° C, which produce no effects in normal individuals, will regularly induce a painful burning sensation. The increase in témperature is usually a result of vasodilatation with increased blood flow. The exact basis for the spontaneous vasodilatation with rise in temperature and the burning sensation is not known. *(Imparato and Riles, pp. 998–1000)*

169. (C)

170. (A)

171. (D) Raynaud's phenomenon and Raynaud's disease have the same recurrent episodes of vasocontriction in the upper extremities initiated by exposure to cold or emotional stress. In 10% to 15% of patients, the legs may be involved as well as the arms. Three sequential phases classically occur—pallor, cyanosis, and rubor. Raynaud's phenomenon may exist as a primary disorder, termed Raynaud's disease, or it may be a secondary manifestation of a more serious vascular disease. The disorders associated with Raynaud's phenomenon include Buerger's disease, scleroderma, thoracic outlet syndrome, atherosclerosis, periarteritis nodosa, and disseminated lupus erythematosus. A critical point in the evaluation of Raynaud's disease is to determine the existence of a more severe disorder. Buerger's disease or thromboangiitis obliterans is an inflammatory process involving the walls of arteries with involvement of neighboring nerve and vein that may terminate into thrombosis of the artery. Both upper and lower extremities may be affected. Heavy tobacco smoking has been almost universally associated with Buerger's disease. *(Imparato and Riles, pp. 994, 996, 997)*

172. (A)

173. (B) The degrees of severity of a frostbite injury have been grouped into four different types analogous to the classification of burn injury. First degree injury consists of edema and redness of the affected part without necrosis of the skin. Formation of blisters occurs in a second degree injury. There is necrosis of the skin in a third degree injury. In a fourth degree injury, gangrene of the extremity develops that requires amputation. *(Imparato and Riles, p. 1000)*

174. (C) Rapid rewarming of injured tissue, using water with a temperature in the range of 40° to 44° for 20 minutes is the most important aspect of treatment of frostbite. Higher temperatures are more injurious than beneficial. A frostbitten part should never be exposed to hot water, an open fire, or an oven, for the loss of sensitivity can result in a thermal injury. *(Imparato and Riles, p. 1000)*

175. (A) Buerger's disease or thromboangiitis obliterans is most often seen in men who smoke greater than 20 cigarettes per day, and are between 20 and 40 years of age. The distribution of the arterial involvement is not the same as in atherosclerotic disease. Smaller, more peripheral arteries, usually in a segmental distribution are involved, similar to the diabetic. *(Imparato and Riles, pp. 994–995)*

176. (D) The principle finding in aortoiliac occlusive disease is diminution or absence of femoral pulses combined with absence of popliteal and pedal pulses. Diabetics most often have occlusive disease of the tibial arteries, although some do also have aortoiliac disease. Patients with Buerger's disease may also have tibial occlusive disease. The femoral and popliteal arteries in these patients should not be affected. Unless patients with abdominal aneurysm have concomitant aortoiliac occlusive disease or arterioemboli from their aneurysm, their peripheral pulses should be intact. *(Imparato and Riles, pp. 958, 967)*

177. (E) In the diabetic, arterial occlusive disease typically involves the popliteal artery and its branches down to the pedal arches. Because of diabetic neuropathy, the patient may not be aware of minor trauma to the foot. Within hours or days of a trivial injury, a virulent necrotizing infection can appear rapidly spreading along musculofascial planes because of the diabetic's extraordinary susceptibility to infection. *(Imparato and Riles, p. 971)*

178. (E) In patients with aortoiliac disease, concomitant coronary artery or cerebral atherosclerosis occurs frequently. It has been found that 10% of persons with aortoiliac disease have small aneurysms as well. A younger group of patients in their fifth or sixth decades has been identified who have hypercoagulability and thrombose their abdominal aortas while only having mild atherosclerosis of the common iliac arteries. *(Imparato and Riles, p. 957)*

179. (C) The perforators adjacent to the medial malleolus are often responsible for the development of stasis ulcers at that level. When they become incompetent, the findings of perforator or deep venous disease are more serious than disease of the superficial system, which is composed of the greater and lesser saphenous veins. Primary varicosities due to valvular weakness or weakness of vein walls are associated with the superficial system, whereas secondary varicosities are present in those patients with other symptoms of deep venous disease (stasis ulcers, brawny edema, dermatitis). *(Greenfield, pp. 1012, 1028)*

180. (E) The term ischemic stroke refers to cerebral infarction occurring as a result of impaired blood flow. Atherosclerosis is the basis of this in the vast majority of patients but it can also occur when the lumen is occluded by emboli, hermatoma, fibromuscular hyperplasia, or arteritis. Injury, trauma, or thoracic aneurysms involving the carotid artery can result in dissection and tearing of the intima. *(Imparato and Riles, p. 974)*

181. (C)

182. (A)

183. (D) The Adson's maneuver that demonstrates the obstruction of the subclavian artery by the scalenus anticus muscle is the most useful test to indicate thoracic outlet syndrome. The Allen's test will show the integrity of the palmar arches. In patients with thoracic outlet syndrome, the radial pulse will decrease or obliterate during the Adson's maneuver, but the radial pulse should be present during the Allen's test. The submersion test is performed for patients who complain of cold-related color and temperature changes to their upper extremities. If the submersion test is positive, patients will show classic color changes of Raynaud's phenomenon, pallor, cyanosis, and rubor. The exercise stress test is most helpful in documenting exercise-induced claudication in patients with femoropopliteal disease. At rest, these patients may show only slightly decreased Doppler pressures and pulses. However, following exercise that produces the symptoms, the drop in pressure and recovery time are proportional to the extent of arterial occlusive disease. The Valsalva maneuver can be used to assess venous, not peripheral arterial disease. *(Imparato and Riles, pp. 944, 997)*

184. (C) Venous valves are the focal point of most of the pathology of venous thrombosis. The sinus in which the valve lies is where the initial thrombus forms. In addition, the loss of valvular function after recannulization of a vein produces venous insufficiency. *(Greenfield, p. 1011)*

185. (C) The most common cause of secondary lymphedema in the United States is malignant disease metastatic to lymph nodes. Surgical removal of lymph nodes, particularly when combined with radiation therapy that produces lymphatic fibrosis, is another common cause. Lymphangitis is most often caused by *Staphylococcus* or beta hemolytic *Streptococcus*. Compression stockings or gloves may help to reduce the edema. *(Greenfield, pp. 1036, 1038)*

186. **(C)** Varicella and diphtheria are not known to cause heart disease. However, rubella, occurring in the first trimester of pregnancy is one of the few infectious diseases known to cause congenital heart disease, usually patent ductus arteriosus. All evidence indicates that mitral stenosis is almost always due to rheumatic fever. Since it is now rare, the most common heart disease in children is congenital heart disease. *(Spencer, p. 771; Spencer and Culliford, p. 855)*

187. **(E)** Obstructive lesions, which occur in pulmonic valvular stenosis, aortic valvular stenosis, and coarctation of the aorta, impede emptying of the involved ventricular chamber. This results in systolic overloading and corresponding hypertrophy of the ventricle. As pressures in the left atrium and left ventricle are normally greater than those in the right atrium and ventricle, a defect in either artrial or ventricular septum results in a shunt of oxygenated blood from the left to the right side of the heart. This causes pulmonary congestion from an increase of pulmonary blood flow and a corresponding decrease in systemic blood flow. Right-to-left shunting produces cyanosis and is seen in tetralogy of Fallot and other types of cyanotic heart disease due to the emptying venous blood into the systemic circulation. *(Spencer, p. 774)*

188. **(D)** Seven malformations will comprise the majority of abnormalities seen in a large pediatric cardiology clinic. Ventricular septal defect with or without pulmonic stenosis is the most common, representing 20% or more of all patients. The other six malformations, each occurring in 10% to 15% of patients are artial septal defect, pulmonic valvular stenosis, patent ductus arteriosus, aortic valvular stenosis, coarctation of the aorta, and transposition of the great vessels. The frequency of the different defects varies with the age of the group evaluated. *(Spencer, pp. 771–772)*

189. **(B)**

190. **(A)**

191. **(A)**

192. **(B)** Cyanosis does not occur in isolated atrial and ventricular septal defects. In atrial and ventricular septal defects, the pressure in the left atrium and

ventricle are greater than those in the right atrium and ventricle. The blood that is shunted is oxygenated. Pulmonary congestion occurs from an increase in pulmonary blood flow and often a corresponding decrease in systemic blood flow occurs. With the increase in blood flow, pulmonary hypertension occurs. Patent ductus also produces this same left-to-right shunt. Cyanotic heart diseases produce a right-to-left shunt of blood. Unoxygenated blood is in the systemic circulation producing arterial hypoxemia and cyanosis. This is due to the combination of an intracardial septal defect with obstruction to the normal flow of blood into the pulmonary artery. The classic example of this is the tetralogy of Fallot a combination of ventricular septal defect and pulmonic stenosis. Venous blood entering the right ventricle is then shunted directly into the aorta to produce cyanosis. In addition to the cyanosis, the malformation decreases the pulmonary blood flow and hence limits the capacity of the lungs to absorb oxygen. With transposition of the great vessels, the aorta originates from the right ventricle and the pulmonary artery from the left ventricle. As a result, venous blood returning through the vena cavae to the right atrium enters the right ventricle and is then ejected directly into the aorta. Oxygenated blood returning from the lungs through the pulmonary veins to the left ventricle is then expelled through the pulmonary artery to the lungs. Cyanosis as well as dyspnea in the newborn are the most prominent symptoms. *(Spencer, pp. 772, 774, 812, 820)*

193. **(E)** Atrial septal defects are among the most common cardiac malformations. Ventricular septal defects occur in 20% to 30% of congenital defects. Patent ductus arteriosus occurs once in every 2000 births and constitutes 10% of all cases of congenital heart disease. Tetralogy of Fallot is one of the most common cyanotic malformations, occurring in more than 50% of all cases of cyanotic heart disease. *(Spencer, pp. 796, 802, 807, 812)*

194. **(E)** Pulmonary congestion in the child with congenital heart disease produces a susceptibility to bacterial infections. Recurrent episodes of pneumonia may occur in the first few years of life. Rubella in the first trimester has been emphasized because of the high incidence of cardiac defects. In the majority of patients with congenital heart disease, there is about a 2%-associated occurrence of congenital heart defects in other members of the same family. Whether it occurred at birth or infancy, cyanosis, its variations in appearance as well as its location, is important in these patients. A decrease in exercise tolerance, exhibited by squatting may be a sign of exertional dyspnea. *(Spencer, pp. 772, 775)*

195. (D) Abnormalities in growth and development are among the most common signs of cardiac disease. Cyanosis may be obvious, and results simply from a decrease in cardiac output with sluggish regional blood flow through the capillary circulation. More oxygen is extracted and a greater amount of reduced hemoglobin is present. Cyanosis and clubbing, a consequence of chronic cyanosis, and polycythemia are often seen in congenital heart disease. Hepatic enlargement is the hallmark of congestive failure in children. *(Spencer, pp. 774, 775, 776)*

196. (B)

197. (A) Congenital aortic stenosis is a common congenital abnormality, representing 8% to 10% of all patients with congenital heart disease. Many children with significant stenotic lesions are asymptomatic and need cardiac catheterization to determine the severity. The most common symptoms are fatigue, dyspnea, angina, and syncope, occurring in 30% to 40% of patients. Coarctation is also a common congenital malformation, occurring in 10% to 15% of patients with congenital heart disease. Most children are asymptomatic or have minimal symptoms despite severe hypertension. The classic combination of hypertension in the upper extremities with absent or decreased pulses in the lower extremities in a child immediately suggests coarctation. *(Spencer, pp. 781–783, 787–788)*

198. (A) Pulmonic stenosis is a common defect, constituting about 10% of all patients with congenital heart disease. It is a spectrum of disorders involving the pulmonary valve cusps, the valve annulus, the pulmonary artery, and the right ventricle. On physical examination, a loud, harsh systolic murmur, heard best in the second left interspace, is characteristic. The murmur is an ejection type murmur with the peak intensity varying along with the degree of stenosis. *(Spencer, pp. 779, 791)*

199. (D) Atrial septal defects, representing 10% to 15% of all cases of congenital heart disease, encompass a variety of malformations involving the atrial septum or pulmonary veins and result in a left-to-right shunt of blood from the systemic to pulmonary circulation. On physical examination, a soft, systolic murmur is heard best in the second or third left intercostal space. The murmur arises at the pulmonary valve from the increased flow of blood. *(Spencer, pp. 796, 797)*

200. (C) Ventricular septal defect (VSD), comprises 20% to 30% of all congenital heart defects. Four major anatomic types of VSD have been recognized, based upon their location in the ventricular septum: (1) perimembranous septal defect, the most common, occurring in 80% of patients; (2) outflow defect anterior to the crista supraventricularis; (3) inflow defects near the tricuspid; and (4) muscular defects in the muscular ventricular system. The two major consequences from VSD are cardiac failure and pulmonary hypertension. A loud harsh pansystolic murmur is usually present along the left sternal border in the third or fourth intercostal spaces, often with a thrill. In addition, basal diastolic murmurs occur rarely from (1) aortic insuffiency from prolapse of an aortic cusp into the underlying septal defect or (2) pulmonic insufficiency from pulmonary hypertension. *(Spencer, pp. 802–803)*

201. (B) Patent ductus arteriosus, which constitutes about 10% of all congenital heart disease, is an important normal fetal pathway connecting the pulmonary artery at its bifurcation to the aorta just beyond the origin of the left subclavian artery and normally closes soon after birth. Through this channel, the embryo's and fetus' life blood bypasses the collapsed lungs, flowing directly from the pulmonary artery to the aorta. The hallmark of patent ductus is the continuous machinery murmur. It is a harsh rasping sound accentuated in systole and diminishing in diastole. It is best heard in the second left intercostal space but is normally widely transmitted over the chest and into the neck. Coarctation of the aorta will produce a systolic murmur over the left hemithorax. *(Spencer, pp. 807–809, 789)*

202. (A) The frequent symptoms of cardiac disease include dyspnea, edema, hepatomegaly, ascites, arrhythmia, angina, syncope, and fatigue. With the exception of angina, symptoms are usually a late sign of advanced cardiac disease. The initial change in most cardiac disease is a rise in intracardiac pressure in the involved chamber followed by cardiac hypertrophy, a manifestation of Starling's law of the heart. Symptoms develop as compensatory mechanisms fail. *(Spencer and Culliford, p. 843)*

203. (D) Angina is the hallmark of coronary artery disease, a symptom of myocardial anoxia with subsequent anaerobic metabolism. Classic angina is described as precordial discomfort appearing with exercise, emotion, or eating, relieved by rest or nitroglycerine. Dyspnea is one of the cardinal symptoms of left heart failure and it is a late sign of heart disease. Syncope occurs with aortic stenosis from the transient decrease in cerebral blood flow. Arrthymias are usually found in patients with mitral stenosis, the older patients with intrinsic disease in the atrioventricular conducting mechanism and in severe cardiac failure. *(Schwartz et al, p. 844)*

204. (E) The majority of heart–lung machines use a simple roller pump that produces an almost non-pulsatile flow of blood. Disposable membrane and bubble oxygenators are used to oxygenate venous blood prior to return to the patient. The blood must be anticoagulated by heparin just prior to bypass. At the end of the bypass procedure, protamine is given to neutralize the heparin. *(Spencer and Culliford, p. 846)*

205. (A) Extracorporeal circulation does produce some trauma. Derangement of normal clotting mechanisms may occur, producing an increased tendency towards bleeding for 18 to 24 hours. A slight degree of renal insuffiency may occur, manifested by a rise in blood urea nitrogen, returning to normal in 2 to 3 days. Reports from Scandinavia and England found a high frequency of transient neurologic abnormalities following perfusion. Multiple organ injury was common in the first two decades of extracorporeal perfusion so that pump times longer than 1 to 3 hours were regularly associated with signs of multiple organ injury. *(Spencer and Culliford, p. 848)*

206. (E) Myocardial preservation can be accomplished by arresting the heart with hyperkalemic hypothermic cardiac arrest. Both crystalloid and blood cardioplegia are widely used with little difference in the two techniques for cardiac arrest periods of 60 to 90 minutes. Continuous topical hyperthermia, constantly irrigating the pericardium with a 4° electrolyte solution, is an important part of the procedure to keep the heart from being rewarmed as the temperature of the perfusate in the pump oxygenator is usually 25° to 30° C. With the combination of periodic infusion of cold blood and hypothermia, the myocardial temperature can easily be kept below 15° C. *(Spencer and Culliford, p. 848)*

207. (C) Stroke is perhaps the most serious complication following extracorporeal circulation, occurring with a frequency of 1% to 2% following open-heart operations. Possible causes of stroke include carotid disease, emboli from the heart or air emboli from incomplete evacuation of air from cardiac chambers. In the majority of patients who suffer stroke, the cause remains unknown, so stroke remains a distressing and serious cause of morbidity following open-heart surgery. Postoperative bleeding, cardiac arrhythmias, renal failure and respiratory insufficiency are all complications, but they can be monitored, followed, and controlled. *(Spencer and Culliford, pp. 849–851)*

208. (C) When the diagnosis of cardiac arrest is considered, it should be either excluded within 30 to 60 seconds, or treatment should be initiated. Depending on the temperature, cerebral anoxia following circulatory arrest produces brain injury within 3 to 4 minutes. Periods of anoxia for 6 to 8 minutes may produce extensive but reversible brain injury, whereas longer periods regularly cause irreversible injury. *(Spencer and Culliford, p. 852)*

209. (B)

210. (C) Dyspnea is the most important symptom in patients with mitral stenosis. This appears whenever mean left atrial pressure exceeds 30 mm Hg long enough to produce significant transudation of fluid into the pulmonary capillaries. At first, it appears with extreme exertion, but it subsequently occurs with lesser degrees of exertion as the stenosis progresses. Other symptoms of advanced disease include chronic cough, orthopnea, paroxysmal nocturnal dypsnea, hemoptysis, and pulmonary edema. Aortic stenosis may present early on as slight dyspnea on exertion. The turning point in the illness is heralded by the appearance of one or more of three symptoms: angina pectorus, syncope, or left ventricular failure. Syncope develops in about one third of patients with aortic stenosis and does not occur in patients with mitral stenosis. *(Spencer and Culliford, pp. 856, 870)*

211. (B) The clinical status of the patient with coronary artery disease is usually in one of five groups. asymptomatic, stable angina of varying severity, unstable angina, acute myocardial infarction, and postinfarction angina. The patient who is asymptomatic and who has angiographically significant disease with little or no angina has the most common clinical problem. Coronary artery bypass, medical therapy, or angioplasty may be indicated for patients who fall into any of these groups. *(Spencer and Culliford, p. 887)*

212. (E) Angina pectoris, occurring most frequently, is a periodic discomfort usually substernal, appearing typically with exertion, after eating, or with extreme emotion. The symptoms subside with sublingual nitroglycerine. There is a constant risk of sudden death with angina pectoris, probably due to an acute disturbance of rhythm with terminal ventricular fibrillation. Myocardial infarction with or without thrombosis of a diseased coronary artery is another frequent and fatal complication. In some patients, congestive heart failure develops and may become the principle disability causing death. *(Spencer and Culliford, p. 885)*

213. (E) Although the best therapy for acute myocardial infarction is rapidly changing, the results from immediate administration of thrombolytic agents, both through IV and intracoronary route has demonstrated a decrease in mortality. Angioplasty may be used in combination with intracoronary thrombolytics to reduce residual stenosis in the once-thrombosed vessel. Patients with triple vessel disease who suffer a massive infarction should probably undergo immediate bypass with insertion of an intraaortic balloon pump prior to their operation. *(Spencer and Culliford, p. 888)*

214. **(A)** With proper technique, combined with the preoperative use of dipyridamole and aspirin, patency 1 month following operation should be in the range of 90% to 95%. In the first 5 years after operation, patency decreases slowly, about 2% to 3% each year so five-year patency rate is in the range of 75% to 80%. Occlusion of the graft during this time is probably due to anastomotic technique, trauma to the vein graft during harvesting, or rarely, postoperative adhesions. *(Spencer and Culliford, p. 890)*

215. **(D)** In the period 5 to 10 years after operation, there is an increase of atherosclerotic disease in vein grafts and the patency rate is probably no better than 50%. For this reason, the use of the internal mammary artery has increased markedly. The 10-year patency rate is near 95% and the internal mammary artery seems to be relatively immune to atherosclerosis. *(Spencer and Culliford, pp. 890, 891)*

216. **(B)** The most common organisms that cause acute pyogenic pericarditis are *Haemophilus influenza* and *Staphylococcus*. In the majority of patients with chronic constrictive pericarditis, the cause is unknown, probably the end-stage viral pericarditis. In recent years, intensive radiation has become a significant cause in some series. *(Spencer and Culliford, pp. 894, 895)*

217. **(D)** Unfortunately, the fixed-rate asynchronous units, the initial pacemakers, stimulated the ventricle at a fixed rate that could possibly compete with the patient's own rhythm and produce ventricular fibrillation. The fixed-rate pacemakers have been supplanted by demand pacemakers, usually triggered from a ventricular electrode. A more complex type is the atrioventricular pacemaker, requiring an electrode in the right atrium as well as the right ventricle. All these have the advantage of coordinating with the patient's own cardiac rhythm and supplying an "atrial kick" when the atrioventricular sequential pacing is employed. Pro-

grammable pacemakers permit adjustment of rate, pulse, amplitude, and duration. *(Spencer and Culliford, p. 897)*

218. **(D)** Pericardiotomy syndrome is fairly common and usually responds to therapy with ibuprofen. A mild postoperative pericardiotomy syndrome consists of fever, a pericardial friction rub, pleural effusion, and a normal white blood count. Although many postoperative patients experience a transient elevated white blood cell count, it is not a part of the pericardiotomy syndrome. *(Spencer and Culliford, p. 889)*

219. **(C)** A left ventricular aneurysm results when a severe transmural infarction destroys virtually all muscular fibers in the area of the infarction and are subsequentially replaced by fibrous tissue. The aneurysm usually enlarges to a moderate degree and then becomes stationary; progressive enlargement and rupture, as usually occurs with atherosclerotic aneurysms, is rare. More than 80% of aneurysms develop in the anterolateral portion of the left ventricle. Lateral or posterior aneurysms are rare. *(Spencer and Culliford, pp. 891–893)*

220. **(B)**

221. **(A)**

222. **(B)** The two life-threatening problems for patients with penetrating cardiac trauma are tamponade and hemorrhage. Tamponade develops rapidly as the normal pericardium can accommodate only 100 to 250 mL of blood. Small wounds, such as those from an icepick or knife, often produce tamponade because the laceration in the pericardium is small. Bullets or large knives threaten immediate death from exsanguination as blood can be expelled through the pericardial laceration into the pleural cavity. The treatment should be control of the hemorrhage through emergency thoracotomy. The key to tamponade is considering the diagnosis in any patient with hypotension and a penetrating thoracic wound and performing a pericardial aspiration. Blunt cardiac trauma usually results from automobile accidents when the steering wheel impacts against the chest. The direct injury may be a cardiac contusion. The contusion varies from simple subepicardial hemorrhage to a full-thickness myocardial contusion. The clinical picture is that of pericarditis with a pericardial effusion and chest pain. *(Spencer and Culliford, pp. 880–881)*

Subspecialty List: Surgery

QUESTION NUMBER AND SUBSPECIALTY
1. Hemostasis
2. Neurogenic shock—characteristics
3. Cardiogenic shock—characteristics
4. Hypovolemic shock—characteristics
5. Septic shock—characteristics
6. Breast carcinoma—characteristics
7. Mammography—indications
8. Breast mass—history
9. Bowel obstruction—physical findings
10. Biliary colic—characteristics
11. Intestinal obstruction—laboratory evaluation
12. Mesenteric occlusion—characteristics
13. Thyroid surgery—risks
14. Thyroid cancer—characteristics
15. Thyroid cancer—characteristics
16. Thyroid mass—evaluation
17. Thyroid cancer—prognosis
18. Primary hyperparathyroidism—characteristics
19. Hypothyroidism—characteristics
20. Surgical anatomy
21. Colon anatomy
22. Crohn's disease—characteristics
23. Crohn's disease—characteristics
24. Ulcerative colitis—characteristics
25. Crohn's disease—characteristics
26. Crohn's disease—characteristics
27. Colitis—causes
28. Pseudomembranous colitis—treatment
29. Crohn's disease—x-ray findings
30. Ulcerative colitis—complications
31. Colitis—treatment
32. Ulcerative colitis—surgical management
33. Diverticulosis—characteristics
34. Lower gastrointestinal bleeding—evaluation
35. Diverticulitis—characteristics
36. Diverticulitis—complications
37. Polyps—malignant potential
38. Hemorrhoidectomy—indications
39. Anal fissure—characteristics
40. Colon cancer—screening
41. Esophageal achalasia—characteristics
42. Esophageal achalasia—treatment
43. Gastroesopageal reflux—complications
44. Esophageal motility—evaluation
45. Diaphragmatic hernias—complications
46. Esophageal cancer—characteristics
47. Pancreas—anatomy
48. Pancreatitis—diagnosis
49. Pancreatitis—treatment
50. Pancreatitis—complications
51. Pancreatitis—evaluation
52. Pancreatitis—characteristics
53. Pancreatic pseudocyst—treatment
54. Pancreatic cancer—characteristics
55. Whipple procedure—characteristics
56. Spleen—physiology
57. Strangulated hernia—characteristics
58. Incarcerated hernia—characteristics
59. Direct hernia—characteristics
60. Indirect hernia—characteristics
61. Sliding hernia—characteristics
62. Femoral hernia—characteristics
63. Hernia repair—complications
64. Brain tumors—characteristics
65. Brain tumors—characteristics
66. Peripheral radiculopathy—characteristics
67. Stomach—physiology
68. Stomach—physiology
69. Stomach—physiology
70. Atrophic gastritis—characteristics
71. Melena—characteristics
72. Gastric ulcers—characteristics
73. Stomach—physiology
74. Duodenal ulcers—characteristics
75. Gastrointestinal bleeding—evaluation
76. Duodenal ulcers—treatment
77. Gastric lymphoma—treatment
78. Chronic gastritis—characteristics
79. Duodenal ulcers—characteristics
80. Stress ulcers—characteristics
81. Chronic gastritis—characteristics
82. Prepyloric ulcers—characteristics
83. Cholelithiasis—physiology
84. Cholelithiasis—characteristics
85. Gallbladder—laboratory evaluation
86. Sclerosing cholangitis—characteristics
87. bile—physiology
88. Gallbladder—physiology
89. Cholelithiasis—treatment

90. Cholelithiasis—characteristics
91. Chronic cholecystitis—evaluation
92. Acute cholangitis—treatment
93. Cholecystitis—characteristics
94. Cholecystitis—characteristics
95. Cholecystitis—characteristics
96. Cholecystitis—characteristics
97. Liver—anatomy
98. Liver—physiology
99. Liver—anatomy
100. Hepatitis—characteristics
101. Hepatitis—characteristics
102. Hepatic metastases—characteristics
103. Hepatocellular carcinoma—characteristics
104. Tumor markers
105. Portal hypertension—causes
106. Cirrhosis—prognosis postshunting
107. Cirrhosis—indications for shunting
108. Liver abcess—characteristics
109. Liver abcess—characteristics
110. Liver abcess—characteristics
111. Liver abcess—characteristics
112. Liver abcess—characteristics
113. Small bowel tumors—characteristics
114. Small bowel tumors—characteristics
115. Carcinoid—characteristics
116. Meckel's diverticulum—characteristics
117. Appendix—physiology
118. Appendicitis—characteristics
119. Appendicitis—characteristics
120. Appendicitis—pathogenesis
121. Appendix—anatomy
122. Right lower quadrant pain—differential diagnosis
123. Appendicitis—in pregnancy
124. Appendicitis—x-ray findings
125. Appendicitis—management
126. Prostatic disease—laboratory evaluation
127. Postrate cancer—treatment
128. Testicular mass—management
129. Scrotal swelling—management
130. Testicular mass—differential diagnosis
131. Urinary tract calculi—pathology
132. Joints—characteristics
133. Joints—characteristics
134. Joints—characteristics
135. Subacromial bursitis—characteristics
136. Bicipital tendonitis—characteristics
137. Supraspinatus tendonitis—characteristics
138. Rotator cuff tear—characteristics
139. Neuropraxia—characteristics
140. Meniscal tears—diagnosis
141. Chondromalacia patella—characteristics
142. Anoxia—complications
143. Aortic occlusion—characteristics
144. Superficial artery occlusion—characteristics
145. Major venous thrombosis—characteristics
146. Major venous thrombosis—characteristics
147. Diabetes mellitus—skin changes
148. Buerger's disease—skin changes
149. Chronic tissue ischemia—characteristics
150. Arterial injury—clincial findings
151. Congenital arteriovenous fistula—characteristics
152. Arterial reconstruction—management
153. Bleeding—management
154. Anterior compartment syndrome—characteristics
155. Stocking neuropathy—diagnosis
156. Arterial occlusive disease—laboratory evaluation
157. Thrombi—characteristics
158. Emboli—characteristics
159. Chronic venous insuffiency—characteristics
160. Embolic disease—treatment
161. Aneurysms—characteristics
162. Abdominal aortic aneurysm—characteristics
163. Atherosclerotic occlusive disease—characteristics
164. Abdominal aortic aneurysms—characteristics
165. Aortoiliac occlusive disease—characteristics
166. Livedo reticularis—symptoms
167. Erythromegalia—symptoms
168. Acrocyanosis—symptoms
169. Raynaud's phenomenon—characteristics
170. Raynaud's disease—characteristics
171. Buerger's disease—characteristics
172. Frostbite—characteristics
173. Frostbite—characteristics
174. Cold exposure—management
175. Buerger's disease—characteristics
176. Aortoiliac disease—characteristics
177. Diabetes—foot care
178. Aortoiliac disease—characteristics
179. Venous stasis ulcers—pathogenesis
180. Ischemic stroke—characteristics
181. Raynaud's disease—diagnosis
182. Thoracic outlet syndrome—diagnosis
183. Femoropopliteal disease—diagnosis
184. Venous valves—characteristics
185. Secondary lymphedema—causes
186. Heart disease in children—causes
187. Congenital heart disease—pathophysiology
188. Congenital heart disease—characteristics
189. Tetralogy of Fallot—characteristics
190. Ventricular septal defect—characteristics
191. Atrial septal defect—characteristics
192. Transposition of the great vessels—characteristics
193. Congenital heart disease—characteristics
194. Congenital heart disease—history
195. Congenital heart disease—physical findings
196. Congenital aortic stenosis—characteristics
197. Coarctation of the aorta—characteristics
198. Pulmonic stenosis—physical findings
199. Atrial septal defect—physical findings
200. Ventricular septal defect—physical findings
201. Patent ductus arteriosus—physical findings
202. Cardiac disease—symptoms
203. Coronary artery disease—symptoms
204. Extracorporeal circulation—characteristics
205. Extracorporeal circulation—complications
206. Myocardial preservation—characteristics
207. Extracorporeal circulation—complications

208. Cerebral anoxia—characteristics
209. Mitral stenosis—characteristics
210. Aortic stenosis—characteristics
211. Clinical cardiac pathology—characteristics
212. Coronary artery disease—characteristics
213. Myocardial infarction—management
214. Coronary artery bypass grafting—complications
215. Coronary artery bypass grafting—characteristics
216. Chronic constrictive pericarditis—characteristics
217. Pacemakers—characteristics
218. Pericardiotomy syndrome—characteristics
219. Ventricular aneurysms—characteristics
220. Blunt cardiac trauma—characteristics
221. Penetrating cardiac trauma—characteristics
222. Blunt cardiac trauma—characteristics

REFERENCES

Adams JT. Abdominal wall, omentum, mesentery, and retroperitoneum. In Schwartz SI, et al (eds) *Principles of Surgery,* 5th ed. New York: McGraw-Hill, 1989, p. 1491.

Bradley EL III, Zeppa R. The pancreas. In Sabiston DC Jr, (ed) *Textbook of Surgery,* 13th ed. Philadelphia: WB Saunders, 1986, p. 1170.

Cohn I Jr, Nance FC. The colon and rectum: anatomy and surgical procedures. In Sabiston DC Jr, (ed) *Textbook of Surgery,* 13th ed. Philadelphia: WB Saunders, 1986, p. 983.

Degowin EL, Degowin RL. *Bedside Diagnostic Examination,* 5th ed. New York: McMillan, 1989.

Duthie RB, Hoaglund FT. Orthopaedics. In Schwartz SI, et al (eds). *Principles of Surgery,* 5th ed. New York: McGraw-Hill, 1989, p. 1879.

Frank IN. Urology. In Schwartz SI, et al (eds) *Principles of Surgery,* 5th ed. New York: McGraw-Hill, 1989, p. 1729.

Greenfield LJ. Venous and lymphatic disease. In Schwartz SI, et al (eds), *Principles of Surgery,* 5th ed. New York: McGraw-Hill, 1989, p. 1011.

Imparato AM, Riles TS. Peripheral arterial disease. In Schwartz SI, et al (eds) *Principles of Surgery,* 5th ed. New York: McGraw-Hill, 1989, p. 933.

Goldberg SM, Nivatvongs S., Rothenberger DA. Colon, rectum, and anus. In Schwartz SI, et al (eds) *Principles of Surgery,* 5th ed. New York: McGraw-Hill, 1989, p. 1225.

Hamilton JD. The liver: viral hepatitis and the surgeon. In Sabiston DC Jr., (ed) *Textbook of Surgery,* 13th ed. Philadelphia: WB Saunders, 1986, p. 1121.

Langer B., Greig PD. The liver: Peritoneovenous shunts for intractable ascites. In Sabiston DC Jr, (ed). *Textbook of Surgery,* 13th ed. Philadelphia: WB Saunders, 1986, p. 1116.

Kaplan EL. Thyroid and parathyroid. In Schwartz SI, et al (eds). *Principles of Surgery,* 5th ed. New York: McGraw-Hill, 1989, p. 1613.

Meyers WC. The liver: Anatomy and physiology. In Sabiston DC Jr, (ed). *Textbook of Surgery,* 13th ed. Philadelphia: WB Saunders, 1986, p. 1053.

Moody FG, McGreevy JM, Miller TA. Stomach. In Schwartz SI, et al (eds). *Principles of Surgery,* 5th ed. New York: McGraw-Hill, 1989, p. 1157.

Morton JH. Abdominal wall hernias. In Schwartz SI, et al (eds). *Principles of Surgery,* 5th ed. New York: McGraw-Hill, 1989, p. 1525.

Pairolero PC, Trastek VF, Payne WS. Esophagus and diaphragmatic hernias. In Schwartz SI, et al (eds). *Principles of Surgery,* 5th ed. New York: McGraw-Hill, 1989, p. 1103.

Rush, BF Jr. Breast. In Schwartz SI, et al (eds). *Principles of Surgery,* 5th ed. New York: McGraw-Hill, 1989, p. 549.

Schwartz SI. Appendix. In Schwartz SI, et al (eds). *Principles of Surgery,* 5th ed. New York: McGraw-Hill, 1989, p. 1315.

Schwartz SI. Gallbladder and extrahepatic biliary system. In Schwartz SI, et al (eds). *Principles of Surgery,* 5th ed. New York: McGraw-Hill, 1989, p. 1381.

Schwartz SI. Hemostasis, surgical bleeding and transfusion. In Schwartz SI, et al (eds) *Principles of Surgery,* 5th ed. New York: McGraw-Hill, 1989, p. 115.

Schwartz SI. Liver. In Schwartz SI, et al (eds). *Principles of Surgery,* 5th ed. New York: McGraw-Hill, 1989, p. 1327.

Schwartz SI. Manifestations of gastrointestinal disease. In Schwartz SI, et al (eds). *Principles of Surgery,* 5th ed. New York: McGraw-Hill, 1989, p. 1061.

Schwartz SI. Spleen. In Schwartz SI, et al (eds). *Principles of Surgery,* 5th ed. New York: McGraw-Hill, 1989, p. 1441.

Shires GT III, Canizaro PC, Carrico CJ. Shock. In Schwartz SI, et al (eds). *Principles of Surgery,* 5th ed. New York: McGraw-Hill, 1989, p. 137.

Silen W, Steer M. Pancreas. In Schwartz SI, et al (eds). *Principles of Surgery,* 5th ed. New York: McGraw-Hill, 1989, p. 1413.

Spencer DC, Chyatt D, Collins WF, et al. Neurologic surgery. In Schwartz SI, et al (eds). *Principles of Surgery,* 5th ed. New York: McGraw-Hill, 1989, p. 1831.

Spencer FC. Congenital heart disease. In Schwartz SI, et al (eds). *Principles of Surgery,* 5th ed. New York: McGraw-Hill, 1989, p. 771.

Spencer FC, Culliford AT. Acquired heart disease. In Schwart SI, et al (eds). *Principles of Surgery,* 5th ed. New York: McGraw-Hill, 1989, p. 843.

Taber's Cyclopedic Medical Dictionary, 15th ed. New York: McGraw-Hill, 1989.

Townsend CM Jr, Thompson JC. Small intestine. In Schwartz SI, et al (eds). *Principles of Surgery,* 5th ed. New York: McGraw-Hill, 1989, p. 1189.

Weinerth JL. The male genital system. In Sabiston DC Jr, (ed). *Textbook of Surgery,* 13th ed. Philadelphia: WB Saunders, 1986, p. 1670.

CHAPTER 4

Pediatrics

Mary S. Andresen, Deborah G. Aragon, Mark A. Colloton,
and Patricia C. Young

Questions

DIRECTIONS (Questions 1 through 3): For each of the items in this section, ONE or MORE of the numbered options is correct. Choose the answer

A if only 1, 2, and 3 are correct,
B if only 1 and 3 are correct,
C if only 2 and 4 are correct,
D if only 4 is correct,
E if all are correct.

1. Which of the following would be included in the differential diagnosis of a child with chronic diarrhea (formless stools for more than 14 days, which may be persistent or intermittent)?

   (1) lactase deficiency
   (2) short bowel syndrome
   (3) celiac disease
   (4) lymphangiectasia

2. The most common malignancy of childhood is acute lymphoblastic leukemia (ALL). Which of the following is/are true in relationship to this disease?

   (1) birth defects are not increased in children of parents previously treated for ALL
   (2) anemia, thrombocytopenia, and neutropenia are common at presentation
   (3) the disease is heterogenous requiring different treatment regimens
   (4) risk of a second malignancy in treated patients is high

3. Transient tachypnea of the newborn is characterized by which of the following?

   (1) uneventful vaginal delivery
   (2) early onset of tachypnea
   (3) cyanosis relieved by minimum O_2
   (4) abnormal blood gases

DIRECTIONS (Questions 4 through 17): Each group of items in this section consists of lettered headings followed by a set of numbered words or phrases. For each numbered word or phrase, select the ONE lettered heading that is most closely associated with it. Each lettered heading may be selected once, more than once, or not at all.

For each cardiac lesion select the physical findings with which it is commonly associated.

(A) decreased and delayed or absent femoral pulses
(B) bounding pulses with respiratory distress in premature infants with systolic murmur, if any, at second left ICS
(C) loud first heart sound with widely split second heart sound
(D) evidence of gross congestive failure without a systolic murmur
(E) systolic murmur along the lower left sternal border not heard in the first days of life

4. secundum atrial septal defect

5. ventricular septal defect

6. persistent ductus arterosus

7. coarctation of aorta

Questions 8 through 11

Dermatological diseases are common in pediatric patients. Match the diagnosis with the **most appropriate** statement.

(A) the pattern of inheritance can be autosomal dominant or recessive
(B) subsides after the first few months of life
(C) slow, but spontaneous involution

(D) a staphylococcal infection
(E) may involve the diaper area

8. neonatal pustular melanosis

9. strawberry hemangiomas

10. seborrheic dermatitis

11. epidermolysis bullosa

Questions 12 through 15

For each age group select the orthopedic problem with which it is commonly associated.

(A) subluxation of radial head
(B) scoliosis
(C) fracture of clavicle
(D) Legg-Calvé-Perthes
(E) slipped capital femoral epiphysis

12. adolescent female

13. newborn

14. 5 to 9 years, male

15. 1 to 4 years

Questions 16 and 17

(A) involves the dorsa of the toes and distal aspect of foot
(B) seen in prepubertal children
(C) both
(D) neither

16. allergic contact dermatitis

17. tinea pedis

DIRECTIONS (Questions 18 through 23): Each of the numbered items or incomplete statements in this section is followed by answers or by completions of the statement. Select the ONE lettered answer or completion that is BEST in each case.

18. An 8-year-old female presents with evidence of polyarthritis. The chart shows that she had a documented beta *Streptococcus* infection 20 days previously. The differential diagnosis includes rheumatic fever. What additional finding would permit you to make the diagnosis of rheumatic fever based on clinical examination? (Modified Jones Criteria)

(A) fever
(B) arthralgia
(C) acute pharyngitis
(D) carditis
(E) erythema multiforme

19. The following is true regarding adolescent gynecomastia.

(A) gynecomastia begins in Tanner Stage II–III and disappears in 1 to 2 years
(B) the underlying mass may be fixed and there may be skin dimpling
(C) gynecomastia is due to excess fatty tissue in an obese patient
(D) gynecomastia is not a painful condition
(E) surgical intervention is not a consideration in treatment of gynecomastia

20. The most common vasculitis in childhood is Henoch–Schonlein purpura (HSP). All the following are true about this condition **EXCEPT**

(A) colicky abdominal pain may be present
(B) a protein-losing enteropathy secondary to intestinal involvement is part of the spectrum of disease
(C) all children with HSP have renal involvement
(D) platelet counts are abnormal, as are coagulation studies
(E) joint, ankle, and knee pain are associated with HSP

21. The most common thrombocytopenia of childhood is ITP. To substantiate the diagnosis, what laboratory test would you order?

(A) clot retraction
(B) bleeding time
(C) platelet count
(D) CBC
(E) ANA antibody test

22. The nevus is a common skin lesion in childhood. Which one of the following types of nevi should be excised?

(A) acquired pigmented nevi
(B) lentigines (macular nevi)
(C) halo nevus
(D) nevus sebaceous
(E) achromic nevi (nevus depigmentosus)

23. A patient is brought into the emergency room after an automobile accident. His skin is cold, clammy, and pale and his neck veins are flat. You notice signs of trauma at the right upper quadrant of the abdomen. What type of shock is this patient likely to have?

(A) cardiogenic shock
(B) hypovolemic shock
(C) simple shock
(D) distributive or vasogenic shock
(E) terminal shock

DIRECTIONS (Questions 24 through 31): For each of the items in this section, ONE or MORE of the numbered options is correct. Choose the answer

A if only 1, 2, and 3 are correct,
B if only 1 and 3 are correct,
C if only 2 and 4 are correct,
D if only 4 is correct,
E if all are correct.

24. A child presents with a history of viral gastroenteritis and has mildly dry mucous membranes. The child's vital signs are normal and the child clinically appears to be less than 5% dehydrated. Which of the following is/are true about the treatment of this child?

    (1) if the child is able to tolerate oral fluids, oral rehydration may be instituted instead of parenteral fluid administration
    (2) commercially available oral electrolyte products are usually recommended, although flat soda, Gatoraid or Jell-O water may be used as well
    (3) if the child has a history of vomiting, clear fluids should be given in small amounts and administered slowly (1 teaspoon every 20 minutes) and amounts of fluid may be increased slowly as tolerated. After 8 hours without vomiting, the child may be gradually returned to a normal diet
    (4) rice water, juice, boiled milk, and tea are acceptable fluids to use in oral rehydration

25. Fever is a common chief complaint in pediatrics. Which of the following is/are true regarding fever(s) in children?

    (1) a child is considered to have a fever if their rectal temperature is 38.0° to 38.5° C
    (2) laboratory tests for a child 3 months of age or younger who has been febrile for 24 hours or greater, who looks clinically well, and has no focal physical findings may be delayed after 6 to 12 hours of close follow-up
    (3) children who are less than 2-years-old, have a fever of 39.4° C or above, have a WBC count of 15,000 mm^3 or above, and have an ESR of 30 mm/hr or above are likely to be bacteremic and may have an underlying disease such as pneumonia or meningitis
    (4) effective treatment for children with fevers include use of acetaminophen or aspirin, alcohol baths, drinking clear liquids, and reduction in the amount of clothes the child wears

26. Animal bites, particularly dog bites, are common in pediatric patients. Which of the following characteristics are true about animal bites?

    (1) the most common organism found in animal bites is *Yersinia pestis*
    (2) hand injuries, and bites older than 24 hours should be sutured
    (3) animal bites that are sutured are less likely to become infected; puncture wounds are more likely to become infected
    (4) other treatment considerations include administration of tetanus toxoid, wound irrigation, and debridement of devitalized tissue

27. Which of the following is/are true about the treatment of burns?

    (1) electrical burns should be followed up in 7 days to assure proper healing
    (2) intact blisters should be opened, cleaned, and debrided
    (3) initial treatment of minor burns should include packing the area in ice to retard heat damage to the skin
    (4) partial thickness burns may be cleaned and dressed with 1% silver sulfadiazine cream or fine mesh impregnated with petrolatum jelly

28. Which of the following should be initiated when treating a patient with a severe head injury?

    (1) establish an airway, remembering to rule out cervical spine injury
    (2) hyperventilate, keeping the Pco$_2$ at 20 to 25 mm Hg, and Pao$_2$ of 90 mm Hg
    (3) elevate the head if shock is not present
    (4) observe for signs of shock but do not introduce IV fluids for treatment as this might increase intracranial pressure

29. Which of the following is/are true about acute asthma attacks?

    (1) asthma is a common pediatric entity and has the physical finding of wheezing, which is found in the majority of children with acute asthma attacks
    (2) injectable and inhaled beta agonist therapy is very helpful in the initial management of an acute asthma attack. Humidified oxygen is a must when dealing with the acute asthmatic
    (3) rectal theophylline suppositories are a helpful way to give a loading dose of theophylline to a vomiting patient with an acute asthma attack. An acceptable serum theophylline level is between 15 and 25 µg/mL
    (4) status asthmaticus is present when a patient fails to have a significant response to initial attempts at bronchodilator therapy

30. Which of the following growth patterns for children is/are correct?

    (1) a newborn may lose up to 15% of birthweight in the first few days of life
    (2) an infant should double his or her birthweight by 5 months of age
    (3) an infant should triple his or her birthweight by 15 months
    (4) for the first 2 months of life, the infant should gain 30 g (1 ounce) per day

31. Failure to thrive is a common pediatric condition that occurs in about 8% of this population. Which of the following statement(s) is/are also true regarding FTT?

    (1) FTT is most commonly seen in children under 2 years of age
    (2) most children with FTT need hospitalization to determine the cause of their growth delay
    (3) FTT may be defined as deceleration of growth velocity leading to a loss of two or more major percentiles on a standard growth chart
    (4) laboratory studies are very helpful in the diagnosis of failure to thrive

DIRECTIONS (Questions 32 through 35): Each group of items in this section consists of lettered headings followed by a set of numbered words or phrases. For each numbered word or phrase, select the ONE lettered heading that is most closely associated with it. Each lettered heading may be selected once, more than once, or not at all.

Match the following types of poisonings with their antidote.

    (A) methylene blue
    (B) oxygen
    (C) atropine sulfate
    (D) naloxone
    (E) syrup of Ipecac

32. carbon monoxide

33. methemoglobin (nitrates)

34. narcotics

35. organophosphates

DIRECTIONS (Questions 36 through 38): Each of the numbered items or incomplete statements in this section is followed by answers or by completions of the statement. Select the ONE lettered answer or completion that is BEST in each case.

36. The most dangerous inflicted injury in terms of morbidity and mortality is

    (A) a skull fracture
    (B) an intrabdominal injury
    (C) a subdural hematoma
    (D) a subgaleal hematoma
    (E) multiple fractures of the extremities

37. Radiologic characteristics of inflicted injuries include all of the following EXCEPT

    (A) spiral fractures
    (B) multiple fractures in different stages of healing
    (C) symmetrical fractures
    (D) fractures of the scapula or sternum
    (E) evidence of subperiosteal bleeding

38. The diagnosis of childhood sexual molestation is most frequently made by

    (A) the child's emotional distress and fearfulness of a physical examination
    (B) the child's detailed explicit account of his/her experience
    (C) physical evidence of perineal trauma; that is, redness, swelling, discharge, abrasions
    (D) laboratory evidence of gonorrhea in cultures of the mouth, anal area, or vaginal discharge
    (E) parental complaints of recent onset of sexualized behaviors, including masturbation, and explicit sexual vocabulary

DIRECTIONS (Question 39): For each of the items in this section, ONE or MORE of the numbered options is correct. Choose the answer

    A if only 1, 2, and 3 are correct,
    B if only 1 and 3 are correct,
    C if only 2 and 4 are correct,
    D if only 4 is correct,
    E if all are correct.

39. In the United States, placing children in foster care can be life saving for abused, neglected, or abandoned children. However, studies indicate there are also certain identifiable difficulties with foster care. These include

    (1) foster care rarely provides comprehensive integrated services for children
    (2) foster parents rarely receive support or guidance

(3) natural parents who retain custody can change a child's placement

(4) frequent placement changes affect how a child forms attachments, learns to trust, and relates to adults and peers

DIRECTIONS (Questions 40 and 41): Each of the numbered items or incomplete statements in this section is followed by answers or by completions of the statement. Select the ONE lettered answer or completion that is BEST in each case.

40 Clinical experience indicates that most infants with polycythemia

(A) are in respiratory distress
(B) develop convulsions
(C) exhibit priapism
(D) are asymptomatic
(E) develop necrotizing enterocolitis

41. In hyaline membrane disease (respiratory distress syndrome)

(A) symptoms usually develop within minutes of birth
(B) females are more commonly affected
(C) chest x-rays show bilateral lung infiltrates
(D) diagnosis cannot be made prenatally
(E) prognosis is not related to birth weight

DIRECTIONS (Questions 42 through 45): Each group of items in this section consists of lettered headings followed by a set of numbered words or phrases. For each numbered word or phrase, select the ONE lettered heading that is most closely associated with it. Each lettered heading may be selected once, more than once, or not at all.

From statistical reviews of reported cases of childhood maltreatment, the abuser is

(A) In 1% of the cases
(B) In 4% of the cases
(C) In 5% of the cases
(D) In 25% of the cases
(E) In 90% of the cases

42. a caretaker related to the child

43. a sibling of the victim

44. an unrelated babysitter

45. a male friend of the mother's

DIRECTIONS (Questions 46 through 60): For each of the items in this section, ONE or MORE of the numbered options is correct. Choose the answer

A if only 1, 2, and 3 are correct,
B if only 1 and 3 are correct,
C if only 2 and 4 are correct,
D if only 4 is correct,
E if all are correct.

46. The health care providers' main responsibilities to abused and neglected children is/are

(1) detection (diagnosis)
(2) prevention
(3) reporting
(4) treatment

47. If a six-year-old female child presents within 72 hours of an alleged sexual attack, laboratory data should include

(1) a wet mount preparation for sperm
(2) acid phosphates
(3) vaginal, rectal, and throat cultures for gonorrhea
(4) pregnancy testing

48. In the case of adoptions, most authorities agree that

(1) adoptions should be accomplished through approved agencies
(2) adoptions of older children, or those of different religious or ethnic heritage than the adoptive parents should be discouraged
(3) the adopted child should be told of his or her adoption as soon as he or she is able to comprehend the situation
(4) adoption should be accomplished as soon after birth as possible, in order to ensure success

49. In unilateral sensorineural hearing loss

(1) the Weber test lateralizes to the unaffected ear
(2) the Weber test follows the pattern found in normal patients
(3) the Rinne test follows the pattern found in normal patients
(4) the Rinne test reveals that bone conduction is greater than air conduction

50. Physical examinations in the newborn

(1) need only be done at designated times
(2) should always be timed and dated on the chart note
(3) should be performed after adequate handwashing. Jewelry need not be removed before the examination
(4) can be stressful in sick infants or if done by an unskilled examiner

SUMMARY OF DIRECTIONS				
A	**B**	**C**	**D**	**E**
1, 2, 3 **only**	**1, 3** **only**	**2, 4** **only**	**4** **only**	**All are** **correct**

51. In the newborn, vital signs are an important component of repeated observations. Accordingly, many nurseries use skin sensors for continuous temperature monitoring. These skin sensors

    (1) should be firmly attached to the skin
    (2) should be applied with nonporous tape
    (3) are more representative of mean body temperature when attached to the upper thigh or arm
    (4) must be used in areas with a low ambient relative humidity to be accurate

52. True polycythemia in children can be caused by

    (1) cyanotic congenital heart disease
    (2) placental dysfunction syndromes
    (3) hemoglobinopathies
    (4) tumors

53. Factors known to affect neonatal bilirubin levels include

    (1) genetics
    (2) perinatal events
    (3) infant feeding practices
    (4) ethnic factors

54. Absolute contraindications to the administration of DTP vaccine include

    (1) viral respiratory infection without fever
    (2) convulsion 24 hours after previous DTP
    (3) family history of epilepsy
    (4) temperature of 105.1°F following previous DTP.

55. Outbreaks of measles virus (rubeola) infection have occurred in the 1980s in the following populations:

    (1) preschool infants younger than 15 months
    (2) college students born after 1960
    (3) previously vaccinated school-aged children
    (4) unimmunized infants aged 2 to 5 years

56. An 18-month-old unimmunized infant who is infected with human immunodeficiency virus (HIV) should receive which of the following vaccines?

    (1) IPV
    (2) MMR
    (3) DPT
    (4) OPV

57. A four-month-old infant born to a mother infected with human immunodeficiency virus (HIV)

    (1) may be infected but asymptomatic
    (2) has a 90% to 95% chance of developing AIDS
    (3) will be ELISA positive for HIV due to transplacental antibody
    (4) cannot be definitely diagnosed as AIDS until 15 months of age

58. Patients at an increased risk of acquiring infection with cytomegalovirus (CMV) include the following:

    (1) toddlers in day care
    (2) neonatal ICU nurses
    (3) parents of toddlers in day care
    (4) renal transplant nurses

59. Which of the following regimens is accepted for therapy of group A streptococcal pharyngitis in a 9-year-old who weighs 75 pounds?

    (1) pen VK 250 mg po tid for 10 days
    (2) pen VK 500 mg po bid for 10 days
    (3) benzathine penicillin 1.2 million U intramuscularly
    (4) pen VK 750 mg po qd for 10 days

60. Which of the following infants should be given varicella–zoster immune globulin (VZIG)?

    (1) an infant whose mother develops varicella one day after delivery
    (2) a 1-day-old infant whose 2-year-old brother develops varicella
    (3) an infant whose mother developed varicella 2 days prior to delivery
    (4) a 1-month-old infant with varicella

DIRECTIONS (Questions 61 through 65): Each group of items in this section consists of lettered headings followed by a set of numbered words or phrases. For each numbered word or phrase, select the ONE lettered heading that is most closely associated with it. Each lettered heading may be selected once, more than once, or not at all.

For each of the following vaccines, select the best description of the biological components.

    (A) live virus vaccine
    (B) killed bacteria
    (C) bacterial toxoid
    (D) purified bacterial capsule
    (E) killed virus vaccine

61. diphtheria vaccine

62. MMR vaccine

63. oral polio virus (OPV) vaccine

64. pertussis vaccine

65. haemophilus influenzae type b

DIRECTIONS (Questions 69 through 76): For each of the items in this section, ONE or MORE of the numbered options is correct. Choose the answer

A if only 1, 2, and 3 are correct,
B if only 1 and 3 are correct,
C if only 2 and 4 are correct,
D if only 4 is correct,
E if all are correct.

66. Diagnostic criteria for the mucocutaneous–lymph node syndrome (Kawasaki's syndrome) include which of the following?

(1) fever greater than 5 days
(2) generalized lymphadenopathy
(3) swelling of the hands and feet
(4) diarrhea and vomiting

67. Risk factors for acute otitis media in the first year of life include

(1) parental history of acute otitis media
(2) male gender
(3) parental or sibling with history of atopy
(4) having a sibling with a history of recurrent otitis media

68. Which of the following is/are true regarding mortality in adolescence?

(1) adolescent males have twice the mortality rate of adolescent females
(2) accidents are the leading cause of death in adolescence
(3) excluding violent causes of death, cancer is the number one killer in adolescence
(4) females outnumber males in completed suicides

69. Normal pubertal growth and development is demonstrated by which of the following?

(1) menarche always occurs after the peak height velocity has been attained
(2) axillary hair precedes pubic hair by about 2 years in both males and females
(3) for males, pubertal development usually begins with testicular enlargement followed by the appearance of pubic hair
(4) for females, appearance of pubic hair usually precedes breast budding

70. The following statement(s) is/are true when speaking of jaundice in the neonate

(1) normally begins on the extremities and spreads proximally

(2) can usually be detected at a level of 6 to 7 mg/dL
(3) with a cephalohematoma, there is no greater risk of jaundice
(4) may be associated with hypothyroidism, galactosemia, and phenylketonuria

71. Criteria that rule out physiologic jaundice of the newborn are

(1) jaundice in the first 24 hours of life
(2) total serum bilirubin concentrations greater than 12.9 mg/dL in a full term infant, or 15 mg/dL in a premature infant
(3) direct serum bilirubin concentration greater than 1.5 to 2 mg/dL
(4) clinical jaundice persisting longer than 1 week in a full-term infant or 2 weeks in a premature infant

72. Juvenile rheumatoid arthritis is characterized by which of the following?

(1) migratory arthritis
(2) daily, constant joint swelling or pain
(3) conjunctivitis
(4) morning stiffness

73. Which of the following is/are true regarding adolescent suicide?

(1) it is higher for boys than girls
(2) victims are often intoxicated with alcohol at the time of death
(3) firearms are the most common method for suicide
(4) the majority of adolescents had previously been referred to a mental health professional

74. Which of the following is/are true about sinusitis in childhood?

(1) common organisms causing infection include *S. pneumoniae*, *B. catarrhalis*, and nontypable *H. influenza*
(2) frontal sinuses are a frequent site of infection in preschool children
(3) sinus headache is an infrequent complaint in children under 5 years of age
(4) the incidence of acute and chronic sinusitis decreases in latter childhood

SUMMARY OF DIRECTIONS				
A	**B**	**C**	**D**	**E**
1, 2, 3 only	1, 3 only	2, 4 only	4 only	All are correct

75. Which of the following is/are true about bacterial meningitis in childhood?

(1) *H. influenzae type B, Streptococcus pneumoniae*, and *Neisseria meningitis* are responsible for most cases of meningitis in the 2-months to 12-year age group

(2) parents of children in day care who are exposed to a child with H. influenzae meningitis should be alerted to the potential of H. influenzae infection in their child

(3) both *N. meningitis* and *H. influenza type B* meningitis have the potential sequelae of hearing loss

(4) the peak incidence of S. pneumoniae meningitis is in the school-aged child

76. Which of the following is/are true about cystic fibrosis (CF)?

(1) probably inherited as an autosomal dominant trait

(2) the gene for CF resides in the middle of the long arm of chromosome 7

(3) diagnosis can be attained via the sweat chloride test, quantitative stool trypsin, and immunoreactive trypsin

(4) recurrent pulmonary infections caused by group A beta hemolytic strep and H. influenzae are common

DIRECTIONS (Questions 77 through 82): Each of the numbered items or incomplete statements in this section is followed by answers or by completions of the statement. Select the <u>ONE</u> lettered answer or completion that is <u>BEST</u> in each case.

77. The Jones criteria for diagnosis of rheumatic fever includes all of the following as *major* criteria **EXCEPT**

(A) carditis
(B) polyarthritis
(C) Syndeham's chorea
(D) erythema chronicum migrans
(E) subcutaneous nodules

78. All the following are true of infant colic **EXCEPT**

(A) colicky crying can occur at any time of the day
(B) colic is more common in males than females
(C) colic begins in the first month of life, usually the first week

(D) colic usually resolves spontaneously by 3 months of age
(E) colic is not felt to be related to gas pains

79. All of the following are true regarding cryptorchidism **EXCEPT**

(A) it is more common in premature than normal-term infants
(B) it is more commonly unilateral than bilateral
(C) it is frequently associated with Fragile X syndrome
(D) it may be easily confused with retractile testes in childhood
(E) cryptorchid testes have an increased rate of testicular cancer

80. All the following are true regarding sports participation by teens **EXCEPT**

(A) epiphyseal injuries, although uncommon, can cause variation in growth
(B) the cardiac abnormality most associated with sudden death is hypertrophic cardiomyopathy
(C) children with Down's syndrome should not be allowed to participate in contact sports until an x-ray evaluation is done of the neck
(D) isometric exercise should be encouraged for teens with mildly elevated blood pressure
(E) swimming is an activity with low likelihood of inducing bronchospasm in an asthmatic

81. Suicide is the third leading cause of death among 15 to 19-year olds in the United States. All the following statements about adolescent suicide are true **EXCEPT**

(A) the method of suicide most commonly used by teenagers is ingestion of medication
(B) leaving a suicide note suggests premeditation and should be considered a sign of serious intent
(C) male adolescents lead female adolescents in the incidence of suicide attempts, but females outnumber males in completed suicides
(D) it is difficult to assess the seriousness of intent by the actual potency or medical lethality of the method

82. The incidence of anorexia nervosa and bulimia has increased in the past two decades; 1 in every 100 16 to 18-year-old females has such an eating disorder. All the following would be an important criterion for the diagnosis of anorexia nervosa **EXCEPT**

(A) intense fear of becoming fat
(B) refusal to maintain body weight over a minimal normal weight for age and height

(C) weight loss of at least 15% of original body weight or, for patients under 18 years of age, if weight loss from original body weight plus weight gain from projected growth charts reaches 15%

(D) absence of a known physical illness that would account for weight loss

DIRECTIONS (Questions 83 through 87): Each group of items in this section consists of lettered headings followed by a set of numbered words or phrases. For each numbered word or phrase, select the ONE lettered heading that is most closely associated with it. Each lettered heading may be selected once, more than once, or not at all.

For each age group select the developmental milestone in personal–social behavior one would look for in an assessment of the child

(A) 28 weeks
(B) 12 months
(C) 18 months
(D) 3 years
(E) 5 years

83. plays with feet and toys; expectant in feeding situations

84. uses spoon with moderate spilling; toilet regulated

85. cooperates in dressing; gives toy; finger feeds

86. dresses without assistance; asks meaning of words

87. uses spoon well; puts on shoes; takes turns

DIRECTIONS (Questions 88 and 89): For each of the items in this section, ONE or MORE of the numbered options is correct. Choose the answer

A if only 1, 2, and 3 are correct,
B if only 1 and 3 are correct,
C if only 2 and 4 are correct,
D if only 4 is correct,
E if all are correct.

88. A normal 18-month-old's language development includes

(1) using plurals and pronouns
(2) pointing to three body parts when asked
(3) repeating three digits
(4) jargon and ten-plus words

89. A normal 4-year-old's language development includes

(1) asks questions: why? how?
(2) knows four-plus colors
(3) beginning concepts of time: past, future
(4) knows opposites

DIRECTIONS (Question 90): Each of the numbered items or incomplete statements in this section is followed by answers or by completions of the statement. Select the ONE lettered answer or completion that is BEST in each case.

90. The average 3-year old can

(A) catch a ball
(B) copy a triangle
(C) knows the days of the week
(D) climb stairs with alternating feet
(E) skips smoothly

DIRECTIONS (Questions 91 and 92): For each of the items in this section, ONE or MORE of the numbered options is correct. Choose the answer

A if only 1, 2, and 3 are correct,
B if only 1 and 3 are correct,
C if only 2 and 4 are correct,
D if only 4 is correct,
E if all are correct.

91. Traditionally, a child's development is divided into the following categories

(1) gross motor
(2) fine motor/adaptive
(3) speech and language
(4) personal–social

92. In differentiating features of a carcinoma and a sarcoma, a sarcoma

(1) is of epithelial tissue origin rather than mesodermal
(2) is generally resistant to radiation sensitivity
(3) metastases common to regional nodes rather than lungs
(4) generally has a poor prognosis

DIRECTIONS (Questions 93 through 96): Each group of items in this section consists of lettered headings followed by a set of numbered words or phrases. For each numbered word or phrase, select the ONE lettered heading that is most closely associated with it. Each lettered heading may be selected once, more than once, or not at all.

(A) tender, swollen tibial tuberosity in an adolescent
(B) obese child with progressive pain and limp
(C) pain and crepitus with examination of patella
(D) incomplete tearing of a muscle or tendon
(E) incomplete tearing of a ligament with associated pain and swelling

93. osteoarthritis

94. mild or moderate sprain

95. Osgood-Schlatter disease

96. slipped capital femoral epiphysis

DIRECTIONS (Questions 97 and 98): Each group of items in this section consists of lettered headings followed by a set of numbered words or phrases. For each numbered word or phrase, select

A if the item is associated with (A) only,
B if the item is associated with (B) only,
C if the item is associated with both (A) and (B),
D if the item is associated with neither (A) nor (B).

(A) stretching of tendon or muscle
(B) stretching of ligament
(C) both
(D) neither

97. sprain

98. strain

DIRECTIONS (Question 99): For each of the items in this section, ONE or MORE of the numbered options is correct. Choose the answer

A if only 1, 2, and 3 are correct,
B if only 1 and 3 are correct,
C if only 2 and 4 are correct,
D if only 4 is correct,
E if all are correct.

99. There are several types of dehydration. Which of the following is/are true regarding the effect of the type on physical signs?

(1) in hyponatremic dehydration, intracellular fluid (ICF) volume is increased
(2) in isonatremic dehydration, the mucous membranes are dry
(3) in hypernatremic dehydration, the extracellular fluid (ECF) volume is decreased
(4) in hyponatremic dehydration, the blood pressure is high

DIRECTIONS (Question 100): Each of the numbered items or incomplete statements in this section is followed by answers or by completions of the statement. Select the ONE lettered answer or completion that is BEST in each case.

100. Down's syndrome involves all the following EXCEPT

(A) the incidence in the general population is 1 in 600 to 800 live births
(B) the presence of an extra number 18 chromosome
(C) increased frequency of congenital heart disease
(D) an association with advanced maternal age
(E) varying degrees of mental retardation

Answers and Explanations

1. **(E)** A careful history is important in the diagnosis of chronic diarrhea. Patients have few, if any, physical findings. Lactase deficiency is related to the low lactase levels in the intestine, which leads to accumulation of lactose. Short bowel syndrome refers to GI problems resulting from extensive small bowel resection. Celiac disease, gluten enteropathy, is believed to be related to a toxic effect of the protein gluten on the wall of the bowel. Definitive diagnosis is made by jejunal biopsy. The osmotic load of the undigested milk sugar lactose is responsible for the associated diarrhea. This lactose deficiency may be seen following protracted diarrhea of various etiologies. Congenital lactase deficiency is rare. Lymphangiectasia is a dysfunction of the intestinal lymphatic system resulting in the loss of lymph into the bowel. It may be seen in Turner or Noonan syndrome.

   The secondary form results from obstruction to lymph flow in disorders such as regional enteritis, scleroderma, retroperitoneal tumors, or lymphomas. *(Avery et al, pp. 432–438)*

2. **(A)** The disease is heterogenous with many different treatment regimens. Anemia, thrombocytopenia, and neutropenia are common findings at the presentation of ALL. Those patients who have survived to become parents have not had an increased incidence of birth defects in their children. The risks of a second malignancy in treated patients remains low. *(Avery et al, pp. 556–558)*

3. **(A)** Infants with TTN usually follow a completely uneventful delivery. There is early onset of tachypnea, and the cyanosis that is observed is relieved by a minimal amount of O_2. The blood gases are normal. The usual course is uneventful with resolution in about 3 days. Hypoxemia, hypercapnia, and acidosis are uncommon. It may be difficult to distinguish TTN from hyaline membrane disease. The distinctive feature of TTN is the sudden recovery versus the often protracted course of hyaline membrane disease. *(Behrman et al, p. 399)*

4. **(C)** In the typical patient with secundum atrial defect there is prominence of the left chest and, on auscultation, the first heart sound tends to be loud. The pathognomonic feature is a widely split second sound. *(Avery et al, p. 367)*

5. **(E)** The murmur of a VSD is typically heard toward the end of the first week of life after the pulmonary vascular resistance has decreased. The murmur occurs at the lower left sternal border. Clinical problems, such as CHF, occur in the first 6 months of life or not at all. *(Avery et al, pp. 328–329)*

6. **(B)** An infant with a persistent ductus arteriosus is typically small and premature, with respiratory distress that does not improve with conventional management. A murmur may not be heard. If it is present, it is typically systolic at the second left intercostal space. Bounding pulses and wide pulse pressure is also found. *(Avery et al, pp. 354–355)*

7. **(A)** The earliest finding in an infant with coarctation of the aorta is decreased and delayed or absent femoral pulses. Although often not identified in the nursery, this finding is important in early identification of the lesion. The usual presentation is at 1 to 3 weeks of life with tachypnea, tachycardia, and pallor with cyanosis. *(Avery et al, pp. 346–348)*

8. **(B)** This is a recently described condition that presents with clusters of easily ruptured vesicopustules on the forehead, neck, and lower back. The lesions have a rim of scale after they rupture and the base may be hyperpigmented. The melanosis gradually subsides over the first few months of life. *(Carpo et al, p. 501)*

9. **(C)** Strawberry hemangiomas are raised from the skin. At birth they may be identified as macular areas of erythema. These hemangiomas grow during the first months of life and eventually involute spontaneously without scarring. Therapy is not advised in the great majority of cases. Occasionally,

the location will necessitate therapy. Prednisone for 6 to 12 weeks is the initial therapy. Radiation and laser therapy are used if the lesion does not respond to steroids but the cosmetic result is poorer. *(Avery et al, p. 1149; Crapo et al, p. 502)*

10. **(E)** Seborrheic dermatitis may be identified in the axillae, neck folds, scalp, and diaper area. The presence of greasy-appearing plaques that are adherent suggests the diagnosis. It is an inflammatory disorder of the sebaceous glands. For severe and persistent lesions, and particularly for lesions in the diaper area, 1% hydrocortisone cream is helpful. *(Crapo et al, pp. 503–504)*

11. **(A)** Epidermolysis bullosa can be either autosomal dominant or autosomal recessive in inheritance. The recessive form is the most severe and can be lethal. The dominant form can range from being a nuisance to a moderate medical problem. Emollients to decrease friction and the prevention of bacterial infection of the blisters are important steps in management of this disease. *(Crapo, et al, p. 503)*

12. **(B)** Idiopathic scoliosis is more common in adolescent females than in males. There appears to be a pattern of inheritance that is multifactorial and an autosomal dominant genetic pattern with variable penetrance. *(Behrman et al, pp. 1350–1356)*

13. **(C)** The most common fracture in the newborn is that of the clavicle, which occurs during labor and delivery. In treating this lesion, immobilization is unnecessary. Pinning the total sleeve to the shirt and gentle handling will reduce the discomfort. *(Behrman et al, p. 389)*

14. **(D)** Legg-Calvé-Perthes disease (avascular necrosis of the femoral head) is more common in males. It occurs in children from 3 to 11 years with the most common age range being 5 to 9. *(Behrman et al, pp. 1350–1356)*

15. **(A)** Subluxation of the radial head (Nursemaid's Elbow) is a very common injury that occurs in children between 1 and 4 years of age. The child presents with refusal to move the arm and holds it slightly flexed at the elbow and pronated at the forearm. The lesion is a tear in the annular ligament at its attachment on the radius. *(Behrman et al, pp. 1350–1356)*

Slipped capital femoral epiphysis (not a correct answer) is most frequently seen in obese adolescents, usually males from 10 to 16 years of age. *(Behrman et al, pp. 1350–1356)*

16. **(C)**.

17. **(D)** Tinea pedis presents as interdigital maceration, scaling and fissures. The scaling occurs primarily on the instep or weightbearing surface. Pruritus is a common symptom. Secondary bacterial infection is common. It is rare before puberty. Allergic contact dermatitis involves the dorsum of the toes and the distal foot. The lesions are erythematous, scaly, and vesicular and are seen in prepubertal children. *(Polin et al, p. 38)*

18. **(D)** The diagnosis of rheumatic fever is based on clinical grounds. The modified Jones' criteria are the classic for diagnosis. Two major manifestations or one major and two minor manifestations strongly suggest rheumatic fever. The major criteria are polyarthritis, carditis, erythema marginatum, subcutaneous nodules, Sydenham's chorea. The minor manifestations are fever, arthralgia, previous rheumatic fever or rheumatic heart disease, an elevated sedimentation rate or C-reactive protein, and a prolonged P–R interval. *(Avery et al, pp. 386–389)*

19. **(A)** Gynecomastia begins in Tanner Stage II–III and disappears in 1 to 2 years. The underlying mass is mobile and there is no skin dimpling that would suggest a cancerous mass. The tissue is breast tissue, not fatty tissue secondary to obesity. Tenderness is a common symptom, as is irritation by clothing, which is relieved by wearing undershirts. Surgical intervention is not a common consideration; however, there are those males who have persistent breast tissue beyond the usual time for resolution and who are having significant psychologic problems with this disorder. Hence, surgery is considered, recommended, and successful. *(Rosenstein et al, pp. 60–61)*

20. **(D)** Colicky abdominal pain is a common presenting symptom but not invariably present. The edema experienced by these patients is thought to be related to a protein losing enteropathy secondary to the intestinal involvement in the disease. All children have renal involvement in HSP. Not all patients have hematuria, but renal biopsy confirms the presence of renal disease in all patients. Platelet counts and coagulation studies are normal. Joint, ankle, and knee pain may be the presenting complaint. *(Avery et al, pp. 445–446)*

21. **(C)** In idiopathic thrombocytopenic purpura, the platelet count is reduced below 20,000/mm³ (some authors say less than 50,000/mm³). Clot retraction, bleeding time, and the tourniquet test are depen-

dent upon platelet function and are abnormal in ITP. The WBC is normal and anemia is usually not present. Although the differential smear may show decreased platelets, the working diagnosis is made by a platelet count and confirmed by bone marrow examination. In adolescents, systemic lupus erythematosus is a consideration in the differential diagnosis of thrombocytopenic purpura. This would make the ANA test appropriate for ruling out that disease, but would not substantiate the diagnosis of ITP. *(Behrman et al, p. 1071)*

22. **(D)** Nevus sebaceous (Jadassohn) usually occurs on the head and is present at birth as a yellowish placque without hair. At puberty, there are changes that histologically reveal hyperplasia of the epidermus. In adulthood, there are frequently malignant changes. The usual recommendation is for removal in early adolescence. Acquired pigmented nevi are benign lesions and need be removed only for cosmetic purposes or because their location causes chronic irritation. A very small number of these nevi become malignant. Lentigines are small round dark macules that appear anywhere on the body. The lesions are benign and may be viewed as normal when the number is small. Halo nevus reflects the disappearance of melanocytes in a common pigmented nevus. These lesions are seen frequently in adolescents and children. Eventually, the lesions disappear. Excision would only be considered if there is something unusual about the nature of the central lesion. Achromic nevi are present at birth. They are areas of macular hypopigmented patches with irregular borders. They represent a focal defect in melanin production. *(Behrman et al, pp. 1393–1395)*

23. **(B)** Hypovolemic shock occurs after a reduction in blood volume caused by factors that include hemorrhage (internal or external), plasma loss via burns, sepsis, nephrotic syndrome, fluid shift due to third spacing, fluid and electrolyte loss, or fluid shift due to endocrine conditions such as diabetes mellitus, diabetes insipidus, hypothyroidism, and adrenal insufficiency. Cardiogenic shock stems from a dysfunction of the heart that may result from myocardial insufficiency or mechanical obstruction to the flow of blood into and out of the heart. Distributive or vasogenic shock is due to decreased intravascular volume secondary to leaky capillaries resulting from conditions such as septic shock, anaphylaxis, or barbiturate intoxication. Clinically, the patient's skin is warm, dry, and flushed initially. Terminal shock is irreversible damage to the heart and brain due to altered metabolism and tissue perfusion. This results in death. *(Barkin, pp. 20–32)*

24. **(A)** Many juices are hypoosmolar and may draw water into the intestinal lumen. Rice water and tea lack carbohydrates and are not acceptable fluids for oral rehydration. Because it contains large amounts of sodium, boiled milk is also not acceptable. *(Barkin, pp. 50–51; Schmitt, pp. 502–505)*

25. **(B)** Rectal temperatures are more accurate than axillary temperatures. Antipyretics may be used with children who are uncomfortable due to fever, or have a temperature of 38.6° C. Antipyretics may be held off until that time. Aspirin should not be used in children who have chickenpox or influenza-like illnesses because of the link with Reyes syndrome. Most providers use no aspirin with children at all. Children under the age of 3 months should have laboratory tests drawn because of the danger of severe underlying disease. Common organisms in bacteremic children include: *Staphylococcus aureus, Streptococcus pneumoniae, Haemophilus influenzae* and *Neisseria meningitides*. Sponging, not alcohol baths, is useful in treating fevers, along with antipyretics and limiting the amount of clothes worn. *(Barkin, pp. 178–183)*

26. **(D)** *Pasteurella multocida* is the most common organism with *S aureus* a secondary organism. Animal bites should be vigorously cleaned, irrigated, and debrided of devitalized tissue. Suturing is determined by functional or cosmetic reasons. Hand injuries, those involving extensive tissue damage, or wounds older than 24 hours duration should not be sutured. Along with puncture wounds, sutured wounds are more likely to become infected. Tetanus prophylaxis is indicated along with antibiotic prophylaxis for those bites considered high risk for infection. *(Barkin, pp. 230–231)*

27. **(D)** Initial treatment of burns includes immersing the burn in cold water or applying cold compresses to the area. Ice may damage tissue or cause hypothermia in severe burns. Treatment of partial-thickness burns is conducted by cleaning; blisters should remain intact and 1% silver sulfadiazine or petrolatum gauze should be applied. The dressings should be changed every 24 hours initially and every 2 to 3 days thereafter. Electrical burns commonly show little tissue damage at first but increased tissue damage with time is common. These burns should be followed daily. *(Barkin, pp. 237–241)*

28. **(A)** Injury to the cervical spine must always be ruled out. Airway management including intubation and oxygen should be initiated, particularly for the acutely unconscious patient. Hyperventilation and elevation of the head of the bed are crucial in the treatment of severe head injury. Shock is anoth-

er important consideration. It should be managed aggressively because cerebral perfusion pressure depends on an adequate blood pressure. Shock must be treated first and fluids are generally administered at two thirds maintenance. *(Barkin, pp. 315–323)*

29. **(C)** Asthma is a common pediatric problem, but children having an acute asthma attack do not always wheeze. Clinicians must conduct a complete history and physical for all children to establish the diagnosis of asthma but some children may need chest x-rays and a CBC to rule out other causes of wheezing and respiratory difficulty. It is important to establish their respiratory status, but pulmonary function tests may not be helpful in children because of their difficulty inspiring and expiring into a machine. Humidified oxygen is a necessity and inhaled and/or injected beta agonists are important initial therapy. Rectal theophylline suppositories have erratic absorption and should not be used. Liquid rectal theophylline preparations may be used in the same dose as oral preparations, but only for a short time. The therapeutic serum theophylline level is 10 to 20 µg/mL. Status asthmaticus is present when a patient fails to respond to epinephrine or beta agonists administered as initial therapy. *(Barkin, pp. 581–588)*

30. **(C)** Infants should gain between 15 and 30 g per day during the first 2 months of life. In the newborn period, they may initially lose up to 10% of their body weight. Infants should double their birthweight at 5 months and triple their birthweight at 12 months. *(Barkin, p. 655)*

31. **(B)** FTT is the deceleration of growing leading to a drop in two percentile lines on a standard growth chart. Generally, the first growth parameter to decline is the weight, followed by the height, and finally, if the malnutrition continues, the head circumference growth will become delayed. There are two types of FTT: organic failure to thrive (OFTT) when a definable medical condition causes the growth delay, and nonorganic failure to thrive (NOFTT) when this organic component is not present. NOFTT is commonly the result of poor parenting skills due to a chaotic lifestyle. Most cases of FTT can be dealt with on an outpatient basis with a team approach of medical provider, dietitian, and social worker. Laboratory tests are not useful in making the diagnosis of FTT; in fact, only 1.4% of the tests ordered were of any help in the diagnostic process. *(Bithony et al, p. 557; Colloton, 10/89)*

32. **(B); 33.(A); 34.(D); 35.(C)** Causes of methemoglobinemia include nitrates, nitrites, and sulfonamides. Organophosphates in pesticides include malathion and parathion. Ipecac is an emetic, not an antidote. *(Barkin, p. 274)*

36. **(C)** Subdural hematoma is the most dangerous inflicted injury, often causing death or serious neurologic sequelae (i.e., seizures, blindness, and/or mental retardation). Subdurals may be associated with skull fractures, but fractures will heal. Intraabdominal injuries are the second most common cause of death in battered children. Because the abdominal wall is flexible, the force of a blow to the abdomen is usually absorbed by the internal organs, thus causing a ruptured liver or spleen, tears of the small intestine, or intramural hematomas. Subgaleal hematomas, although unsightly, usually resolve within a month, leaving no residual. Extremity fractures, if properly treated, heal without deformity or residual deficit in function. *(Behrman et al, p. 81)*

37. **(C)** Bone trauma is found in 10% to 20% of physically abused children. Inflicted fractures of the shaft of bones are usually spiral rather than transverse, and spiral fractures of the femur prior to the age of walking are usually inflicted. Multiple bony injuries at different stages of healing imply repeated assaults and are diagnostic of nonaccidental trauma. Fractures of the scapula or sternum are so unusual that they should arouse suspicion of inflicted injury. Many inflicted injuries result from pulling on an extremity. This force tears the periosteum from the bone, thus causing subperiosteal bleeding. By 4 to 6 weeks after the injury, calcification occurs. Rare bone diseases such as scurvy and syphilis may radiologically resemble nonaccidental bone trauma, but the bony changes are symmetrical. *(Behrman et al, p. 81)*

38. **(B)** Most frequently, children do not disclose sexual molestation for long periods of time. Therefore, at the time they present to the health care provider they are not having acute emotional distress. Also, because of the delay in disclosure, physical findings are usually absent. Positive cultures for gonorrhea are confirmatory evidence of sexual activity, but in and of themselves do not make the diagnosis. Parental assessments of a child's emotional state and behavioral changes are also supportive of the diagnosis, but do not make it. The diagnosis most often rests on the graphic history offered by the victim. This can include descriptions of sexual behaviors not commensurate with a child's development or experience level. *(Behrman et al, p. 82)*

39. **(E)** Foster care is typically provided by local welfare authorities for children who have been neglected and abused. For many children this gives them an environment for physical and emotional safety. However, for others it becomes another episode of deprivation. The United States does not have a comprehensive and well-integrated system for foster care. Foster care is usually managed by

individual counties, rather than by state or national authorities, allowing for wide variations in policies. Understaffed and underbudgeted welfare departments do not have the means to develop well-integrated child-oriented foster care programs, to offer support and guidance for foster parents, nor to screen foster parents and children adequately to anticipate problems that may result in another change of placement. The legal system also has been slow to respond to permanent planning for children, making it possible for repeated placement changes. (*Behrman et al, pp. 48–49*)

40. (D) Most polycythemic infants are asymptomatic. This increases the importance of routine hematocrit testing for all newborns. The physical examination is normal except for a plethoric appearance and occasionally cyanosis. Symptoms of hyperviscosity that may occasionally be present include: respiratory distress, convulsions, congestive heart failure, priapism, and renal vein thrombosis. (*Avery and Taeusch, p. 609*)

41. (A) Sometimes referred to as respiratory distress syndrome, hyaline membrane disease occurs after the onset of breathing in infants with lung immaturity and deficiency of pulmonary surfactants. Onset of symptoms occurs within minutes of birth, but often they are not recognized as significant for some hours. Duskiness, tachypnea, grunting, and significant retractions are characteristic. Increasing cyanosis, often relatively unresponsive to increased inspired oxygen concentrations, is a necessary feature of the disease. Hyaline membrane disease is nearly twice as common in males as in females. Earliest x-ray findings show a fine miliary mottling of the lungs, with central consolidation. The air-filled tracheobronchial tree stands out in relief against the opacified hila. The miliary reticulogranularity of the lung parenchyma is usually present within minutes of birth. Approaches to prenatal diagnosis are the demonstration of a deficiency of alveolar surfactant. The relationship between a low lecithin–sphingomyelin ratio and clinical respiratory distress provides the ability to predict with a greater than 90% accuracy which infants are at risk. Because the phospholipids that are most surface-active are saturated, a measure of the concentration of dissaturated phosphatidylcholine allows greater accuracy in studies on amniotic fluid. The chances for survival of infants with hyaline membrane disease who require ventilation are directly related to their birthweights. Those who are born after 34 weeks and require ventilation have a greater than 90% chance of survival, those born between 28 and 33 weeks have a 75% chance of survival, and those between 26 and 28 weeks, a 50% chance of survival. (*Avery and Taeusch, pp. 133–145*)

42. (E); 43.(A); 44.(B); 45.(C) The abuser is a related caretaker in 90% of cases, a male friend of the mother in 5%, an unrelated babysitter in 4%, and a sibling in 1%. These statistics are apt to change as do social conditions, that is, currently, women are more likely to be involved in abuse but this difference disappears in families in which the mothers work and fathers are the primary caretakers. There is also, presently a trend for increased reporting of abuse in day care settings. (*Behrman et al, p. 80*)

46. (A) Physicians, physician assistants, and all health care providers must be able to recognize abused children and confirm the diagnosis. Recognition during the first 6 months of life is extremely important because the risk of a fatal outcome is highest in this age group. Prevention should be provided at all contacts with the parents by offering support, anticipatory guidance, and asking questions that allow parents to express any difficulties they are experiencing. All 50 states have laws requiring that health care providers report suspected cases of child abuse and neglect to a local child protective agency. Physician assistants, without specific training in psychiatry or mental health rarely provide direct treatment for abused children and their families. (*Behrman et al, p. 79*)

47. (A) In the vagina, sperm are motile for 6 hours and nonmotile for 72 hours or longer. The presence of sperm substantiates the victim's story. Acid phosphatase is present for 24 hours and confirms ejaculation. Gonorrhea cultures are positive less than 5% of the time, but are evidence that confirm the victim's history. When the cultures are positive, the alleged perpetrator will also need to be cultured. Pregnancy testing is not contributory (therefore, not indicated) in a child of this age, but in a postmenarchial child, medication to prevent pregnancy should be given. (*Behrman et al, p. 83*)

48. (B) Adoptions accomplished through approved agencies are preferred to independent adoptions, as they tend to have more adequate assessment of the psychosocial setting of the prospective adoptive family. Although, in general, adoptive placement should be made as soon after birth as possible, adoptions of older children, or across religious or ethnic lines are appropriate and reasonable alternatives to having adoptable children languish in institutions or temporary homes. The adopted child should be told of his/her adoption as soon as reasonably good verbal facility and comprehension have been achieved, usually about ages 3 to 4. (*Behrman et al, p. 48*)

49. (B) In sensorineural hearing loss, the Weber test lateralizes to the healthy ear. The affected inner ear or nerve is less able to receive vibrations arriving by any route, including bone. The sound is, therefore, heard in the better ear. On the Rinne test, air conduction lasts longer than bone conduction because the affected inner ear or nerve is less able to perceive vibrations arriving by either route. Therefore, the normal pattern prevails. *(Bates, p. 211)*

50. **(C)** A one-time physical examination of the newborn is useless, except for identifying gross congenital malformations. Observations and physical examinations of newborns need to be a "running appraisal" of findings over time. This is to assess the baby's condition and adaptation to extrauterine life, rather than assessments just at previously designated times, namely, admission and discharge. In the newborn, physical examinations are highly time dependent; that is, what is normal at 5 minutes of age is not normal at 3 hours, especially in regard to respiration and color. For this reason, all chart notes need to be specifically timed and dated. Particularly when performed by the unskilled on a premature sick infant, the physical examination can have adverse results, such as decreased body temperature, decreased skin perfusion, and decreased oxygenation. Handwashing to the elbows after removal of rings, bracelets, and watches should be performed immediately before and after touching the infant with no handling of fomites in the period during which the infant is handled. Nosocomial infections are one of the results of casual "baby-to-baby" examinations. *(Avery and Taeusch, p. 55)*

51. **(B)** In the normal newborn, care should be taken with assessment of even routine vital signs. A normal core temperature does not necessarily indicate an optimal environmental temperature for the infant. An infant who is chilled and vasoconstricted after a bath may have a normal core temperature, but a suboptimal environmental temperature. Skin sensors are widely used for continuous monitoring. It is essential to have the temperature sensor attached firmly to the skin. Porous tape needs to be used to avoid overheating. The usual site has been the upper abdominal wall, although the upper thigh or arms is preferred as more representative of mean body temperature. A high relative humidity is important, in servocontrolled incubators to prevent a paradoxically low-core temperature. When radiant heaters are used, the ambient humidity should be at least 40%. *(Avery and Taeusch, p. 55)*

52. **(E)** An increased hematocrit may reflect a relatively decreased plasma volume or an absolute increase in RBC mass. True polycythemia is due to an increased RBC mass. Polycythemia occurs with arterial hypoxemia (cyanotic heart disease, pulmonary disorders); tumors (renal, hepatic, cerebellar);

and abnormal hemoglobin (increased oxygen affinity). Neonatal polycythemia is generally due to fetal hypertransfusion or to one of the placental dysfunction syndromes. Hypertransfusion occurs with delayed umbilical cord clamping or in twin-to-twin transfusions, where one twin becomes polycythemic and the other anemic. *(Avery and Taeusch, p. 608)*

53. **(E)** Genetic (parents' and infant's blood types) and ethnic factors are known to affect neonatal bilirubin levels. With Rh and ABO incompatibility, hemolysis of infant blood cells and subsequent release of bilirubin occurs. Serum bilirubin values appear to be significantly higher in apparently normal Chinese, Japanese, Korean, and American Indian babies. Some perinatal events associated with increased bilirubin include delayed cord clamping and traumatic delivery (breech, vacuum extraction, difficult forceps). Delayed clamping of the cord is believed to result in higher peak bilirubin concentrations because the infant has a larger red cell mass and thus a greater capacity to produce bilirubin. Traumatic deliveries may produce bruising in an infant and the resorption of red cells from hemorrhagic sites will result in hyperbilirubinemia. Surveys indicated that between one in 50 and one in 200 breast-fed infants will develop hyperbilirubinemia. This is usually of late onset (after the third day). Bilirubin concentrations instead of falling, as is the usual course in a normal term infant, continue to rise often until the end of the second week, and with continued nursing may gradually decline to normal over a period of 1 to 4 months. *(Avery and Taeusch, pp. 626–627)*

54. **(C)** The contraindications to DPT are previous severe reactions to DPT including encephalopathy within 7 days, convulsion within 3 days, persistent high-pitched crying for 3 or more hours within 48 hours, collapse or shock-like state within 48 hours, temperature of 40.5°C or greater unexplained by another cause, and an immediate severe or anaphylactic reaction. Although some practitioners elect to defer immunization, a nonfebrile respiratory illness is not a contraindication to DPT. A family history of seizure is not a contraindication to vaccination. *(Red Book, p. 321)*

55. **(E)** Outbreaks in children less than 5 years have occurred both in unimmunized children and in children too young for immunization (less than 15 months). Outbreaks in college aged and junior high school students were the focus in many outbreaks; the majority were in previously vaccinated students. *(Markowitz et al, pp. 75–81)*

56. **(A)** An unimmunized child should be caught up as rapidly as possible, and DTP, OPV, and MMR may be given at one visit. However, a patient infected

with HIV should receive inactivated polio virus (IPV) instead of oral polio vaccine (OPV). MMR, a live viral vaccine, is indicated because complications have not occurred in HIV-infected children, no killed-virus vaccine is available, and because measles is devastating in children with HIV. *(Red Book, p. 114, Table 19)*

57. **(B)** The diagnosis of AIDS is difficult in an infant less than 15 months of age due to the presence of maternal antibody, but is appropriate when certain indicator diseases are present. Infants may be asymptomatic at birth, but 50% of cases of congenital AIDS present within the first year. The best current estimate is that 50% of infants born to HIV-infected women will also develop infection. *(Fallon et al, pp. 4, 10)*

58. **(B)** CMV infection occurs readily in day care, probably due to frequent contact with urine and saliva, and the infected children transmit virus to their parents. Nurses who practice good personal hygiene acquire CMV infection no more frequently than do their peers in the community. *(Balfour et al, p. 1909; Pass et al, p. 1414)*

59. **(A)** Streptococcal pharyngitis may be successfully treated with penicillin given intramuscularly or orally, two, three, or four times per day. Failure rates are unacceptably high (more than 20%) when dosed only once per day. *(Red Book, p. 391; Gerber et al, pp. 153–155)*

60. **(B)** Varicella zoster immune globulin (VZIG) should be given to a newborn infant of a mother who had chickenpox within 5 days before delivery or within 48 hours after delivery. VZIG does not modify established varicella. A newborn exposed to a sibling with varicella is not considered to be at high risk for complicated varicella because transplacental maternal antibody will usually protect the infant. *(Red Book, p. 460)*

61. **(C); 62.(A); 63.(A); 64.(B); 65.(D)** MMR and OPV are attenuated live virus vaccines. Diphtheria and tetanus toxoids are together with formalin-treated killed whole *B pertussis* organisms in DTP vaccine. Purified polysaccharide from the capsule of *H influenzae* type b is given alone in PRP vaccine, or covalently linked to a bacterial toxoid as in PRP-D vaccine. *(Red Book, p. 9)*

66. **(B)** Diagnostic criteria for Kawasaki syndrome are *fever for 5 days or longer*; and four of the five following: *conjunctival injection, rash, mucus membrane changes* such as cracked dry lips, injected pharynx or strawberry tongue, *extremity changes* such as redness and swelling of palms and soles, or desquamation, and cervical lymphadenopathy. Other

illness that may mimic Kawasaki syndrome, for example, streptococcal infection, must be excluded. Diarrhea and vomiting and generalized lymphadenopathy, although occasionally seen in children with Kawasaki's syndrome, are not diagnostic criteria. *(Bell, pp. 20–26)*

67. **(C)** In this longitudinal study in Boston, neither parental history of otitis media nor familial history of atopy (asthma, hay fever, or eczema) were found to be significant. Male gender, having a sibling, sharing a room with a sibling, having a sibling with a history of recurrent acute otitis media, no breastfeeding, taking a bottle to bed, parental smoking, and health care in an urban health center did correlate with increased risk of AOM. *(Teele et al, p. 85)*

68. **(A)** Most deaths of adolescents are violent and preventable. Following accidents, homicide, and suicide, cancer is the next leading cause of death. Males outnumber females in completed suicides by 3:1 but females outnumber males in suicide attempts by 3:1. *(Neinstein, pp. 77, 641)*

69. **(B)** Axillary hair in girls and boys occurs approximately 2 years *after* the development of pubic hair. The sequence of pubertal development usually occurs with the appearance of breast buds followed by the growth spurt, although a small percentage of girls (16%) develop pubic hair prior to breast enlargement. Alteration in the sequence of pubertal development may be a diagnostic clue to endocrine pathology. *(Copeland et al, p. 23)*

70. **(C)** Jaundice progresses in a cephalocaudal manner, with the extremities the last to be affected. Jaundice is visible clinically usually at 6 or 7 mg/dL. Cephalohematomas are reservoirs of RBC that can act as an increased source of bilirubin. Jaundice is associated with all these syndromes (hypothyroidism, galactosemia, and PKU) and they should be included in the differential diagnosis. *(Merenstein et al, pp. 325, 327–328)*

71. **(E)** All these are true. Jaundice in the first 24 hours is always abnormal. In a normal newborn, these levels are excessive. A direct quotient greater than 1.5 to 2 mg/dL warrants a more thorough investigation for hepatic damage. Jaundice appearing after the first week of life suggests breast milk jaundice, sepsis, hepatobiliary abnormalities, or hemolytic anemia. *(Merenstein et al, p. 325; Behrman et al, p. 405)*

72. **(C)** Migratory arthritis is associated with rheumatic fever. Conjunctivitis occurs with Reiter's syndrome. Juvenile rheumatoid arthritis is characterized by mono, pauci, or polyarticular joint swelling constantly and daily for at least 6 weeks. It

is almost always possible to elicit a history of morning stiffness. *(Rennebohm, pp. 185–186)*

73. **(A)** Choices 1, 2, and 3 are correct. Unfortunately, only a minority (30% to 45%) of teens who are suicide victims had ever been referred for mental health evaluation. In one series, only 2 of 27 were in treatment at the time of suicide. *(Brent, pp. 269–270)*

74. **(B)** These organisms are usually recovered from sinus aspirates. Frontal sinuses are rarely a site of infection until age 6 to 10. Sinus headaches are infrequent in children 5 years or younger. Acute and chronic sinusitis increases in latter childhood. *(Behrman et al, p. 874)*

75. **(A)** These are the most common organisms in this age group. Children in day care settings are at a higher risk for secondary cases of meningitis. Hearing loss does occur as a sequelae with both *H influenzae* and *N meningitides*. The peak incidence of *S pneumoniae* meningitis occurs in infants 3 to 5 months of age. *(Behrman et al, p. 569)*

76. **(A)** Pulmonary infections are more common with *S aureus* and *P aeruginosa*. *P aeruginosa* is responsible for a chronic low-grade infection that progresses. The patients colonized with *P aeruginosa* may require recurrent hospitalizations for intensive inhalation therapy and antibiotics. *(Behrman et al, pp. 926–935)*

77. **(D)** Erythema chronicum migrans is the cutaneous manifestation of Lyme disease. This rash develops at the site of the tick bite and develops into an expanding erythematous annular lesion with central clearing of approximately 16 cm. The rash of rheumatic fever is erythema marginatum that occurs over the trunk and inner surfaces of arms and legs. The rash is barely red, slightly raised, nonpruritic, and spreads in wavy lines or rings with sharp margins. *(Behrman et al, p. 541)*

78. **(B)** Colic does not have any sexual predilection. It is important to realize that colicky crying can occur at any time of the day, although it frequently occurs at the same time each day. Although parents frequently attribute colic to gas pain, there is no evidence to support this. The cause of colic is not elucidated but is felt to relate to a settling-in process to extrauterine stimuli. *(Schmitt, pp. 441–442)*

79. **(C)** In Fragile X syndrome the testes are large. Fragile X syndrome is also associated with mental retardation. Cryptorchid testes are associated with many congenital and chromosomal abnormalities. *(Behrman et al, pp. 267, 1164)*

80. **(D)** Isometric exercises such as weight lifting should be discouraged because this form of exercise produces a marked increase in both systolic and diastolic blood pressures. X-rays should be done on Down's syndrome patients to rule out atlantoaxial subluxation. Activities such as swimming, which does not induce bronchospasm, should be encouraged for asthmatics. *(Hulse et al, pp. 7–9)*

81. **(C)** Female adolescents lead male adolescents in the incidence of suicide attempts. Males outnumber females in completed suicides. *(Behrman et al, p. 437)*

82. **(C)** Weight loss would be at least 25% of original body weight or, for patients under 18 years of age, if weight loss plus weight gain projected from growth chart reaches 25%. A weight loss of at least 15% is itself not an important criteria for diagnosing anorexia nervosa. *(Behrman et al, p. 443)*

83. **(A); 84.(C); 85.(B); 86.(E); 87.(D)** At 28 weeks, the toddler usually plays with feet and toys and is expectant in feeding situations. By 18 months, the infant uses a spoon with moderate spilling and is toilet regulated. By 12 months, the infant cooperates in dressing, gives toy and finger feeds. By 5 years, the child dresses without assistance and asks the meaning of words. By 3 years, the child uses a spoon well, puts on shoes, and takes turns. *(Lewis, p. 163)*

88. **(C)** There are age-related norms established for articulation of speech and development of language and concepts. The correct response to this "K" question is C because 2 and 4 are correct answers. An 18-month-old child has attained sufficient maturation in his/her language development to be able to point to three body parts (2) and to have jargon and ten-plus words (4). Numbers 1 and 3 are incorrect responses because using plurals and pronouns (1) and repeating three digits (3) are 3-year-old skills. *(Kaye et al, pp. 35–36)*

89. **(B)** Using the established age-related norms for development of language and concepts, the correct response to this "K" question is B. Numbers 1 and 3 are correct responses because a 4-year-old has attained the language skills necessary to ask questions such as why and how and is beginning to understand concepts of time: past, future. Numbers 2 and 4 are incorrect responses because knowing four-plus colors and opposites are 5-year-old skills. *(Kaye et al, p. 36)*

90. **(D)** A 3-year-old has attained the skill of climbing stairs with alternating feet, making D the correct choice. Knowing the days of the week is a 4- to

5-year-old skill; catching a ball and skipping smoothly are 5 to 6-year-old skills; copying a triangle is a 6 to 7-year-old skill. *(Kempe et al, p. 32)*

91. **(E)** Development follows a dynamic sequential pattern with the timetable varying not only in normal versus abnormal persons, but also reflecting individual differences among children. It is helpful to divide development into categories as above, making E the correct response. In the infant, assessment of development is dependent primarily on motor and reflex parameters. Later, language and visual motor perception assume greater relative importance. *(Kaye et al, pp. 24–26)*

92. **(C)** In comparing a carcinoma and a sarcoma, there are clear differentiating features. The correct response to this "K" question is C because numbers 2 and 4 are correct statements and numbers 1 and 3 are false. Number 2: A sarcoma is generally resistant to radiation as opposed to a carcinoma, which is often sensitive including some cures. Number 4: A sarcoma generally has a poor prognosis in contrast to a carcinoma, which is variable. Number 1: epithelial tissue origin applies to carcinoma, and sarcoma is of mesodermal origin; Number 3: metastases to regional nodes applies to carcinoma, with lungs being the primary site for metastases of a sarcoma. *(Kempe et al, p. 624)*

93. **(C); 94.(E); 95.(A); 96.(B)** Osteoarthritis is manifested when the physical examination of the patellofemoral compartment of the knee joint yields pain and crepitus (C). A mild or moderate sprain is diagnosed by incomplete tearing of a ligament (E) as opposed to a strain, which involves the tendon. Complete tearing can result in instability of the joint. Osgood–Schlatter disease is suspected in an adolescent with knee pain and is demonstrated on physical exam by a tender, swollen tibial tuberosity (A). Slipped capital femoral epiphysis should be suspected in an obese child with pain and/or limp; greater than 40% of the children so affected are indeed obese. Additionally, it is important to always examine the hip joint in any child complaining of knee pain as pain can be referred. The D

choice does not relate to any of the numbered items and is, therefore, an incorrect response. *(Bates, pp. 450–451; Kempe et al, pp. 613, 616)*

97. **(B); 98.(A)** Soft tissue trauma may be divided into several categories according to the anatomical area that has been injured. A sprain is the stretching of a ligament. A strain is defined as stretching of a tendon or muscle. In either of these injuries there may be some degree of tissue tearing. *(Kempe et al, p. 616)*

99. **(A)** The correct response to this K question is A as 1, 2, and 3 are true statements. Number 1, hyponatremic dehydration or loss of sodium in excess of water produces an increase in intracellular fluid (ICF) volume. Number 2, an isonatremic dehydration, where there is a proportionate loss of water and sodium, mucous membranes are dry on physical examination. Number 3, hypernatremic dehydration, loss of water in excess of sodium, produces a decrease in extracellular volume. Number 4 is a false statement because in hyponatremic dehydration, the blood pressure is very low. *(Behrman et al, p. 196)*

100. **(B)** The appropriate answer is B, which is the only incorrect choice given. Down's syndrome involves the presence of an extra number 21 chromosome and has been the best recognized and most frequent human chromosomal syndrome. A applies to Down's syndrome in that the incidence is indeed 1 in 600 to 800 live births. Actually, among all conceptuses, greater than twice this frequency occurs but more than one half of these are spontaneously aborted during early pregnancy. C, frequency of congenital heart disease, is associated with Down's syndrome, primarily septal defects, especially of the endocardial cushion. D, associated with advanced maternal age, is correct with the reason for the correlation unknown. The major thought has to do with some aspect of aging of the oocyte. E is a correct statement, as all children with Down's syndrome exhibit some degree of mental retardation, albeit there is a wide variability of severity. *(Behrman et al, pp. 254–255)*

REFERENCES

Avery ME, First LR (eds). *Pediatric Medicine*, 1st ed. Baltimore, MD: Williams and Wilkins; 1989.

Avery ME, Taeusch HW. *Scaffer's Diseases of the Newborn*, 5th ed. Philadelphia, PA: WB Saunders; 1984.

Balfour CN, Balfour HH Jr. Cytomegalovirus is not an occupational risk for nurses in renal transplant and neonatal nurses: Results of a prospective study. *JAMA.* 256:1909–1014, 1986.

Barkin RM. *Emergency Pediatrics*, 2nd ed. St. Louis, MO: C. V. Mosby; 1987.

Bates. *A Guide to Physical Examination and History Taking*. Philadelphia, PA: JB Lippincott, 1987.

Behrman RE, Vaughn VC. *Nelson Textbook of Pediatrics*, 13th ed. Philadelphia, PA: Saunders; 1987.

Bell DM. Kawasaki update: More answers, fewer questions. *Contemp Pediatr.* 2: 20–36, 1985.

Bithony WG, Rathbun J. Failure to thrive, In: Levine M, Crocker A, et al. (eds). *Developmental–Behavioral Pediatrics*. Philadelphia, PA: W. B. Saunders; 1983.

Brent, DSA. Suicide and suicidal behavior in children and adolescents. *Pediatr Rev.* 10:269–275, 1989.

Colloton M. Investigating failure to thrive. *J Am Acad Phys Assist.* October 1989.

Copeland KC, Brochman RR, Rauk JL. Variations in normal sexual development. *Pediatr. Rev* 8:18–26, 1986.

Crapo JD, Hamilton MA, Edgman S (eds). *Medicine & Pediatrics in One Book*. Philadelphia, PA: Hanley & Belfus; St. Louis, MO: C. V. Mosby; 1988.

Dajani AS, Asmar BI, Thirumoorthi MC. Systemic *Haemophilus influenzae* disease: An overview. *J Pediatr.* 94:355–364, 1979.

Fallon J, Eddy J, Wiener L, Pizzo PA. Human immunodeficiency virus infection in children. *J Pediatr.* 114:1–30, 1989.

Gerber MA, Randolph MD, DeMae K, et al. Failure of once-daily penicillin V therapy for streptococcal pharyngitis. *Am J Dis Child.* 143:153–155, 1989.

Handbook of Common Poisonings in Children, 2nd ed. Evanston, IL: American Academy of Pediatrics; 1983.

Hulse E, Strong W. Participation evaluation for athletics. *Pediatr Rev.* 9:1–10, 1987.

Kaye R, Oski FA, Barness LA. *Core Textbook of Pediatrics*, 2nd ed. Philadelphia, PA: J. P. Lippincott; 1982.

Kempe CH, Silver HK, O'Brien D, Fulginiti VA. *Current Pediatric Diagnosis & Treatment*, 9th ed. CN: Appleton & Lange; 1987.

Lewis M. *Clinical Aspects of Child Development*. Philadelphia, PA: Lea & Febiger; 1982.

Markowitz LE, Preblud SR, Orenstein WA, et al. Patterns of transmission in measles outbreaks in the United States, 1985–1986. *N Engl J Med* 320:75–81, 1989.

Merenstein GB, Gardner SL. *Handbook of Neonatal Intensive Care*, 2nd ed. St. Louis, MO: C. V. Mosby Company; 1989.

Neinstein L. *Adolescent Health Care. A Practical Guide*. Baltimore–Munich: Urban & Schwarzenberg; 1984.

Pass RF, Huffo C, Ricks R, et al. Increased rate of cytomegalovirus infection among parents of children attending daycare centers. *N Engl J Med.* 314:1414–1418, 1986.

Polin RA, Ditmar MF. *Pediatric Secrets*. Philadelphia, PA: Hanley & Belfus; St. Louis, MO: C. V. Mosby; 1989.

Rennebohm RM. Rheumatic diseases of childhood. *Pediatr Rev.* 6:183–190. 1989.

Report of the Committee of Infectious Diseases (*The Red Book*), 21st ed. Elk Grove Village, IL: American Academy Pediatrics; 1988.

Rosenstein BJ, Fosarelli PD. *Pediatric Pearls: The Handbook of Practical Pediatrics*. Chicago, London, Boca Raton: Year Book Medical Publishers; 1989.

Schmitt BD. Colic: Excessive crying in newborns. *Clin Perinatol.* 12:441–450, 1985.

Schmitt BD. *Your Child's Health*. Toronto: Bantam Books; 1987.

Teele DW, Klein JO, Rosner B, et al. Epidemiology of otitis media during first seven years of life in greater Boston: A prospective, cohort study. *J Infect. Dis.* 160:83–94, 1989.

Subspecialty List: Pediatrics

CHAPTER 5

Emergency Medicine

Kevin T. Fitzpatrick

Questions

DIRECTIONS (Questions 1 through 3): Each of the numbered items or incomplete statements in this section is followed by answers or by completions of the statement. Select the ONE lettered answer or completion that is BEST in each case.

1. The most common form of shock in the initial phase of multisystem trauma is

    (A) hypovolemic shock
    (B) septic shock
    (C) neurogenic shock
    (D) cardiogenic shock
    (E) burn shock

2. Using the rule of nines, calculate the body surface area (BSA) involvement of an adult with a circumferential burn injury involving the left leg and right arm.

    (A) 9% BSA
    (B) 18% BSA
    (C) 27% BSA
    (D) 36% BSA
    (E) 70% BSA

3. Alcohol is involved in what percent of fatal single vehicle accidents?

    (A) 10%
    (B) 20%
    (C) 40%
    (D) 60%
    (E) 100%

DIRECTIONS (Questions 4 through 7): Each group of items in this section consists of lettered headings followed by a set of numbered words or phrases. For each numbered word or phrase, select the ONE lettered heading that is most closely associated with it. Each lettered heading may be selected once, more than once, or not at all.

Match the type of shock with its characteristic physical findings.

(A) hypotension without tachycardia, peripheral vasodilatation
(B) hypotension, tachycardia, distended neck veins
(C) near normal blood pressure, tachycardia, wide pulse pressure
(D) tachycardia, peripheral vasocontriction, narrow pulse pressure
(E) tachycardia, edema due to loss of plasma volume

4. hypovolemic shock

5. septic shock

6. cardiogenic shock

7. neurogenic shock

DIRECTIONS (Questions 8 through 17): For each of the items in this section, ONE or MORE of the numbered options is correct. Choose the answer

    A if only 1, 2, and 3 are correct,
    B if only 1 and 3 are correct,
    C if only 2 and 4 are correct,
    D if only 4 is correct,
    E if all are correct.

8. Potentially lethal chest trauma includes

    (1) hemothorax
    (2) open chest wounds
    (3) cardiac tamponade
    (4) pneumothorax

9. Characteristics of Boerhaave's syndrome include

    (1) sudden onset of severe chest pain
    (2) esophageal reflux associated with postural changes
    (3) often precipitated by forceful vomiting
    (4) gradual onset of dull epigastric pain

SUMMARY OF DIRECTIONS				
A	**B**	**C**	**D**	**E**
1, 2, 3 only	**1, 3 only**	**2, 4 only**	**4 only**	All are correct

10. Common causes of hypovolemic shock in the trauma patient include

   (1) femur fractures
   (2) pelvic fractures
   (3) hemothorax
   (4) closed head injury

11. Compartment syndromes often result from crush injuries or fractures of an extremity. Early signs and symptoms include

   (1) pulselessness
   (2) decreased sensation
   (3) poor capillary refill
   (4) pain

12. Emergency care of the major burn patient includes

   (1) administration of prophylactic IV antibiotics
   (2) vigorous administration of IV fluids
   (3) application of ice to affected areas
   (4) fiberoptic bronchoscopy to diagnose inhalation injury

13. Radiographic findings suggestive of aortic transection include

   (1) widened mediastinum
   (2) abnormal aortic contour
   (3) depression of left mainstem bronchus
   (4) left hemothorax

14. Treatment of flail chest injuries include

   (1) positioning patient on the affected side
   (2) positioning patient away from affected side
   (3) placement of sand bags on flail segment
   (4) intubation and positive pressure ventilation in patients with respiratory distress

15. Signs and symptoms of acute pancreatitis include

   (1) severe epigastric pain
   (2) rapid onset of pain
   (3) radiation of pain to the back
   (4) nausea and vomiting

16. Cardinal signs of a felon (infection of the finger tuft) include

   (1) fingers held in flexion
   (2) intense pain upon passive extension of the finger

   (3) sensitivity upon palpation along the course of the tendon sheaths
   (4) uniform swelling of the finger

17. A boutonniere deformity is characterized by

   (1) avulsion of the extensor digitorum communis tendon from its insertion on the middle phalanx
   (2) avulsion of the extensor digitorum communis tendon from its insertion on the distal phalanx
   (3) the proximal interphalangeal joint becomes markedly flexed and the distal interphalangeal joint extended
   (4) loss of extension in the distal phalangeal joint

DIRECTIONS (Questions 18 and 19): Each of the numbered items or incomplete statements in this section is followed by answers or by completions of the statement. Select the ONE lettered answer or completion that is BEST in each case.

18. Which spinal nerve supplies sensation to only the middle finger?

   (A) C5
   (B) C6
   (C) C7
   (D) C8
   (E) T1

19. Sensation to the skin of the legs and feet is derived from lumbar and sacral nerves. Which spinal nerve supplies sensation to the lateral aspect of the foot?

   (A) L3
   (B) L4
   (C) L5
   (D) S1
   (E) S2

DIRECTIONS (Questions 20 and 21): For each of the items in this section, ONE or MORE of the numbered options is correct. Choose the answer

   A if only 1, 2, and 3 are correct,
   B if only 1 and 3 are correct,
   C if only 2 and 4 are correct,
   D if only 4 is correct,
   E if all are correct.

20. Clinical features of acute diverticulitis often include

   (1) crampy abdominal pain
   (2) persistent vomiting
   (3) left lower quadrant pain
   (4) left flank pain

21. Radiographic findings suggestive of small bowel obstruction include

    (1) free intraperitoneal air seen best under the diaphragm on the upright KUB
    (2) air fluid levels within the bowel loops
    (3) a large amount of gas within the large bowel
    (4) distended loops of small bowel, proximal to the point of obstruction

DIRECTIONS (Question 22): Each of the numbered items or incomplete statements in this section is followed by answers or by completions of the statement. Select the <u>ONE</u> lettered answer or completion that is <u>BEST</u> in each case.

22. A 35-year-old male presents to the ER with a 2-hour history of severe epigastric pain. He reports the sudden onset of this discomfort. The patient denies vomiting. He reports a long history of intermittent abdominal pain relieved by antacids. The patient is lying on the stretcher, avoiding all movement. The abdomen is diffusely tender with muscular rigidity and guarding. The most likely diagnosis is

    (A) acute cholecystitis
    (B) perforated duodenal ulcer
    (C) acute appendicitis
    (D) acute diverticulitis
    (E) cholelithiasis

DIRECTIONS (Questions 23 through 25): For each of the items in this section, <u>ONE</u> or <u>MORE</u> of the numbered options is correct. Choose the answer

    A if only **1, 2, and 3** are correct,
    B if only **1 and 3** are correct,
    C if only **2 and 4** are correct,
    D if only **4** is correct,
    E if <u>all</u> are correct.

23. Common causes of small bowel obstruction include

    (1) adhesions from previous abdominal surgery
    (2) abdominal wall or internal hernias
    (3) intussusception
    (4) mesenteric lymphadenopathy

24. Common features of ruptured ectopic pregnancy include

    (1) sudden onset of abdominal and pelvic pain
    (2) history of scant or missed menstrual period
    (3) evidence of intraabdominal bleeding
    (4) unilateral, tender adnexal mass

25. Proper care of the patient with acute abdominal pain includes

    (1) nasogastric suctioning
    (2) serial physical examinations

    (3) careful attention to intravascular volume replacement
    (4) adequate anesthesia

DIRECTIONS (Question 26): Each of the numbered items or incomplete statements in this section is followed by answers or by completions of the statement. Select the <u>ONE</u> lettered answer or completion that is <u>BEST</u> in each case.

26. Murphy's sign is best described as

    (A) referred pain from the abdomen to the shoulder or scapula
    (B) rebound tenderness often seen in peritonitis
    (C) pain with palpation of the RUQ upon deep inspiration, pain causes patient to halt inspiratory effort
    (D) abdominal pain elicited by gently rocking the pelvis
    (E) a fetal position assumed by the patient with abdominal pain

DIRECTIONS (Questions 27 through 30): Each group of items in this section consists of lettered headings followed by a set of numbered words or phrases. For each numbered word or phrase, select the <u>ONE</u> lettered heading that is most closely associated with it. <u>Each lettered heading may be selected once, more than once, or not at all.</u>

Match the following pain patterns and location with the most likely diagnosis

    (A) sudden, severe midepigastric pain that progresses to diffuse abdominal discomfort.
    (B) sudden, severe right upper quadrant pain with radiation to the right scapular and shoulder region.
    (C) severe epigastric pain with radiation to the back.
    (D) vague midabdominal pain that localizes to the right lower quadrant.

27. perforated duodenal ulcer

28. acute cholecystitis

29. appendicitis

30. acute pancreatitis

DIRECTIONS (Question 31): For each of the items in this section, <u>ONE</u> or <u>MORE</u> of the numbered options is correct. Choose the answer

A if only <u>1, 2, and 3</u> are correct,
B if only <u>1 and 3</u> are correct,
C if only <u>2 and 4</u> are correct,
D if only <u>4</u> is correct,
E if <u>all</u> are correct.

31. Sources of emboli causing acute arterial occlusions can include

    (1) endocardium secondary to myocardial infarction
    (2) embolized atheromatous material from abdominal aortic aneurysms
    (3) left atrium secondary to atrial fibrillation
    (4) arterial arteriosclerotic stenosis with secondary thrombosis

DIRECTIONS (Questions 32 and 33): Each of the numbered items or incomplete statements in this section is followed by answers or by completions of the statement. Select the <u>ONE</u> lettered answer or completion that is <u>BEST</u> in each case.

32. A 60-year-old male presents to the ER with hematemesis. Past medical history is significant for cirrhosis. Physical examination is significant for disorientation, ascites, and splenomegaly. The most likely diagnosis is

    (A) UGI bleeding secondary to perforated duodenal ulcer
    (B) UGI bleeding secondary to erosive gastritis
    (C) UG bleeding secondary to Mallory Weiss tears
    (D) UGI bleeding secondary to gastroesophageal varices
    (E) UGI bleeding secondary to Boerhaave's syndrome

33. Proper treatment of soft tissue abcesses in an otherwise healthy individual consists of which of the following?

    (A) application of hot packs
    (B) observation and close follow-up
    (C) administration of broad spectrum antibiotics
    (D) incision, drainage, and local wound care
    (E) application of topical antibiotics

DIRECTIONS (Questions 34 through 37): For each of the items in this section, <u>ONE</u> or <u>MORE</u> of the numbered options is correct. Choose the answer

A if only <u>1, 2, and 3</u> are correct,
B if only <u>1 and 3</u> are correct,
C if only <u>2 and 4</u> are correct,
D if only <u>4</u> is correct,
E if <u>all</u> are correct.

34. Which of the following statements are true regarding pilonidal abcesses?

    (1) commonly have a chronic waxing and waning course
    (2) arise from fistulous communications with the rectosigmoid colon
    (3) require wide excision for definitive treatment
    (4) during acute episodes frank abscess formation can be readily appreciated over the presacral area

35. Which of the following statements regarding infected sebaceous cysts are true?

    (1) results from obstructed secretory glands
    (2) results from infected hair follicles within the dermis
    (3) requires excision of the cyst capsule to prevent recurrence
    (4) responds well to oral antibiotics

36. A paronychia is characterized by

    (1) an infection localized around the nail base
    (2) often tracks proximally along the tendon sheath
    (3) often accompanied by subungal abscess
    (4) an infection localized to the finger tuft

37. Proper care following venomous snake bite includes

    (1) application of a tourniquet proximal to wound
    (2) application of ice to affected part
    (3) immobilize affected part
    (4) perform a cruciate incision above the bite, followed by suctioning of the subcutaneous tissues

DIRECTIONS (Questions 38 through 41): Each group of items in this section consists of lettered headings followed by a set of numbered words or phrases. For each numbered word or phrase, select the <u>ONE</u> lettered heading that is most closely associated with it. <u>Each lettered heading may be selected once, more than once, or not at all.</u>

Match the following KUB findings with the corresponding most likely abdominal process.

    (A) free air beneath the diaphragm
    (B) loss of psoas shadow

(C) dilated loops of small bowel with air fluid level

(D) lower rib fractures

(E) essentially normal KUB

38. small bowel obstruction

39. retroperitoneal abscess

40. duodenal ulcer perforation

41. hemoperitoneum

DIRECTIONS (Question 42): Each of the numbered items or incomplete statements in this section is followed by answers or by completions of the statement. Select the ONE lettered answer or completion that is BEST in each case.

42. The most common cause of large bowel obstruction in the adult is which of the following?

(A) diverticulitis

(B) abdominal wall hernias

(C) carcinoma

(D) sigmoid volvulus

(E) adhesions

DIRECTIONS (Questions 43 through 46): For each of the items in this section, ONE or MORE of the numbered options is correct. Choose the answer

A if only 1, 2, and 3 are correct,
B if only 1 and 3 are correct,
C if only 2 and 4 are correct,
D if only 4 is correct,
E if all are correct.

43. Epistaxis from the anterior inferior septal plexus of blood vessels is usually adequately controlled by

(1) compression of the mobile portion of the nose for 5 to 10 minutes

(2) compression of the bleeding site with a pledgett impregnated with a topical vasoconstrictor

(3) cauterization with silver nitrate

(4) packing the anterior nasal cavity with ¼ inch petroleum gauge

44. Clinical findings in orbital blowout fractures include

(1) history of direct orbital injury

(2) impaired extraocular movement

(3) dysplasia

(4) numbness of the upper lip

45. Factors that mediate wound infection in the acute setting include

(1) the degree of bacterial contamination

(2) body part involved

(3) amount of devitalized tissue in the wound

(4) past medical history

46. Early signs and symptoms suggestive of inhalation injury in the burn victim include

(1) singed nasal hair

(2) carbonaceous sputum

(3) darkened oral or nasal mucosa

(4) patchy infiltrates on chest radiograph

DIRECTIONS (Question 47): Each of the numbered items or incomplete statements in this section is followed by answers or by completions of the statement. Select the ONE lettered answer or completion that is BEST in each case.

47. Burn shock is best described as

(A) hypovolemia due to loss of plasma volume into the extravascular spaces

(B) hypovolemia due to widespread thermal lysis of blood vessels

(C) cardiogenic shock due to myocardial depression

(D) hypovolemia due to bleeding from the burn wound

(E) heart failure due to renal failure and volume overload

DIRECTIONS (Questions 48 and 49): For each of the items in this section, ONE or MORE of the numbered options is correct. Choose the answer

A if only 1, 2, and 3 are correct,
B if only 1 and 3 are correct,
C if only 2 and 4 are correct,
D if only 4 is correct,
E if all are correct.

48. Which of the following statements regarding chemical burns is true?

(1) burned areas should be copiously lavaged with tap water

(2) dry chemical agents should be brushed from the skin prior to lavage

(3) all clothing, as it may retain caustic agents, should be removed from the patient

(4) acid and alkaline burns are best treated by application of a neutralizing agent to the surface of the burn wound

SUMMARY OF DIRECTIONS				
(A)	**(B)**	**(C)**	**(D)**	**(E)**
1, 2, 3 only	1, 3 only	2, 4 only	4 only	All are correct

49. Which of the following statements regarding escharotomy is true?

    (1) it is used to prevent compartment syndromes in circumferential burn wounds
    (2) it is associated with significant blood loss
    (3) it is used to relieve respiratory distress
    (4) it requires general anesthesia

DIRECTIONS (Question 50): Each of the numbered items or incomplete statements in this section is followed by answers or by completions of the statement. Select the ONE lettered answer or completion that is BEST in each case.

50. The most effective method of providing anesthesia for repair of finger lacerations, fractured phalanx or abscess drainage is

    (A) topical anesthetics
    (B) bier block
    (C) digital block
    (D) intramuscular analysis
    (E) ice packs

DIRECTIONS (Question 51): For each of the items in this section, ONE or MORE of the numbered options is correct. Choose the answer

    A if only 1, 2, and 3 are correct,
    B if only 1 and 3 are correct,
    C if only 2 and 4 are correct,
    D if only 4 is correct,
    E if all are correct.

51. Without epinephrine, lidocaine is toxic in doses exceeding 4.5 mg/kg. Symptoms of lidocaine toxicity include

    (1) apprehension
    (2) disorientation
    (3) nausea
    (4) excitement

DIRECTIONS (Questions 52 and 53): Each of the numbered items or incomplete statements in this section is followed by answers or by completions of the statement. Select the ONE lettered answer or completion that is BEST in each case.

52. Which is the most commonly fractured bone?

    (A) distal tibia
    (B) clavicle
    (C) distal radius
    (D) ribs
    (E) mandible

53. The best method of restoring adequate intravascular volume in the hypovolemic patient is

    (A) central venous lines, namely, suclavian, jugular lines
    (B) saphenous vein cutdowns
    (C) large peripheral IVs
    (D) fluid boluses via the infusion part of pulmonary artery catheters
    (E) administration of antidiuretic hormone

DIRECTIONS (Questions 54 and 55): For each of the items in this section, ONE or MORE of the numbered options is correct. Choose the answer

    A if only 1, 2, and 3 are correct,
    B if only 1 and 3 are correct,
    C if only 2 and 4 are correct,
    D if only 4 is correct,
    E if all are correct.

54. Chest tubes are indicated in a variety of emergency conditions including hemothorax, tension pneumothorax, open thoracic wounds, etc. General principles of chest tube insertion include

    (1) insert chest tube no lower than the 5th intercostal space
    (2) place the tube over the superior aspect of the rib
    (3) insert chest tube between the anterior to midaxillary line
    (4) after puncturing the pleura, placed a gloved finger through the pleura to check for adhesed lung

55. Signs and symptoms of airway compression include

    (1) altered mental status
    (2) hoarseness
    (3) gurgling, snoring
    (4) abnormal chest wall motion

DIRECTIONS (Questions 56 through 63): Each group of items in this section consists of lettered headings followed by a set of numbered words or phrases. For each numbered word or phrase, select the ONE lettered heading that is most closely associated with it. Each lettered heading may be selected once, more than once, or not at all.

Match the following types of fractures with their common complications

    (A) femoral shaft fractures
    (B) femoral neck fractures
    (C) open tibial fractures
    (D) supracondylar humeral fracture
    (E) scapular fractures

56. osteomyelitis

57. Volkmann's ischemic contracture

58. avascular necrosis

59. fat emboli syndrome

Questions 60 through 63

Spinal cord lesions can produce a variety of clinical manifestations. Match the following cord syndromes with their clinical characteristics.

    (A) anterior cord syndrome
    (B) Brown–Sequard syndrome
    (C) nerve root syndrome
    (D) complete cord syndrome
    (E) disc herniations

60. flaccid paralysis below cord lesion

61. complete paralysis, loss of pain perception with preservation of light touch, proprioception, and temperature sensation

62. hemisection of the cord resulting in loss of proprioception, vibration, and light touch on the side of the lesion, loss of pain and temperature on the contralateral side

63. typically occurs as a cervical injury with motor deficits that are more severe than sensory deficit

DIRECTIONS (Question 64): For each of the items in this section, ONE or MORE of the numbered options is correct. Choose the answer

    A if only 1, 2, and 3 are correct,
    B if only 1 and 3 are correct,
    C if only 2 and 4 are correct,
    D if only 4 is correct,
    E if all are correct.

64. Clinical signs of lumbar disc herniation include

    (1) reduction of deep tendon reflex
    (2) sciatic pain with straight leg raising
    (3) muscle weakness
    (4) low back pain made worse by valsalva

DIRECTIONS (Question 65): Each of the numbered items or incomplete statements in this section is followed by answers or by completions of the statement. Select the ONE lettered answer or completion that is BEST in each case.

65. A 65-year-old male presents to the ER with anorexia, malaise, shaking, chills, and watery diarrhea. Chest x-ray demonstrates small alveolar infiltrates.

Sputum samples are somewhat watery with Gram stains demonstrating a few polymorphonuclear leukocytes and no predominant bacterial species. Temperature is 103°F. The most likely diagnosis is

    (A) Klebsiella pneumonia
    (B) Lyme disease
    (C) Legionnaire's disease
    (D) mycoplasma pneumonia
    (E) viral meningitis

DIRECTIONS (Questions 66 through 68): For each of the items in this section, ONE or MORE of the numbered options is correct. Choose the answer

    A if only 1, 2, and 3 are correct,
    B if only 1 and 3 are correct,
    C if only 2 and 4 are correct,
    D if only 4 is correct,
    E if all are correct.

66. Phenytoin is often used intravenously for the treatment of status epilepticus. Side effects include

    (1) hypotension
    (2) tachycardia
    (3) bradycardia
    (4) tachypnea

67. Proper treatment of the adult with acute asthma includes

    (1) β-adrenergic agonists (epinephrine, terbutaline)
    (2) sedation
    (3) supplemental O_2
    (4) mucolytic agents

68. Clinical manifestation of diabetic ketoacidosis include

    (1) hypotension
    (2) a "fruity" odor to the patients breath
    (3) tachycardia
    (4) nausea

DIRECTIONS (Question 69): Each of the numbered items or incomplete statements in this section is followed by answers or by completions of the statement. Select the ONE lettered answer or completion that is BEST in each case.

69. The most common precipitating factor in the development of diabetic ketoacidosis is

    (A) omission of daily insulin
    (B) misuse of oral hyperglycemia medications
    (C) pancreatitis
    (D) infection
    (E) inappropriately high doses of insulin

DIRECTIONS (Question 70): For each of the items in this section, ONE or MORE of the numbered options is correct. Choose the answer

A if only 1, 2, and 3 are correct,
B if only 1 and 3 are correct,
C if only 2 and 4 are correct,
D if only 4 is correct,
E if all are correct.

70. Symptoms of cocaine toxicity include

(1) seizures
(2) hallucinations
(3) dysrhythmias
(4) vertical nystagmus

DIRECTIONS (Questions 71 through 72): Each of the numbered items or incomplete statements in this section is followed by answers or by completions of the statement. Select the ONE lettered answer or completion that is BEST in each case.

71. A male multisystem trauma patient is found to have a "free-floating" prostate on rectal exam and blood is noted at the urinary meatus. The initial step in evaluating these findings is

(A) intravenous pyelogram
(B) pelvic CT scan
(C) retrograde urethrogram
(D) insertion of a foley catheter to obtain a urine sample
(E) insertion of suprapubic catheter

72. The proper rate and sequence of ventilation and chest compression in one-person CPR is

(A) One ventilation per 15 compressions at a rate of 80 to 100 compressions per minute
(B) Two ventilations per 7 compressions at a rate of 80 to 100 compressions per minute
(C) One ventilation per 7 compressions at a rate of 80 to 100 compressions per minute
(D) Two ventilation per 15 compressions at a rate of 80 to 100 compressions per minute
(E) Three ventilations per 15 compressions at a rate of 80 to 100 compressions per minute

DIRECTIONS (Questions 73 and 74): For each of the items in this section, ONE or MORE of the numbered options is correct. Choose the answer

A if only 1, 2, and 3 are correct,
B if only 1 and 3 are correct,
C if only 2 and 4 are correct,
D if only 4 is correct,
E if all are correct.

73. True statements regarding the Heimlich maneuver include

(1) airway obstruction can be relieved by subdiaphragmatic compression forcing an artificial cough
(2) proper hand position is in the midline abdomen below the xiphoid process and above the umbilicus
(3) each thrush should be separate and distinct
(4) proper hand position is in the midline atop the xiphoid process

74. Characteristics of a ruptured Achille's tendon include

(1) the acute onset of severe lower calf pain
(2) loss of plantar flexion of the foot
(3) common in males aged 40 to 50
(4) loss of dorsiflexion

DIRECTIONS (Question 75): Each of the numbered items or incomplete statements in this section is followed by answers or by completions of the statement. Select the ONE lettered answer or completion that is BEST in each case.

75. A young athlete comes to the Emergency Department with complaints of a dull ache in the upper third of the calf. The pain was mild at first but over the last week has increased, with pain present at rest. Initial radiography is negative. This history suggests

(A) ruptured Achilles tendon
(B) lower extremity fascial hernia
(C) shin splints
(D) Osgood–Schlatter disease
(E) fibular stress fracture

DIRECTIONS (Question 76): For each of the items in this section, ONE or MORE of the numbered options is correct. Choose the answer

A if only 1, 2, and 3 are correct,
B if only 1 and 3 are correct,
C if only 2 and 4 are correct,
D if only 4 is correct,
E if all are correct.

76. Which of the following statements regarding pediatric fractures is/are correct?

(1) the most common site of fractures in children is at the epiphysical plate
(2) metaphyseal fracture alignment is, as a rule, less important in children than in adults

(3) the strongest element of a child's bone is the periosteum

(4) Salter type II fractures, which involve a metaphysis fracture and epiphyseal plate slip, usually require open reduction and are at risk for bone growth arrest.

DIRECTIONS (Questions 77 through 80): Each group of items in this section consists of lettered headings followed by a set of numbered words or phrases. For each numbered word or phrase, select the <u>ONE</u> lettered heading that is most closely associated <u>with</u> it. <u>Each lettered heading may be selected once, more than once, or not at all.</u>

Match the following fractures and dislocations with their anatomical description

(A) comminuted

(B) subluxation

(C) compression

(D) diastasis

(E) avulsion

77. disruption of the interosseous membrane connecting two joints

78. caused by impaction of one bone upon another

79. disruption of a joint with partial contact remaining between the two bones that make up the joint

80. any fracture where there are more than two segments

Answers and Explanations

1. **(A)** The most common form of shock in the initial stages of multisystem trauma is hypovolemic shock from hemorrhage. Neurogenic shock can occur from spinal injuries that result in a loss of peripheral vascular sympathetic tone. Cardiogenic shock can occur with severe chest trauma and is characterized by shock that is unresponsive to fluid resuscitation accompanied by high central venous pressures. Septic shock occurs as a result of bacterial infection, usually late in the trauma patient's hospital course. *(Committee on Trauma, ACS, pp. 62–64)*

2. **(C)** The "rules of nines" is a method for calculating the BSA involvement of burn injuries. The system divides various parts of the body into multiples of nine (Fig. 5–1). Bear in mind that the full BSA value for an extremity is assigned only for circumferential injuries. For example, if only the anterior surface of the arm were involved, this would constitute 4.5% BSA. BSA for various body parts varies in adults and children. *(Moylan, p. 448)*

3. **(D)** Alcohol is involved in greater than half of all drownings, fires, falls, pedestrian injuries, assaults, and suicides. The use of alcohol is one of the major predisposing factors to an individual sustaining a traumatic injury. *(Waller, pp. 307–347)*

4. **(D)** *Hypovolemic shock* produces peripheral vasocontriction as central organ systems are preferentially perfused. Tachycardia results from an effort to maintain adequate perfusion. A narrow pulse pressure is often noted. *(Committee on Trauma, ACS; pp. 62–64)*

5. **(C)** *Septic shock* produces a hyperdynamic cardiac output with a wide pulse pressure, near-normal blood pressure, and tachycardia. This frequently results from gram-negative septicemia secondary to exotoxin release. *(Committee on Trauma, ACS; pp. 62–64)*

6. **(B)** *Cardiogenic shock* results from cardiac failure; distention of the neck veins are a classic characteristic. Hypotension and tachycardia are common findings. Cardiogenic shock can arise from infarctions occurring at the time of the traumatic event, cardiac contusions, and direct cardiac injury. *(Committee on Trauma, ACS; pp. 62–64)*

7. **(A)** *Neurogenic shock* occurs when spinal trauma causes a loss of peripheral vascular sympathetic tone, resulting in vasodilatation with hypotension and bradycardia. Isolated head injuries do not cause shock in the adult. Infants and small children can lose sufficient intravascular volume with a head injury for hypovolemic shock to occur. *(Committee on Trauma, ACS; pp. 62–64)*

8. **(A)** Hemothorax can result in significant blood loss and hypoxemia. Open chest wounds can cause equilibration between atmospheric and intrathoracic pressure, thus resulting in impaired gas exchange. Cardiac tamponade commonly results from penetrating chest injuries. Even small amounts of blood trapped within the pericardium can restrict cardiac filling. Pneumothorax is usually well-tolerated by the healthy adult. *(Committee on Trauma, ACS; pp. 94–95)*

9. **(B)** Boerhaave's syndrome is rupture of the esophagus, which can occur from instrumentation, trauma, or spontaneously. Pain at the site of perforation is often sudden and severe. This condition is often precipitated by forceful vomiting. Esophageal reflux associated with postural changes is most characteristic of hiatal hernia. *(Skinner, pp. 817–820)*

10. **(A)** Isolated head injury does not cause hypovolemic shock. For symptomatic hypovolemia to occur, an adult must lose up to 35% of total blood volume. The cranial vault cannot accommodate this amount of volume. Pelvic and femur fractures are often associated with significant bleeding that can often be unappreciated due to the expandability of surrounding soft tissues. Hemothorax can cause significant blood volume loss. *(Committee on Trauma, ACS; p. 136)*

Figure 5-1. The percentage of body area is calculated by the rule-of-nines.

wound further damages compromised skin tissue. *(Moylan, p. 445)*

13. **(E)** Aortic rupture results from stresses caused by unequal rates of horizontal deceleration. These stresses are greatest at fixation points of the arch, such as the great vessels. Most aortic tears occur at the isthmus. Definitive diagnosis is achieved by aortography. The clinician must have a high index of suspicion for this entity, as the radiographic findings listed are suggestive, not diagnostic. *(Peyton and Wolfe, pp. 184–185)*

14. **(D)** Flail chest occurs when multiple contiguous ribs are fractured, resulting in a free-floating segment of chest wall. Normal respiratory motion of the chest is impaired. The main pathophysiological event is contusion of the lung beneath the bony injury. Sand bags do nothing to address this problem. Positioning the patient onto the affected side is impractical in the multiple-injury patient. In patients with respiratory distress secondary to flail chest and contusion of the underlying lung, intubation and positive pressure ventilation are indicated. *(Committee on Trauma, ACS; p. 15)*

15. **(E)** The majority of patients suffering from acute pancreatitis have associated gallstone disease or alcohol abuse. The pain of this condition has a rapid onset and quickly becomes severe, deep, and unremitting. The pain often radiates towards the back or around the costal margins. *(Beal, p. 887)*

16. **(E)** A felon is a localized infection of the finger tuft (Fig. 5–2). These infections have no way to spontaneously decompress as they are trapped between the septa that attach the skin to bone. As the infection spreads, it travels along the tendon sheath. The patient is forced to assume a flexed position for comfort. This tendon sheath involvement causes discomfort upon passive extension. *(Hoppenfeld, p. 88)*

17. **(B)** A boutonniere deformity (Fig. 5–3) results from separation of the extensor tendon from its insertion on the middle phalanx. Pain is demonstrated by palpation of the middle phalanx. Avulsion of the extensor tendon from the distal phalanx (answer 2) results in inability to extend the tip of the finger and is characteristic of a mallet finger deformity. *(Hoppenfeld, p. 87)*

11. **(C)** Compartment syndromes develop from an increase in pressure within fascial planes, causing local ischemia. Decreased sensation from nerve compression and local pain as well as tense swelling and weakness are early signs and symptoms. Pulselessness and decreased capillary refill are late signs associated with compartment syndromes. *(Committee on Trauma, ACS; pp. 189–190)*

12. **(C)** Major burn victims require vigorous volume resuscitation to combat burn shock. Fiberoptic bronchoscopy is the key to definitive diagnosis of inhalation injury. Prophalatic IV antibiotics are contradicted, as this will merely encourage the development of resistant organisms. Ice to the burn

Figure 5-2. An infection (a felon) of the finger tufts.

Figure 5-3. A boutonniere deformity.

18. **(C)** C5 supplies sensation to the lateral aspect of the arm. C6 supplies sensation to the lateral forearm, thumb and index finger. C7 supplies the middle finger (See Fig. 4). C8 supplies ring and little finger, medial palm. *(Galli et al, p. 73)*

19. **(D)** (See Fig. 5). The L3 dermatome covers the anterior thigh. The L4 dermatome covers the medial aspect of the leg. The L5 dermatome covers the lateral leg and dorsum of the foot while the SI dermatome involves the lateral aspect of the foot. *(Hoppenfeld, p. 230)*

20. **(B)** Diverticulitis is an inflammatory process within diverticula, most commonly affecting the sigmoid colon in older adults. Sigmoid involvement accounts for the characteristic left lower quadrant pain. Persistent vomiting is not a common feature. Flank pain would be more indicative of renal disease. *(Beal, p. 888)*

21. **(C)** The abdominal radiograph of a small bowel obstruction will often reveal air fluid vessels within distended loops of small bowel, proximal to the point of obstruction. Free air denotes perforation of the stomach, or small or large bowel. Minimal gas will be found in the large bowel, or beyond the point of obstruction. *(Beal, p. 880)*

22. **(B)** The sudden onset of abdominal pain and signs of peritonitis occurring in a patient with a history of dyspepsia are keys to the differential diagnosis.

Figure 5-4. The C7 neurologic level.

Figure 5-5. Sensation of the foot.

Acute cholecystitis is often accompanied by nausea and vomiting; patients are also quite restless in the early stages. Appendicitis begins with rather dull pain that gradually worsens. Patients with acute diverticulitis often give a history of episodic LLQ pain. The pain occurs rather suddenly but is usually localized to the LLQ. *(Beal, p. 884)*

23. **(A)** Intraabdominal adhesions and abdominal hernias are the most common causes of small bowel obstruction. In children, intussuseption is frequently encountered. Mesenteric lymphadenopathy would not, in and of itself, cause the bowel to obstruct. *(Beal, p. 891)*

24. **(E)** A ruptured ectopic pregnancy requires prompt diagnosis and rapid surgical intervention. Sudden sharp pain occurs at the time of rupture. Vital signs will change in relationship to the degree of intraabdominal bleeding. Rupture commonly occurs 6 to 12 weeks following conception. Nausea and vomiting are often present. *(Beal, p. 890)*

25. **(A)** Nasogastric suctioning acts as both a treatment and diagnostic maneuver in the patient with acute abdominal pain. NG suctioning relieves gastric dilatation and helps lessen the likelihood of aspiration. Suctioned material can be examined for occult blood. Serial abdominal exams provides a wealth of data regarding the progression or regression of an abdominal process. Many abdominal diseases cause significant third-space volume loses, necessitating careful attention to intravascular volume status. Providing a patient with analgesia prior to the establishment of a definitive diagnosis is extremely dangerous, as it renders further serial exams and patient reports meaningless. *(Beal, pp. 875–885)*

26. **(C)** Murphy's sign is caused by the descent of the liver and gallbladder during deep inspiration coming into contact with the examiner's fingers during right subcostal palpation. If the gallbladder is inflammed, pain will be produced, halting the inspiratory effort. This is pathognomic for cholecystitis. *(Beal, p. 885)*

27. **(A)** *Perforated duodenal ulcer*—pain begins suddenly, located in the midepigastic region. As peritonitis progresses, generalized abdominal pain is noted. This can cause a rigid or "board-like" abdomen on exam. There may be "free air" noted on plain radiographs of the upright abdomen. *(Beal, pp. 880–883)*

28. **(B)** *Acute cholecystitis* often begins suddenly with rapidly increasing pain. Pain is referred to the right shoulder and scapular area as subdiaphragmatic irritation triggers the phenic nerve. Nonvisualization of radionucleotide in the gallbladder during HIDA scan is diagnostic. *(Beal, pp. 880–883)*

29. **(D)** *Appendicitis* has rather vague and variable initial symptoms. However, over time pain usually localizes to the RLQ. Anorexia or even aversion to food is frequently seen. Fever of greater than 101°F is uncommon. *(Beal, pp. 887–889)*

30. **(C)** In *acute pancreatitis*, patients usually complain of the rapid onset of deep unrelenting midepigastric pain with radiation to the back. Patients may often give a history of intermittent dull epigastric pain. Alcoholism and cholelithiasis are the most frequent causes. *(Beal, pp. 886–887)*

31. **(E)** Acute arterial occulsion can be either intrinsic or extrinsic. Intrinsic occlusion is more common, resulting from embolic or thrombotic events. Extrinsic occlusions are usually the result of trauma. Common sources for emboli in addition to those described include valvular vegetation and thrombosis secondary to congestive heart failure and cardiomyopathies. *(Simmerman and Fogarty, pp. 696–697)*

32. **(D)** Bleeding from gastroesophageal varices is a result of portal hypertension due to a relative or absolute obstruction of splenic blood flow. Cirrhosis resulting from acute alcoholic hepatitis is a common cause of portal hypertension. Cirrhosis is commonly associated with variceal bleeding, encephalopathy, and ascites. Splenomegaly is a common finding. Emergency endoscopy should be performed on all patient with UGI bleeding, as other causes of bleeding may be present. *(Brown and Busuttil, pp. 788–789)*

33. **(D)** Definitive care of soft tissue abcesses is achieved through incision and drainage. Antibiotics in the healthy individual are unnecessary. Packing gauze should be placed into the wound to permit drainage and prevent premature closure of the skin edges. *(Warren, p. 981)*

34. **(B)** Pilonidal abscesses are presacral soft tissue infections usually chronic in nature. These do not communicate with the rectosigmoid. It is often easy to overlook the subtle appearance of these abscesses in the perisacral area. As multiple septations occur within the abscess cavity, wide excision is required for resolution. *(Warren, p. 988)*

35. **(B)** Sebaceous cysts arise from occluded secretory glands within the dermis. These require excision of the cyst capsule to prevent recurrence. Oral antibiotics are of little help in resolving infected sebaceous cysts, as the abcess cavity is avascular and does not permit antibiotic penetration. *(Warren, p. 992)*

36. **(B)** A paronychia is commonly seen as a "run around" or "hangnail" infection. It does not localize, as the infectious process has room to spread around the base of the nail. Infection that involves the finger tuft or track along the tendon sheath is more indicative of a felon. *(Warren, p. 993)*

37. **(B)** Management of snake bite involves lessening the absorption of venom. This is best accomplished by application of a tourniquet proximal to the wound. Care is taken that arterial inflow is not compromised; the tourniquet should *not* be taken down at intervals. The limb should be immobilized. Ice should *not* be applied. Cruciate incisions heal poorly; a single, linear incision is sufficient to allow for adequate drainage. *(Rammings, pp. 358–360)*

38. **(C)** Dilated small bowel with air–fluid levels is indicative of small bowel obstruction. The dilation is seen proximal to the point of obstruction with decompressed bowel distal to the lesion. *(Beal, pp. 883–884)*

39. **(B)** The psoas muscle is a posterior retroperitoneal structure. This paired set of muscles is usually easily discerned on plain abdominal radiographs. Loss of this shadow may be indicative of a mass effect obscuring the psoas outline. *Beal, pp. 883–884)*

40. **(A)** Free intraabdominal air is indicative of perforation of a hollow viscus, that is, the small or large bowel or stomach. It is best seen in an upright film where air will accumulate under the diaphragm. *(Beal, pp. 883–884)*

41. **(D)** Hemoperitoneum is a difficult diagnosis to make based on a plain x-ray alone. Associated injuries such as lower rib fractures indicate that the patient's abdomen has been subjected to great force. Such findings would lead the clinician to strongly suspect liver or spleen injuries. *(Beal, pp. 883–884)*

42. **(C)** Carcinoma of the colon is the most common cause of large bowel obstruction in the adult. Diverticulitis can also cause large bowel obstruction, and patients often give a history of intermittent left lower quadrant pain. Sigmoid volvulus is a less common cause of large bowel obstruction. It is seen most often in elderly persons with poor bowel habits and chronic constipation. *(Beal, p. 896)*

43. **(E)** All the methods are acceptable and will control the majority of cases with anterior nasoseptal bleeding. Posterior nasal bleeding as seen in patients with hypertension or atherosclerosis is much more difficult to control and may require extensive packing and the use of occlusive balloons. These are managed in step-wise fashion from compression to cauterization and, finally, packing. *(Snow, p. 1412)*

44. **(E)** Orbital blowout fractures occur when external forces increase intraorbital pressure, fracturing the orbital floor and entrapping extraoccular musculature. Inspection of the orbital rim may reveal a stepoff. Numbness of the upper lip suggests compression of the infraorbital nerve. Diplopia is a common finding. Orbital x-rays will often show clouding of the maxillary sinus. *(Georgiade and Manstein, p. 406)*

45. **(E)** The blood supply and ability of certain areas of the body to resist bacteria will greatly affect the propensity for wound infection. Past medical history that is significant for immunosuppressive disorders will also affect wound outcome. Foreign bodies and devitalized tissue within the wound will predispose the development of infection. *(Lammers, pp. 478–530)*

46. **(A)** Singed nasal hair, carbonaceous sputum, darkened oral or nasal mucous membranes, and history of burns in an enclosed space are highly suggestive for the presence of an inhalation injury. Bronchoscopy is used for definitive diagnosis. Even with the most severe inhalation injury, early chest x-rays appear normal. *(Herndon et al, p. 157)*

47. **(A)** Burn shock results from increased capillary permeability that permits the loss of plasma volume and macromolecules from the intravascular to the extravascular spaces. This transmigration of fluid leads to extensive edema formation and hypovolemia. Formulas for aggressive fluid resuscitation are designed to combat this phenomenon. All burn patients with injuries to greater than 20% BSA are at risk for significant plasma volume loss. *(Demling, p. 189)*

48. (A) Prolonged lavage with tap water is the most effective treatment of liquid chemical burns. Application of neutralizing agents produces an exothermic reaction, thus worsening tissue damage. Clothing that may retain noxious agents should be removed. *(Luteman and Curreri, p. 233)*

49. (B) Eschar is the thick, nonelastic material that forms on the surface of a full-thickness burn wound. In patients with circumferential chest or extremity burns, compartment pressures can rise beneath the eschar. This process compromises breathing and/or arterial inflow. The treatment is to make a longitudinal incision through the eschar to relieve compartment pressures. This procedure is accompanied by little blood loss and is relatively painless. *(Monafo and Freedman, pp. 247–248)*

50. (C) Digital blocks are accomplished by the injection of local anesthesia (without epinephrine) into nerves on the lateral and medial aspects of the digit. Bier block is the IV introduction of anesthesia into the limb that is occluded by an inflated BP cuff. This method is useful in soft tissue procedures on the hand and forearm. Topical anesthetics and intramuscular analgesia are ineffective in providing proper patient comfort. *(Simmon and Brenner, p. 108)*

51. (E) All these symptoms, which can be easily overlooked, can be prodromes to the onset of convulsions due to lidocaine toxicity. The severity of toxic reactions is dependent on the rapidity of drug absorption and the susceptibility of the patient. The use of lidocaine with epinephrine will allow for less rapid absorption and the use of higher doses. *(Simmon and Brenner, p. 87)*

52. (B) The most commonly fractured bone is the clavicle. Overall clavicular fractures account for 5% of all fractures in all age groups. These fractures are usually treated with a figure of eight clavicular wrap. *(Simmon and Brenner, p. 218)*

53. (C) Flow through a catheter is adversely affected by its length. Long indwelling central venous lines such as subclavian, jugular, or pulmonary artery catheters do not have the flow characteristics necessary for volume resuscitation. These types of lines are time-consuming to place and carry with them significant morbidity. The proper method of volume replacement is via two or more short-length, large bore peripheral IVs. *(Committee on Trauma, ACS; p. 16)*

54. (E) Chest tubes should be placed no lower than the 5th intercostal space to avoid injury to the diaphragm. Placement of the tube medial to the anterior axillary line increases the risk of lacerating the internal mammary vessels. The tube should be placed over the rib to avoid the intercostal neurovascular bundle. *(Committee on Trauma, ACS; p. 108)*

55. (E) It is important to recognize the somewhat subtle signs that may indicate airway obstruction. Agitation can often be attributed to intoxication when in actuality it heralds impending respiratory obstruction. A good test of airway patency is the patient's ability to converse with the examiner. A conversant patient indicates that the airway is patent and brain perfusion is adequate. *(Committee on Trauma, ACS; p. 33)*

56. (C) *Osteomyelitis* is infection of the bone, which often becomes chronic. Destruction of bone is often the consequence of this condition. This is most often the result of an open or "compound" fracture. This complication can be prevented by meticulous wound care designed to remove all foreign and devitalized material. *(Adams, p. 54)*

57. (D) Volkmanns ischemic contracture results from brachial artery injury in the setting of supracondylar humeral fracture. Ischemic damage to the flexion muscles of the forearm result in a flexion contraction of the hand and wrist. Other injuries that result in compartment syndromes may yield the same ischemic injury. *(Adams, p. 143)*

58. (B) Avascular necrosis is boney necrosis secondary to insufficient blood supply. It usually occurs in a fracture near the articular surface of a bone, especially if the terminal fragment is devoid of soft tissue attachments. This may occur following fracture of the femoral neck. Other common sites include navicular, scaphoid and talar fractures. *(Adams, p. 60)*

59. (A) Fat emboli syndrome is an uncommon but serious complication of long bone fractures, mainly at the femur or tibia. It usually occurs 2 days following injury and is characterized by alterations in mental status and/or respiratory insufficiency. Patients will often demonstrate a petechial rash. The etiology remains unclear; however, it is postulated that fat globules or released fatty acids play a role. *(Adams, p. 54)*

60. (D) Complete cord syndrome is characterized by complete flaccid paralysis and loss of all sensation below the level of injury. Deep tendon reflexes are absent. Injuries to the C1–C4 level result in respiratory arrest due to the respiratory muscle paralysis. *(Galli et al, p. 12–19)*

61. (A) Anterior cord syndromes occur most commonly in hyperflexion injuries of the cervical spine. Clinically, there is immediate, complete paralysis and loss of sensation below the lesion. Light touch, proprioception, and vibratory sense are spared, as they are controlled through the intact dorsal columns. These patients have a much better prognosis for recovery then do those with complete cord lesions. (Galli et al, pp. 12–19)

62. **(B)** Brown-Sequard Syndrome results from functional or anatomic hemisecton of the spinal cord. The consequence is loss of proprioception, vibration, and light touch on the ipsilateral side of the injury and loss of pain and proprioception on the contralateral side. (Galli et al, pp. 12–19)

63. **(C)** Nerve root syndrome commonly occurs in the cervical region and results from isolated nerve root injuries. Unilateral facet dislocations and disc herniations are the most common causes. (Galli et al, pp. 12–19)

64. **(E)** Lumbar disc herniation results from herniation of the central nucleus pulposus causing nerve root compression with sciatica and lower extremity symptoms. The pain of lumbar disc herniation is worsened by coughing, sneezing, and the valsalva maneuver. It is associated with flattening of the lumbar curve and muscle spasm. Nerve root compression, most commonly L4–L5 or L5–S1, often results in muscle weakness and neurologic deficits. (Galli et al, p. 256)

65. **(C)** Legionnaire's disease is suggested by the presence of a constellation of symptoms including fever, respiratory symptoms, toxemia, constitutional symptoms, diarrhea, and a typically nonproductive cough.

   Mycoplasma pneumonia accounts for 25% of all community-acquired pneumonia. Symptoms include upper and lower respiratory tract complaints, fever, cough, and headaches. The treatment of choice is erythromycin.

   Klebsiella pneumonia is seen most commonly in immunosuppressed individuals as a necrotizing lobar pneumonia. The entity is frequently associated with lung abscess and empyema. Klebsiella often has a rapid onset associated with pleuritic chest pain, shortness of breath, and rigors.

   Lyme disease is a tick-borne illness characterized by malaise, fatigue, fever, myalgia, lymphadenopathy, and malar rash. (Zwanger, p. 257; Pavikrishnan, p. 253)

66. **(B)** Phenytoin should always be given intravenously when intervening in acute neurologic emergencies. Intramuscular injection leads to uncertain absorption and pain. Phenytoin slows conduction through the AV node leading to bradycardia and hypotension. All patients receiving IV

phenytoin should be closely followed by EKG monitoring. (Sacks, p. 567)

67. **(B)** Beta-adrenergic agonists are the preferred medications for the treatment of asthmatics. Theophylline should be withheld for the more refractory case. Mucolytic agents are contraindicated as they may further bronchospasm. Sedation is contraindicated as it may lead to further respiratory compromise. (Sherman, p. 278)

68. **(E)** The osmotic diuresis and loss of intracellular water seen in diabetic ketoacidosis produces total body fluid depletion resulting in hypotension and reflex tachycardia. Ketone bodies are oxidized to acetone, causing the characteristic sweet or fatty odor to the breath. Nausea, vomiting, and abdominal pain are common occurrences, due in part to gastric dilatation and paralytic ileus. (Ragland, pp. 490–491)

69. **(D)** The most common precipitating factor in diabetic ketoacidosis is infection. All ketoacidotic patients must be thoroughly screened for the presence of an occult infectious process. Stressors, such as infection, cause the production of counterregulatory hormones such as glucagon, catecholamines, and cortisol. Stress hormone production, and their resultant antiinsulin effect, in conjunction with a relatively insufficient supply of insulin, set the stage for the development of ketoacidosis. (Ragland, pp. 490–491)

70. **(E)** Neurologic findings in cocaine toxicity range from apprehension and restlessness to twitching and generalized seizures, coma, and areflexia. Cardiac toxicity can lead to a wide range of dysrhythmias. It has been postulated that coronary artery vasospasm causes the myocardial infarctions seen in cocaine abusers. (Gerkin, p. 121)

71. **(C)** A "high-riding" or "free-floating" prostate on rectal exam, or blood at the urinary meatus is indicative of urethral injury. IVPs or pelvic CT scans are less then optimal imaging modalities to assess this entity. Insertion of a foley catheter is contraindicated as a partial urethral tear may be completed. Retrograde urethrograms should be performed to assess the integrity of the urethra prior to catheterization. (Ahlering, p. 663)

72. **(D)** The proper sequence of one person CPR as proposed by the American Heart Association is 15 compressions alternating with 2 ventilations. Two-person CPR is performed using five compressions to one ventilation. (Albarran-Sotelo, p. 47)

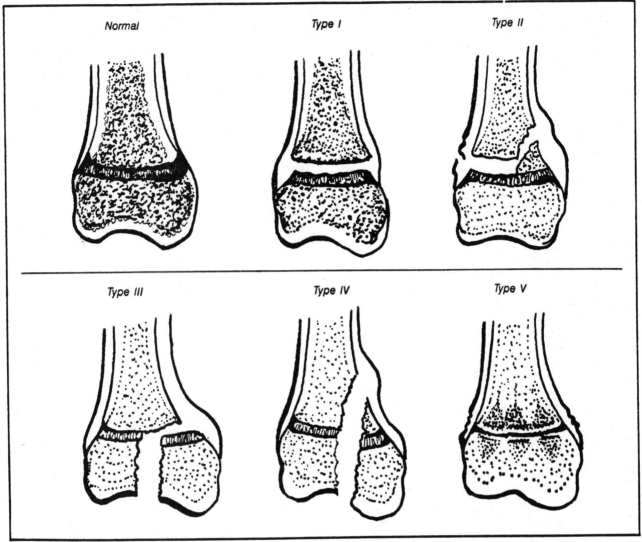

Figure 5-6. The Salter-Harris classification system used in epiphyseal injuries.

73. (A) The Heimlich maneuver is performed with the rescuer either kneeling astride the recumbent victim or standing behind the upright victim. Sharp, abdominal thrusts designed to quickly raise intra-abdominal pressures are applied. Care is taken to maintain hand placement below the xiphoid process to lessen the risk of rib fracture. *(Albarran-Sotelo, p. 58)*

74. (A) The most common site of Achilles tendon rupture is approximately 2 inches above the point of calcaneal attachment. This injury is common among sedentary men aged 40 to 50 years, but is also seen in athletes. Patients will often complain of agonizing lower calf pain and demonstrate an inability to plantar flex the foot. Partial tears are often misdiagnosed as some plantar flexion is preserved. *(Simon, p. 407)*

75. (E) The fibula is the most common site of stress fractures. It is commonly seen in young athletes, military recruits, and dancers. Early radiographs are often negative but in 10 to 14 days, a fine transverse line will often be seen, tracing the fracture site. The entity is commonly misdiagnosed as shin splints, which are more often characterized by pain on the anteriomedial surface of the distal leg. Fascial hernias are easily diagnosed by the presence of a reducible mass when the muscle is relaxed. Osgood–Schlatter disease is a painful condition of the tibial tuberosity seen in adolescents. *(Simon, p. 392)*

76. (A) Children's bones are more porous than adult's. The periosteum is the strongest element, with the epiphyseal plate the weakest. The epiphysis is the "growth plate" of young bones. Salter classification III and IV fractures have a high risk of growth arrest. As a general rule metaphyseal fractures in children require less alignment then those in adults (Fig. 5–6). *(Simon, p. 19)*

77. **(D)** Diastasis is a disruption of the interosseus membrane of a joint. This presents as a joint injury with edema and tenderness, as in a superior ankle dislocation. *(Simon, pp. 4–5, 402)*

78. **(C)** Compression fractures occur as a result of axial loading of one bone upon another. Most commonly seen in the spinal vertebrae of elderly with complaints of pain and occasionally radicular nerve pain. *(Simon, pp. 4–5)*

79. **(B)** Subluxation involves a partial dislocation of a joint in that there is continued contact of the bones. The clinical presentation is similar to a dislocation. *(Simon, pp. 4–5)*

80. **(A)** Comminuted fracture by definition implies more than two bone fragments. Variation of this is the butterfly fracture where a "v" shaped fragment is seen or a segmented fracture where there are two transverse fractures with a piece or segment of bone between. *(Simon, pp. 2–3)*

REFERENCES

Adams JC. Complications of Fractures. *In Outline of Fractures*. Churchill Livingston; Edinburgh: 1987.

Ahlering T, Weintraub P, Weinburg A, Skinner D. Urologic surgery and trauma. In Civetta E, ed. Critical Care. London: JB Lippincott; 1988.

Albarran-Sotelo R, Flint L, Kelly K, eds. Instructor's Manual for Basic Life Support. Washington, D.C.: American Heart Association; 1987.

Beal JM. The acute abdomen. In: Sabiston DS, ed. *Textbook in Surgery*. Philadelphia, PA: WB Saunders; 1981.

Brown SL, Busuttil RW. Portal hypertension. In Moore W, ed. *Vascular Surgery; A Comprehensive Review*. New York: Grune & Stratton; 1983.

Committee on Trauma. *Advanced Trauma Life Support Program of the American College of Surgeons*. Chicago, IL: ACS; 1989.

Demling R. Fluid resuscitation. In: Bostwick JA, ed. *The Art and Science of Burn Care*. Rockville, MD: Aspen Publishers; 1987.

Diethelm AG. The acute abdomen. In: Sabiston DC, ed. *Textbook of Surgery*. Philadelphia, PA: WB Saunders; 1986.

Galli RL, Spraite DW, Simon RR. *Emergency Orthopedics of the Spine*. Norwalk, CT: Appleton & Lange; 1989.

Georgiade DG, Manstein ME. Maxillofacial trauma. In: Moylan JA, ed. *Trauma Surgery*. Philadelphia, PA: JB Lippencott; 1988.

Gerkin RD. Cocaine. In Tintinalli, ed. Emergency Medicine. A Comprehensive Study Guide. New York: McGraw-Hill; 1985.

Herndon DJ, Thompson PB, Brown M, Traber DL. Diagnosis, pathophysiology and treatment of inhalation injury. In: Boswick JA, ed. *The Art and Science of Burn Care*. Rockville, MD: Aspen Publishers; 1987.

Hoppenfeld S. *Physical Examination of the Spine and Extremities*. New York: Appleton-Century-Crofts; 1976.

Lammers RL. Principles of wound management. In: Roberts JR, Hedges JR, eds. *Clinical Procedures in Emergency Medicine*. Philadelphia, PA: WB Saunders; 1985.

Luteman A, Curreri P. Chemical burn injury. In: Boswick JA, ed. *The Art and Science of Burn Care*. Rockville, MD: Aspen Publishers; 1987.

Monafo WW, Freedman BM. Electrical and lightning injury. In: Boswick JA, ed. *The Art and Science of Burn Care*. Aspen Publishers: Rockville, MD; 1987.

Moylan JA. Burn injury, In: Moylan JA, ed. *Trauma Surgery*. Philadelphia, PA: JB Lippincott; 1988.

Pavikrishnan KP. Viral and mycoplasma pneumonias in adults. In: Crome JE, Ruiz RL, eds. *Emergency Medicine, A Comprehensive Study Guide*. New York: McGraw-Hill; 1988.

Peyton RB, Wolfe WG. Traumatic thoracic aneurysm. In: Moylan JA, ed. *Trauma Surgery*. Philadelphia, PA: JB Lippencott; 1988.

Ragland G. Diabetic ketoacidosis in adults. In: Krome JE, Ruiz RL, eds. *Emergency Medicine, A Comprehensive Study Guide*. New York: McGraw-Hill; 1988.

Rammings KP. Bites and stings. In Sabiston DC, ed. *Textbook of Surgery*. Philadelphia, PA: WB Saunders, 1986.

Sacks C. Seizures and status epiletieus in adults. In: Krome JE, Ruiz RL, eds. *Emergency Medicine, A Comprehensive Study Guide*. New York: McGraw-Hill; 1988.

Sherman S. Acute asthma in adults. In: Krome JE, Ruiz RL, eds. *Emergency Medicine, A Comprehensive Study Guide*. New York: McGraw-Hill; 1988.

Simmerman JJ, Fogarty TJ. Acute arterial occlusions. In: Moore W, ed. *Vascular Surgery, a Comprehensive Review*. New York: Grune & Stratton; 1983.

Simmeon RR, Brenner BE. Anesthesia and regional blocks. In: Simmon RR, Brenner BE, eds. *Emergency Procedures and Techniques*. Baltimore, MD: Williams & Wilkins; 1987.

Simmon RR, Brenner BE. Orthopedic Procedures. In Simmon RR, Brenner BE, eds. *Emergency Procedures and Techniques*. Baltimore, MD: Williams & Wilkins; 1987.

Simon R, Koenigknecht SJ. Emergency Orthopedics, The Extremities. Norwalk, CT: Appleton & Lange; 1987.

Skinner DB. Perforation of the esophagus: Spontaneous (Boerhaave's syndrome), traumatic and following esophagoscopy. In Sabiston DC, ed. *Textbook of Surgery*. Philadelphia, PA: WB Saunders; 1986.

Snow JB. Surgical disorders of the ears, nose, paranasal sinuses, pharynx, and larynx. In Sabiston DC, ed. *Textbook of Surgery*. Philadelphia, PA: WB Saunders; 1986.

Urbaniak JR. Replantation of amputated digits and hands. In Sabiston DC, ed. *Textbook of Surgery*. Philadelphia, PA: WB Saunders; 1986.

Waller JA. Alcohol and unintentional injury. In: Kissin B, Begleiter H, eds. *The Biology of Alcoholism*, vol 4. New York: Plenum; 1976.

Warren T. Incision and drainage of cutaneous abscesses and soft tissue infections. In: Roberts JR, ed. *Clinical Procedures in Emergency Medicine*. Philadelphia, PA: WB Saunders; 1985.

Zwanger M. Legionnaire's disease. In: Krome JE, Ruiz RL, eds. *Emergency Medicine, A Comprehensive Study Guide*. New York: McGraw-Hill; 1988.

Subspecialty List: Emergency Medicine

Internal Medicine: Acquired Immunodeficiency Syndrome

Joan Alfiero

Questions

DIRECTIONS (Questions 1 through 4): Each group of items in this section consists of lettered headings followed by a set of numbered words or phrases. For each numbered word or phrase, select the ONE lettered heading that is most closely associated with it. Each lettered heading may be selected once, more than once, or not at all.

For each disease process, select the drug of choice with which it is treated.

(A) amphotericin B 3
(B) ganciclovir (DHPG) 4
(C) trimethoprim/sulfamethoxazole (Bactrim/Septra) 1
(D) acyclovir
(E) pyrimethamine and sulfadiazine 2

1. pneumocystic carinii pneumonia (PCP) C
2. toxoplasmic encephalitis E
3. cryptococcal meningitis A
4. cytomegalovirus (CMV) chorioretinitis B

DIRECTIONS (Question 5): Each of the numbered items or incomplete statements in this section is followed by answers or by completions of the statement. Select the ONE lettered answer or completion that is BEST in each case.

5. All the following statements regarding PCP are true **EXCEPT**

(A) the definitive diagnosis is made by obtaining pneumocysts on silver stain of sputum, bronchial washings, or lung tissue
(B) it is the leading cause of death in AIDS patients
(C) it occurs in 80% to 90% of all AIDS patients

(D) Treatment failure is defined as lack of clinical improvement after 3 days
(E) Most AIDS patients will survive their first episode of PCP

DIRECTIONS (Questions 6 through 9): Each group of items in this section consists of lettered headings followed by a set of numbered words or phrases. For each numbered word or phrase, select

A if the item is associated with (A) only,
B if the item is associated with (B) only,
C if the item is associated with both (A) and (B),
D if the item is associated with neither (A) nor (B).

(A) cryptococcal meningitis 6 +7 -8 - 9
(B) toxoplasmic encephalitis 7 -8 - 9
(C) both
(D) neither

6. computerized tomography (CT) of the head is usually normal

7. presenting symptoms of headache, fever, and altered sensorium

8. cerebrospinal fluid (CSF) may show normal protein and glucose as well as absence of pleocytosis

9. chronic suppressive therapy is required to prevent recurrences

DIRECTIONS (Questions 10 through 14): Each of the numbered items or incomplete statements in this section is followed by answers or by completions of the statement. Select the ONE lettered answer or completion that is BEST in each case.

10. All the following statements regarding the drug Pentamidine are true EXCEPT

   (A) it may cause sterile abcesses when administered intramuscularly
   (B) it may be used orally
   (C) It is used as prophylaxis for PCP in aerosolized form
   (D) dysglycemia is one of the most common side effects
   (E) it may cause renal dysfunction

11. All the following statements about patterns of HIV infection in the United States are true EXCEPT

   (A) the cumulative incidence of AIDS cases is disproportionately higher in blacks and Hispanics than in whites
   (B) the highest risk of HIV infection in pediatric patients occurs in children born to women who themselves are at risk of HIV infection
   (C) the percentage of reported AIDS cases in New York and San Francisco compared to the total United States population has gradually increased over time
   (D) it is estimated that as of December 1988, 1.0 to 1.5 million people have been infected with HIV

12. Which one of the following tests is used initially to evaluate the presence of HIV infection in a patient?

   (A) HIV antibody status by ELISA
   (B) HIV serum p24 antigen status
   (C) HIV antibody status by Western Blot
   (D) T-lymphocyte subset studies
   (E) In vitro culture of HIV from patient's blood

13. HIV-infected patients are at increased risk for all the following CNS diseases EXCEPT

   (A) progressive multifocal leukoencephalopathy (PML)
   (B) primary CNS lymphoma
   (C) cryptococcoma
   (D) bacterial meningitis
   (E) TB meningitis

14. Which one of the following statements is true about pediatric HIV infection?

   (A) a positive HIV antibody status in a neonate reflects the presence of HIV infection
   (B) symptoms of HIV infection are often seen in the first 6 weeks of life

   (C) chronic lymphocytic infiltrative pneumonia (LIP) and chronic parotid enlargement are commonly seen in children
   (D) Kaposi's sarcoma is frequently diagnosed in children, but is difficult to treat.
   (E) neurologic involvement, principally progressive encephalopathy, has been described in 10% to 20% of pediatric AIDS cases

DIRECTIONS (Questions 15 through 25): For each of the items in this section, ONE or MORE of the numbered options is correct. Choose the answer

A if only 1, 2, and 3 are correct,
B if only 1 and 3 are correct,
C if only 2 and 4 are correct,
D if only 4 is correct,
E if all are correct.

15. Retrosternal pain or burning on swalllowing in an HIV infected patient may be due to

   1. candidiasis
   2. cytomegalovirus (CMV)
   3. herpes simplex virus (HSV)
   4. oral hairy leukoplakia

16. Administration of AZT (zidovudine) in HIV-infected patients is often associated with

   1. significant sustained increase in CD4 (T helper cells)
   2. suppression of P24 antigenemia, if present
   3. increase in serum BUN and creatinine
   4. anemia and neutropenia

17. The incidence of new HIV infection in groups at recognized risk between 1985 and present has shown

   1. a decline in the percent of homosexuals/bisexuals
   2. an increase in the percent of hemophiliacs
   3. an increase in the percent of IV-drug users
   4. elimination of the category of persons with no known risk factor

18. Prior to developing AIDS, an HIV-infected patient may present with which of the following

   1. absence of symptoms
   2. symptoms of fatigue, fever, night sweats, and weight loss
   3. a history of previous acute mononucleosis-like syndrome
   4. persistent generalized lymphadenopathy

19. Mycobacterium avium intracellulare (MAI)

1. often infects the bone marrow causing pancytopenia
2. can be present in any organ in the body
3. often produces symptoms of chronic fever, diaphoresis, and weight loss
4. is a multiresistant organism whose therapy typically involves a multidrug regimen

20. Which of the following would be **LEAST** appropriate in the evaluation of an HIV-infected patient with profuse diarrhea?

1. stool for ova and parasites
2. colonoscopy with biopsy
3. stool for acid-fast bacteria (AFB)
4. barium enema

21. Neurologic syndromes seen in HIV-infected patients include which of the following disorders?

1. aseptic meningitis
2. myelopathy
3. dementia
4. peripheral neuropathy

22. The risk of HIV transmission

1. for blood recipients decreases if blood is donated by a family member
2. for homosexual men increases when practicing receptive anal intercourse
3. for blood recipients decreased dramatically in 1987 when routine screening of blood for HIV antibodies became available
4. by sexual contact increases in the presence of genital ulcers

23. The risk of HIV transmission to health-care workers

1. is greatly reduced when universal precautions are implemented
2. is lower than the risk of hepatitis B virus (HBV) transmission
3. is approximately 0.5% following a single needlestick exposure to blood from an HIV-infected patient.
4. has been documented from exposure to body fluids other than blood, such as feces, sputum, urine, or vomitus.

24. Which of the following statements regarding herpes virus infections in AIDS patients are true?

1. isolation of CMV from the lung is uncommon and warrants initiation of antiviral treatment.
2. prompt administration of antiviral treatment for active HSV infection reduces morbidity and risk of serious complications.
3. in treatment of mucocutaneous HSV, topical acyclovir reduces the formation of new lesions as well as the risk of dissemination.
4. disseminated varicella zoster virus (VZV) infection warrants hospitalization and treatment with high-dose IV acyclovir.

25. AIDS-associated Kaposi's sarcoma

1. may present in the lung as nodular infiltrates
2. is seen primarily in IV drug users
3. may respond to alpha-interferon administration
4. when treated with radiotherapy is associated with a high-response rate and an improved prognosis

Answers and Explanations

1. **(C)** Trimethoprim/sulfamethoxazole is the drug of choice in treating *P carinii* pneumonia (PCP); dosing is based on the trimethoprim component at 15 to 20 mg/kg/day in divided doses. If patients have a history of intolerance to sulfonamides or trimethoprim, pentamidine is the second-line drug for PCP treatment. Trimethoprim/sulfamethoxazole is associated with a high frequency of adverse reactions that include rash, leukopenia, thrombocytopenia, nausea, vomiting, or nephritis. A change in treatment to Pentamidine may be warranted if the side effects become severe. *(Masur and Kovacs, pp. 419–424)*

2. **(E)** Standard treatment of an acute episode of toxoplasmic encephalitis is the combination of pryimethamine at 75 to 100 mg daily and sulfadiazine at 6 to 8 g daily. This combination blocks folic acid metabolism of the proliferative form of *Toxoplasma gondii* and is synergistic against the organism. Corticosteroids are often indicated to manage increased intracranial pressure from mass effects. Associated with this treatment is a high frequency of toxic side effects, most commonly bone marrow suppression and rash. Folinic acid should be added to the therapy at doses of 10 to 30 mg daily in an effort to prevent bone suppression; should hemotologic toxicity arise, the dose may be increased to 50 mg daily. In the advent of severe toxicity, sulfadiazine should be discontinued, as it is more often responsible for the toxicity; clindamycin, an investigational agent, may be substituted. Anecdotal reports of response suggests a promising role for this drug; however, definitive recommendations regarding dose and duration await clinical trials. *(Israelski and Remington, pp. 437–441)*

3. **(A)** Standard treatment for cryptococcal meningitis is amphotericin B at 0.4 to 0.6 mg/kg per day IV. The side effects of amphotericin B commonly include high fever, rigors, nausea, vomiting, hypotension, and renal dysfunction. Cerebrospinal fluid (CSF) cultures should become sterile during initial therapy, and CSF cryptococcal antigen titers usually fall with therapy. Fluconazole, an oral triazole antifungal agent, appears to be a promising alternative but is presently an investigational agent available for compassionate use in the advent of treatment failure or intolerance to amphotericin B. *(Grant and Armstrong, pp. 459–462)*

4. **(B)** Ganciclovir, or DHPG, is the recommended treatment of CMV chorioretinitis. Initial treatment consists of 5 mg/kg, intravenously, bid for 14 to 21 days with duration of "induction therapy," dependent on degree of response determined by follow-up ophthalmologic exams. Maintenance treatment 5 to 7 days a week at 6 mg/kg once daily is required in an effort to prevent recurrence of lesions, as it has been shown that, with cessation of therapy, retinal lesions usually recur. The toxicity of ganciclovir includes bone marrow suppression (particularly neutropenia and thrombocytopenia), rash, headache, confusion, nausea, and vomiting, and may be the limiting factor in determining dose and duration of maintenance treatment. *(Drew, pp. 495–501)*

5. **(D)** Absense of clinical improvement after 5 to 7 days of treatment indicates therapeutic failure and the need for switching to alternate therapy. The addition of high-dose corticosteroid therapy to conventional agents may be successful in improving patients who fail treatment. PCP, which occurs in 80% to 90% of all AIDS patients, is the leading cause of death in these patients. Most (approximately 60%) survive their first episode of PCP due to early detection and effective treatment. Clinical presentation is characterized by fever, shortness and breath, and cough. Chest x-ray may reveal diffuse patchy infiltrates; however, it may be normal in up to 30% of patients. A definitive diagnosis of PCP is made only by obtaining pneumocysts on silver stain of sputum, bronchial washings, or lung tissue. *(Hopewell, pp. 409–416; Masur and Kovacs, pp. 421–426; MMWR, No. S-4)*

6. **(A)** CT of the head is usually normal in cryptococcal meningitis, although in rare circumstances, a ring-enhancing lesion can be demonstrated if a cyptococcoma is present. Diagnosis of cryptococcal

meningitis requires isolation of *Cryptococcus neoformans* from CSF. A head CT has become indispensable for diagnosis and management of patients with toxoplasmic encephalitis. The study most often reveals multiple hypodense, ring-enhancing lesions more frequently seen in the basal ganglia and corticomedullary junction. Double-dose contrast gives maximal enhancement of lesions and is, therefore, preferable to single-dose studies. Magnetic resonance imaging is more sensitive and may demonstrate lesions not picked up by CT scan, but there are no findings pathognomonic for toxoplasmosis. Definitive diagnosis is made by demonstration of *T gondii* (cysts or tachyzoites) in brain tissue obtained by biopsy. This procedure is recommended for patients with presumptive toxoplasmic encephalitis based on head CT or MRI who have not responded to empiric therapy within 3 to 4 weeks. *(Israelski and Remington, pp. 431–435; Grant and Armstrong, pp. 457–459)*

7. **(C)** Clinical presentation of toxoplasmic encephalitis, the most common CNS infection in AIDS patients, includes fever and headache in more than one half of patients, altered mental status and focal neurologic deficits in 60% of patients, and seizures in one third of patients. Hemiparesis is the most common focal finding, but patients may also present with ataxia, visual field loss, and cranial nerve palsies. Less commonly, toxoplasma may involve retina, lung, heart, abdomen, and testes. Cryptococcal meningitis, the second most common opportunistic infection of the CNS associated with AIDS, presents with fever, (often low grade), headache, and altered mental status. Less frequently seen are focal neurologic deficits, seizures, meningismus, and photophobia. Extracranial disseminated disease occurs in up to 50% of patients. *(Israelski and Remington, pp. 429–431; Grant and Armstrong, pp. 457–459)*

8. **(C)** In toxoplasmic encephalitis, CSF may be completely normal or may show mild pleocytosis and elevated protein. Although the presence of IgG toxoplasma antibodies in serum does not predict the development of toxoplasmic encephalitis in patients, its absence argues strongly against the presence of disease in a patient with intracerebral lesions. Production of toxoplasma-specific antibodies in the CSF may be useful in diagnosing active CNS infection. The CSF of patients with cryptococcal meningitis may reveal normal glucose and protein with absence of pleocytosis. Latex agglutination detects cryptoccal polysaccharide antigen in serum and CSF, a positive titer indicating active disease. Less commonly, an India-ink stain of CSF may reveal organisms with their typical large capsules. CSF cryptoccal antigen titers are serially followed to determine response to therapy; however, serum titers may remain high and cannot be correlated with clinical improvement. *(Israelski and Remington, pp. 431–436; Grant and Armstrong, pp. 457–459)*

9. **(C)** Duration of initial treatment of toxoplasmic encephalitis is approximately 6 weeks, providing there is steady improvment of intracerebral lesions on neuroradiographic imaging. Chronic suppressive therapy is required indefinitely to prevent recurrence of lesions or development of new lesions. Although the combination of pyrimethamine and sulfadiazine is highly active against the proliferative form of *T gondii*, it is not effective against the dormant cyst. Therefore, if therapy is withdrawn, relapse may occur in up to 80% of cases. Pyrimethamine at 25 to 50 mg daily and sulfadiazine at 2 to 4 g daily, both taken orally with folinic acid, appears to be an adequate suppressive regimen. Recurrences may still present on suppressive treatment, requiring reinitiation of high-dose therapy. Initial management of cryptococcal meningitis usually consists of daily amphotericin B until a total of 750 to 1000 mg is reached, depending upon patient response, CSF cultures, and CSF cryptococcal antigen titers. Maintenance therapy with two to three times weekly infusions of amphotericin B is begun immediately to prevent relapse; treatment may eventually be tapered to 100 mg weekly. Monitoring includes CBC, renal function, and electrolytes, as well as periodic CSF and serum cultures and antigen titers. Dosage may need to be altered if renal dysfunction occurs. *(Israelski and Remington, pp. 431–436; Grant and Armstrong, pp. 459–462)*

10. **(B)** Pentamidine, one of the treatments for PCP, is not available orally. Intramuscular administration of pentamidine is no longer used due to the high incidence of sterile abcess formation; thus, once-daily IV infusion (4mg/kg in 100 mL D5W) is the preferred route of administration. Adverse effects of pentamidine include renal dysfunction. (elevation of blood urea nitrogen and serum creatinine); hypoglycemia, which may be followed by hyperglycemia, orthostatic hypotension; leukopenia; thrombocytopenia; nausea; and metallic taste. Most of these side effects are reversible after the medication is discontinued; however, the dysglycemia may be permanent and necessitate insulin. Aerosolized pentamidine is presently used for PCP prophylaxis at a suggested regimen of 300 mg once monthly. Prophylaxis appears to be effective both primarily in patients with fewer than 250 CD4 lymphocytes per mm[3], and secondarily in patients who have had one or more episodes of PCP. The aerosolized form of pentamidine is associated with few adverse effects because it is not administered systemically; the most common is bronchospasm. This can be easily reversed with inhalation of a bronchodilater. *(Masur and Kovacs, pp. 419–426)*

11. **(C)** The cumulative incidence of reported AIDS cases in the United States is disproportionately higher in blacks and Hispanics. Although 80% of the population in the United States is composed of whites, 59% of all persons with AIDS are white. Conversely, whereas blacks and Hispanics compose 12% and 6% of the United States population, they make up 27% and 13% of all AIDS cases, respectively. The geographic distribution of AIDS cases throughout the United States has shifted with time. The percent of AIDS cases in New York and San Francisco, although disproportionately larger than other areas in the United States, has gradually decreased since 1983; these other areas have, however, seen an increase in cases. The proportion of adult AIDS cases in women has increased over time. The highest risk of HIV infection in children occurs in those born to women who are at risk of HIV infection. Women at increased risk should be counseled, tested for HIV antibody status, and advised of the risk of HIV transmission to fetus should pregnancy arise. As of December 1988, 1.0 to 1.5 million people have been infected with HIV. Using an extrapolation method, projections have been made estimating 365,000 diagnosed AIDS cases in the United States by 1992. *(MMWR, No. S-4)*

12. **(A)** The first step in evaluating the presence of HIV infection is the HIV antibody status using the enzyme-linked immunosorbent assay (ELISA) technique. HIV antibodies may be detected by this screening method 1 to 2 months after the onset of acute illness. If this test is found to be positive, it is confirmed by the more specific Western Blot (WB) method of HIV antibody detection. HIV serum p24 antigen may be detected by ELISA in the period prior to antibody seroconversion but is less sensitive than antibody status and may be present in the serum for only a brief period of time. Persistent p24 antigenemia or the reappearance of antigenemia is associated with poor clinical outcome and more rapid progression to AIDS. In-vitro culture of HIV is used in clinical trials and in research, but is rarely indicated in routine practice. T-lymphocyte subset studies are routinely used only in known HIV infected patients. Major subsets include CD4 (T-helper) cells and CD8 (T-suppresor) cells. A decrease in absolute number of CD4 cells generally correlates with a decline in function of the immune system and an increase in risk of opportunistic infection. *(Tindall et al, pp. 329–338)*

13. **(D)** Progressive multifocal leukoencephalopathy (PML) results from destruction of oligodendrocytes by the JC papovirus, a DNA "slow" virus. Neurologic deterioration occurs with diminished mental acuity, visual impairment, cranial nerve and motor dysfunction and, in terminal stages, altered consciousness. Neuroradiographic imaging reveals hypodense white matter lesions with irregular borders without contrast enhancement or mass effect. At present, there is no known treatment of this infection. Primary CNS lymphoma commonly presents with symptoms of confusion and memory loss as well as hemiparesis, seizures, headache, aphasia, or cranial nerve palsies. Single or multiple lesions that are frequently hypodense and contrast enhancing are seen on CT or MRI scanning of the head; these lesions may be indistinguishable from toxoplasmosis. Treatment for primary CNS lymphoma involves whole brain irradiation; however, survival is not significantly improved. HIV-infected patients are at increased risk for all forms of tuberculosis, both pulmonary and extrapulmonary; the latter includes TB meningitis. To date, there are no studies documenting an increased risk of bacterial meningitis in HIV-infected patients. Cryptococcoma is discussed briefly in question 6. *(Price and Brew, pp. 359–365)*

14. **(C)** HIV may be transmitted from mother to neonate during intrauterine life as well as during delivery. HIV antibodies cross the placenta; thus, the positive HIV antibody status of the infant may reflect the presence of maternal antibodies. Symptoms of HIV infection, fever, chronic diarrhea, and thrush may appear as early as 5 months of age. There is often a decrease in weight gain and linear growth, and an increase in infections such as otitis media and pneumonia. Staphylococcal and gramnegative infections begin to occur. Chronic lymphocytic infiltrative pneumonia (LIP) and chronic parotid enlargement are common in children. LIP appears on chest x-ray as interstitial, usually bilateral, infiltrates. PCP is the most common opportunistic infection in children but others include mycobacterium avium-intracellulare (MAI), toxoplasmosis, viral, cryptococal, and other fungal infections. Kaposi's sarcoma occurs rarely in children, but lymphomas are seen frequently. Neurologic involvement, primarily progressive encephalopathy, has been described in more than half of pediatric AIDS cases. *(Grossman, pp. 533–541)*

15. **(A)** Symptoms of dysphagia (difficulty swallowing), odynophagia (pain or burning on swallowing), and retrosternal pain are associated with esophagitis. The most common cause of esophogitis is *Candida albicans*, with most, but not all, patients having both oral thrush and esophageal candidiasis. An empiric trial of antifungal therapy, usually ketoconizole at 200 mg daily, is indicated in patients with oral thrush and esophogeal complaints. If symptoms fail to improve on ketoconizole, endoscopy is warranted to look for other etiologic agents. These include HSV and less commonly, CMV. The clinical picture of esophagitis may be complicated by simultaneous presence of multiple infectious

agents. Definitive diagnosis should be made by endoscopically-directed biopsy of the esophogeal mucosa. HSV esophagitis usually responds to a course of oral acyclovir at 200 mg 5 times daily, but may also require maintenance therapy at 200 mg 2 to 3 times daily to prevent recurrence. CMV esophagitis should be treated with IV ganciclovir (DPHG), and although initial response is often favorable, relapses are common. Oral hairy leukoplakia caused by Epstein–Barr virus (EBV) produces a white thickening of the oral mucosa, particularly the tongue. The lesions can range in size from a few millimeters to much of the dorsal surface of the tongue. Oral hairy leukoplakia does not extend into the esophagus or cause esophogeal symptoms. *(Drew, pp. 498–505; Greenspan et al, pp. 373–380)*

16. **(C)** AZT (zidovudine) was found in a multicenter trial in 1986 to prolong survival as well as reduce the frequency and severity of opportunistic infection in patients with AIDS and severe ARC. Since September 1986, AZT has been available for clinical use in patients with AIDS or HIV-infected patients with CD4 lymphocyte counts of less than 200. The present recommended dose of AZT is 200 mg orally every 4 hours, although alternate dosing is being studied in clinical trials. AZT is commonly associated with bone marrow suppression, particularly anemia and neutropenia, especailly in patients with CD4 counts of less than 100. Also reported are headaches, nausea, myalgias, and insomnia. Serum BUN and creatinine usually remain unaffected. After initiation of AZT, there appears to be a rise in the CD4 lymphocyte count that quickly reaches a plateau and may decrease back to baseline; it is likely that the latter is due to overall myelosuppression secondary to AZT. Continuous rise in CD4 count is not often demonstrated; however, if AZT therapy is discontinued, CD4 has been shown to drop. Similarly, p24 antigenemia is suppressed by AZT and will rebound following discontinuation of AZT. These clinical data support the laboratory observation that AZT therapy is a suppressive and not a curative regimen in treatment of HIV infection. Recent evidence has demonstrated that AZT is indicated in patients with CD4 counts between 200 and 500; patients taking AZT showed slower progression to AIDS and great stability in immunologic parameters when compared to patients receiving placebos. *(Richman, pp. 397–403*

17. **(B)** Trends of newly diagnosed HIV infections in the United States in groups at recognized risk have changed over time. Evidence indicates a decrease in the incidence of new infections in homosexual men, reflecting reduced high-risk sexual behavior in this population. The risk of new infection in hemophiliacs has decreased dramatically with the development in 1984 of heat treatment of clotting factor concentrates. The incidence of new infection in IV-drug users and their heterosexual partners appears to be increasing. Seroprevalence in IV-drug users is strongly associated with the number of persons with whom needles are shared, and the use of shooting galleries. Effective interventions for behavior change are difficult but essential in an attempt to persuade IV-drug users to not share needles or to clean needles and drug paraphernalia with bleach. The incidence of new HIV infection in people with no known risk factors remains between 3% and 6%; however, 75% are reclassified into known-risk categories following additional questioning. *(MMWR No. S-4; Wofsy, pp. 307–312)*

18. **(E)** HIV infection can be viewed as a spectrum of illnesses from the totally asymtomatic patient to the patient with full-blown AIDS. The majority of patients with HIV infection are without symptoms or signs of clinical disease. Primary HIV infection associated with HIV seroconversion is described as a mononucleosis-like syndrome with symptoms of headache, fever, malaise, myalgias, arthralgias, sore throat, lymphadenopathy, diarrhea, and maculopapular rash. The illness is sudden in onset, usually lasting 3 to 14 days and may be accompanied by aseptic meningitis. Prior to developing AIDS, an HIV-infected patient may present with chronic symptoms of fatigue, fever, night sweats, and weight loss. Persistent generalized PGL involving two or more extrainguinal sites is a common finding in HIV-infected patients. *(Abrams, pp. 343–351)*

19. **(E)** Mycobacterium avium-intracellulare (MAI) is the most common bacterial complication found in AIDS patients and causes widely disseminated infection. MAI frequently produces symptoms of chronic fever, diaphoresis, and weight loss; also associated are diarrhea and chronic abdominal pain with hepatosplenomegaly. It often infects bone marrow, causing pancytopenia. Anemia may be profound enough to require chronic transfusions. MAI may be found in virtually any organ in the body including spleen, liver, lymph nodes, lungs, kidneys, adrenals, and gastrointestinal tract. Treatment with a multidrug regimen has anecdotally improved symptoms, although it has not altered the progression of the disease or dissemination of the organism seen at autopsy. MAI is a multiresistant organism, but it may be inhibited by achievable concentrations of ansamycin, clofazimine, ciprofloxacin, ethambutol, rifampin, ethionamide, and cycloserine. Multiple regimens using combinations of these drugs have been used with no clear consensus on appropriate drugs or dosages. *(Jacobson, pp. 468–471)*

20. **(D)** Diarrhea accompanied by weight loss and abdominal cramps are common presenting symptoms in HIV-infected patients. Although AIDS wasting syndrome (HIV infection without superimposed enteric infection) is frequently seen in AIDS patients, intestinal infection should first be excluded. Initial evaluation should include stool culture for routine bacterial pathogens including *Salmonella, Shigella, Camphylobacter,* and *Yersinia.* Therapy is directed at each specific organism and should be of 1 to 2 weeks duration. Stool examination for ova and parasites may reveal *Giardia lamblia and Entamoeba histolytica,* which are associated with acute enteritis. *Cryptosporidium* and *Isospora belli,* two atypical parasitic infections common in patients with AIDS, are easily identified by examination of stool with acid-fast stain. In patients with cryptosporidiosis, symptoms develop insidiously and become more severe with deterioration of the immune system. Symptoms may include voluminous (1 to 25 L daily) diarrhea, weight loss of more than 10% total body weight, severe abdominal pain, and dehydration. The biliary tract may become involved causing nausea and vomiting. There is currently no effective treatment of cryptosporidium and management is aimed at supportive care. Isosporiasis is diagnosed less frequently than cryptosporidiosis but the symptoms are indistinguishable. Other chronic causes of enteritis include mycobacterium avium-intracellulare (also demonstrated on acid-fast stain), CMV, and Kaposi's sarcoma, all of which require histopathologic examination of tissue obtained from biopsy via colonoscopy. Barium enema would be least helpful in diagnosing the etiology of diarrhea in HIV-infected patients. *(Cello, pp. 393–394; Chaisson, pp. 480–481; Soave, pp. 485–493)*

21. **(E)** Aseptic meningitis may occur acutely with seroconversion or later in the course of HIV infection in both symptomatic and asymptomatic patients. Progressive vacuolar myelopathy is a common complication of HIV infection that presents with progressive gait disturbance and ataxia, often followed by bowel and bladder dysfunction. It is often accompanied by dementia but may occur in relative isolation. AIDS dementia complex is characterized by cognitive, motor, and behavioral abnormalities. This is the most common CNS disorder associated with HIV infection and is considered to eventually affect the majority of AIDS patients. Peripheral neuropathy can be seen at any stage of HIV infection and presents both sensory and motor dysfunction. The sensory symptoms are more common and include numbness, "burning," and pain usually beginning in the toes and feet. *(Price and Brew, pp. 359–369)*

22. **(C)** In 1983, the self-deferral program of volunteer blood donors who thought they may be at risk for HIV infection was begun in an attempt to reduce HIV transmission through blood transfusions. However, it was not until April 1985 that HIV-antibody testing of donated blood was instituted. This dramatically decreased risk of HIV transmission to blood recipients. Although blood recipients often wish to have blood donated by family members, this does not decrease the risk of HIV transmission as risk factors for HIV infection in family members are usually not known or not admitted. Sexual transmission is responsible for the majority of AIDS cases; thus, safer sex practices have become essential. Receptive anal intercourse carries the greatest risk of infection to homosexual men and female partners of bisexual men. The use of latex condoms with or without nonoxynol-9 (a spermicide displaying HIV viricidal acitivty) reduces the risk of HIV transmission. The presence of genital ulcers increases the risk of HIV transmission, likely on the basis of increased contact with blood at the ulcer site. *(MMWR, No. S-4; Jaffe and Lifson, pp. 299–306; Wofsy, pp. 307–319)*

23. **(A)** The risk of HIV transmission to health care workers has been evaluated and demonstrated to be approximately 0.5% (1 in 200) following a single needlestick exposure to HIV-infected blood. Although the incidence of transmission is low, the magnitude of risk emphasizes the need for effective infection control procedures. Universal precautions, treating all blood and body fluids as though infected with HIV, reduces the risk of occupational exposure. Protective measures include handwashing before and after patient contact, proper disposal of sharp objects, no recapping of needles, use of gloves when handling blood or body fluids/tissues, and use of goggles and gowns when splatter of body fluids is anticipated. The use of masks is necessary only with procedures during which there is aerosolization of body fluids or with contagious airborne diseases. No cases of HIV transmission to health care workers from contact with body fluids other than blood have been documented. The potential for HBV transmission to health care workers after accidental exposure is much greater than HIV transmission. Studies demonstrate that 10% to 30% of health care workers have serologic evidence of past or present HBV exposure. Twelve thousand health care workers become infected with HBV each year, of which 700 to 1200 become chronic carriers. *(MMWR, No. S-6; Gerberding, pp. 321–328)*

24. **(C)** CMV infection in AIDS patients is quite common and can cause several clinical illnesses, most frequently chorioretinitis, gastrointestinal disease, and pneumonia. Culture of CMV from pulmonary secretions or lung tissue is common, but its isolation does not always indicate active disease. Many patients with pulmonary disease and CMV isolation from the lung have concomitant infections, thereby raising doubt as to whether CMV is a true pulmonary pathogen. CMV is considered a possible pathogen when CMV-infected cells are seen histopathologically in tissue specimens. Therapy with ganciclovir (DHPG) should be considered when CMV is felt to be documented as a pulmonary pathogen and the patient's clinical course is deteriorating HSV infection, common in HIV-infected patients, may cause oral, genital, and anorectal lesions, as well as esophogitis and other organ involvement. The severity of illness depends upon the degree of immunosuppression in the patient and site of infection. Prompt administration of therapy, acyclovir, for active infection reduces morbidity and the risk of serious complications. Topical acyclovir, although reducing virus shedding, does not reduce formation of new lesions or risk of dissemination. Recurrent VZV infection manifesting as shingles occurs commonly in immunosuppressed HIV-infected patients. Dissemination of VZV to lung, liver, and CNS has been associated with a high mortality rate. This life-threatening disease process warrants hospitalization and treatment with high-dose IV acyclovir. *(Drew, pp. 495–509)*

25. **(B)** Kaposi's sarcoma (KS) is the most frequent AIDS-associated malignancy and is seen primarily in homosexual men. Unlike classic KS, which presents as relatively indolent cutaneous lesions, KS in AIDS patients is often aggressive and can be found as cutaneous lesions, visceral lesions, or both. Cutaneous KS can appear on any body surface but is commonly seen on the face and in the oral cavity. KS may cause pulmonary disease, gastrointestinal disease leading to gastric outlet obstruction, or GI bleeding, and cause lymphatic obliteration leading to severe lymphedema. Pulmonary KS may be seen on chest x-ray as nodular infiltrates, with or without pleural effusions, and patients often present with shortness of breath, hemoptysis, and dyspnea. Definitive diagnosis of Kaposi's sarcoma is readily made by biopsy. Radiotherapy is effective palliative treatment for KS lesions; however, progression and dissemination are not altered with treatment and prognosis is not improved. Multiple cytotoxic chemotherapeutic agents have been used in treatment of visceral KS with varying response rates. Most of these agents, including vincristine, vinblastine, adriamycin, methotrexate, and bleomycin, have been associated with severe toxicities. Alpha-interferon administered parenterally has proven effective against KS, particularly in patients with early disease who do not yet have marked depletion of CD4 cells. *(Mitsuyasu, pp. 511–523)*

Subspecialty List:
Acquired Immunodeficiency Syndrome

Question Number and Subspecialty

REFERENCES

Abrams DI. The pre-AIDS syndromes. Asymptomatic carriers, thrombocytopenic purpura, persistent generalized lymphadenopathy, and AIDS-related complex. *Infect Dis Clin North Am.* 2(2): 343-351, 1988.

Cello JP. Gastrointestinal manifestations of HIV infection. *Infect Dis Clin North Am.* 2(2): 387-396, 1988.

Centers for Disease Control. *AIDS and Human Immunodeficiency Virus Infection in the United States: 1988 Update. MMWR.* Vol. 38, No. S-4, 1989, pp. 1-38.

Centers for Disease Control. *Guidelines for Prevention of Transmission of Human Immunodeficiency Virus and Hepatitis B Virus to Health Care Workers and Public Safety Workers. MMWR.* Vol. 35, No. S-6, 1989, pp. 1-37.

Chaisson RE. Infections due to encapsulated bacteria, Salmonella, Shigella, and Campylobacter. *Infect Dis Clin North Am.* 2(2): 475-484, 1988.

Drew WL. Perpesvirus infections. How to use granciclovir and acyclovir. *Infect Dis Clin North Am.* 2(2): 495-501, 1988.

Gerberding JL. Occupational health issues for providers of care to patients with HIV infection. *Infect Dis Clin North Am.* 2(2): 321-328, 1988.

Grant IH, Armstrong D. Fungal infections in AIDS. Cryptococcus. *Infect Dis Clin North Am.* 2(2): 457-464, 1988.

Greenspan JS, Greenspan D, Winkler JR. Diagnosis and management of the oral manifestations of HIV infection and AIDS. *Infect Dis Clin North Am.* 2(2): 373-385, 1988.

Grossman M. Children with AIDS. *Infect Dis Clin North Am.* 2(2): 419-428, 1988.

Israelski DM, Remington JS. Toxoplasmic encephalitis in patients with AIDS. *Infect Dis Clin North Am.* 2(2): 429-445, 1988.

Jacobson MA. Mycobacterial diseases. Tuberculosis and Mycobacterium avium complex. *Infect Dis Clin North Am.* 2(2) 464-474, 1988.

Jaffe HW, Lifson AR. Acquisition and transmission of HIV. *Infect Dis Clin North Am.* 2(2): 299-306, 1988.

Masur H, Kovacs JA. Treatment and prophylaxis of *Pneumocystis carinii* pneumonia. *Infect Dis Clin North Am.* 2(2): 419-428, 1988.

Price RW, Brew B. Management of the neurologic complications of HIV infection and AIDS. *Infect Dis Clin North Am.* 2(2): 359-372, 1988.

Richman DD. The treatment of HIV infection. Azidothymidine (AZT) and other new antiviral drugs. *Infect Dis Clin North Am.* 2(2): 397-407, 1988.

Soave R. Cryptosporidiosis and isosporiasis in patients with AIDS. *Infect Dis Clin North Am.* 2(2): 485-493, 1988.

Tindall B, Cooper DA, Donovan B, Penny R. Primary human immunodeficiency virus infection. Clinical and serologic aspects. *Infect Dis Clin North Am.* 2(2): 329-341, 1988.

Wofsy CB. Prevention of HIV transmission. *Infect Dis Clin North Am.* 2(2): 307-319, 1988.

Internal Medicine: Dermatology

Heidemarie C. Watts

Questions

DIRECTIONS (Questions 1 through 11): Each of the numbered items or incomplete statements in this section is followed by answers or by completions of the statement. Select the ONE lettered answer or completion that is BEST in each case.

1. All the following are considered elevated lesions **EXCEPT**

   (A) plaques
   (B) macules
   (C) wheals
   (D) pustules
   (E) scales

2. Differential diagnosis of scaly feet must include all **EXCEPT**

   (A) pityriasis rubra pilaris
   (B) tinea pedis
   (C) dyshidrotic eczema
   (D) tinea versicolor
   (E) contact dermatitis

3. The differential diagnosis of papulosquamous lesions on the trunk includes

   (A) guttate psoriasis
   (B) secondary syphilis
   (C) erythema nodosum
   (D) A and B
   (E) all of the above

4. The most common skin cancer is

   (A) squamous cell carcinoma (SCC)
   (B) primary melanoma
   (C) actinic keratosis (AK)
   (D) keratoacanthoma
   (E) basal cell carcinoma (BCC)

5. Chronic urticaria management includes

   (A) oral H 1 and 2 antihistamines
   (B) identification and removal of possible causes
   (C) complete blood count (CBC) and differential
   (D) routine skin testing and/or biopsy
   (E) avoidance of epinephrine except with respiratory distress

6. Pityriasis rosea manifestations include all **EXCEPT**

   (A) prodromal symptoms such as malaise
   (B) a heralds patch
   (C) pruritus
   (D) scaly oval papulosquamous lesions
   (E) resolution of rash within less than 2 weeks

7. The drug of choice in treating uncomplicated erysipelas is

   (A) tetracycline
   (B) cephalothin
   (C) vancomycin
   (D) penicillin
   (E) nafcillin

8. Feature(s) that distinguish discoid lupus erythematous (DLE) from subacute systemic lupus erythematous (SCLE) is/are

   (A) primary therapy
   (B) clincial findings
   (C) laboratory findings
   (D) immunopatholgy
   (E) none off the above

9. A necrotic skin ulcer is most commonly associated with the bite of a

   (A) gypsy moth
   (B) brown recluse spider
   (C) scabies
   (D) black widow spider
   (E) scorpion

10. Target lesions are pathognomonic of

    (A) erythema marginatum
    (B) erythema multiforme
    (C) erythema annulare
    (D) erythema nodosum
    (E) erythema gyratum repens

11. The factor **NOT** exacerbating acne vulgaris is

    (A) cosmetics
    (B) emotional stress
    (C) topical steroids
    (D) mechanical stress
    (E) food

DIRECTIONS (Questions 12 through 24): Each group of items in this section consists of lettered headings followed by a set of numbered words or phrases. For each numbered word or phrase, select the ONE lettered heading that is most closely associated with it. Each lettered heading may be selected once, more than once, or not at all.

Questions 12 to 15

Select the viral skin problem for each of the cutaneous lesions.

   (A) verruca vulgaris
   (B) herpes zoster
   (C) *Molluscum contagiosum*
   (D) coxsackie
   (E) erythema infectiosum

(12) grouped vesicles, unilateral along a dermatome

(13) slapped face appearance

(14) grayish vesicles in the mouth, on the hands and feet

(15) dome-shaped papules with central umbilication

Questions 16 through 20

Match the appropriate diagnostic test with the listed diagnosis.

   (A) syphilis
   (B) erythrasma
   (C) herpes simplex
   (D) tinea versicolor

   (E) scabies
   (F) ecthyma

(16) KOH (potassium hydroxide)

(17) Tzanck smear

(18) dark-field

(19) Wood's light

(20) mineral oil scrape

Questions 21 through 24

For each characteristic nail change select the most likely associated disease or disorder.

   (A) transverse ridges (Beau's lines)
   (B) koilonychia
   (C) whitening (Terry nails)
   (D) green
   (E) pitting

21. cirrhosis

22. alopecia areata

23. iron deficiency

24. hyperthyroidism

DIRECTIONS (Questions 25 through 27): Each group of items in this section consists of lettered headings followed by a set of numbered words or phrases. For each numbered word or phrase, select

   A if the item is associated with (A) only,
   B if the item is associated with (B) only,
   C if the item is associated with both (A) and (B),
   D if the item is associated with neither (A) nor (B).

25. Therapy for severe Rhus dermatitis (poison ivy/oak) include

    (A) systemic corticosteriods
    (B) desensitization

26. Curative Kaposi's sarcomas therapies may include

    (A) excisional surgery
    (B) chemotherapy

27. Eczematous dermatitis resulting from endogenous factors include

    (A) nummular dermatitis
    (B) dermatophytid

DIRECTIONS (Questions 28 through 36): For each of the items in this section, ONE or MORE of the numbered options is correct. Choose the answer

A if only 1, 2, and 3 are correct,
B if only 1 and 3 are correct,
C if only 2 and 4 are correct,
D if only 4 is correct,
E if all are correct.

28. Course and prognosis of toxic epidermal necrolysis (TEN) is highly dependent on

1. systemic corticosteriods
2. management of fluids and electrolytes
3. topical skin care
4. hospitalization

29. Which of the following cutaneous changes occur with renal insufficiency?

1. generalized pruritus
2. Muehroke's nails
3. Kyrle's disease
4. lichen planus-like dermatosis

30. Drugs most likely associated with erythema nodosum:

1. bromides
2. sulfonamides
3. oral contraceptives
4. salicylates

31. Skin manifestations suggestive of malignant disease are

1. dermatitis herpetiformis
2. Sweet's syndrome
3. purpura
4. leukocytoclastic vasculitis

32. Mongolian spots usually

1. disappear in childhood
2. are a malignancy indicator
3. occur in the lumbosacral area
4. are present in more than 30% of whites

33. Bullae on lower extremities include the following diagnosis

1. pemphigus vulgaris
2. epidermolysis bullosa acuisita (EBA)
3. bullous diabeticorum
4. bullous pemphigoid

34. Atopic dermatitis is a chronic skin disorder associated with

1. elevated serum IgE
2. family history of atopic dermatitis
3. allergic rhinitis and/or asthma
4. geographic tongue

35. Varicella (chickenpox)

1. has an average incubation period of 14 days
2. cannot be transmitted through blood transfusions
3. is usually treated symptomatically
4. occurs only in children and young adults

36. Viral disease(s) occuring in children

1. rubella
2. rubeola
3. kawasaki
4. scarlet fever

Answers and Explanations

1. **(B)** Macules are flat, nonpalpable lesions marked by pigment alteration and vary in sizes and shapes. Cafe-au-lait spots and vitiligo are examples of macules.

The incorrect answers are A: Plaques are palpable raised plateau-like lesions of variable sizes and thickness. The scaly psoriatic plaques are an example of these. C: Wheals are inflamed, flat-topped papules or plaques formed by transient and superficial edema. They may appear as small papules or involve areas as large as the entire back; an example of these would be the wheals in urticaria (hives). D: Pustules are palpable vesicles filled with exudate that may contain bacteria as in folliculitis or they may be sterile as in the lesions of pustular psoriasis. E: Scales are palpable results of abnormal shedding or the accumulation of the stratum corneum. An increased rate of cell production appearing as scaly plaques in psoriasis or the scaling with a dermatophyte infection such as tinea versicolor are examples. *(Fitzpatrick, pp. 22–37)*

2. **(D)** Tinea versicolor is a superficial fungal infection characterized by scaly hypo-pigmented and hyperpigmented macules involving the trunk and the proximal extremities. A positive KOH (potassium hydroxide) with the pathognomonic spaghetti and meatballs (very short hyphea and spores) is diagnostic for this.

The incorrect answers are A: Pityriasis rubra pilaris is a chronic disorder, both familial and acquired. It manifests itself with reddish scaly plaques and keratotic follicular papules affecting the entire body including the oral mucosa. Most commonly involved are the palms and soles. B: Tinea pedis may manifest itself with erythema, scaly plaques, and/or maceration on the feet. Pruritus may accompany the cutaneous symptoms. The diagnosis of tinea pedis can usually be confirmed by a positive KOH (long hyphea) and/or a dermatophyte culture. C: Scaling and fissuring may be present on the feet and hands with chronic dyshidrosis. It is often accompanied by secondary bacterial infection. E: Scaly feet secondary to shoe contact dermatitis can be very difficult to diagnose because of the insidious onset of the reaction. The lesions usually appear to be on the dorsal aspect of the feet. One method of establishing the diagnosis is to place a piece of the suspected shoe material as a patch test on the skin of the back. *(Epstein, pp. 154; Fitzpatrick, pp. 517–519, 697–698, 1371, 1378–1379, 2197–2200, 2222–2223)*

3. **(D)** Guttate psoriasis manifests with erythematous papulosquamous macules, papules, and plaques scattered over most of the body. Greater than 50% of all patients report a preceding streptococcal infection. These patients may go on to develop chronic psoriasis. Secondary syphilis skin lesions may include macules, papules, papulosquamous and follicular eruptions, with or without scaling scattered over the body. The lesions represent a tissue reaction to the *Treponema pallidum* carried to the site by the blood and the lymphatics. The nontreponemal serologic test RPR should be done to rule out secondary syphilis. If positive, a fluorescent treponemal pallidum absorption test (FTA-ABS) should follow to confirm the diagnosis.

The incorrect answers are C and E: Erythema nodosum usually presents with erythematous tender nodules on the anterior shins. They may also appear in areas containing subcutaneous fat. Spontaneous resolution usually occurs in 3 to 6 weeks. Bedrest, identification, and elimination of underlying causes are usually sufficient. *(Fitzpatrick, pp. 463–481, 1142–1143, 2405–2425; Lynch, pp. 198, 231–233)*

4. **(E)** Basal cell carcinoma (BCC) is the most common malignant skin cancer in light-skinned people. The predominant occurrence is on sun-exposed areas seldom observed before age 40. It rarely metastasizes unless treatment to eradicate is not initiated promptly once the diagnosis has been made. Treatment modalities include excisional, electro or cryo surgery or radiation.

The incorrect answers are A: SCC is a skin cancer that develops mostly because of exposure to sunlight and other chemical agents; that is, arsenic, coal tar, creosote oil. Exposure to x-rays and gamma rays with resulting SCC is experimentally and epidemiologally evident. Treatment of SCC includes electro, chemo and excision surgery. Radiation therapy may be used where surgical excision may be cosmetically objectionable. B: Primary cutaneous malignant melanoma is the leading fatal illness arising in the skin with an expected increase of incidence every year. It is a highly visible tumor and occurs principally during the productive years except for the lentigo maligna melanoma, which is predominantly seen in the elderly. Sun exposure has been implicated in the etiology of primary melanoma. Recognition of precursor lesions such as lentigo maligna, congenital melanocytic nevi, and the dysplastic nevi and changes in their variegation is crucial for the survival rate to improve. Surgical excision with the margin of these varying according to the depth of the tumor is the definitive therapy. C: Actinic keratosis (AK), a precancerous lesion, presents on sun-exposed areas in almost 100% of the elderly white population. It may also be found on other fair-skinned people from teens and other adults. AK may progress into a SCC without therapy. Treatment may include topical chemotherapy, cryotherapy, curettage and electrodesiccation and surgical excision. D: A keratoacanthoma is a fast growing benign skin tumor believed to arise from the hair follicles. It resembles the SCC during the active growth phase with sunlight, chemical carcinogens, trauma and genetic predelection being factors in this. Forms of therapy include topical or intralesional injections of 5-fluorouracil, curettage, surgical excision, and waiting for spontaneous regression. *(Fitzgerald, pp. 733–743, 747–756, 759–771, 766–772, 947–963)*

5. **(D)** Skin testing in chronic urticaria should be done only if a particular antigen is known to cause the patient's reaction. Uncommon causes include inhalants. The majority of patient's cannot demonstrate a sensitivity to foods while on a double-blind food challenge. Skin biopsies are only indicated in patients who exhibit signs and symptoms of urticarial vasculitis that may include angioedema, macular erythema, palpable purpura within wheals and general features of malaise, fever, myalgias, lymphadenopathy, hepatomegaly and splenomegaly.

The incorrect answers are A, B, C, and E: A thorough history and physical with the evaluation of certain laboratory tests including a CBC with differential, an erythrocyte sedimentation rate, and urinalysis is necessary. The yields of these tests are low, but a finding of eosinophilia may indicate a drug reaction or IgE-medicated allergic disorder, an elevated erythrocyte sedimentation rate may suggest necrotizing vasculitis. Physical examination in

all patients should include a test for physical urticaria such as stroking the skin with a brisk stroke to identify dermatographism, a localized cold or warm stimulus for cold or heat urticaria. Running in place may elicit cholinergic urticaria and a special instrument, usually found with dermatologist's equipment may reproduce solar urticaria. Avoidance of aspirin and other nonsteroidal antiinflammatory drugs, as well as alcohol, excessive heat, and exertion should be prescribed. Antihistamines at low doses should be administered until tolerance increases. Should this fail, an antihistamine of another class, then a combination may be used. A combination of H 1 and 2 may be beneficial in treating some urticarial patients. Systemic corticosteroids are not useful in treating chronic urticaria. Epinephrine should be given only during an acute attack with laryngeal edema symptoms. *(Epstein, pp. 100–102; Fitzpatrick, pp. 1289–1290, 1303)*

6. **(E)** The duration of the secondary lesions in pityriasis rosea (PR) averages 2 to 10 weeks. PR is thought to be caused by an infectious agent but not to be contagious. Structures resembling mycoplasma have been detected on primary plaque. It is regarded as unusual to have recurrent PR. The disease is self-limiting and treatment is symptomatic.

The incorrect answers are A, B, C, and D: Prodromal symptoms of PR such as general malaise, headaches, and gastrointestinal distress appear to occur frequently. The herald patch is the primary lesion in 50% to 90% of cases. It is usually oval or round with fine scaling at the borders and can be found anywhere on the body. The secondary, symmetrical, papulosquamous lesions may appear over the following 7 to 10 days. Most patients will have oval lesions following the skin lines, in particular on the trunk forming the classic "Christmas tree" pattern. These are usually limited from the neck down the trunk, ending at the wrists and midthighs. Pruritus (itching) may range from severe in 25% to moderate in 50% of patients. It appears to be absent in about 25%. Therapy is symptomatic and ultraviolet radiation has shown to be of benefit. *(Epstein, pp. 116–117· Fitzpatrick, pp. 982–990)*

7. **(D)** Penicillin is the drug of choice in the treatment of erysipelas, which is usually a group A streptococcal skin infection. Erysipelas, a superficial cellulitis, most often occurs in infants and older adults. The source is commonly the upper respiratory tract.

The incorrect answers are as follows, A: As many as 40% of group A streptococci may be resistant to the tetracyclines. B: Cephalothin may be substituted in the very ill patient with a questionable penicillin allergy. C: In the case of an immediate type of reaction, the very ill patient may be treated with vancomycin. E: Nafcillin should be used in the patient with a suspected severe staphylococcal infection. *(Fitzpatrick, pp. 2104–2113)*

8. **(E)** The incorrect answers are as follows, A: Because DLE often produces permanent scarring, it is imperative to treat these disfiguring lesions aggressively during the acute inflammatory stage. Topical therapy with potent fluorinated corticosteroid ointments such as betamethasone or fluocinomide are used as primary therapy. Systemic corticosteroids or aminoquinoline antimalarials are not indicated in patients with uncomplicated DLE. Whereas the primary therapy in SCLE will require some form of systemic therapy, that is, aminoquinoline antimalarials to induce and maintain remission, topical treatment has been found to be unsuccessful. B: Scarring lesions confined primarily to the skin on the face and neck are seen in DLE. The lesions in DLE are characterized by thick scaling, erythematous papules and plaques and prominent follicular dilation and hyperkeratosis. Most lesions expand and gradually heal with central scarring and depigmentation. This is in contrast to SCLE lesions characteristically affecting the trunk and upper extremities. Usually, they have easily detachable scales that tend to enlarge and coalesce, but heal without scarring. Diffuse nonscarring alopecia, photosensitivity, excessive fatigue, and joint pain should arouse the clinician's suspicion towards the diagnosis of SCLE. Other differentials, namely, psoriasis, dermatomyositis, or erythema multiforme should also be considered. Skin biopsies may be helpful in the diagnosis. C: Laboratory values in DLE are usually not helpful in contrast to the majority of SCLE patients that show antinuclear antibodies by indirect immunofluorescence testing of their serum. Also, with SCLE antibodies to the Ro/SSA antigen are present in greater than 60%. D: Patients rarely if ever have immune deposits in their clinically normal skin with uncomplicated DLE. Although 40% to 50% of SCLE lesions do not have immune deposits on direct immunofluorescence examination, the absence of this finding cannot exclude this diagnosis. *(Fitzpatrick, pp. 1817–1827; Lynch, pp. 219–220)*

9. **(B)** The brown recluse spider, often called the fiddleback spider because of the violin-shaped figure on its thorax, bites when humans accidentally disturb its habitat. The initial bite is often painless with the wound starting as a small erythematous papule over the first 6 to 12 hours progressing to a blister and/or skin necrosis. The resultant necrotic skin ulcer heals slowly and may require a skin graft. Therapy for the bite remains controversial, with dapsone, antibiotics, corticosteroids, and antihistamines recommended.

The incorrect answers are as follows. A: The gypsy moth (*Lymantria dispar*) a caterpillar species may cause irritation with its histamine-containing hairs. The lesions in this case may appear as grouped vesicles and/or bullae. C: Papules and vesicles are the most common lesions of scabies, but the burrow is the most characteristic and diagnostic feature. D: The black widow spider, also called the "hourglass" spider, has a neurotoxin venom. This produces minimal local reactions. Generalized pain may occur within 1 to 8 hours. Characteristically, the crampy abdominal pain may be associated with pain in the flanks, chest, or confused with acute appendicitis, renal colic, or acute myocardial infarction. Nausea and vomiting accompany most bites. E. Scorpions are of primary medical interest in tropical or desert areas such as the southwestern United States, Mexico, and the Middle East. Their venom induces complex cardiac arrhythmias. It is not known whether the venom's effect on platelets or other venom proteins induce ulcerative skin lesions. *(Fitzpatrick, pp. 2496–2505)*

10. **(B)** Erythema multiforme is an acute, self-limited eruption of the skin and the mucous membranes. The target or iris lesion, the most characteristic feature of this disease, develops abruptly and symmetrically on extensor surfaces as well as on the palms and soles.

The incorrect answers are as follows. A: Erythema marginatum is a specific skin manifestation of rheumatic fever. The lesion may begin as an erythematous papule or blotch, spreading peripherally. Lesions may appear on the trunk and the limbs with some pigmentary changes. C: Eruptions with erythema annulare centrifugum begin as erythematous or urticaria-like papules. These spread to form large rings with central clearing. Etiology appears to be related to underlying disease. D: Erythematous, tender nodules usually on the anterior shins are typical lesions of erythema nodosum. New lesions may be accompanied by fever, chills, and malaise. Numerous etiologies are attributed to this disease. Spontaneous resolution usually occurs. E: The lesions of erythema gyratum repens are rapidly growing scaly, erythematous, concentric bands that may involve the entire body. Underlying malignancy appears to be etiology of this condition. *(Fitzpatrick, pp. 555–556, 1010–1012, 1142–1143, 1859–1860)*

11. **(E)** Food does not appear to be an exacerbating factor with acne vulgaris. However, some patients cling to the belief that their flare-ups are associated with certain foods and, in particular, with the ingestion of chocolate. Although there is no scientific evidence for this, it is better to eliminate those dietary agents in these cases.

The incorrect answers are as follows. A: Various cosmetics have been found to exacerbate acne, in particular thick, greasy ones such as actor's make-up. The use of water-based cosmetic may be of benefit. B: Just as emotional stress can worsen diseases such as hypertension, diabetes, and others, it can exacerbate acne as well. C: Topical corticosteroids, in particular fluorinated, may exacerbate acne and should not, therefore, be used as therapy. Severe acne that does not respond to antibiotics may, however, benefit from such a regimen. D: Repetitive trauma to the skin such as rubbing can exacerbate acne or produce acneiform lesions. Sports equipment, clothing, namely, belts, etc., and excessive scrubbing of the skin are examples. *(Epstein, p. 44–48; Fitzpatrick, pp. 674–678; Lynch, pp. 112–113)*

12. **(B)** The most distinctive feature of herpes zoster is the localization of the rash. Its characteristic rash is nearly always unilateral, does not cross the midline, and is limited in most cases to the area of skin supplied by a single sensory dermatome. The trigeminal nerve, in particular the ophthalmic division, and the trunk (T3–L2) are the most frequently affected. Lesions rarely occur below the elbows or knees. *(Fitzpatrick, p. 2323)*

13. **(E)** Erythema infectiosum, or Fifth disease is a mild, febrile exanthematous disease of viral etiology. There is usually little or no prodrome. It has been determined that the human parvovirus B19 is the causative agent. Fifth disease begins as a low-grade fever, with or without conjunctivitis, upper respiratory infection, itching, and nausea and vomiting. In many cases, this vague early period is followed by a confluent erythema over the cheeks. This rash is the so-called "slapped face" appearance. It is not untypical for signs and symptoms to occur, then abate, only to reappear especially in times of stress. This may happen for a period of weeks. *(Harrison's, pp. 685–686)*

14. **(D)** It has been determined that Coxsackie A16 virus is the causative agent in hand-foot-and-mouth disease. Classically, the rash appears in the mouth after a short prodromal stage. The prodrome consists of low-grade fever and malaise. The most frequent finding is that of ulcerative oral lesions. Initially, they begin as erythematous papules, 2 to 8 mm across. These progress to form gray, thin-walled vessicles surrounded by a zone of erythema. These lesions continue to progress to form shallow yellow to gray ulcerations with an erythematous halo. The cutaneous lesions may occur simultaneously or shortly after the oral lesions. They are characterized by an erythematous papule or macule, 2 to 10 mm across. From the center arises a gray, round vessicle often surrounded by a red areola. Typically, the lesions run parallel to skin lines. *(Fitzpatrick, pp. 2297–2298)*

15. **(C)** *Molluscum contagiosum* virus is a pox virus. *M contagiosum* is a benign viral disease of the mucous membranes and skin. It generally affects children. In adults, it may be transmitted by sexual contact. The lesions are individual, discrete, smooth pearly to fresh colored, dome-shaped papules. Often, these lesions have a central umbilication and a mildly erythematous base. Deep to the ulceration there is an easily expressable, white curd-like core. *(Fitzpatrick, p. 2351)*

16. **(D)** Tinea versicolor is a superficial recurring fungal infection of the stratum corneum. It is caused by pityrosporum orbiculare (*Malassezia furfur*). The fungus is readily identified in 10% KOH preparation. It typically shows a "spaghetti and meatball" appearance when viewed under a microscope. *(Fitzpatrick, pp. 2199–2200)*

17. **(C)** HSV infections may be rapidly diagnosed by obtaining cells from the base of the lesion and making a smear on a glass slide. This slide is then stained with Wright's stain or Giemsa's stain, and examined for multinucleated giant cells. This is a Tzanck preparation. In a number of studies there was only a 60% correlation between culture-documented HSV and the appearance of multinucleated giant cells. This stresses the importance of obtaining a positive culture result in order to confirm the diagnosis. *(Fitzpatrick, p. 2310)*

18. **(A)** Syphilis is a communicable disease caused by *Treponema pallidum*. The diagnosis of primary syphilis may be made by detecting the organism in early lesions. Serum from moist lesions or scrapings of the base of dry lesions when viewed with a dark field microscope may reveal characteristic movements of *T pallidum*. These include corkscrew rotation, a gentle bending like a bamboo pole, and a spiral spring shortening and lengthening. *(Fitzpatrick, p. 2403)*

19. **(B)** Erythrasma is a common superficial bacterial infection of the skin. It is caused by corynebacterium species. It typically involves the skin of the intertriginous areas and is characterized by well-defined but irregular reddish brown patches. Examination under a Wood's lamp shows a characteristic coral-red florescence, and confirms the diagnosis. *(Fitzpatrick, pp. 2179–2120)*

20. **(E)** The mineral oil technique of Muller and colleagues is excellent for isolating the mite that causes scabies. In this technique, a drop of sterile mineral oil is placed on a sterile scalpel blade. The oil is then applied to the surface of a burrow or papule. The burrow or papule is then scraped vigorously to remove the entire top of the papule. Tiny

flecks of blood will appear in the oil and when viewed under the microscope should reveal mites, ova, and/or feces. *(Fitzpatrick, p. 46)*

21. **(C); 22.(E); 23.(B); 24.(A)** Changes in the nails and nailbed can often aid in establishing a diagnosis. In a patient with cirrhosis for example, Terry's nails can often be found. These are nails in which the proximal end of the nail has a white appearance as a result of nailbed changes, although the distal 1 to 2 mm show a normal pink color. This is felt to be related to hypoalbuminemia. Patients with alopecia areata may often experience pitting of their nails. Characteristically, the pits form transverse rows on the nail plate surface. In severe hair loss disorders, namely, alopecia totalis, the entire surface of the nail may be involved. Koilonychia or spoon nail may be found in normal individuals, but may occur following trauma (especially chronic trauma) to the proximal nail fold. It also may be present in iron deficiency anemia. In addition to being spoon shaped, the nail may be soft. Beau's lines or transverse depressions in the nails may be seen in association with toxemia from hyperthyroidism. *(Fitzpatrick, pp. 656–658)*

25. **(A)** A large-dose, short-term regimen of systemic corticosteroids, that is, 60 to 100 mg daily tapered over 2 to 3 weeks should be used for severe rhus dermatitis mainly to suppress development of further lesions. Anecdotal experiences have also shown "rebound effects" such as a recurrence of the rash with low and short systemic therapy. Topical fluorinated steroids may be of benefit in patients with minimal cutaneous reaction but is not effective during the blistering stage.

The incorrect answer is B: Desensitization to urushiol (the oil contained in the leaves of the plant) to increase tolerance has not been very successful. *(Epstein, pp. 119–121; Fitzpatrick, pp. 1381–1382)*

26. **(D)** Neither surgery nor chemotherapy are considered curative with Kaposi's sarcaoma. Although tumors may initially respond to therapy, the relapse rate is very disappointing; in particular with AIDS patients, it is almost 100%. Most clinicians agree treatment must be directed at the immunorestoration. *(Fitzpatrick, pp. 1083–1085)*

27. **(B)** Dermatophytid reactions are secondary, inflammatory responses of the skin at a side distant from the associated fungal infection. "Id" lesions are culture and KOH negative. It is suspected that the id response may involve a local immunologic reaction to systemically absorbed fungal antigens. Once the dermatophyte infection is treated, the dermatophytid disappears.

The incorrect answer is A: Many factors are proposed as etiologic agents. The pathogenic role of bacteria has not been substantiated. Frequently, dry skin is associated with it, in particular during the winter months. This does not exclude exacerbation in the summer months. Frequent bathing, some topical medication, substances such as wool or soaps, and nutritional factors have been suggested as the cause without supporting evidence in nummular dermatitis. *(Fitzpatrick, pp. 1370–1371, 1409, 2201)*

28. **(E)** 1, 2, 3, and 4. TEN is a severe reaction of the skin to multiple etiologies. Some of the precipitating factors are viral, bacterial, and/or fungal infections, neoplastic disease, idiopathic, and drug allergies, which are the most frequent. Some of the most common ones are nonsteroidal inflammatories, antibiotics, phenolphthalein, barbiturates, and many others. Onset of TEN is acute with symptoms of skin tenderness, malaise, and fever preceding a morbilliform rash concentrated on the face and extremeties, within a few hours to a couple of days. The lesions may vesiculate before the rash becomes confluent. These vesicles become large, flaccid bullae that rupture easily and result in denuded areas. Mucous membranes such as the lips, mouth, eyes, and genital areas, are usually severely involved. Among other complications are high fever, leukocytosis, electrolyte imbalance, pulmonary edema, and renal failure. Therapy consists of high doses of corticosteroids, fluid, and electrolyte therapy and proper eye and skin care. The disease carries a greater than 30% mortality. *(Fitzpatrick pp. 566, 1360–1361; Lynch p. 101)*

29. **(B)** 1. 86% of uremic patients present with generalized pruritus. Because they are frequently on multiple medications, a drug reaction with generalized pruritus is not uncommon. Xerosis (dry skin) also contributes to pruritus and is usually relieved by topical emollients. 3. Kyrle's disease, hyperkeratosis follicularis et parafollicularis in cutem penetrans, presents clinically with often pruritic papules and nodules with a central keratin plug. Topical tretinoin therapy may flatten the lesions and decrease pruritus.

The incorrect answers are the following. 2: Muehrcke's lines are paired, white, parallel bands observed in patients with hypoalbuminemia. 4. Lichen planus lesions are tiny flat-topped, polygonal papules with central umbilication and semitransparent scales known as Wickham's striae. Lichen planus-like dermatosis may develop as a result of drug therapy, namely, antimalarials. Treatment of lichen planus is complex. Systemic corticosteriods alleviates symptoms in most cases. *(Fitzpatrick, pp. 658, 969–973, 1977–1979)*

30. **(A: 1, 2, and 3.)** Tender, erythematous subcutaneous nodules, usually located on the anterior shins in erythema nodusum, are most frequently caused by the use of oral contraceptives. Hypersensitivity to drugs other than bromides, sulfonamides, halogens, tetracycline, penicillin, and 13-cisretinoic acid.

The incorrect answer is 4: In severe or recurrent cases nonsteroidal antiinflammatory drugs such as acetylsalic acid, indomethacin, or naproxen are commonly used as therapy. Systemic steroids are necessary for the more severe cases only. *(Fitzpatrick, pp. 1360–1361)*

31. (E) 1. Dermatitis herpetiformis is associated with intestinal lymphoma. Cutaneous lesions are pruritic grouped papules, vesicles, and crusts, in a symmetric distribution most commonly on the elbows, knees, buttocks, and the shoulders. 2. Sweet's syndrome consists of painful, red, raised plaques and nodules mostly on the face and extremities. It is most commonly associated with leukemia. 3. The most common cause of idiopathic thrombocytopenic purpura (ITP) is lymphoma. The diagnosis of ITP may precede the most common associated lymphoma, Hodgkin's disease. Purpura may also be seen secondary to bone marrow infiltration by leukemia or carcinoma. 4. Leukocytoclastic vasculitis can be a presenting sign in squamous cell carcinoma of the bronchus and malignant lymphoma. *(Fitzpatrick, pp. 1918–1920, 1927)*

32. (B) 1. Mongolian spots are congenital and usually disappear, depending on the size, within a few years. Mongolian spots may persist into adulthood, with a 3% to 4% incidence in the Japanese. 3. Mongolian spots are congenital and almost always located in the lumbosacral area and on the buttocks. When seen on the face it may be confused with the nevus of Ota. One point of difference in the pigmentation of the mongolian spot is a blue–black macule of varying sizes, whereas the nevus of Ota has a characteristic mottling with blue and brown spots. The nevus of Ota is not congenital and may persist through life. Laser therapy offers hope to decrease the color intensity with both.

The incorrect answers are C: 2. Reference is made to the fact that one patient with mongolian spots on the nose was found to have metastatic melanoma of the liver and lymph nodes. 4. Mongolian spots are observed in more than 90% of the Asiatic and Amerindian races, less frequently in blacks, and in less than 10% of whites. *(Fitzpatrick, pp. 853–856)*

33. (E) 1. Pemphigus vulgaris may present with flaccid bullae commonly involving the scalp, umbilicus, and other parts of the body including the mucous membranes. Delay of diagnosis may be life threatening. 2. EBA, a chronic blistering disease, is characterized by blister formation over joint surfaces. Extensor surfaces of the lower legs and the mucous membranes may also be involved. In general, these bullae are tense. 3. Spontaneous bullae may appear in diabetics usually on the extremities, especially on the feet. In general, the bullae heal without scaring over several weeks. 4. Large tense bullae in bullous pemphigoid are characteristic of this disease. The most common sites include the inner thighs, flexor surfaces of the forearms, axillae, abdomen, and other areas of the body, including the mucous membranes. this disease occurs predominantly in the sixth, seventh, and eighth decades of life. *(Fitzpatrick, pp. 572–573, 580–581, 589, 2075–2076)*

34. (E) 1. During the course of atopic dermatitis there is an increased level of serum IgE. Eosenophilia is commonly associated with exfoliative dermatitis. 2. To establish the diagnosis, a personal or family history of atopic dermatitis should be present. 3. At least 50% of patients with atopic dermatitis develop allergic rhinitis or asthma. Hyperreactivity in the bronches have been described by atopic dermatitis patients even without overt asthma. 4. More than 60% of atopic dermatitis patients have a personal hsitory of geographic tongue. This term describes the process of changing shapes on the surface of the tongue. *(Epstein, pp. 67–68; Fitzpatrick, pp. 1201, 1385, 1390–1393; Lynch, p. 238)*

35. (B) Varicella is an acute, highly contagious disease that occurs most often in childhood, but can occur at any age, worldwide. The average incubation period is 14 or 15 days with the main route of transmission through the respiratory tract. Presenting signs and symptoms may include a prodromal with a generalized pruritic rash following. Characteristic lesions progressing from erythematous macules to papules. Vesicles and crusts at different stages throughout the disease may present. Constitutional symptoms are usually mild in normal children. Varicella may be associated with more extensive skin lesions, high fever, severe malaise, pneumonia and other life-threatening complications in adults, and immunologically compromised patients of any age. Treatment is usually symptomatic. *(Fitzpatrick, pp. 2314–2340; Lynch, p. 84)*

36. (A) 1. Rubella (German measles) is a common viral infection in children and young adults. The rash appears first on the face, then generalizes with discrete erythematous macules and papules clearing within 2 to 4 days, followed by fine desquamation. This is in contrast to rubeola, which persists. 2. Rubeola (measles) is also a highly contagious viral disease in children. Three distinct phases are present in measles: (1) an asymptomatic incubation period of about 10 to 12 days; (2) prodromal period with fever, chills, malaise, coryza, conjunctivitis, and cough; (3) onset of the rash, erythematous macules and papules starting on the face, then spreading downward. Koplik's spots usually appear in the mouth 24 to 48 hours prior to the rash. The average clinical course is about 10 days. Symptomatic therapy is usual unless complications such as encephalitis warrants antibiotic treatment. 3. Kawasaki, a viral illness, has a list of six criteria to establish the diagnosis. (a) The disease begins with a high fever not responding to antipyretics. The fever must last for at least 5 days to be considered compatible with this disease. At the second stage, fever may fluctuate over the next week or two. Often myringitis and/or diarrhea may follow. A cough may be present as the third manifestation. (b) Conjunctival injection and uveitis may be present in 70% of the children. (c) Fissuring red lips and a hypertrophic tongue, as well as small mucosal ulcerations, may accompany the illness. (d) Palms and soles that turn bright red and peel as the fever declines are the fourth manifestation of Kawasaki. (e) A skin eruption is the fifth manifestation; there are several kinds of eruptions—a red, confluent rash with papules or pustules in the diaper area, a scarlatiniform rash, and a third type presenting with large annular, brownish lesions such as those associated with erythema multiforme. (f) Cervical adenitis is the sixth manifestation. There are many more signs and symptoms then those mentioned, such as abdominal pain and, most troublesome of all, cardio-

vascular disease. No specific form of treatment is available.

The incorrect answer is 4: Scarlet fever presents with a diffuse erythematous eruption, having a sandpaper quality, a sequela of a group A streptocci infection in the pharynx. Desquamation usually occurs within 4 to 6 days lasting several weeks. Other clinical findings include enlarged tonsils, strawberry tongue, and generalized lymphadenopathy. It occurs usually in children, only rarely in adults. Early penicillin therapy prevents development of suppurative and nonsuppurative sequelae. *(Fitzpatrick, pp. 2108–2111, 2289–2290, 2291–2295, 2376–2382)*

REFERENCES

Epstein E. *Common Skin Disorders*, 2nd ed. Oradell, NJ: Medical Economic Company Inc.; 1983.

Fitzpatrick TB, Eisen AZ, Wolff K, Freedburg IM, Austen KF. *Dermatology in General Medicine*, 3rd ed. New York: McGraw-Hill; 1987.

Isselbacher KJ, Adams RD, Braunwald E, Petersdorf RG, Wilson JD, eds. *Harrison's Principles of Internal Medicine*, 11th ed. New York: McGraw-Hill; 1987.

Lynch PJ. *Dermatology for the House Officer*, 2nd ed. Baltimore, MD: Wilkins; 1987.

Subspecialty List: Dermatology

Question Number and Subspecialty

1. Skin lesions—elevated
2. Scaly feet—differential
3. Papulosquamous lesions—differential
4. Skin cancer—frequency
5. Chronic urticaria—treatment
6. Pityriasis rosea—characteristics
7. Erysipelas—treatment
8. Lupus erythematosus—discoid vs. systemic
9. Insect bites—characteristics
10. Erythema multiforme—characteristics
11. Acne vulgaris—exacerbating factors
12. Herpes zoster—characteristics
13. *Erythema contagiosum*—characteristics
14. Coxsackie-characteristics
15. *Molluscum contagiosum*—characteristics
16. Tinea veriscolor—laboratory evaluation
17. Herpes simplex—laborabory evaluation
18. Syphilis—laboratory evaluation
19. Erythrasma—laboratory evaluation
20. Scabies—laboratory evaluation
21. Cirrhosis—nail characteristics
22. Alopecia areata—nail characteristics
23. Iron deficiency—nail characteristics
24. Hyperthyroidism—nail characteristics
25. Rhus dermatitis (poison ivy/oak)—treatment
26. Kaposi's sarcoma—treatment
27. Eczematous dermatitis—characteristics
28. Toxic epidermal necrolysis—characteristics
29. Renal insufficiency—cutaneous changes
30. Erythema nodosum—causes
31. Malignancy—skin changes
32. Mongolian spots—characteristics
33. Bullae—differential diagnosis
34. Atopic dermatitis—characteristics
35. Varicella—characteristics
36. Viral disease in children—characteristics

Internal Medicine: Renal

Robert Howell

Questions

DIRECTIONS (Questions 1 through 3): Each group of items in this section consists of lettered headings followed by a set of numbered words or phrases. For each numbered word or phrase, select the ONE lettered heading that is most closely associated with it. Each lettered heading may be selected once, more than once, or not at all.

1. excretion via nephrons

2. would not be obtained by increasing plasma oncotic pressure

3. active transport and oncotic pressure in the peritubular capillaries

(A) urea, creatinine, and BUN
(B) edema
(C) enhanced proximal tubular reabsorption
(D) distal convuluted tubule

DIRECTIONS (Questions 4 and 5): Each of the numbered items or incomplete statements in this section is followed by answers or by completions of the statement. Select the ONE lettered answer or completion that is BEST in each case.

4. Which of the following areas compose most of the renal mass?

(A) cortex and medulla
(B) renal pyramids and nephrons
(C) renal pelvis and capillary network
(D) medullary rays and glomeruli
(E) renal pelvis and nephrons

5. The glomerulus includes all below EXCEPT

(A) a capillary network lined with endothelial cells
(B) a central region of mesongial cells
(C) the visceral layer of Bowman's epithelium
(D) the parietal layer of Bowman's capsule
(E) cells of the dense convoluted tubule

DIRECTIONS (Questions 6 through 26): For each of the items in this section, ONE or MORE of the numbered options is correct. Choose the answer

A if only 1, 2, and 3 are correct,
B if only 1 and 3 are correct,
C if only 2 and 4 are correct,
D if only 4 is correct,
E if all are correct.

6. The thick ascending limb of the loop of Henle absorbs sodium chloride rapidly and causes

(1) a decreased osmolality and tubular fluid concentration of sodium chloride to drop to 30 mmol/L
(2) the voltage across the lumen to become positive
(3) the tubular fluid to become dilute
(4) concentration of fluid in the distal loop when it passes through this region

7. The concentration of urine depends largely on

(1) the loop of Henle
(2) large osmotic pressure gradient between the papilla and cortex
(3) the countercurrent system
(4) nephrons

8. Renal prostaglandins

(1) promote water excretion
(2) increase the effect of arginine vasopressin
(3) limit the effect of arginine vasopressin
(4) promote water absorption

9. 50% to 70% of body weight is composed of water that is

(1) two thirds intracellular fluid
(2) one third extracellular fluid

(3) regulated by the amount of solvent in each compartment

(4) not dependent on the amount of adipose tissue

10. The formation of urine

(1) helps to maintain volume and composition of body fluids

(2) provides a template for erythropoietin

(3) provides for elimination of metabolic wastes

(4) is inversely proportional to the cardiac output

11. The kidney

(1) is regulated by hormones

(2) manufactures hormones

(3) aids in the conversion of hormones

(4) filters approximately 180 L of extracellular fluid per 24 hours

12. Which has been converted by the kidney to its active form?

(1) parathyroid hormone

(2) antidiuretic hormone

(3) aldosterone

(4) 1.25-dihydroxycholecalciferol

13. Hematuria

(1) is not painful except when there is passage of large clots in the ureter or urethra

(2) occurs in sepsis and other systemic disorders

(3) occurs in acute interstitial nephritis

(4) occurs in cystic and inflammatory disease

14. Benign recurrent hematuria of childhood is associated with

(1) microscopic hematuria

(2) gross hematuria

(3) normal renal imaging and biopsy

(4) progressive disease

15. Occlusive disease of the renal arteries leading to ischemia and renal hypoperfusion are

(1) indicators of prerenal syndrome

(2) associated with hyperreninemia

(3) clinically different

(4) associated with polyuria

16. Forms of hypertension that may be corrected by surgery are

(1) renovascular hypertension

(2) pheochromocytoma

(3) unilateral renal parenchymal disease

(4) primary hyperaldosteronism

17. The **MOST** correct statements concerning intravenous pyelograms (IVP) and arteriography are

(1) IVPs are not a good screening test for suspected renovascular hypertension

(2) IVPs are most accurate in the child and least accurate in the atherosclerotic adult

(3) arteriography is by far the only accurate measure of renal occlusive vascular disease

(4) arteriography allows for single injections

18. Calcium stones compose 75% to 85% of virtually all stones in the United States. These include

(1) uric acid stones

(2) cystine stones

(3) strupite stones

(4) magnesium apatite stones

19. Evaluation of the patient with stones includes

(1) 24-hour urine collection

(2) serum electrolytes

(3) serum and urine calcium and uric acid

(4) serum and urine creatinine

20. In the patient with hyperchloremic acidosis, you will find

(1) decreased serum bicarbonate

(2) sulfate and phosphate excreted normally

(3) increased reabsorption of chloride ions

(4) renal excretion of acid is reduced

21. In adult polycystic kidney disease you would find

(1) cortical and medullary cysts

(2) renal failure as a newborn

(3) hepatic cysts and intracranial aneurysms

(4) reduced bicarbonate absorption

22. The statement/statements most accurately associated with scleroderma (progressive systemic sclerosis) in renal tissue would be

(1) renal failure is associated with 40% to 50% of all deaths

(2) renal involvement is rarely the presenting symptom

(3) closely resembles accelerated nephrosclerosis

(4) petechial hemorrhages and wedge-shaped cortical infarts

23. The **LEAST** likely symptom associated with acute pyelonephritis would be

(1) nausea and vomiting with fever and chills

(2) leukocytosis

(3) CVA tenderness or pain on deep abdominal palpation

(4) cystitis

24. **WHICH** of the following is associated with systemic lupus erythematosus?

(1) multisystem disease, etiology unknown
(2) involves deposition of circulating immune complexes
(3) hematuria
(4) proteinuria

25. Select the statement or statements that best describe diabetes mellitus and the kidney

(1) lesions include papillary necrosis
(2) associated with progressive renal failure
(3) mild asymptomatic proteinuria
(4) mortality rate lower and ideal candidates for long-term dialysis

26. The normal range of the serum osmolality is 285–295 mOsm/L and is calculated: (1 mOsm glucose = 180 mg/L; 1 mOsm BUN = 28 mg/L)

(1) $2 \, (Na^+ mmol/L) + glucose \, mmol/L + BUN \, mmol/L$

(2) $2 \, (Na^+ mOsm/L) + \dfrac{glucose \, mOsm/L}{1.8 \, mmol} + \dfrac{BUN \, mOsm/L}{28 \, mmol}$

(3) $2 \, (Na^+ meg/L) + \dfrac{glucose \, mg/dL}{1.8} + \dfrac{BUN \, mg/dL}{2.8}$

(4) $2(Na^+ meg/L) + glucose \, meg/L + BUN \, meg/L$

Answers and Explanations

1. **(A)** Nephrons in the kidney are chiefly responsible for the excretion of waste products in our blood. These waste products include urea, creatinine, and blood urea nitrogen (BUN). These products develop from the breakdown of proteins and high-energy molecules. Potassium is an electrolyte that easily passes through the membrane of the nephron and is not considered waste. *(Hruska, pp. 728–736)*

2. **(B)** Plasma oncotic pressure is measured within the intravascular space of each vessel. The oncotic pressure is dependant upon total amount of the solute and type. Intracellular fluids move from a region of low concentration of solute to higher concentrations. Therefore, as we increase the oncotic pressure, these fluids move into the intravascular space, limiting formation of edema. *(Hruska, pp. 728–736)*

3. **(C)** Active transport is energy-assisted movement across the cell membrane. In this case, it is across the wall of the nephron. Oncotic pressure, as discussed in Answer 2, moves fluids into the lumen of the vessel or nephron. Therefore, active transport combined with increasing oncotic pressure, provides for enhanced proximal tubular reabsorption in the nephron. This is achieved by removing fluid from efferent and afferent arterioles that encircle the proximal tubule. *(Hruska pp. 728–736)*

4. **(A)** Morphologically, the kidney can be viewed as having a renal pelvis where blood vessels and ureters arise. The small renal pelvis leads into the renal medulla. The medulla is surrounded by the more superficial renal cortex. Part of the medulla and cortex is composed of the many different sizes of nephrons. The medulla and cortex make up most of the renal mass. The loop of Henle and collecting tubules transverse the medulla. The proximal and distal tubules are in the cortex. *(Hruska, p. 728)*

5. **(E)** The glomerulus is a tuft of capillaries surrounded by Bowman's capsule, the principal filtering constituent of the nephron. The glomerulus does not contain cells of the dense, convoluted tubule. The glomerulus is composed of a capillary network lined with endothelial cells. It also has a central region of mesangial cells. It forms the visceral layer

6. **(E)** The loop of Henle lies between the proximal and distal convoluted tubules. The thick ascending limb rises toward the collecting ducts that later form the ureters. This limb of the loop absorbs sodium chloride, quickly causes a decreased serum osmolality, and the tubular fluid concentration of sodium drops to 30 mmol/L. The voltage across the lumen becomes positive because of the addition of Na^+ and flux of H^+. The tubular fluid becomes dilute due to Na^+ loss. However, the concentration of fluid increased in the distal loop when it passes through this region. *(Hruska pp. 733–734)*

7. **(E)** The ability to concentrate the urine is a primary characteristic of the kidney; it is needed to prevent dehydration. This ability is shared by the nephrons, the sodium countercurrent system, the large osmotic gradient between the papilla and cortex, and the loop of Henle. The chief operative ion in water conservation is sodium (Na^+). *(Hruska, pp. 734–735)*

8. **(B)** Renal prostaglandins act on renal mass to regulate water and salt excretion. The chemical action of prostaglandins is to limit the effect of arginine vasopressin. By limiting arginine vasopressin, vasodilatation is limited and water excretion is promoted. In response to decreased intravascular volume prostaglandins mediate renin release. This is altered in hypertension. *(Hruska, p. 736)*

9. **(A)** Water constitutes 50% to 70% of body weight. Distribution of water is chiefly into two areas of the body, namely, the intracellular and extracellular fluid. The percentage attributed to each region is dependent on the amount of adipose (fat) tissue, which has a certain percentage of water. Two thirds of body water is located in intracellular fluid, and one third in extracellular fluid. Extracellular fluid is further divided into plasma and interstitial por-

tions. The total amount of water is regulated by the amount of solvent in each compartment. *(Coe, p. 737)*

10. **(B)** Chiefly, the formation of urine permits elimination of metabolic wastes and helps to maintain the volume and composition of body fluids. Urine does not act as a template for erythropoietin. The filtrates from the glomerulus enter Bowman's Capsule and pass through the tubullar portion of the nephron; about 1L is excreted as urine and the rest of the 180 L of filtrate is reabsorbed into the body each day. *(Andreoli, p. 502)*

11. **(E)** The kidney filters approximately 180 L of extracellular fluid each day as indicated in Answer 10. Kidney function is, in part, regulated by hormones such as aldosterone, secreted by the adrenal cortex, which partially regulates sodium reabsorption. Antidiuretic hormone is released by the neurohypophysis and causes the renal tubular pores to become extremely permeable to water. Erythropoietin, red blood cell precursor, is formed in the kidney and after transport to bone marrow, actively causes the production of red blood cells. Vitamin D is converted to its active metabolite form, 1,25-dihydroxycholecalciferol, in the kidney along with 24,25-dihychroxycholecalciferol by hydroxylation of 25-hydroxycholecaldiferol. *(Andreoli, pp. 502–503)*

12. **(D)** Parathyroid hormone (PTH) arises in the parathyroid gland. Antidiuretic hormone (ADH) is made in the neurohypophysis and is active once released. Vitamin D (25-hydroxyvitamin D) is converted to its active form in the kidney. Its active metabolite, 1,25-dihydroxycholecalciferol, or another metabolite, 24, 25-dihydroxycholecalciferol, are produced from the hydroxylation of 25-hydroxycholecalciferol. Vitamin D acts with PTH to maintain the level of ionized calcium in extracellular fluid. Vitamin D is best known for enhancing the intestinal absorption of calcium. Aldosterone is secreted in its active form from the adrenal cortex. *(Andreoli, pp. 502–503; Kalhr, p. 518)*

13. **(E)** Hematuria, the presence of blood in the urine, may be occult or gross. It may result from trauma, bleeding disorders, infections, stones, glomerular disease, or neoplasms. It generally denotes structural genitourinary disease. Its relationship to voiding, onset, and red cell morphology may indicate location and type of lesion. It is usually not painful except when large clots are produced. It can also accompany parasite infections, arteriovenous malformations and drug reactions. *(Andreoli, p. 503)*

14. **(A)** Benign recurrent hematuria of childhood is associated with microscopic or gross hematuria. Renal imaging and biopsy is usually normal. It is usually not associated with progessive disease that leads to renal failure. *(Andreoli, p. 503)*

15. **(A)** Occlusive disease of the renal arteries is associated with renal tissue ischemia that may lead to renal infarcts. It is also associated with hypoperfusion. These occlusive disease states are associated with hyperreninemia and are indicators of prerenal syndromes. But the effects of ischemia and hypoperfusion are clinically different and, generally, they are not accompanied by polyuria. *(Andreoli, pp. 503–504)*

16. **(E)** Surgically correctable lesions of hypertension save the patient from a lifetime of antihypertensive therapy. Patient history, physical examination, and diagnostic testing should indicate the surgically correctable cause. Because of the relative frequency of some of these lesions and the lasting benefits of correction, early recognition and treatment is desirable. These lesions include Cushing's syndrome, renovascular hypertension, pheochromocytoma, coarctation of the aorta, primary hyperaldosteronism, and unilateral renal parenchymal disease. *(Foster, pp. 1041–1058)*

17. **(B)** IVPs are not a good screening test for suspected renovascular hypertension. Arteriography is by far the only accurate measure of renal occlusive vascular disease. Arteriography permits multiple injections and projections. IVPs are least accurate in the child are most accurate in the atherosclerotic adult. *(Foster, p. 1048)*

18. **(A)** In the United States, the four principally identified stones are calcium, uric acid, cystine, and struvite. Calcium stones account for 75% to 85% of this group. Magnesium apatite stones are not identified as medically significant. In most cases of calcium stones, urinary calcium excretion exceeds approximately 300 mg per day. Hyperthyroidism, excessive milk intake, excessive vitamin D intake, and renal tubular acidosis cause this rise. *(Coe, p. 1211)*

19. **(E)** Evaluation of the patient with stones includes obtaining stones for analysis, evaluation of the urine, acid, and creatinine. It is important to do a complete history and physical examination. Laboratory findings, x-ray, and imaging are also important diagnostic tools. *(Coe, p. 1213)*

20. **(E)** Hyperchloremic acidosis results from impared renal excretion of acid and decreased serum bicarbonate. Sulfate and phosphate are excreted normally and increased reabsorption of chloride ions is also found. This form of metabolic acidosis is due to renal insufficiency and results in an increase in the normal ion gap. *(Coe, p. 1208)*

21. (B) Cortical and medullary cysts are found in adult polycystic kidney disease. Additionally, hepatic and intracranial aneurysms ("berry") are found during work-up. It is an autosomal dominant disease that also can involve the pancreas. Uremia develops slowly and these patients generally live longer than those with other causes of renal insufficiency. (Coe, p. 1206)

22. (E) Scleroderma (progressive systemic sclerosis) is associated with 40% to 50% of all death resulting from renal failure. It closely resembles accelerated nephrosclerosis, usually appears in the third to fifth decade, and renal involvement is rarely the presenting symptom. It is a multiorgan disease that also attacks the heart, lungs, colon, jejunum, and ileum. Dysphagia occurs in 90% of patients. There are petechial hemorrhages, wedge-shaped cortical infarcts in the kidney, and diffuse thickening of the skin, with telangiectasia and variable pigmentation. *(Hollenberg, p. 1202)*

23. (D) Acute pyelonephritis is associated with nausea and vomiting, fever, chills, leukocytosis, contravertebral angle tenderness, or paid on deep abdominal palpation. The patient may or may not have cystitis, and can be suffering from headache or malaise. *(Harrison's pp. 1191–1192)*

24. (E) Systemic lupus erythematosis also has multisystem involvement. It is an inflammatory autoimmune disorder, and its etiology remains unclear. There is deposition of immune complexes in capillaries of the attacked organ. Blacks are highly susceptible. The patient complains of fever, weight loss, and anorexia. Some have the "butterfly" rash and alopecia. There is protein uria and hematuria in laboratory finding, and there may be mildly elevated liver function indicated on the liver tests. *(Harrison's, pp. 1183–1184)*

25. (A) Diabetes mellitus and its effect on renal mass may lead to a mild asymptomatic proteinuria or papillary necrosis as well as progressive renal failure. The mortality rate is higher and diabetics are not good long term candidates for dialysis. Diabetic nephropathy, intercapillary glomerulosclerosis (also known as Kimmelstiel-Wilson disease) occurs in about 25% of patients with diabetes. This is characterized by diffuse or discrete nodules that rarely involves every glomerulus. Patients with long-term diabetes are likely to present with intercapillary glomerulosclerosis, arteriolar nephrosclerosis, and pyelonephritis. *(Harrison's, pp. 1187–1188)*

26. (B) The normal range for serum osmolality is 285 to 295 mOsm/L. It is calculated by

$$2(Na^+ \text{ mmol/L}) + \text{glucose mmol/L} + \text{BUN mmol/L}$$
OR

$$2(Na^+ \text{mmol/L}) + \frac{\text{glucose mg/dL}}{18} + \frac{\text{BUN mg/dL}}{2.8}$$

Here, 1 mOsm of glucose = 180 mg/L; 1 mOsm of BUN = 28 mg/L. The serum osmolality is a measure of the number of solute particles present (expressed as osmoles) per kilogram of water. A solution with high osmolality will have more particles and less water than a solution with lower osmolality. *(Andreoli, p. 536)*

REFERENCES

Andreoli TE. Approach to the Patient with Renal Disease. Smith LH, Wyngaarden JB, eds. *Cecil's Textbook of Medicine.* WB Saunders; 1988.

Bikle DD. Vitamin D. In: Smith LH, Wyngaarden JB (eds.) *Cecil's Textbook of Medicine.* WB Saunders; 1988.

Coe, FL. Principles of the renal regulation of fluids and electrolytes. In: De Vita Jr VT, Du Pont HL, Kelley WN, et al, eds. *The Textbook of Internal Medicine.* JB Lippincott; 1989.

Coe FL, Favus MJ. Nephrolithiasis, Peterdorf RG, In: Isselbacker KJ, Braunwald E, Fauci AS, Martin JB, Wilson JD, eds. *Harrison's Principles of Internal Medicine,* 11th ed. New York: McGraw-Hill; 1987

Coe FL, Kathpolia S. Hereditary tubular disorders. In: Isselbacker KJ, Braunwald E. Fauci AS, Martin JB, Wilson JD, eds. *Harrison's Principles of Internal Medicine,* 11th ed. New York: McGraw-Hill; 1987.

Foster JH. Surgically correctible hypertention. Schwartz SI, Shires GT, Spencer FC, et al (eds). *Principles of Surgery,* 5th ed, New York: McGraw-Hill; 1989.

Glassock RJ, Brenner BM. Glomerulopathies associated with multisystem diseases. In: Isselbacker KJ, Braunwald E, Fauci AS, Martin JB, Wilson JD, eds. *Harrison's Principles of Internal Medicine,* 11th ed. New York: McGraw-Hill; 1987.

Hollenberg NK. Vascular injury to the kidney. In: Isselbacker KJ, Braunwald E, Fauci AS, Martin JB, Wilson JD, eds. *Harrison's Principles of Internal Medicine,* 11th ed. New York: McGraw-Hill; 1987.

Hruska KA. Structure and Function of the Kidney. In: De Vita Jr VT, Dupont HL, Kelley NN, et al, eds. *The Textbook of Internal Medicine.* JB Lippincott; 1989.

Kalhr, S. Structure and Function of the Kidney. In Smith LH, Wyngaarden JR, eds. *Cecil's Textbook of Medicine.* Philadelphia, PA: WB Saunders, 1988.

Krupp MA. Fluid and electrolyte disorders. In: Krupp MA, Schroeder SA, Tierney Jr LM, eds. *Current Medical Diagnosis and Treatment.* Norwalk, CT: Appleton & Lange; 1989.

Stamm WE, Turck M. Urinary tract infection, pyelonephritis, and related conditions. In: Isselbacker KJ, Braunwald E, Fauci AS, Martin JB, Wilson JD, eds. *Harrison's Principles of Internal Medicine,* 11th ed. New York: McGraw-Hill; 1987.

Subspecialty List: Renal Medicine

Questions and Subspecialty
1. Physiology
2. Physiology
3. Physiology
4. Anatomy
5. Anatomy
6. Physiology
7. Physiology
8. Physiology
9. Physiology
10. Physiology
11. Physiology
12. Physiology
13. Hematuria—characteristics
14. Hematuria—benign type in childhood
15. Renal artery disease—characteristics
16. Hypertension—surgically correctable
17. Intravenous pyelograms and arteriography—comparison
18. Urinary calculi
19. Urinary calculi—laboratory evaluation
20. Hyperchloremic acidosis—characteristics
21. Polycystic kidney disease
22. Renal scleroderma
23. Acute pyelonephritis—findings
24. Systemic lupus erythematosus—characteristics
25. Diabetes mellitus—effect on kidney
26. Serum osmolality—calculation

Internal Medicine: Pulmonary

Ricky D. Miller , William Reynolds

Questions

DIRECTIONS (Questions 1 through 5): Each group of items in this section consists of lettered headings followed by a set of numbered words or phrases. For each numbered word or phrase, select the ONE lettered heading that is most closely associated with it. Each lettered heading may be selected once, more than once, or not at all.

Select the most probable initial presentation of symptoms for the pneumonias listed below.

(A) 50-year-old black male developed cough productive of yellow sputum, a single shaking chill, temperature of 103°F. Examination revealed rales at the right base. Chest x-ray shows a right lower lobe infiltrate.

(B) 35-year-old white female presents with a 2-day history of fever up to 100°F, headache, and malaise followed by a frequent harsh cough productive of scant sputum. On examination, you notice left bullous myringitis, minimal scattered rhonchi, and chest x-ray reveals moderate diffuse infiltrates.

(C) 45-year-old oriental alcoholic thin female presents with sudden onset of severe chills, fever, SOB, and cough productive of red mucoid sticky sputum. Patient appears toxic and cyanotic. Vital signs: temperature:102°F, respiration:28, pulse:120, blood pressure:90/62. You appreciate minimal rales and dullness in the right upper lobe with decreased breath sounds. Chest x-ray reveals right upper lobe consolidated with bulging fissure.

(D) Ill-appearing 25-year-old white male presents with dyspnea, nonproductive cough. Vital signs; temperature:103.5°F, respiration:38, pulse:140, blood pressure:100/60. Physical exam reveals a thin, dyspneic male with scattered mild rhonchi and peripherial cyanosis. Chest x-ray reveals diffuse interstial pnuemonia.

(E) A 35-year-old male returns from a vacation at the beach with anorexia, malaise, and a minimal cough that is nonproductive. The patient's wife states that he has a continuous fever of 103.7°F. Vital signs: temperature:103.8°F, respiration:22, pulse:55, blood pressure:110/84. Exam reveals slightly dry oral membranes, rales over the right base with sharp stabbing pain upon inspiration. Chest x-ray shows a right lower lobe pneumonia.

(1) Legionnares' disease
(2) pneumococcal pneumonia
(3) Klebsiella pneumonia
(4) *Pneumocystis carinii* pneumonia
(5) mycoplasmal pneumonia

DIRECTIONS (Questions 6 through 30): Each of the numbered items or incomplete statements in this section is followed by answers or by completions of the statement. Select the ONE lettered answer or completion that is BEST in each case.

6. A 50-year-old male presents with a history of persistant cough, hemoptysis, and weight loss, and states he has had "several lung infections" over the past 3 to 4 months. The patient is a 30 pack-year smoker and also complains of right shoulder and chest pain. The patient is afebrile, pale, and dyspneic with exertion. The chest x-ray suggests mediastinial widening and perihilar adenopathy.

Which of the following diagnosis is most consistent with the given history?

(A) bronchiectasis
(B) chronic obstructive pulmonary disease
(C) chronic bronchitis
(D) asthma
(E) bronchogenic carcinoma

7. A patient presents with a history of dyspnea on exertion and chronic cough worse with arising in the mornings. During exam you notice decreased breath sounds, increased anterior–posterior diameter and increased expiratory phase during respiration. The patient is a 42 pack-year smoker. On chest x-ray, hyperinflation of the lungs is noted with flattened diaphrams. Arterial blood gases reveal PaO_2: 68, $PaCO_2$: 40. The FeV1 and vital capacity are less than predicted values.

    Which is the most likely diagnosis?

    (A) emphysema
    (B) pneumonia
    (C) congestive heart failure
    (D) chronic bronchitis
    (E) bronchogenic carcinoma

8. In the above patient, which of the following would improve pulmonary function and longevity?

    (A) Oxygen at 2 L per minute by nasal cannula
    (B) aminophyllin intravenously; loading dose followed by oral theophyllin
    (C) antibiotics for suppressive therapy
    (D) exercise reconditioning
    (E) none of the above

9. Which of the following tests is least helpful in the diagnosis of bronchogenic carcinoma?

    (A) sputum cytology
    (B) bronchoscopy and biopsy
    (C) ventilation–perfusion scan
    (D) pulmonary function test
    (E) CAT scan

10. Which of the following is the best screening exam for carcinoma of the lung?

    (A) CAT scan
    (B) bronchoscopy
    (C) sputum cytology
    (D) chest x-ray with previous comparison
    (E) arterial blood gases

11. Which of the following is the most common cause for chronic obstructive pulmonary disease?

    (A) air pollution
    (B) recurrent infection
    (C) smoking
    (D) asthma
    (E) trauma

12. Which of the following is in the correct order for frequency of occurrence in bronchogenic carcinoma, starting with the most frequent and progressing to the least frequent cell type?

    (A) adenocarcinoma, small cell anaplastic carcinoma, large cell carcinoma, epidermoid carcinoma.
    (B) epidermoid carcinoma, adenocarcinoma, large cell carcinoma, small cell anaplastic carcinoma.
    (C) small cell anaplastic carcinoma, large cell carcinoma, epidermoid carcinoma, adenocarcinoma.
    (D) small cell anaplastic carcinoma, adenocarcinoma, large cell carcinoma, epidermoid carcinoma.
    (E) large cell carcinoma, small cell carcinoma, adenocarcinoma, epidermoid carcinoma.

13. A 19-year-old female is involved in an automobile accident; she is hospitalized with a fractured femur; her past medical history is unremarkable. The patient suddenly develops dyspnea, cough, and anxiety with retrosternal lateralized chest pain. Vital signs are pulse:120, respiration:32, blood pressure:120/80, temperature:100.1°F. Chest x-ray shows mild bilateral atelectasis and the EKG is normal. The most likely diagnosis is which of the following?

    (A) pneumonia
    (B) myocardial infarction
    (C) pulmonary embolism
    (D) costochondritis with hyperventilation
    (E) unrecognized pneumothorax

14. The most common cause of hemoptysis is which of the following?

    (A) tuberculosis
    (B) trauma
    (C) bronchogenic carcinoma
    (D) bronchitis
    (E) pulmonary embolism

15. Deep regular respirations with periods of apnea best describe which of the following?

    (A) Cheyne–Stokes respiration
    (B) Biots breathing
    (C) Kussmaul respiration
    (D) stridulous breathing
    (E) apnea

16. A 21-year-old thin male presents to your office with a sudden onset of vague chest pain radiating to the left shoulder, dyspnea, and cough. He states that his past medical history is unremarkable except for smoking. The onset of the above symptoms occurred while playing basketball. Vital signs are unremarkable except for a pulse of 110 and a respiratory rate of 28. You note decreased breath sounds, hyperresonance, and decreased vocal fremitus on the left thorax. At this time which of the following appears to be the most likely diagnosis?

(A) mycoplasmal pneumonia
(B) work-induced asthma
(C) spontaneous pneumothorax
(D) bronchial carcinoma
(E) aortic stenosis with angina

17. During your examination of the above patient the x-ray returns to reveal air in the pleural space with visable retracted lung border, there is no pleural effusion. Treatment should consist of which of the following?

(A) nitroglycerine IV
(B) epinephrine subcutaneously
(C) further investigation with a CAT scan of the chest
(D) aspiration of the air with a large needle or chest tube
(E) endotracheal intubation

18. The most sensitive test for the diagnosis of a pulmonary embolism is which of the following?

(A) CAT scan of the chest
(B) EKG
(C) arterial blood gases
(D) ventilation–perfusion scan
(E) chest x-ray

19. A 22-year-old female presents to the Emergency Department with extreme shortness of breath after jogging. No past medical history is immediately available. Vital signs are pulse:120, respiration:32, temperature:98.7°F, blood pressure:130/84. Exam reveals a lethargic and confused patient; there are diffuse expiratory wheezes and a prolonged expiratory phase. Hyperresonance to percussion is noted. Which is the most likely diagnosis?

(A) pneumothorax
(B) bronchial asthma
(C) bronchiolitis
(D) pulmonary edema
(E) pneumonia

20. Site of insertion for a thoracentesis is determined by which of the following?

(A) ultrasound, chest x-ray, enter on the superior margin of the rib
(B) percussion, chest x-ray, enter on the inferior margin of the rib
(C) percussion, ultrasound, enter on the inferior margin of the rib
(D) percussion, chest x-ray, enter on the superior margin of the rib.
(E) ultrasound, chest x-ray, enter on the inferior margin of the rib.

21. Which of the following factors may precipitate an asthma attack?

(A) anxiety
(B) air pollution
(C) exercise
(D) beta-adrenergic blocking agents
(E) all of the above

22. Which agent provides the most rapid effect and best therapeutic index in the treatment of asthma?

(A) inhaled beta-adrenergic agonist medication
(B) subcutaneous epinephrine
(C) intravenous aminophyllin
(D) hydrocortisone
(E) oral aminophyllin

23. A 13-year-old male presents with a 5-day history of a nonproductive cough, slight midchest pain worse with coughing. The patient has been eating well and has noted only a low-grade fever. Physical exam reveals mild diffuse rhonchi during expiration and the chest x-ray is normal. The CBC is also normal. Based on this history and physical examination, the most likely diagnosis is which of the following?

(A) pneumonia
(B) spontaneous pneumothorax
(C) asthma
(D) bronchitis
(E) cystic fibrosis

24. The treatment of the above patient would NOT include which of the following?

(A) postural drainage
(B) cough suppressant
(C) antibiotic
(D) avoidance of inhaled irritants
(E) increase in fluid intake

25. Of the following which is the best of all clinical respiratory measurements for assessing the progress of different types of pulmonary fibrotic diseases?

(A) arterial blood gases
(B) vital capacity
(C) inspiratory reserve volume
(D) total lung capacity
(E) tidal volume

26. A child is brought to your office with high fever, difficulty swallowing, and drooling over the past several hours. On exam you notice an ill-appearing child with inspiratory stridor, breath sounds that are equal bilaterally, and symmetrical chest movement. Which of the following is the most likely diagnosis?

    (A) epiglottitis
    (B) bacterial pharyngitis
    (C) viral croup
    (D) foreign body aspiration
    (E) pneumonia

27. Of the following which would be the best and safest way to approach the above child?

    (A) direct visualization of the pharynx with a tongue blade
    (B) obtain a lateral soft tissue x-ray prior to exam
    (C) direct visualization with the aid of a laryngoscope
    (D) obtain a bronchoscopy as soon as possible
    (E) obtain a rapid strep screen by blindly swabbing the oropharynx

28. A 2-year-old patient is brought to the Emergency Department by his mother with sudden onset of choking, gagging, coughing, and wheezing. The patient was last seen playing on the floor with several small toys. Vital signs are respiration:28, pulse: 120, temperature:98.6°F. Exam reveals decreased breath sounds over the right lower lobe with inspiratory rhonchi and a localized expiratory wheeze. Chest x-ray shows normal inspiratory views but expiratory views show localized hyperinflation with mediastinal shift to the left. Which of the following is the most likely diagnosis?

    (A) viral croup
    (B) subglottic tumor
    (C) foreign body aspiration
    (D) epiglottitis
    (E) asthmatic bronchitis

29. In the above patient, which of the following would be the correct way to progress in the treatment in this case?

    (A) chest physiotherapy
    (B) cool-mist therapy with racemic epinephrine
    (C) bronchoscopy as soon as possible
    (D) intubation as soon as possible
    (E) start antibiotics with antitussives

30. A 28-year-old female presents with sudden onset of shortness of breath, circumoral and carpopedal dysesthesia (tingling sensation), and carpopedal spasm. She complains of vague chest pain. Review of systems is unremarkable except for recent in-

crease in stress at work. Vital signs are respiration:32, pulse:82, blood pressure:110/70, temperature:98.6°F. EKG is normal. Exam reveals tachypnea, although the patient's breath sounds are normal, and the exam is otherwise normal. Which of the following is the most likely diagnosis?

    (A) pneumonia
    (B) primary pulmonary hypertension
    (C) asthma
    (D) hyperventilation
    (E) myocardial infarction

DIRECTIONS (Questions 31 through 50): For each of the items in this section, ONE or MORE of the numbered options is correct. Choose the answer

    A if only 1, 2, and 3 are correct,
    B if only 1 and 3 are correct,
    C if only 2 and 4 are correct,
    D if only 4 is correct,
    E if all are correct.

31. The most commonly encountered endocrine syndromes found in lung cancer are

    (1) inappropriate antidiuretic hormone secretion
    (2) Cushing's syndrome
    (3) gynecomastia
    (4) hypothyroidism

32. Which of the following tests are best used to differentiate between restrictive and obstructive pulmonary disease?

    (1) total lung capacity
    (2) ventilation–perfusion scanning
    (3) forced expiratory volume in 1 second divided by the forced vital capacity
    (4) chest x-ray

33. Which of the following are physical findings consistent with a consolidated pneumonia?

    (1) rales
    (2) increased vocal fremitus
    (3) dullness with percussion
    (4) decreased whispered pectoriloquy

34. Treatment for a patient found to have a pulmonary embolism should include which of the following?

    (1) aggressive fluid therapy
    (2) oxygen therapy
    (3) antibiotic treatment
    (4) heparin therapy

35. Which of the following might indicate that a trial of corticosteriods would be worthwhile in a patient with chronic obstructive pulmonary disease (COPD)?

(1) improved forced expiratory volume after 1 second GREATER than 20% after inhalation of a bronchodilator.
(2) A history of fluctuation in the severity of pulmonary symptoms.
(3) The finding of a prominent wheeze or "noisy" chest on physical examination.
(4) finding of eosinophilia of the blood or sputum on microscopic examination.

36. Which of the following clinical manifestations would you NOT expect to find in a patient with primary pulmonary hypertension?

(1) dyspnea
(2) chest pain resembling angina
(3) hoarseness
(4) clubbing

37. Which of the following could be used to determine if there is partial airway obstruction above or below the tracheal bifurcation?

(1) stridor
(2) pulmonary function tests
(3) chest x-ray
(4) ventilation—perfusion scanning

38. Initial treatment of COPD should include

(1) bronchodilators
(2) elimination of smoking
(3) instruction on bronchial hygiene
(4) corticosteroids

39. Finding consistent with a severe bronchial asthma attack would include which of the following?

(1) chest silent to auscultation
(2) PaCO$_2$ < 35 mm Hg normal (35 to 45)
(3) PaCO$_2$ > 45 mm Hg normal (35 to 45)
(4) Loud generalized wheezes to auscultation

40. A 60-year-old male presents to your office with a history of asthma, new onset hypertension, and angina. The patient notes no change in his stable angina pattern. On exam you notice moderate expiratory wheezes and the patient states he has noted worsening of his asthma over the past week. There are no rales, jugular venous distention, or pedal edema noted on exam. His medications include Theodur (theophylline), 200 mg bid; Ventolin (albuterol) inhaler, 2 puffs qid; nitroglycerine patch, 10 cm^2 applied daily; and Inderal (propanolol), 40 mg bid recently added for control of hypertension. Vital signs are blood pressure: 160/100, pulse: 52, respi-

ration: +30; the patient is afebrile. Appropriate management of this patient should include which of the following?

(1) epinephrine, 0.3 mL of 1:1000 solution subcutaneously
(2) obtain a theophyllin level
(3) increase propanolol for better control of hypertension
(4) discontinue propanolol and start a calcium channel blocking agent

41. A 54-year-old male is brought to the Emergency Room by ambulance after a fall from 10 feet. The patient presents in acute respiratory distress. Vital signs are pulse: 110, blood pressure: 94/60, respiration: 38. Exam reveals marked decrease in breath sounds on the right, with dullness. Stat portable chest x-ray reveals a large air–fluid level on the right. Initial treatment of this patient should include which of the following?

(1) establish two large-bore IVs with lactated Ringer's solution
(2) obtain blood for a CBC and type and crossmatching for possible blood transfusion
(3) placement of a right-sided chest tube
(4) perform an immediate thorocotomy in the Emergency Department

42. Which of the following will deliver oxygen in a concentration of 40% or above?

(1) face mask with oxygen reservoir
(2) nasal cannula at 2 L/min
(3) face mask without oxygen reservoir at 10 L/min
(4) mouth-to-mouth ventilation

43. Respiration is stimulated by which of the following?

(1) arterial PH
(2) exercise
(3) arterial PCO$_2$
(4) arterial PO$_2$

44. While rotating through the neonatal intensive care, a term neonate is admitted to the unit after resuscitation with the diagnosis of meconium aspiration. Which of the following should be initiated in the management of this child?

(1) chest physiotherapy and suctioning of the oropharynx
(2) transcutaneous monitoring of the PO$_2$
(3) chest x-ray
(4) fluid restriction

45. Which of the following are risk factors for the development of hyaline membrane disease?

(1) female sex of child
(2) prematurity
(3) vaginal delivery
(4) maternal diabetes

46. The initial evaluation of hemoptysis should include which of the following?

(1) Gram stain of sputum
(2) apply a tuberculin skin test
(3) chest x-ray
(4) immediate bronchoscopy

47. A thoracentesis is performed on a patient with a pleural effusion on chest x-ray. The fluid obtained is cloudy with a protein greater than 3.5 g/dL and a specific gravity of 1.020. The differential diagnosis for this patient would include which of the following?

(1) bacterial infection
(2) severe anemia
(3) rheumatoid arthritis
(4) liver disease

48. Which of the following statements are true concerning a pulmonary abscess?

(1) they are frequently caused by aspiration related to altered consciousness
(2) anaerobic bacteria are the primary organism recovered
(3) cultures can reveal multiple bacterial organisms
(4) they are uncommon in edentulous patients

49. Which of the following pneumonias is not likely to be complicated by the formation of a pulmonary abscess?

(1) *Klebsiella pneumoniae*
(2) *Staphylococcus aureus*
(3) *Streptococcus pyogens*
(4) pneumococcal pneumonia

50. Which of the following would you expect in a fresh water near-drowning patient?

(1) hypoxia
(2) pulmonary edema
(3) acidosis
(4) marked electrolyte abnormalities

Answers and Explanations

1. **(E)** Legionella pneumonia (Legionnaires' disease) is rare in children and is responsible for several percent of the adult-acquired pneumonias. It is most commonly seen in summer and fall. The clinical presentation consists of anorexia, malaise, and weakness in 100% of the cases. Usually, a nonproductive, "nontroublesome" cough is noted initially, progressing to a cough productive of watery, often bloody sputum. The temperature curve is continuous (nonspiking), and relative bradycardia occurs in 60% of patients; pleuritic pain is noticed by 33% of patients. Laboratory exam frequently reveals abnormal liver function tests; hyponatremia and hypophosphatemia each occur in 50% of cases. Unilobar infiltrates occur in 66% and multifocal infiltrates occur in 33% of cases. Erythromycin is the drug of choice for treatment. *(Eisenberg and Copass, pp. 203–210)*

2. **(A)** The classical presentation of pneumococcal pneumonia is an abrupt onset characterized by a single shaking chill (80% of patients), a rapidly rising temperature and cough (75% of cases) productive of yellow-green to rusty or bloody sputum. Leukocytosis is typical, sputum Gram stain reveals gram-positive diplococci, often intracellular. X-ray reveals lobar infiltrates. *(Eisenberg and Copass, pp. 203–210)*

3. **(C)** Klebsiella pneumonia usually occurs in patients with underlying conditions such as alcoholism, chronic obstructive airway disease, or diabetes. Primary Klebsiella pneumonia occurs in males 80% to 90% of the time and most are middle-aged or older patients. Approximately 66% of patients have coexistant alcoholism. Typically, the sputum is described as a nonputrid homogeneous thick mixture of blood and mucus, often brick red in color. On exam, the patient appears acutely ill, febrile, dyspneic, and often cyanotic. Lung exam may reveal decreased breath sound with few rales, despite evidence of consolidation on chest x-ray. Bulging fissures and abscess formation occur more frequent in Klebsiella pneumonia than is any other type. *(Beeson et al, pp. 1565–1568)*

4. **(D)** *Pneumocystis carinii* pneumonia is an acute interstitial plasma cell pneumonia, although rare in the general population, it occurs in about 60% of AIDS patients and is a major cause of death in patients with this syndrome. Clinical onset is abrupt, with high fever, tachypnea, mild cough, and cyanosis. Pulmonary physical findings may be slight and disproportionate to the degree of illness. Arterial blood gases usually reveal severe hypoxemia. Morphological demonstration of the organism requires samples of the parenchymal compartments. Open lung biopsy, bronchoalveolar lavage, transbronchial biopsy, and transthoracic aspiration yields organisms in 80% of cases. *(Krupp et al, p. 916)*

5. **(B)** Mycoplasmal pneumonia is the most common pneumonia in adults under age 40. Fever, headache, and malaise predate the cough by 2 to 4 days. The cough is persistent, hacking, and sputum is scant and sometimes bloodtinged. The temperature rarely exceeds 102°F. Bullous myringitis occurs in 10% of cases and the chest exam may be normal regardless of radiographic evidence of pneumonia. Cultures are not readily available and cold agglutinins are present in 50% of patients. Drugs of choice for mycoplasmal pneumonia are tetracycline and erythromycin. *(Eisenberg and Copass, pp. 203–210)*

6. **(E)** The clinical manifestations of bronchogenic carcinoma can vary, and many patients are asymptomatic when the pulmonary lesion is discovered. Cough usually productive of scant sputum is a common symptom, hemoptysis occurs frequently secondary to ulceration in the pulmonary lesion. Frequently, because of a significant smoking history, patients with carcinoma also have obstructive pulmonary disease and dyspnea with exertion. Weight loss is also a common complaint of bronchogenic carcinoma but generally occurs with more extensive disease beyond the time the neoplasm is limited to the lung. Chest pain may be due to pleural involvement but must also suggest metastatic disease. Pulmonary infections occur distal to the bronchial obstruction and can mask the tumor. Any atypical or recurrent pulmonary infections should

suggest carcinoma. Chest x-ray may demonstrate hilar and mediastinial lymph node involvement, pleural effusion, rib metastasis, elevation of a diaphram, tracheal compression or distortion, and pericardial effusion. Although pulmonary diseases, particularly at end stages, present with similar symptoms the entire history, physical, laboratory, and roentgenographic findings must be correlated to form the correct diagnosis. Asthma and chronic obstructive pulmonary disease usually reveal hyperinflation of the lungs and flat diaphrams. Bronchiectasis shows coarse lung markings and even honeycombing due to the abnormal dilatation of the bronchial tree. Chronic bronchitis has been used in various ways, sometimes referring to a simple smoker's cough and at other times to severe COPD. It is usually described as a productive cough that is present on most days for at least 3 months of the year. *(Beeson et al, pp. 457–460)*

7. **(A)** Emphysema denotes a disease characterized pathologically by destruction of interalveolar septa, including blood vessels, and coalescence of air spaces to form abnormal cystic bullous areas in the lung that do not exchange air. The disease is inherited and signs and symptoms manifest usually in the third and fourth decades; smoking can lower the age of onset by 10 to 20 years. Emphysema has an insidious onset of progressive dyspnea on exertion and cough. Sputum production may occur but is not characteristic. In advanced disease, symptoms of cor pulmonale may be present. In general, there is increased A–P diameter, hyperinflation of the lungs with depressed diaphragms, and depressed diaphragmatic motion. Hyperresonance of the chest, decreased breath sounds, and an increased expiratory phase with occasional wheezing is present. The PaO_2 is often maintained in the 60 to 70 range and the $PaCO_2$ is normal to elevated until the disease is far advanced. Pulmonary function testing is usually very helpful; the FEV1 and vital capacity are decreased. *(Krupp et al, pp. 152–153)*

8. **(E)** All the answers may help the patient symptomatically, but there is no effective way, over the long term, to improve pulmonary function test and longevity in emphysema. *(Krupp el al, pp. 152–157)*

9. **(D)** Pulmonary function tests are helpful in determining restrictive from obstructive pulmonary diseases but does not aid in the diagnosis of pulmonary carcinoma. Sputum cytology can yield a diagnosis in 40% to 60% of cases, and bronchoscopy with biopsy can not only give one a direct view of the lesion, but yields positive results in 75% to 80% of cases of pulmonary neoplasm. CAT scan is helpful in the visualization and location of a pulmonary lesion and is also helpful in the determination of metastases. Ventilation–perfusion scanning is a sensitive test for the examination for regional lung function and may be helpful in the diagnosis of pulmonary carcinoma. *(Beeson et al, pp. 460–461; Krupp et al, pp. 160–162)*

10. **(D)** All the examinations, except arterial blood gases, are helpful in the diagnosis of pulmonary carcinoma (see answer to question 9). However, the chest x-ray when compared to previous films is the least expensive and less invasive examination, therefore, it is the best screening exam for bronchogenic carcinoma. *(Krupp et al, pp. 160–162)*

11. **(C)** COPD results from some combination of chronic obstructive problems and pulmonary emphysema; both disorders are closely related to cigarette smoking. It is generally believed that emphysema results from the effect of proteolytic enzymes on lung tissue. When there is a very severe congenital deficiency of serum antiproteolytic activity, it is likely that emphysema will develop even if the subject does not smoke. This deficiency results in 0.5% to 2% of cases of COPD. The development of emphysema depends on prolonged exposure to noxious irritants, usually cigarette smoke. *(Beeson, et al, pp. 414–415)*

12. **(B)** The frequency of different cell types of bronchogenic carcinoma varies in the literature. In general, epidermoid carcinoma occurs with the greatest frequency and constitutes approximately 40% to 50% of pulmonary neoplasms. Adenocarcinoma (bronchogenic and bronchioloalveolar), large cell carcinoma, and small cell anaplastic carcinoma occur at similar rates between 15% to 20%. *(Beeson et al, pp. 458–459)*

13. **(C)** People at risk for pulmonary embolism are those at hypercoagulable states. This may arise from the use of birth control pills, local stasis, immobilization that may be the result of an accident or illness, fractures, obesity, and congestive heart failure. Emboli that cause clinically significant pulmonary insult commonly arise in the ileofemoral and pelvic venous beds. Signs and symptoms often begin abruptly, and include dyspnea, cough, anxiety, and chest pain (frequently pleuritic in nature). Hemoptysis may occur; tachycardia and tachypnea are common in this illness. A low-grade fever, hypotension, and cyanosis are also signs of pulmonary embolism. The presence of a deep venous thrombosis aid in the rapid clinical diagnosis. Radiographic evidence of consolidation may be present in cases of pulmonary embolism. *(Mills, p. 535; Beeson et al, pp. 442–444)*

14. **(D)** Hemoptysis is the expectoration of blood or bloody sputum. Some of the important causes of hemotysis include pneumonias, pulmonary emboli, bronchogenic carcinoma, mitral stenosis, COPD, tuberculosis, and other granulomatosis diseases. However, the most common cause of hemoptysis is bronchitis. *(Friedman, p. 136)*

15. **(A)** Cheyne–Stokes respiration is the most common form of periodic breathing. Periods of apnea alternate regularly with series of respiratory cycles. In each cycle, the rate and amplitude of successive respirations increase to a maximum, then decrease progressively until the series is terminated with an apneic period. Kussmaul respiration is applied to deep, regular sighing respirations, regardless of rate. This pattern of breathing is seen in diabetic ketoacidosis, uremia, peritonitis, severe hemorrhage, and pneumonia. Biots breathing is an uncommon variant of Cheyne–Stokes respiration in which periods of apnea alternate irregularly with series of breaths of equal depth. This is most often seen in meningitis. Stridulous breathing is a high-pitched whistling or crowing sound with respirations when the air passes over a partly closed glottis. This occurs with edema of the vocal cords (i.e., infection), neoplasm, abscess of the pharnyx, and foreign body in the pharynx. Apnea is simply the absence of respiration. *(DeGowin and DeGowin, pp. 270–281)*

16. **(C)** Spontaneous pneumothorax is more likely to occur in young, thin, tall individuals. The patient usually complains of chest pain, dyspnea, cough, usually during exertion. Physical exam reveals decreased breath sounds, increased resonance, and decreased fremitus on the involved side. There may be deviation of the trachea and heart to the side opposite that of involvement. Distention of the neck veins may be visible if the pneumothorax is under tension and hypotension may occur. *(Friedman, pp. 124–125)*

17. **(D)** The description of the x-ray confirms the diagnosis of pneumothorax. Aspiration of the air to allow reexpansion of the lung must occur. This is most quickly achieved by aspiration with a large-bore needle but, frequently, chest tubes are required. Cough should be suppressed, pain control is manditory, and bed rest is required. Endotracheal intubation is not required in this patient; CAT scan delays the needed treatment, and the other choices are not beneficial in the treatment of a pneumothorax. *(Krupp, et al, pp. 172–173)*

18. **(D)** The ventilation–perfusion scan is the most sensitive screening procedure for embolization, because the perfusion of the embolized area is pro-foundly impaired with minimal impairment of ventilation. A negative study of good technical quality excludes angiographically detectable pulmonary embolism. Chest x-rays are abnormal in most patients with pulmonary embolization with infarction; the abnormalities are, however, often nonspecific. EKGs are often normal or may show nonspecific changes. Clinically significant embolization is almost always associated with hypoxemia; however, this may be obscured by reflex hyperventilation and hypocapnia. Pulmonary angiography allows direct visualization of the vascular tree and is the procedure of choice for establishing the diagnosis. Nonetheless, this procedure has obvious limitations, and because of the controversy in this area, the choice of this procedure was not included in the answers. *(Mills et al, p. 535; Beeson et al, pp. 444–445)*

19. **(B)** With the history of acute onset of dyspnea during exertion and the findings of hyperresonance, expiratory wheezes, and prolonged expiratory phase, the obvious diagnosis is bronchial asthma. There are many aggravating activities and substances for the exacerbation of asthma including: infection, drugs, exertion, cold, inhaled irritants, and emotional stress. During an asthma attack, bronchospasm and hypersecretion of mucus results in airway obstruction and air trapping. Most patients with asthma are hypocapnic as a result of reflex hyperventilation. However, with progressive airway obstruction, fatigue, and increasing retention of carbon dioxide, mental status changes can occur, and is evidence of a severe, possibly life-threatening episode. *(Mills et al, pp. 529–530)*

20. **(D)** The site for a thoracentesis is determined by percussion to find the air–fluid level in the chest, and chest x-ray, to confirm level of fluid and rule out other problems. The puncture should be made superior to the rib to avoid the nerve and vessels that are inferior to each rib. Ultrasound does not aid in the location for thoracentesis. A post-tap chest x-ray should also be obtained to rule out a traumatic pneumothorax. *(Bope et al, p. 261)*

21. **(E)** All the choices may aggravate or stimulate an asthma attack. Inhaled allergens typically produce immediate "Type I," IgE-mediated, allergic reaction in the airway, although "Type III," IgG-mediated reactions may also occur in some patients. The parasympathetic nervous system also plays a part in the asthmatic response. Cholinergic stimulation induces mediator production in the mast cell and causes contraction of bronchial smooth muscle. Vigorous exercise produces bronchoconstriction in some asthmatic patients. Furthermore, beta-adrenergic blockers as well as indomethacin, aspirin, and certain yellow coloring agents may induce asth-

ma. Asthma-like reactions to inorganic chemicals and organic dusts are noted frequently. The role of emotional stress is difficult to assess, but clearly some subjects have exacerbations of their disease during stress. *(Beeson et al, pp. 403–408)*

22. **(A)** Therapy for asthma can include all the choices, but inhaled beta-adrenergic agonist provides the most rapid effect, therefore, the best therapeutic index. Use of epinephrine is contraindicated in patients with known cardiac disease and is not recommended in patients more than age 50. Aminophyllin, IV and oral, have a slower onset of action and therapeutic levels must be maintained and monitored. Hydrocortisone also has a delayed onset of action and its uses should be limited if possible. *(Beeson el al, pp. 408–410)*

23. **(D)** Bronchitis may be acute or chronic, caused by any number of infectious agents, or due to chemical or mechanical irritants. There is generally a dry hacking nonproductive cough for 4 to 5 days, after which it is likely that the cough will become productive. Fever is usually mild, the chest x-ray can rule out pneumonia and other pulmonary problems, and the white blood cell count is normal to slightly elevated. Diffuse rhonchi may be heard during forced expiration; however, the lungs may sound clear. *(Kempe et al, p. 350)*

24. **(B)** Treatment of bronchitis is aimed at clearing the bronchial tree; chest physiotherapy and increased fluid intake in highly recommended. Avoidance of any substance that might aggravate bronchial irritation is paramount (cigarette smoke, etc.). Antibiotics should be employed if there is evidence of bacterial infection. The use of cough suppressants does not aid in the clearance of the respiratory tract and may aggravate clearing the respiratory tract, and in most cases should be avoided. *(Kempe et al, p. 350)*

25. **(B)** Vital capacity is the sum of the inspiratory reserve volume, the tidal volume, and the expiratory reserve volume. Any factors that reduce the ability of the lung to expand also reduce the vital capacity. Therefore, fibrotic lung diseases such as tuberculosis, emphysema, chronic asthma, lung cancer, chronic bronchitis, and fibrotic pleurisy can all reduce pulmonary compliance and reduce the vital capacity. For this reason, the vital capacity is the most important of clinical respiratory measurements in the assessment of the progression of these diseases. Arterial blood gases are helpful in the determination, objectively, of the oxygenation of the blood, but are not reliable in the assessment of progression in fibrotic diseases. Changes in tidal volume may not become apparent until late in the

disease process. *(Krupp et al, p. 126; Guyton, pp. 470–472)*

26. **(A)** Epiglottitis is the most serious form of croup affecting children from ages 3 to 6 years old. The most common pathogen is *Haemophilus influenzae* Type B, although beta-hemolytic streptococci and pneumoncocci have been implicated in rare cases. The onset is usually abrupt over a period of a few hours and patients present with high fevers, respiratory distress signaled by stridor, difficulty in swallowing, and severe sore throat signaled by drooling. Many patients have a muffled voice due to inflammation of the epiglottic and arytenoid cartilages. *(Kempe et al, pp. 344–345; Mills et al, pp. 372–373)*

27. **(B)** When epiglottitis is suspected, the mouth or neck should not be examined without first obtaining a soft tissue lateral neck x-ray, which would show edema and swelling of the epiglottis. The patient should be kept calm. If epiglottitis is noted on x-ray, orotracheal or nasotracheal intubation should be performed in the operating room, as an emergency tracheostomy may be needed. Visualization with a tongue blade or laryngoscope has been associated with abrupt laryngeal spasm, obstruction, and death. Chloramphenicol is the antibiotic of choice for epiglottitis. *(Kempe et al, pp. 344–345; Mills et al, pp. 372–373)*

28. **(C)** Foreign body aspiration presents in children usually from ages 4 months through 6 years; frequently there is a history of playing with small objects. The aspiration of the foreign body classically precipitates an acute episode of choking, gagging, coughing, and wheezing. The chest x-ray results in this question are classic for foreign-body aspiration. *(Kempe et al, pp. 347–348)*

29. **(C)** The treatment of foreign-body aspiration is hospitalization with immediate bronchoscopy to remove the foreign body. Chest physiotherapy should not be used for fear of completely obstructing the airway. Cool mist therapy and antibiotics would not, of course, be helpful, and intubation in this patient is not required, as the foreign body is causing only local effects. *(Kempe et al, pp. 347–348)*

30. **(D)** Hyperventilation usually occurs in young people without other evidence of cardiopulmonary disease, often in the presence of a recent emotional upset. Circumoral and carpopedal dysesthesias and spasm may occur. Frequently, anxiety exceeds the evidence for cardiopulmonary disease. Arterial blood gases are usually not needed but will show an increase in pH and a decrease in $PaCO_2$. Patients

usually rapidly improve and reassurance is essential. *(Friedman, pp. 124–125)*

31. **(A)** In lung carcinoma, the most commonly encountered endocrine syndromes are inappropriate antidiuretic hormone secretion, Cushing's syndrome, and gynecomastia. Small cell anaplastic carcinoma is especially associated with the development of these syndromes, suggestive of hormone overproduction. Small cell anaplastic carcinoma cell may be of neural crest-cell derivation and may have the potential for secreting many different chemical mediators. Hypothyroidism is not commonly encountered as a result of carcinoma of the lung. *(Beeson et al, pp. 459, 1103)*

32. **(B)** The term *restrictive ventilatory disorder* denotes a pattern of abnormalities in lung function. The word *restrictive* is employed to indicate a restriction of or limitation to the amount of gas within the lungs. Thus, ventilatory disorders are characterized by reduction in lung volume. The hallmark of restriction is a decrease in the vital capacity. Obstructive ventilatory disorder denotes the constellation of abnormalities that resolves from airway obstruction, regardless of its cause. Obstructive disorders are detected principally by the tests of the behavior of the respiratory system under dynamic conditions. The FeV1/Fvc (Forced expiratory volume in 1 second divided by the forced vital capacity) is the most widely used, although tests of maximal flow-volume relationships are increasingly being used. *(Beeson et al, pp. 416–417, 427–428)*

33. **(A)** Patients with pneumonia may present in a variety of clinical presentations. However, findings disclosed by proper physical examination of the lungs should aid in the formulation of the differential diagnosis. Vocal fremitis is increased in consolidated pneumonias and by inflammation surrounding other pulmonary lesions by transmitting bronchotracheal air vibration with greater efficiency than do the air-filled pulmonary alveoli. Consolidated pulmonary tissue has increased density verses normal lung tissue, therefore yielding impaired resonance, dullness, and flatness to percussion. This consolidated tissue also transmits whispered syllables distinctly, even when the pathological process is too small to produce bronchial breathing. Rales refer to sounds in the lungs from the movements of fluids or exudates in the airways. Although there are different types of rales, they sound like clicks or small bubbles and occur in bronchiectasis, pneumonia, consolidation, infarction, bronchitis, and TB. *(DeGowin and DeGowin, pp. 296–319)*

34. **(C)** The treatment of a patient with a pulmonary embolism should include bed rest, analgesics, and oxygen, as indicated. Anticoagulation should begin as soon as possible if no contraindication exists. Hemoptysis from pulmonary infarction is not a contraindication to anticoagulation. Usually after heparin is used acutely, coumadin therapy is continued for 6 weeks unless there is chronic disease that may predispose the patient to repeated thrombus formation. Antibiotics are not indicated unless a septic infarct is suspected. *(Beeson et al, pp. 447–449)*

35. **(E)** The use of corticosteroids in COPD should be reserved for patients with potential reversibility of the disease. Some clues that a reversible component exist include: (1) improvement in the FeV1, after inhalation of a bronchodilator, of greater than 20%; (2) history of considerable fluctuation in severity of symptoms or of acute attacks of wheezing dyspnea not brought on by exertion; (3) prominent wheeze or "noisy" chest on physical exam; (4) normal chest x-ray except for hyperinflation; (5) eosinophilia of the blood or sputum; (6) allergy skin test, or high serum IgE levels; (7) associated vasomotor rhinitis or nasal polyps; or (8) normal pulmonary diffusing capacity measurement. If no improvement of the FeV1 is noted with a trial of a corticosteroid, the drug should be gradually tapered and discontinued. *(Beeson et al, pp. 416–417)*

36. **(D)** Because of the marked increase in pulmonary vascular resistance and pulmonary arterial pressure, there are a variety of clinical manifestations of primary pulmonary hypertension. Most frequently, dyspnea during exertion, fatigue, and weakness are noted. Substernal discomfort and even angina can be experienced during exertion; this is thought to be caused by right ventricular ischemia. Hoarseness may also be experienced due to compression of the left recurrent laryngeal nerve by the enlarged left pulmonary artery. Occasionally, cyanosis is noted but clubbing is absent in this disease. If clubbing is present, it should prompt further investigation for the cause of pulmonary hypertension. Syncope in primary pulmonary hypertension is an ominous sign suggesting an abrupt fall in cardiac output and may result in sudden death. In almost every patient, an accentuated P_2 is noted with auscultation of the heart. *(Beeson et al, pp. 298–300; DeGowin and DeGowin, p. 368)*

37. **(E)** The presence of partial airway obstruction below the tracheal bifurcation characteristically causes a localized wheeze over the site of obstruction and hyperinflation of the distal lung. Chest x-rays may be able to see the hyperinflation as well as the site of any foreign body or mass that is causing the obstruction. Inspiratory stridor is the hallmark of partial obstruction above the bifurcation. Pulmonary function testing reveals a relatively constant forced expiratory flow over a large portion of the FVC (forced vital capacity) in obstruction above the tracheal carina. Areas of localized decrease in airflow as seen in obstruction below the carina can be detected by ventilation–perfusion test. *(Beeson et al, pp. 418–419)*

38. **(A)** Because all patients with COPD should be regarded as having potentially reversible disease on initial exam, several measures should be instituted immediately. Bronchodilators should be given and drug levels monitored. Smoking and exposure to other pulmonary irritants should be avoided. A health care provider (MD, PA, RN, or RT) should provide the patient with instruction on bronchial hygiene and chest physical therapy. If it is found that the above measures do indeed improve pulmonary function by an appropriate amount, then at that time use of corticosteroids should be continued. *(Beeson et al, pp. 416–417)*

39. **(B)** Physical findings in a severe asthma attack with marked bronchospasm and dyspnea can be associated with a diminution of wheezing and breath sounds. This may lead to a silent chest, an especially serious finding that suggests impending respiratory failure. Arterial blood gas findings in mild to moderate asthma usually reveal normal to low $PaCO_2$ levels. As the bronchospasm worsens, hypoxia and CO_2 retention occur and, in severe episodes, the $PaCO_2$ rises to high levels. This elevation in $PaCO_2$ indicates a desparate situation and usually requires prompt and aggressive intervention. *(Beeson et al, pp. 407–408; Mills et al, p. 529)*

40. **(C)** The patient presented has a somewhat complicated past medical history including asthma, which by the history and exam has worsened in the recent past. The patient appears, however, not to be in acute respiratory distress. The patient has recently been started on propanolol for treatment of hypertension. Because propanolol can accentuate bronchospasm and the patient appears to be at a therapeutic level (pulse rate, 52) without normalization of the blood pressure, consideration should be given to discontinuing this medication and beginning another antihypertensive. The use of epinephrine is contraindicated in patients more than age 50 and patients with a history of coronary artery disease. Anytime a patient on theophylline presents with worsening of symptoms, a serum theophylline level should be obtained so that proper dosage is maintained *(Beeson el al, pp. 408–410)*

41. **(A)** Blunt or penetrating trauma to the chest wall may result in intrapleural bleeding or hemothorax. The patient in question presents with a classical history and physical findings consistent with a hemothorax in the right chest. Hypotension, shock, or even cardiopulmonary arrest may be present depending on blood loss and other injuries sustained. Emergency treatment should consist of the placement of at least two large-bore IVs; blood work should include CBC and the sending of clotted blood for type and crossmatching. A chest tube should be placed for the evacuation of the hemothorax and for treatment of a pneumothorax if present. The patient in question may indeed need surgery, but the above measures should be performed prior to thorocotomy. Every effort should be made to perform the thorocotomy in a well-prepared O.R. by a trained cardiothoracic surgeon. *(Mills et al, pp. 255–256)*

42. **(B)** All the choices are effective methods of oxygen delivery and all health care providers should know the concentrations of O_2 delivered by each. A face mask with an oxygen reservoir at 6 L/min will provide an oxygen concentration at 60%. A nasal cannula at 2 L/min will provide O_2 at 28% to 30%. Mouth-to-mouth ventilation provides O_2 at 17%, and a face mask without an oxygen reservoir at 10 L/min will provide O_2 at a 60% concentration. *(Jaffe et al, pp. 35–36)*

43. **(E)** There are many factors involved in the control and stimulation of respiration. The most important factor in the control of ventilation under normal conditions is the PCO_2 of arterial blood. Increases in the PCO_2 is a strong stimulus to increase respiration and, similarly, decreases in PCO_2 will cause a decrease in respiration. The role of hypoxia to stimulate respiration in the day-by-day control of respiration is small, as the PO_2 can be reduced by large amounts without stimulating an increase in respiration. However, patients with COPD have chronic CO_2 retention and the pH of their cerebrospinal fluid has returned to normal, thus depressing the stimulation of respiration previously discussed. In these people, the hypoxic drive to ventilate becomes very important and treatment of these patients with high concentration of O_2 will act as a negative feedback and depress and possibly stop respiration. Reductions in the blood pH also stimulates respiration. Clinically, this response is difficult to differentiate from an accompanying rise in PCO_2, but animal models have demonstrated the response to pure acidosis convincingly. Exercise also increases respiration promptly for unclear reasons. During exercise the arterial PO_2, PCO_2, and pH remain relatively constant, yet respiration increases at times to very high levels. *(West, pp. 124–125)*

44. **(E)** The management of infants with meconium aspiration must be closely observed for respiratory complication and they must undergo treatment to prevent these complications. Chest physiotherapy and suctioning on a regular basis is suggested early, and continued if signs of respiratory distress is encountered. Chest x-ray is important to help determine which child will develop respiratory distress and, because mechanical ventilation is often required, 10% to 20% of infants will develop pneumothorax or pneumomediastinum. Transcutaneous monitoring of the PO_2 early in the management of these infants aids in the assessment of the severity of the infant's condition. Fluid restriction is important to prevent cerebral and pulmonary edema during resuscitation. The response to asphyxiation may include the inappropriate secretion of antidiuretic hormone for 3 to 4 days after the insult. *(Cloherty and Stark, pp. 203–205, 319–320)*

45. **(C)** The advances in the prevention of hyaline membrane disease are closely related to the identification of risk factors for the development of the disease. Prenatal risk factors for hyaline membrane disease include: prematurity, maternal diabetes, and a history of hyaline membrane disease in siblings. Also, male sex children, second-born twins, and caesarean delivery without labor, are additional risk factors for hyaline membrane disease. *(Cloherty and Stark, p. 168)*

46. **(A)** The initial approach to evaluating hemoptysis involves several simple studies that can be instituted in almost any clinical setting. Studies should include: determination if the sputum is blood streaked or if gross blood is present, a Gram stain, a chest x-ray, a tuberculin skin test, and sputum cytology examination. These studies will aid in the determination for the direction of further studies or referrals. A bronchoscopy may be needed after the above tests are performed, but is not indicated as an initial study for the evaluation of hemoptysis. *(Driscoll et al, p. 252)*

47. **(B)** The patient in this question has an exudative pleural effusion. An exudative effusion is defined as having a protein content of greater than 3 g/dL, is cloudy, and has a specific gravity greater than 1.016. The differential for an exudative plueral effusion include: bacterial and viral infections, TB, neoplasms, post-myocardial infarction, pulmonary infarction, rheumatoid arthritis, and SLE (lupus). Severe anemia and liver disease can cause a pleural effusion, but the effusion is a transudative that is clear, specific gravity less than 1.016, and has a protein content less than 2.5 g/dL. *(Driscoll et al, p. 206)*

48. **(E)** By far the most important factor in the formation of a pulmonary abscess is aspiration, usually related to altered consciousness. Altered consciousness can be caused by a variety of conditions such as alcoholism, stroke, drug use, seizure, or other serious illness. Lung abscess formation is rare in an edentulous person and, if present, suggests the possibility of bronchogenic carcinoma. In 60% of cases only anaerobic bacteria are found, and there are generally an average of three organisms per case. *(Beeson et al, pp. 436–437)*

49. **(D)** Abscess formation may be a complication of pneumonias caused by *S aureus*, *S pyogenes*, and *K pneumoniae*. Pneumococcal pneumonia is rarely associated with lung abscess formation unless other organisms are involved. *(Beeson et al, pp. 436–437)*

50. **(A)** As expected, there are many major complications in the near-drowning patient. Initially, the pulmonary effects must be evaluated and dealt with quickly. These include hypoxia, acidosis, and pulmonary edema that occurs in up to 75% of patients. Renal abnormalities have been reported, but significant electrolyte disturbances are usually not present. *(Eisenberg and Copass, pp. 456–459)*

REFERENCES

Cecil Textbook of Medicine, 18th ed. Philadelphia, PA: WB Saunders; 1988.

Bope CT, Driscoll CE, et al. *Handbook of Family Practice*. Chicago, IL: Year Book Medical Publishers; 1986.

Cloherty JP, Startk AR. *Manual of Neonatal Care*, 2nd ed. Boston, MA: Little Brown; 1986.

Degowin EL, Degowin RL. *Bedside Diagnostic Examination*, 5th ed. New York: Macmillan; 1987.

Eisenberg MJ, Copasus MK. *Emergency Medical Therapy*, 3rd ed. Philadelphia, PA: WB Saunders; 1988.

Friedman HH. *Problem Oriented Medical Diagnosis*, 3rd ed.

Guyton AC. *Textbook of Medical Physiology*, 7th ed. Philadelphia, PA: WB Saunders; 1986.

Jaffe AS. *Textbook of Advanced Cardiac Life Support System*, 2nd ed.

Kempe CH. *Current Pediatric Diagnosis and Treatment*, 9th ed. Appleton & Lange, 1987

Krupp MA, et al. *Current Medical Diagnosis and Treatment*, ed. Norwalk, CT: Appleton & Lange; 1989.

Mills J. Current Emergency Diagnosis and Treatment, 2nd ed. Norwalk, CT: Appleton & Lange, 1985.

West JB. *Respiratory Physiology*, 4th ed. Baltimore, MD: Williams & Wilkins; 1990.

Wyngaarden JP, Smith LH. *Cecil Textbook of Medicine*, 18th ed. Philadelphia, PA: WB Saunders; 1988.

Subspecialty List: Pulmonary

Question Numbers and Subspecialty
1. Legionnaires' disease—characteristics
2. Pneumococcal pneumonia—characteristics
3. *Klebsiella pneumonia*—characteristics
4. *Pneumocystis carnii* pneumonia—characteristics
5. Mycoplasmal pneumonia—characteristics
6. Bronchogenic carcinoma—characteristics
7. Emphysema—characteristics
8. Emphysema—treatment
9. Bronchogenic carcinoma—laboratory evaluation
10. Lung carcinoma—laborabory evaluation
11. Chronic obstructive pulmonary disease—causes
12. Bronchogenic carcinoma—pathology
13. Pulmonary embolism—characteristics
14. Hemoptysis—causes
15. Cheyne—Stokes respiration—characteristics
16. Spontaneous pneumothorax—characteristics
17. Spontaneous pneumothorax—treatment
18. Pulmonary embolism—laboratory evaluation
19. Bronchial asthma—characteristics
20. Thoracentesis—procedure
21. Asthma—exacerbation
22. Asthma—treatment
23. Bronchitis—characteristics
24. Bronchitis—treatment
25. Pulmonary function tests
26. Epiglottitis—characteristics
27. Epiglottitis—evaluation
28. Foreign body aspiration—characteristics
29. Foreign body aspiration—treatment
30. Hyperventilation—characteristics
31. Lung cancer—associated endocrine syndromes
32. Restrictive vs. obstructive pulmonary disease
33. Pneumonia—physical findings
34. Pulmonary embolism—treatment
35. Chronic obstructive pulmonary disease—steroid indications
36. Pulmonary hypertension—characteristics
37. Airway obstruction—anatomic differential
38. Chronic obstructive pulmonary disease—treatment
39. Bronchial asthma—characteristics
40. Asthma—management
41. Hemopneumothorax—management
42. Oxygen therapy
43. Respiratory physiology
44. Meconium aspiration—management
45. Hyaline membrane disease—risk factors
46. Hemoptysis—evaluation
47. Thoracentesis—differential diagnosis
48. Pulmonary abcess—characteristics
49. Pulmonary abcess—differential diagnosis
50. Near drowning—characteristics

Internal Medicine: Infectious Diseases

William K. Chapman, Jr.

Questions

DIRECTIONS (Questions 1 through 10): Each group of items in this section consists of lettered headings followed by a set of numbered words or phrases. For each numbered word or phrase, select the ONE lettered heading that is most closely associated with it. Each lettered heading may be selected once, more than once, or not at all.

1. A mono-spot test on a patient returns positive. During your work-up of this patient you would expect to find all the following **EXCEPT**

    (A) elevated liver function tests
    (B) hepatosplenomegaly
    (C) lymphadenopathy
    (D) atypical lymphocytes on the differential
    (E) pharyngitis

2. All the following are true in case of Lyme disease **EXCEPT**

    (A) there is an expanding erythematous annular lesion
    (B) the treatment of choice is trimethoprim/sulfamethoxazole
    (C) it is the most commonly reported tick-borne disease in the United States
    (D) it is a disease of stages if left untreated
    (E) if arthritis develops, it primarily affects the knee joint

3. You have taken a long awaited 2-week vacation to Acapulco, but have developed "turista" 3 days into your trip. Which of the following are true concerning your condition?

    (A) you probably became infected by drinking a bottle of local Mexican beer
    (B) you can expect your symptoms to continue through your entire vacation
    (C) your symptoms may not have occurred if you had started your trip by taking doxycycline 100 mg daily for 3 days

    (D) bismuth subsalicylate (Pepto Bismol) may make your symptoms worse
    (E) there is a good chance that your symptoms are being caused by one of the Salmonella serotypes

4. In the case of *Giardia lamblia,* stools can be characterized by all the following **EXCEPT**

    (A) mushy in recurrent cases
    (B) blood is not present
    (C) pus is not present
    (D) there is little odor
    (E) they tend to be greasy and float

5. In a suspected case of food-borne botulism, you would expect to find all of the following **EXCEPT**

    (A) the patient had eaten home-canned vegetables 24 hours prior
    (B) muscle twitching as the first neurological manifestation
    (C) impending respiratory failure if not treated promptly
    (D) The patient is afebrile
    (E) an alert, oriented individual, even in severe cases

6. Delta hepatitis is a relatively new hepatic condition. All the following are true regarding this disease **EXCEPT**

    (A) it is a defective RNA virus
    (B) IV drug users are at increased risk
    (C) it exists only as a coninfecting disease with hepatitis B
    (D) there is high infectivity rate among the homosexual population
    (E) its presence in chronic active hepatitis B can indicate a poor prognosis

7. Hepatitis B vaccine is recommended to all the following EXCEPT

   (A) infants born to a hepatitis B surface antigen (HB$_s$Ag) positive mother
   (B) established hepatitis B infectious individuals
   (C) promiscuous male homosexuals
   (D) persons receiving an accidental needle-stick from HB$_s$Ag positive blood
   (E) health care professionals exposed regularly to blood

8. Of all hepatitis infections, hepatitis B (HBV) has the "alphabet soup" of lab values. All the following are true regarding these values EXCEPT

   (A) the surface antibody indicates past infection and is considered protective
   (B) the core antibody I$_g$G indicates infection even if the surface antigen is negative
   (C) the E antigen in the presence of the surface antigen can indicate a greater likelihood for chronic disease
   (D) the surface antigen is the first evidence of acute infection
   (E) the core antigen is usually not detected in the serum by conventional lab methods

9. Two consecutive tuberculin skin tests are read in the same individual as negative and positive, respectively. He or she is considered a "true" converter. The following are true of a converter EXCEPT

   (A) the tests were given within 2 years of each other
   (B) the first test was 7 mm induration and the second test was 14 mm induration
   (C) the person is considered newly infected
   (D) chemoprophylaxis is not necessary if he or she is less than 25-years old and has a negative chest x-ray
   (E) treatment should be provided prophylactically if he/she is a child less than 3-years old

10. Childhood tuberculosis differs from adult tuberculosis in all the following EXCEPT

    (A) hilar lymphadenopathy is the hallmark of childhood tuberculosis
    (B) the child older than 3-years has a lower resistance to tuberculosis infection than does an elderly person
    (C) the dose of isoniazid is larger for the child
    (D) the child has a recurrent nonproductive cough
    (E) caseation and cavity formation occur uncommonly in the child

DIRECTIONS (Questions 11 through 22): Each group of items in this section consists of lettered headings followed by a set of numbered words or phrases. For each numbered word or phrase, select

   A if the item is associated with (A) only,
   B if the item is associated with (B) only,
   C if the item is associated with both (A) and (B),
   D if the item is associated with neither (A) nor (B).

Questions 11 through 13

   (A) Kawasaki's disease
   (B) toxic shock syndrome

11. bilateral, nonpurulent conjunctival injection
12. bacterial etiology believed to be the cause
13. coronary artery involvement in some cases

Questions 14 through 16

   (A) Lyme disease
   (B) Rocky Mountain spotted fever

14. Bell's palsy is a neurological complication
15. tetracycline is the treatment of choice
16. vesicular lesions may develop as the disease progresses

Questions 17 through 20

   (A) Salmonella gastroenteritis
   (B) Shigella

17. bloody stools are a common finding
18. antimicrobial treatment is generally unnecessary in uncomplicated cases
19. associated with sexual transmission
20. antibiotics do not shorten the course of the illness

Questions 21 through 22

   (A) hepatitis B
   (B) hepatitis non-A, non-B

21. blood transfusions have been implicated as a cause
22. associated with chronic active disease

DIRECTIONS (Questions 22 and 23): For each of the items in this section, ONE or MORE of the numbered options is correct. Choose the answer

A if only 1, 2, and 3 are correct,
B if only 1 and 3 are correct,
C if only 2 and 4 are correct,
D if only 4 is correct,
E if all are correct.

23. Which of the following diseases are associated with desquamation of the skin?

(1) scarlet fever
(2) toxic shock syndrome
(3) scalded skin syndrome
(4) Kawasaki's disease

24. A patient you have seen for the first time presents with a petechial rash. She gives you a history of a possible tick bite 2 weeks earlier. You suspect Rocky Mountain spotted fever (RMSF). What other important findings may aid you in your diagnosis of RMSF?

(1) she lives in North Carolina
(2) the patient responds favorably to a 10-day course of erythromycin
(3) her lab values show thrombocytopenia
(4) the disease is transmitted by the vector, *Rickettsia rickettsii*

25. Looking under the laboratory microscope you notice a "face and two large eyes" staring back at you. Realizing this is actually a *Giardia lamblia* trophozoite, you also know this protozoa

(1) is not associated with sexual transmission
(2) primarily affects the large intestine
(3) causes pus-laden stools
(4) can cause malabsorption

26. Infant botulism differs from food-borne botulism in that

(1) there is toxin production in vivo
(2) constipation is common
(3) the ingestion of honey has been implicated as a cause
(4) it primarily affects those 6 to 12 months of age

27. Malaria is relatively uncommon in the United States. Individuals traveling abroad may return with the disease. You suspect a patient to have malaria. You base this on

(1) the patient's complaint about cyclic episodes of chills, fever, and sweating
(2) his/her recent trip to Zimbabwe without prior chemoprophylaxis

(3) splenomegaly during your physical examination
(4) a normal to low leukocyte count

28. Hepatitis A (HAV) differs in many aspects from the other viral hepatic infections. Which of the following are true regarding HAV?

(1) there is no known chronic carrier state
(2) dark urine and clay-colored stools are first noticed after jaundice occurs
(3) the patient can show antibodies to HAV without ever having clinically apparent disease
(4) the IgM antibody indicates past infection and persisting immunity

29. Fever of unknown origin is a diagnostic dilemma. Other than viral and bacterial causes, what other diseases are uncovered during the work-up?

(1) juvenile rheumatoid arthritis
(2) factitious fever
(3) leukemia
(4) thyrotoxicosis

30. The tuberculin skin test is a useful diagnostic aid for the detection of tuberculosis. Which of the following are true regarding this test?

(1) the preferred method is a subdermal injection of 0.1 mL of 25 tuberculin units (TU) of PPD
(2) a palpable erythematous area of 10 mm or more read at 48-hours posttest is considered a positive test
(3) the tine test is preferred over the Mantoux test
(4) a 5- to 9-mm reaction is doubtful for diagnosis and may be due to other mycobacterium species

31. Recommendations for treating cases of tuberculosis prophylactically include

(1) isoniazid is the drug of choice
(2) therapy should be given for 6 to 12 months
(3) multiple drug therapy may be needed in the Southeast Asian population
(4) treatment should be given to close contacts of infected individuals, such as small children

32. Current treatment recommendations for initial uncomplicated pulmonary and extrapulmonary tuberculosis are

(1) isoniazid daily for 12 months
(2) rifampin and isoniazid daily for 9 months
(3) ethambutol and streptomycin daily for 6 months in isoniazid-resistant cases
(4) isoniazid and rifampin daily for 6 months, with pyrazinamide added during the first 2 months

33. Which of the following are true regarding infectious mononucleosis?

(1) it is caused by a member of the herpes group of viruses
(2) rupture of the spleen, either spontaneously or following trauma, may occur
(3) elevated liver function in almost all cases
(4) petechial rash associated with concurrent ampicillin therapy

Answers and Explanations

1. (B) Frequently, the individual with mononucleosis presents with fever, sore throat, lymphadenitis, and malaise. The spleen is enlarged in more than 50% of cases, more than twice that of hepatomegaly. On examination, there may be percussion tenderness over the liver, but without associated hepatomegaly. Laboratory values reveal elevated liver function tests in almost all cases. There is an increase in atypical lymphocytes noted on the differential, usually greater than 10%. *Braunwald et al, p. 701; Wyngaarden et al, p. 1787; Berkow, pp. 2127–2128; Mandell et al, p. 974; Krupp et al, p. 848)*

2. (B) Lyme disease is the leading cause of tick-borne disease in the United States. After the bite of the infected tick, a characteristic expanding annular rash develops, called erythema chronicum migrans. The rash may resolve spontaneously and advance to a second stage that includes neurologic and cardiac sequelae. A third stage may develop involving arthritis, which primarily affects the large joints, mostly the knees. The treatment of choice is, in order of preference, tetracycline, penicillin, and erythromycin. *Braunwald et al, pp. 658–659; Wyngaarden et al, pp. 1726–1727; Berkow, p. 1251; Mandell et al, pp. 1346–1347; Krupp et al, p. 892; Abramowicz, p. 59)*

3. (C) Traveler's diarrhea is most often caused by an enterotoxigenic strain of *Escherichia coli*. Bottled, carbonated beverages are considered safe to drink, as well as is fruit that can be peeled. Bismuth subsalicylate (Pepto Bismol) provides symptomatic relief. Antiperistaltic drugs have no value in treatment. The symptoms resolve in from 1 to 5 days and rarely last 2 to 3 weeks. Prophylactic therapy should begin the day of the trip with either doxycyline 100 mg qd for 3 days or trimethoprim/sulfamethoxazole qd for 3 to 5 days. *Braunwald et al, pp. 506; Wyngaarden et al, pp. 1656–1657; Berkow, p. 786; Mandell et al, pp. 650–651; Abramowicz, p. 98–99)*

4. (D) The stools of one infected with *lamblia* are generally foul-smelling, greasy in appearance, and float in the water. Blood or pus is not present. With recurrent cases, the stools tend to be mushy. *Braunwald et al, p. 800; Berkow, p. 205; Mandell et al, p. 1554; Krupp et al, p. 914)*

5. (B) Botulism is food poisoning caused by the ingestion of the toxin *Clostridium botulinum*. It primarily affects the neuromuscular system. The three types are food-borne, wound, and infant botulism. Home-canned foods are the most common source of contamination. In adults, the first neurological manifestation is blurred vision. Ptosis may even occur. The person is afebrile, and remains alert and oriented throughout the course of the illness. As the illness progresses, neuromuscular block may result in respiratory failure. *Braunwald et al, p. 562; Wyngaarden et al, p. 1633; Berkow, pp. 783–784; Mandell et al, p. 1361; Krupp et al, p. 872)*

6. (D) Delta hepatitis, also known as the delta agent, is a defective RNA virus that replicates only in the presence of the hepatitis B virus (HBV). It cannot exist as an isolated infecting organism. It is associated with a superinfection, which is more severe than infection with HBV alone. This can result in severe chronic hepatitis and cirrhosis. High-risk groups include IV drug users, dialysis patients, and those receiving multiple transfusions. Male homosexuals have shown evidence of delta hepatitis, but the virus has not permeated the homosexual community and the incidence is low. *(Braunwald et al, pp. 1327–1332; Wyngaarden et al, p. 823; Berkow, p. 860; Mandell et al, p. 1012; Krupp et al, p. 398; Peicher and Schiff, pp. 30–33)*

7. (B) Hepatitis B vaccine gives hepatitis B surface antibody response to approximately 90% of those vaccinated. The vaccine can be given before or after exposure. Preexposure vaccination should be given to those at risk of coming in contact with hepatitis B, such as health care workers who may come into contact with infectious blood or blood products. Postexposure vaccination should be given to those who have been accidentally stuck with a needle contaminated with hepatitis B surface antigen (HB$_s$Ag) positive blood, or to infants born to HB$_s$Ag positive mothers. The vaccine is ineffective for those with currently active disease. *(Braunwald et al, p. 1334; Wyngaarden et al, p. 826; Berkow, p. 863; Mandell et al, p. 1020; Krupp et al, p. 400)*

8. (B) Hepatitis B surface antigen (HB$_s$Ag is the first serologic marker of hepatitis B (HBV) infection. It usually occurs during the incubation period and disappears during the recovery phase. The HBV surface antibody (anti-HB$_s$) develops after clinical recovery. It represents past HBV infection. The HBV core antigen (HBcAg) represents the viral inner core. It is not detectable in serum by conventional lab methods, but only by specialized techniques. The HBV core antibody (anti-HB$_c$) is a marker of acute, persistent, or past infection. The anti-HB$_c$(IgM) will be positive for 6 to 18 months after infection, and the anti-HB$_c$(IgG) will remain as the indicator of past infection. There is a "window" period in HBV. This occurs during the transition from the disappearance of HB$_s$Ag and the appearance of anti-HB$_s$. Anti-HB$_c$ (IgM) will be the only indicator of infection during this time. The HBV$_e$ antigen (HB$_e$Ag) is only found in HB$_s$Ag positive serum. Its presence in the serum, along with HB$_s$Ag, for more than 10 weeks, correlates with ongoing viral replication and may be a predictor of chronic disease. *(Braunwald et al, pp. 1325–1327; Berkow, pp. 859–860; Krupp et al, pp. 397–398)*

9. (D) A true converter is one who has 2 consecutive tuberculin skin tests given within 2 years of each other, the first one being read as negative, that is, less than 10 mm induration, and the second one being read as positive, that is, greater than 10 mm induration. The size of the induration must exceed 6 mm between the two readings. The conversion must also not be as a result of the "booster" effect. A conversion is an indicator that a new infection has occurred. In any recently infected person, chemoprophylaxis is recommended if the individual is less than 35-years old and has a negative chest x-ray. Household contacts, especially children under 3-years old, are at increased risk for developing the disease and should be treated prophylactically also. *(Braunwald et al, p. 632; Wyngaarden et al, p. 1683; Berkow, p. 114; Mandell et al, p. 1389; Krupp et al, p. 147).*

10. (B) Childhood tuberculosis (TB) differs in several ways from TB in the adult. The child's symptoms may be mild or nonspecific. Some symptoms, such as a persistent, nonproductive cough, are associated with bronchial compression, due to enlarged hilar lymph nodes. When seen on a chest x-ray, enlarged hilar lymph nodes are considered the hallmark of childhood TB. The child that is less than 3-years old and elderly persons are particularly sensitive to becoming infected with TB. Rarely, a child will develop progressive primary TB, which may result

in caseation and cavity formation. *(Wyngaarden et al, pp. 1683–1685; Berkow pp. 113–115; Mandell et al, pp. 1386–1390; Behrman and Vaughan, p. 631; Farer et al, p. 148)*

11. (C); 12.(B); 13.(A) Kawasaki's disease is a disease of unknown etiology. It consists of an exantham, fever, lymphadenopathy, and polyarteritis. The coronary arteries may become involved, including the formation of aneurysms. The disease is also associated with mucous membrane changes, which include pharyngeal injection fissured lips and injected, non purulent conjunctiva. *Braunwald et al, p. 1444; Wyngaarden et al, p. 2324; Berkow, p. 2050; Mandell et al, p. 1599; Krupp et al, p. 820, Chapel et al, p. 209)*

Toxic shock syndrome is believed to be caused by a strain of *S aureus* that produces a toxin, thus causing the symptoms. Initial presenting symptoms include the sudden onset of fever, rash, pharyngitis, and nonpurulent conjunctivitis. There may also be headache, lethargy, and hypotension. There is no known coronary artery involvement. *(Braunwald et al, p. 541; Wyngaarden et al, p. 1598; Berkow, p. 73; Mandell et al, p. 1107; Krupp et al, p. 858; Chapel et al, p. 202, 209)*

14. (A); 15. (C); 16. (D) Lyme disease begins with the tick bite from *Ixodes dammini*, which transmits the spirochete *Borrelia burgdorferi*. The classic rash, erythema chronicum migrans, begins as a macular or maculopapular lesion that expands leaving centralized clearing. This occurs within 1 month of the tick bite in most patients and can resolve spontaneously. Within a week to months a second stage of the disease can occur, which includes cardiac and neurologic complications. Bilateral Bell's palsy may occur, as well as severe fatigue, peripheral neuropathy, and meningitis. Early manifestations of the disease are treated with tetracycline 250 mg qid for 10 to 21 days, or amoxicillin 250 mg tid for 10 to 21 days. *(Braunwald et al, p. 659; Wyngaarden et al, pp. 1727–1728; Berkow, pp. 1252–1253; Mandell et al, pp. 1347–1348; Abramowicz, p. 59; Petri, pp. 95–99; Chapel et al, p. 218)*

Rocky Mountain spotted fever (RMSF) is transmitted by the bite of the dog tick, *Dermacentor variabilis* or the wood tick, *D andersoni*. The rash of RMSF typically begins as a macular or maculopapular lesion, but progresses to form petechial lesions. The lesions may coalesce to form large hemorrhagic areas. In RMSF, the treatment of choice is either chloramphenicol 50 mg/kg or tetracycline 25 mg/kg divided equally at 6 to 8 hours intervals. *(Braunwald et al, p. 751; Wyngaarden et al, p. 1743; Berkow, p. 151; Mandell et al, p. 1085; Krupp et al, p. 853; Petri, pp. 99–101; Riley and Walker, pp. 172–189.*

17. (C); 18.(A); 19.(B); 20.(A) *Salmonella* gastroenteritis is usually transmitted by infected meat, poultry, eggs, egg products, and raw milk. Infections affecting the intestinal tract are manifested by watery stools, with occasional blood and mucus. The disease is usually self-limited in uncomplicated cases and does not necessarily warrant antibiotic use. Treatment with antibiotics may actually prolong the time in which *Salmonella* resides in the intestinal tract. *(Braunwald et al, p. 598; Wyngaarden et al, p. 1645; Berkow, pp. 88–91; Mandell et al, p. 1261, 1266; Krupp et al, p. 865; Dupont et al, pp. 98–136)*

Shigella is usually transmitted by the stools of infected individuals, particularly the fecal–oral route. There is increasing incidence in the day-care centers, and in homosexuals practicing anilingus. It can also be obtained from contaminated water and sanitation facilities. Shigellosis begins with infrequent, voluminous watery stools. This later progresses to frequent stools with decreased volume, often containing mucus, pus, and blood. Treatment is recommended even in uncomplicated cases, as this shortens the duration of symptoms and eradicates the organisms. If left untreated, *Shigella* may cause a worsening of diarrhea, leading to dehydration. Infants are at greater risk for developing further complications. *(Braunwald et al, pp. 600–601; Wyngaarden et al, pp. 1646–1647; Dupont et al, pp. 98–136; Mandell et al, p. 1271; Krupp et al, p. 868)*

21. (C) Hepatitis B infection used to make up the majority of cases associated with posttransfusion hepatitis. With the advent of blood screening by blood banks, now less than 5% of postransfusion hepatitis cases are hepatitis B. The remainder of posttransfusion hepatitis cases are mostly hepatitis non-A, non-B, constituting approximately 90% of all cases. *(Braunwald et al, p. 1330; Wyngaarden et al, pp. 823–824; Berkow, pp. 806–861; Mandell et al, p. 1002; Krupp et al, pp. 398–400; Peicher and Schiff, p. 33)*

22. (C) Approximately 10% of hepatitis B infected individuals will still have detectable HB$_s$Ag in their blood after 6 months. A small percentage (about 3%) of these will remain HB$_s$Ag positive for years. They may be asymptomatic carriers or develop chronic active disease. This is also confirmed by liver biopsy and failure of liver function tests to return to normal. Approximately 40% to 50% of those with posttransfusion hepatitis non-A, non-B will develop chronic active disease. This too, like hepatitis B, is confirmed by failure of the liver function tests to return to normal, and liver biopsy. Unlike hepatitis B, the HB$_s$Ag will not be detectable in the serum. *(Braunwald et al, p. 1333, Wyn*

gaarden , pp. 823–824; Berkow, p. 859,861; Mandell et al, pp. 1016–1017; Krupp et al, pp. 398–400; Peicher and Schiff, p. 33)

23. (E) Scarlet fever is associated with group A *Streptococcus*. Along with other symptoms there is also a rash and fever. When the fever subsides, the upper layer of the epidermis desquamates where the rash was present.

Toxic shock syndrome is believed to be caused by a toxin-producing strain of *S aureus*. There is a fever, rash, and often hypotension associated with this disease. Desquamation of the epidermis, particularly of the palms and soles, occurs 1 week from the onset of symptoms. Scalded skin syndrome is associated with a coagulase-positive strain of staphylococci, which produces an epidermal toxin causing the skin to slough. This condition is seen most often in infants and young children.

Kawasaki's disease is a disease of unknown etiology, which consists of an exanthem, fever, lymphadenopathy, and polyarteritis. One to two weeks after the onset of symptoms, desquamation occurs to the palms, soles, and periungal areas. *(Braunwald et al; Wyngaarden et al; Krupp et al; Mandell et al; Berkow; Chapel)*

24. (B) Rocky Mountain spotted fever (RMSF) has a high incidence of occurrence in the South Atlantic states, with a high percentage of the cases occurring in North Carolina, South Carolina, Georgia, and Maryland. The disease is transmitted by the bite of the wood tick, *Dermacentor andersoni*, and the dog tick, *D variabilis*. Both these ticks act as vectors of the disease-causing organism, *rickettsii*. Clinically, the patient presents with a macular or maculopapular rash the develops into petechial lesions. Lab values often reveal a normal CBC, increased AST, ALT, and LDH. Thrombocytopenia is present in about one third of the patients. The treatment of choice is either cloramphenicol or tetracycline. *(Braunwald et al, p. 750; Wyngaarden et al, pp. 1743–1744; Berkow, pp. 151, 157; Mandell et al, pp. 1084–1085; Riley and Walker, pp. 172–189)*

25. (D) Giardia lamblia is spread from host-to-host by fecal-oral transmission. It has been associated with sexual transmission, particularly homosexuals practicing analingus. It primarily affects the duodenum and jejunum. Malabsorption may occur, possibly from mechanical blockage of the intestinal mucosa. Regardless of frequency, the stools are free from pus or blood, but may contain mucus. *Braunwald et al, p. 800; Wyngaarden et al, p. 1883; Berkow, p. 205; Mandell, et al, pp. 1553–1554, Krupp, et al, p. 914; Dupont, et al, pp. 98–137)*

26. (A) Botulism is food poisoning caused by the ingestion of the toxin *Clostridium botulinum*. It primarily affects the nervous system. In infant botulism, the ingestion of *C botulinum* spores alone can result in the disease because of toxin production in vivo. Most cases of infant botulism occur between 1 and 6 months of age, but most frequently between ages 2 and 3 months. Honey has been found to have *C botulinum* spores; therefore, it is not recommended for infants less than 12-months old. Constipation may be one of the first presenting complaints in infants. (*Braunwald et al, pp. 562–563; Wyngaarden et al, p. 1634; Berkow, p. 784; Mandell et al, pp. 1361–1362; Krupp et al, p. 872*)

27. (E) Malaria is endemic to many areas of Africa, South America, and Oceania. It is a protozoan parasitic disease caused by one of the four species from the genus *Plasmodium*. It is transmitted most commonly by the bite of an infected *Anopheles* mosquito. After returning from an endemic area, an infected individual will have recurring episodes of chills, fever, and sweating. On examination, splenomegaly is common. Herpes labialis, hepatomegaly, mild icterus, and edema may be present also. Lab findings may show a normal to low leukocyte count, decreased platelets, and an increased sedimentation rate. Demonstration of a parasite on stained blood smears is diagnostic. (*Braunwald et al, pp. 778–782; Wyngaarden et al, pp. 1857–1859; Berkow, p. 207; Mandell et al, pp. 1515–1518; Krupp et al, pp. 900–901*)

28. (B) Hepatitis A virus (HAV) is transmitted by the fecal–oral route. Compared to hepatitis B, it has a much shorter incubation period. The prodromal symptoms are varied, but include dark colored urine and clay colored stools prior to the onset of jaundice, which is the start of the clinical phase. The posticteric phase follows this, lasting 2 to 12 weeks. Lab indicators show a positive HAV antibody of the IgM class (anti-HA(IgM) during an acute infection. During the disappearance of anti-HA (IgM), the anti-HA (IgG) remains as the only serologic marker of past infection and persisting immunity. Passive immunization is possible through immune globulin injections. Exposure to the virus without clinically apparent symptoms can produce antibodies as well. Unlike hepatitis B, there is no known chronic carrier state. (*Braunwald et al, pp. 1325–1330; Wyngaarden et al, p. 821; Berkow, pp. 860–861; Mandell et al, pp. 830–835; Krupp et al, p. 397; Peicher and Schiff, pp. 23–24*)

29. (E) The definition of fever of unknown origin varies in regard to the degree of fever and the length of time the fever is present. A definition derived from various sources is a rectal temperature greater than 101° F for 2 to 3 weeks duration without an identifiable cause, after 1 week of intensive investigation.

Bacterial and viral infections are the usual causes of FUO in about 50% of cases. Of these, viral infections are the presumed etiology in most cases. The remaining causes are categorized into collagen vascular diseases, such as juvenile rheumatoid arthritis or SLE; neoplasms, such as leukemia or lymphoma; miscellaneous causes, which include factitious fever, thyrotoxicosis, and pulmonary emboli, to name a few. (*Braunwald et al, pp. 52–55; Wyngaarden et al, pp. 1524–1525; Berkow, p. 2046; Mandell et al, pp. 339–345; Krupp et al, p. 815*)

30. (D) The tuberculin skin test may be given as a screen for tuberculosis or to individuals who are suspected of harboring the disease. The preferred method of administration is 0.1 mL of 5 tuberculin units (TU) of PPD subdermally, most commonly on the volar aspect of the forearm. This is known as the Mantoux test. The multipuncture, or tine test, is used for large scale screenings, as in schools. A positive reaction is when an area of palpable induration, not erythema, of 10 mm or more at the site tested 48 to 72 hours posttest. Induration of 5 mm to 9 mm is considered nondiagnostic and can be caused by other species of nontuberculous *Mycobacterium*. (*Braunwald et al, p. 630; Wyngaarden et al, p. 1684; Berkow, p. 116; Mandell et al, p. 1389; Behrman and Vaughan, p. 630; Farer et al, pp. 148–150*)

31. (E) Isoniazid is the drug of choice for prophylactic treatment of tuberculosis. It is given in a daily dose of 300 mg for 6 to 12 months. Because of isoniazid resistant strains of *mycobacterium*, the Southeast Asian population may need multiple drug therapy for prophylactic treatment. The risk of developing tuberculosis is particularly high in close contacts of newly infected individuals, and also within 2 years after the development of a positive tuberculin skin test. The risk of developing serious tuberculosis infections, including meningitis, is particularly high among infants and adolescents. (*Braunwald et al, p. 632; Wyngaarden et al, p. 1683; Krupp et al, p. 147; Abramowicz p. 129–132*)

32. (C) Isoniazid alone for 12 months can be given prophylactically for the treatment of tuberculosis (TB), but not to treat initial uncomplicated TB. The current treatment preferred is isoniazid and rifampin daily for 6 months, with pyrazinamide added during the first 2 months. Alternatively, isoniazid and rifampin may be given daily for 9 months. In isoniazid-resistant cases, isoniazid, rifampin, and ethambutol are given for 9 months, with pyrazinamide added during the first 2 months. (*Braunwald et al, p. 631; Wyngaarden et al, p. 1683; Krupp et al, p. 147; Abramowicz p. 129–132*)

33. **(A)** Infectious mononucleosis is caused by the Epstein-Barr virus, a herpes group virus. Clinically, there is pharyngitis, lymph-adenitis, and splenomegaly. Rupture of the spleen may occur, either spontaneously or following trauma, but is infrequent. Elevated liver function tests is the norm. With ampicillin therapy, there may be an associated erythematous macular or maculopapular rash. *(Braunwald et al, pp. 701–702; Wyngaarden et al, pp. 1786–1787; Berkow, pp. 2127–2128; Mandell et al, pp. 974–975; Krupp et al, p. 848)*

REFERENCES

Abramowicz, M, ed. *Handbook of Antimicrobial Therapy,* New Rochelle, NY: The Medical Letter, 1988; 129–132.

Abramowicz, M, ed. Treatment of Lyme disease. *Med Letter.* 1989; 31:57–59.

Behrman RE, Vaughan VC III, eds. *Nelson Textbook of Pediatrics*, 13th ed. Philadelphia, PA: WB Saunders, 1987.

Berkow, R, ed. *The Merck Manual of Diagnosis and Therapy,* 15th ed. Rahway, NJ: Merck & Co; 1987.

Braunwald E, Isselbacher KJ, Petersdorf RG, Wilson JD, Martin FB, Fauci AS, eds. *Harrison's Principles of Internal Medicine,* 11th ed. New York, NY: McGraw Hill, 1987.

Chapel TA, Riley HD Jr, Russo G, Septimus E. Cutaneous signs of infection. *Patient Care.* 1988; 22:185–218.

Dupont HL, Edelman R, Kimmey M. Infectious diarrhea from A to Z. *Patient Care.* 1987;21:98–137.

Farer LS, Reichman LB, Stead WW. TB today: Don't count it out. *Patient Care.* 1987;21:141–165.

Krupp MA, Schroeder SA, Tierney LM Jr, eds. *Current Medical Diagnosis and Treatment.* Norwalk, CT: Appleton & Lange; 1987.

Mandell GL, Douglass RG Jr, Bennett JE, eds. *Principles and Practice of Infectious Disease,* 2nd ed. New York: Wiley; 1985.

Peicher J, Schiff ER. Acute viral hepatitis. *Hosp Med,* June 1988;23–41

Petri WA Jr. Tick-borne diseases. *Am Fam Physic.* 1988;37(6):95–103.

Riley HD Jr, Walker DH. Is it Rocky Mountain spotted fever? *Patient Care.* 1988;22:172–189.

Wyngaarden JB, Smith LH, eds. *Cecil Textbook of Medicine,* 18th ed. Philadelphia, PA: WB Saunders; 1988.

Infectious Disease Subspecialty List:

Question Numbers and Subspecialties

1. Infectious mononucleosis
2. Lyme disease
3. Travelers diarrhea
4. Parasitic infection
5. Botulism
6. Hepatitis
7. Hepatitis
8. Hepatitis
9. Tuberculosis
10. Tuberculosis
11. Kawasaki's disease/toxic shock syndrome
12. Kawasaki's disease/toxic shock syndrome
13. Kawasaki's disease/toxic shock syndrome
14. Lyme disease/Rocky Mountain spotted fever
15. Lyme disease/Rocky Mountain spotted fever
16. Lyme disease/Rocky Mountain spotted fever
17. Salmonella/Shigella
18. Salmonella/Shigella
19. Salmonella/Shigella
20. Salmonella/Shigella
21. Hepatitis
22. Hepatitis
23. Desquamating rashes
24. Rocky Mountain spotted fever
25. *Giardia Lamblia*
26. Infant botulism
27. Malaria
28. Hepatitis A
29. Fever of unknown origin
30. Tuberculin skin testing
31. Tuberculosis treatment
32. Tuberculosis treatment
33. Infectious mononucleosis

Internal Medicine: Cardiology

Deborah H. Lawrason

Questions

QUESTIONS AND ANSWERS

DIRECTIONS (Questions 1 through 32): For each of the items in this section, ONE or MORE of the numbered options is correct. Choose the answer

  A if only 1, 2, and 3 are correct,
  B if only 1 and 3 are correct,
  C if only 2 and 4 are correct,
  D if only 4 is correct,
  E if all are correct.

1. Prolongation of the Q–T interval can be due to

   (1) hyperkalemia
   (2) hereditary syndrome
   (3) digitalis
   (4) quinidine toxicity

2. Factors that can raise high-density lipoprotein are

   (1) exercise
   (2) cessation of cigarette smoking
   (3) therapy with gemfibrozil
   (4) elimination of caffeine from diet

3. Sick sinus syndrome includes the following rhythm disturbances

   (1) alternating slow atrial and ventricular rates with rapid atrial tachyarrhythmias
   (2) persistent sinus bradycardia
   (3) sinus arrest or exit block
   (4) a combination of SA or AV conduction abnormalities

4. Thromboembolism is a complication of

   (1) mitral regurgitation
   (2) pulmonic stenosis
   (3) mitral stenosis
   (4) aortic stenosis

5. Torsade de pointes, a pleomorphic ventricular tachycardia, can be seen with

   (1) severe bradycardia
   (2) quinidine

   (3) disopyramide
   (4) hypokalemia

6. Which of the following are necessary in a cholesterol reducing diet?

   (1) weight reduction in an obese individual
   (2) saturated fat of less than 10% of calories
   (3) cholesterol of less than 300 mg/day
   (4) total fat intake of less than 30% of total calories

7. The following statements are true regarding variant angina (Prinzmental's angina)

   (1) occurs at rest
   (2) transient ST-segment elevations on electrocardiogram
   (3) caused by vasospasm
   (4) beta-adrenergic therapy is treatment of choice

8. The following foods have high cholesterol content·

   (1) soybeans
   (2) coconuts
   (3) salmon
   (4) liver

9. The following therapeutic steps are used in the treatment of chronic congestive heart failure

   (1) digoxin
   (2) low sodium diet
   (3) vasodilators
   (4) diuretics

10. The following drugs affect serum potassium levels

   (1) captopril
   (2) diltiazem
   (3) hydrochlorothiazide
   (4) atenolol

SUMMARY OF DIRECTIONS

A	B	C	D	E
1, 2, 3 only	1, 3 only	2, 4 only	4 only	All are correct

11. In Mobitz type II second-degree AV block

    (1) every atrial impulse is conducted to a ventricle
    (2) a nonconducted P wave is preceded by sinus beats with constant PR intervals
    (3) atria and ventricle have independent pacemakers
    (4) a permanent pacemaker may be necessary

12. The following are associated with Wolff–Parkinson–White syndrome

    (1) delta wave
    (2) prolonged QRS
    (3) short PR intervals
    (4) paroxysmal atrial tachycardia

13. Electrocardiographic finding in atrial fibrillation include

    (1) grossly irregular P waves
    (2) atrial rate 250–350 beats/minute
    (3) ventricular rate 100–160
    (4) sawtooth contour to P waves

14. Precipitating causes of angina pectoris are

    (1) exercise
    (2) cold environment
    (3) walking after large meal
    (4) stress

15. In addition to medical therapy, the following non-drug therapies should be recommended for treating hypertension

    (1) weight reduction diet
    (2) reducing alcohol consumption to less than 2 oz daily
    (3) dietary sodium restriction
    (4) low cholesterol, low-fat diet

16. Inverted T waves can be seen with

    (1) myocardial ischemia
    (2) left ventricular hypertrophy
    (3) subendocardial infarction
    (4) hyperkalemia

17. In congestive heart failure, the following features may be seen on a chest roentgenogram

    (1) increased size and shape of cardiac silhouette
    (2) pulmonary vascular redistribution

    (3) pleural effusions
    (4) Kerley's lines

18. High output heart failure can be caused by

    (1) anemia
    (2) thyrotoxicosis
    (3) pregnancy
    (4) hypertension

19. Which of the following is/are true of one-man cardiopulmonary resuscitation for adults?

    (1) ratio of compressions to breaths is 15:2
    (2) ratio of compression to breaths is 5:1
    (3) rate of compressions is 80–100 times per minute
    (4) rate of compression is at least 100 times per minute

20. Which of the following statements is/are true regarding HDL cholesterol

    (1) removes cholesterol from peripheral tissues
    (2) transports cholesterol to peripheral cells
    (3) low HDL cholesterol (35 mg/daily) is a risk factor for coronary heart disease
    (4) cigarette smoking raises HDL

21. When performing cardiopulmonary resuscitation for small children

    (1) the ratio is 5 compressions to 1 breath
    (2) the rate of compressions is 80–100 times per minute
    (3) depress the sternum 1 to 1½ inches
    (4) use the heel of one hand

22. The following adverse effects are associated with beta-adrenergic blocking agents

    (1) peripheral vasospasm
    (2) fatigue
    (3) insomnia, nightmares
    (4) bronchospasm

23. Complications of hypertension are

    (1) dissecting aortic aneurysm
    (2) myocardial infarction
    (3) cerebral hemorrhage
    (4) aortic stenosis

24. Which of the following is/are true in regards to abdominal aortic aneurysms

    (1) pain located in hypogastrium and lower back
    (2) rupture of an aneurysm results in hypotension and shock
    (3) majority of abdominal aortic aneurysms are asymptomatic
    (4) surgery recommended for aneurysms 3 cm in width or wider

25. Clinical manifestations of thoraic aortic aneurysms is/are

(1) dysphagia
(2) chest pain
(3) tacheal deviation
(4) cough

26. Causes of sudden cardiac death include

(1) hypertrophic obstructive cardiomyopathy
(2) aortic stenosis
(3) coronary heart disease
(4) acute heart failure

27. A new loud systolic murmur in a patient with an acute myocardial infarction can be the result of

(1) left ventricular aneurysm
(2) ventriculoseptal defect
(3) pericarditis
(4) rupture of papillary muscle

28. A mechanical prosthetic heart valve

(1) has an excellent record of durability
(2) is associated with increased incidence of thromboembolism
(3) requires patients to receive anticoagulation therapy
(4) has limited durability

29. The following is/are true regarding an atrial septal defect

(1) results in a left-to-right shunt
(2) most common ASD is ostium secundum type
(3) usually asymptomatic in early life
(4) often diagnosed in early infancy

30. Indications for cardiac pacing include

(1) first-degree AV block
(2) asymptomatic bundle branch block
(3) asymptomatic sick sinus syndrome
(4) symptomatic bradycardia

31. Causes of atrial fibrillation include

(1) rheumatic heart disease
(2) thyrotoxicosis
(3) coronary heart disease
(4) pulmonary emboli

32. Adverse reactions associated with nitroglycerin administration are

(1) headache
(2) hypotension
(3) flushing
(4) nausea and vomiting

DIRECTIONS (Questions 33 through 58): Each of the numbered items or incomplete statements in this section is followed by answers or by completions of the statement. Select the ONE lettered answer or completion that is BEST in each case.

33. Mitral regurgitation may result from abnormalities of all of the following structures EXCEPT

(A) mitral annulus
(B) left atrium
(C) papillary muscles
(D) chordae tendinae
(E) mitral leaflets

34. In severe aortic stenosis, all the following are indications for valve replacement EXCEPT

(A) angina
(B) dyspnea on exertion
(C) palpitations
(D) congestive heart failure
(E) syncope

35. All the following physical findings are characteristic of an aortic regurgitation murmur EXCEPT

(A) wide pulse pressure
(B) diastolic murmur
(C) waterhammer pulse
(D) loud S_1
(E) bisferious pulse

36. The earliest symptom of left-sided heart failure is

(A) orthopnea
(B) pedal edema
(C) paroxysmal nocturnal dyspnea
(D) dyspnea on exertion
(E) fatigue

37. All the following are causes of pericarditis EXCEPT

(A) Dressler's syndrome
(B) trauma
(C) uremia
(D) neoplasm
(E) liver disease

38. All the following statements are true of hypertrophic cardiomyopathy EXCEPT

(A) dyspnea is the most common
(B) systolic ejection murmur is present
(C) associated with sudden death
(D) symptoms increase with exertion
(E) left ventricular hypertrophy is present on echocardiogram

39. All the following medications can aggravate hyperlipidemia **EXCEPT**

   (A) captopril
   (B) thiazide diuretic
   (C) oral contraceptives
   (D) anabolic steroids
   (E) progestins

40. Features of mitral valve prolapse include all the following, **EXCEPT**

   (A) midsystolic clicks
   (B) nonspecific ST–T changes on EKG
   (C) mid-to-late crescendo systolic murmur
   (D) majority of patients are asymptomatic
   (E) S_4 gallop

41. Elevated levels of the following lipoprotein increase the risk of coronary heart disease

   (A) chylomicrons
   (B) triglycerides
   (C) LDL
   (D) VLDL
   (E) HDL

42. All of the following are contraindications to stress testing, **EXCEPT**

   (A) unstable angina
   (B) congestive heart failure
   (C) severe hypertension
   (D) severe aortic stenosis
   (E) premature ventricular contractions

43. The most common cause of mitral stenosis is

   (A) lupus
   (B) bacterial endocarditis
   (C) trauma
   (D) rheumatic fever
   (E) congenital

44. All the following are used in the management of unstable angina **EXCEPT**

   (A) bed rest
   (B) nitrates
   (C) beta-adrenergic blockers
   (D) calcium-channel blockers
   (E) digoxin

45. The most useful cardiac enzyme test for myocardial necrosis is

   (A) creatine kinase —MM
   (B) creatine kinase —MB
   (C) glutamic oxaloacetic transferase
   (D) lactic dehydrogenase
   (E) alkaline phosphatase

46. The major cause of cardiogenic shock is

   (A) perforation of the interventricular septum
   (B) acute myocardial infarction
   (C) atrioventricular block
   (D) pulmonary embolism
   (E) severe bradycardia

47. The standard endocarditis prophylaxis recommendation for dental procedures or surgery of the upper respiratory tract is

   (A) penicillin V 1.0 g orally on the day before procedure and 1.0 g 1 hour after procedure
   (B) penicillin V 2.0 g orally 6 hours before procedure and 1.0 g 6 hours later
   (C) penicillin V 2.0 g orally 1 hour before procedure and 1.0 g 1 hour later
   (D) penicillin V 2.0 g orally 1 hour before procedure and 1.0 g 6 hours later
   (E) penicillin V 1.0 g orally 1 hour before procedure and 1.0 g 6 hours later

48. The following electrocardiogram (Figure 6–1) shows

   (A) left ventricular hypertrophy
   (B) anterolateral ischemia
   (C) acute true posterior wall myocardial infarction
   (D) a normal electrocardiogram
   (E) incomplete right bundle branch block

49. The following electrocardiogram (Figure 6–2) shows

   (A) sinus tachycardia
   (B) supraventricular tachycardia
   (C) ventricular tachycardia
   (D) left bundle branch block
   (E) Wolf–Parkinson–White syndrome

50. The following electrocardiogram (Fig. 6–3) demonstrates:

   (A) acute anterior wall myocardial infarction
   (B) old inferior wall myocardial infarction
   (C) left bundle branch block
   (D) early repolarization
   (E) pericarditis

51. The following electrocardiogram (Figure 6–4) demonstrated

   (A) alternating sinus and paced beats
   (B) intermittent bundle branch block
   (C) ventricular escape beats
   (D) premature atrial contractions
   (E) ventricular bigeminy

Figure 6-1.

Figure 6-2.

Figure 6–3.

52. The following electrocardiogram (Figure 6–5) shows

    (A) atrial fibrillation
    (B) atrial flutter with 2:1 block
    (C) sinus tachycardia
    (D) multifocal atrial tachycardia
    (E) atrial flutter with 4:1 block

53. Absolute contraindications to thrombolytic therapy include all the following **EXCEPT**

    (A) history of cerebrovascular disease
    (B) history of significant gastrointestinal bleeding
    (C) severe uncontrolled hypertension
    (D) diabetes
    (E) recent history of severe trauma

Figure 6–4.

Figure 6–5.

54. Following percutaneous transluminal coronary angioplasty (PTCA), 20% of patients will develop signs of restenosis after

(A) 6 months
(B) 8 months
(C) 10 months
(D) 12 months
(E) 24 months

55. The most common cause of syncope is

(A) seizure
(B) arrhythmia
(C) vasovagal hypotension
(D) transient ischemic attack
(E) hypoglycemia

56. The major side effect of bile acid sequestrants such as cholestryramine is

(A) gastrointestinal
(B) myositis
(C) flushing
(D) rash
(E) reversible liver damage

57. Renovascular hypertension should be suspected with all the following clinical features **EXCEPT**

(A) severe, rapidly accelerating hypertension
(B) presence of an abdominal bruit

(C) onset of hypertension before age 30, particularly in slender, white women
(D) headaches, sweating, and palpitations
(E) onset of hypertension after renal trauma

58. Precipitating causes of heart failure include

(A) systemic infarction
(B) arrhythmias
(C) inappropriate reduction of therapy
(D) dietary sodium excesses
(E) all of the above

DIRECTIONS (Questions 59 through 80): Each group of items in this section consists of lettered headings followed by a set of numbered words or phrases. For each numbered word or phrase, select the ONE lettered heading that is most closely associated with it. Each lettered heading may be selected once, more than once, or not at all.

Questions 59 through 62

(A) aortic stenosis
(B) mitral regurgitation
(C) both
(D) neither

59. pansystolic murmur

60. radiates to axilla

61. bicuspid valve

62. murmur reduced during valsalva maneuver

Questions 63 through 65

(A) increases myocardial oxygen supply
(B) decrease myocardial oxygen demand
(C) both
(D) neither

63. propranolol

64. diltiazem

65. nitroglycerin

Questions 66 through 69

(A) affects serum lipids
(B) affects serum potassium levels
(C) both
(D) neither

66. captopril

67. hydrocholorothiazide

68. diltiazem

69. clonidine

Questions 70 through 73

For each of the antihypertensive drugs listed below, select the mechanism of action with which it is associated

(A) calcium channel blockers
(B) beta-adrenergic blockers
(C) angiotensin-converting enzyme inhibitor
(D) alpha-adrenergic receptor blocker
(E) vasodilator

70. enalapril

71. verapamil

72. metoprolol

73. prazosin

Questions 74 through 77

For each of the heart sounds listed below, select the appropriate origin of the sound

(A) S_1
(B) S_2
(C) S_3
(D) S_4
(E) Opening snap

74. caused by closure of aortic and pulmonic valves

75. associated with atrial contraction in a hypertrophied heart

76. caused by closure of mitral and tricuspid valve

77. heart with left ventricular failure

Questions 78 through 80

Match the congenital heart defect with the appropriate description

(A) atrial septal defect
(B) ventricular septal defect
(C) coarctation of the aorta
(D) patent foramen ovale
(E) patent ductus arteriosis

78. most common congenital malformation in infants and children

79. Cause of surgically correctable hypertension

80. Patient may remain asymptomatic until over the age of forty

Answers and Explanations

1. **(C)** Prolongation of the Q–T interval is associated with two hereditary syndromes. In the Romano–Ward syndrome, affected individuals have prolonged Q–T intervals, normal hearing, and an autosomal dominant inheritance pattern. In Jervall and Lange–Nelson syndrome, the patients have prolonged Q–T intervals, congenital deafness, and autosomal recessive inheritance pattern. Prolongation of the Q–T interval may occur with Type Ia antiarrhythmic drugs, such as quinidine, procainamide, and disopyramide. Hyperkalemia and digitalis will cause shortening of the Q–T interval. *(Braunwald, pp. 699, 749)*

2. **(A)** High-density lipoprotein removes cholesterol from the tissues. There is an inverse relationship between high-density lipoprotein and coronary artery disease. Exercise, cessation of cigarette smoking, and medical therapy with gemfibrozil all raise the HDL level. Gemfibrozil is a lipid regulating drug that lowers serum triglyceride and total serum cholesterol and also increases HDL. Caffeine use is not a factor in raising or lowering the HDL. *(Braunwald, pp. 1161–1162, 1170–1171)*

3. **(E)** Sick sinus syndrome is the result of sinus node dysfunction. The rhythm disturbances include bradycardia–tachycardia syndrome, persistent sinus bradycardia, sinus arrest or exit block, or a combination of SA or AV conduction abnormalities. A patient can have more than one of these conductive disturbances. Patients with symptomatic sick sinus syndrome (such as syncope, dizziness) generally require a permanent pacemaker. *(Braunwald, p. 667)*

4. **(B)** Thromboembolism is a complication of mitral valve disease due to dilation of the left atrium and increased left atrial pressures. With left atrial enlargement, there is a predisposition to atrial fibrillation. *(Braunwald, pp. 1026, 1027)*

5. **(E)** Torsade de pointes is a rapid pleomorphic ventricular tachycardia in which the amplitude and polarity of QRS complexes continuously change and appear to be rotating around an isoelectric baseline. Torsade de pointes occurs in the setting of prolonged ventricular repolarization. The most common causes are potassium depletion, severe bradycardia, and type Ia antiarrhythmics, such as quinidine and disopyramide. *(Braunwald, pp. 698–699)*

6. **(E)** The National Cholesterol Education Program has recommended that the first step in lowering cholesterol is dietary treatment. Cholesterol can be reduced by following a diet with a cholesterol intake of less than 300 mg/day, a total fat intake of less than 30% of the total calories. Weight reduction is recommended in the obese individual to help lower cholesterol. *(National Cholesterol Education Program, pp. 1–7)*

7. **(A)** Prinzmetal's variant angina occurs while the patient is at rest. It is caused by spasm of the major coronary artery. The spasm is usually superimposed upon a fixed atherosclerotic coronary stenosis, but it can also occur in individuals with coronary arteries that are free of significant narrowing. During episodes of vasospasm, there is transmural myocardial ischemia that leads to ST-segment elevation. Long-acting nitrates and calcium channel blockers are used to prevent vasospasm. *(Braunwald, pp. 1360–1361)*

8. **(D)** Cholesterol is found only in foods from animal origin (such as meats, whole milk, cheeses, butter, eggs, ice cream, lard). Soybeans have polyunsaturated fats, which are found in foods of plant origin and decrease cholesterol. Salmon contains omega-3 fatty acids, which are polyunsaturated fats and decrease cholesterol. Saturated fats will raise cholesterol. Saturated fats are generally derived from foods of animal origin. The exceptions are coconut oil and palm oil, which come from plant sources but are highly saturated. *(Braunwald, pp. 1167–1168)*

9. **(E)** When treating chronic heart failure, simple therapeutic means, such as restricting sodium intake and diuretics, are often the first line of therapy. If the symptoms or physical signs of heart failure continue, vasodilators and/or a digitalis glycoside may be used. Vasodilators are used to reduce the heart's workload. Digitalis helps to improve cardiac contractility. (*Braunwald, pp. 485–488*)

10. **(B)** Captopril is a potassium-sparing agent. It is an angiotensin-converting enzyme inhibitor and blocks the formation of angiotensin II, which stimulates aldosterone production. By decreasing aldosterone production, serum potassium levels may increase. Hydrochlorothiazide is a diuretic that can lower serum potassium levels. Hypokalemia can cause muscle weakness, polyuria, leg cramps, or increased ventricular ectopy. Diltiazem, a calcium channel blocker, and atenolol, a beta-adrenergic blocking agent, do not affect serum potassium levels. (*Braunwald, pp. 870, 877*)

11. **(C)** In first-degree AV block, every atrial impulse is conducted to the ventricle. In second-degree AV block, every atrial impulse is not conducted to the ventricles. A nonconducted P wave is preceded by sinus beats with constant PR intervals in Mobitz type II second-degree AV block. Adams–Stokes syncope and complete AV block (atria and ventricle have independent pacemakers) are often preceded by Mobitz type II second-degree AV block and a permanent pacemaker is necessary. (*Braunwald, pp. 702–706*)

12. **(E)** The classical electrocardiographic findings in Wolff–Parkinson–White syndrome are a short PR interval (less than 0.12 seconds), delta wave (initial slurring of the QRS complex), and wide QRS (greater than 0.12 seconds). These findings are caused by preexcitation of the ventricles. In Wolff–Parkinson–White syndrome, patients possess an accessory pathway that originates in one of the atria and terminates in one of the ventricles. The most common arrhythmia associated with Wolff–Parkinson–White syndrome is paroxysmal atrial tachycardia. The tachycardia is based upon a circus movement involving the myocardium, accessory pathway, and atrial myocardium. (*Braunwald, pp. 202–203, 605–606*)

13. **(B)** In atrial fibrillation, the P waves are grossly irregular due to disorganized atrial depolarization. There is no effective atrial contraction. The atrial rate may be 350 to 600 beats per minute with a ventricular response of 100 to 160 beats per minute. In atrial flutter, the P waves are regular, with a sawtooth appearance. The atrial rate in atrial flutter is 250 to 350 beats per minute. (*Braunwald, pp. 660, 672–673*)

14. **(E)** In angina, chest pain is related to an increase in myocardial oxygen demand that can occur with exercise, walking after a large meal, and exposure to cold weather. Stress causes a rise in heart rate and blood pressure, which also increases myocardial oxygen demand. Moreover, angina can occur during episodes of coronary vasoconstriction as a result of a transient decrease in myocardial oxygen supply. (*Braunwald, pp. 1316–1317*)

15. **(A)** Weight loss can be effective in lowering blood pressure and may delay or avoid the need for medical therapy. It has been shown that heavy alcohol consumption increases the risk of developing hypertension. It is recommended that alcohol be limited to less than 2 ounces per day. Dietary sodium restriction will help reduce blood pressure. Moderate sodium restriction can be accomplished by following simple guidelines such as not adding salt to food during cooking or at the table and avoiding obviously high-sodium foods (i.e., processed foods). High cholesterol levels have little effect on blood pressure. A low cholesterol, low-fat diet will reduce the risk of developing coronary heart disease. (*Braunwald, pp. 837, 865–867*)

16. **(A)** Inverted T waves are caused by a number of conditions including myocardial ischemia, subendocardial infarction, and left ventricular hypertrophy. A high serum potassium causes tall and peaked T waves. As the hyperkalemia worsens, the PR interval is prolonged and the QRS can widen. (*Clinical Synopsia-CIBA, pp. 27–30*)

17. **(E)** A chest roentgenogram in a patient with congestive heart failure may show an enlarged cardiac silhouette, pulmonary vascular redistribution, pleural effusions, and Kerley's lines. Pulmonary vascular redistribution is a result of interstitial and perivascular edema developing in the lung bases that leads to compression of the vessels in the lower lobes. With constriction of the lower lobe vessels, dilation of the vessels to the upper lobes occurs. With increased pulmonary, and capillary pressures, pulmonary edema develops and may lead to pleural effusions or Kerley's lines. Kerley's lines are sharp, linear densities caused by edema. (*Braunwald, p. 483*)

18. **(A)** High output heart failure can occur with anemia, thyrotoxicosis, and pregnancy. With these conditions, the cardiac output is markedly elevated and the heart must pump an abnormally large volume. If the heart cannot adapt to the higher demands imposed by hypermetabolic or hyperkinetic states, then cardiac decompensation will occur. Hypertension can lead to a low cardiac output failure. (*Braunwald, pp. 778–790*)

19. (B) In cardiopulmonary resuscitation, one must open the airway and provide rescue breathing and artificial circulation. Artificial circulation is done by external chest compressions at a rate of 80 to 100 times per minute in an adult. Chest compressions are done at least 100 times per minute in an infant. The ratio of chest compressions to breaths is 15:2 in one-man CPR. In two-man CPR, the ratio is 5 compressions to one breath. *(JAMA, p. 2905)*

20. (B) HDL-cholesterol removes cholesterol from peripheral tissues and carries it to the liver. In the liver, HDL is broken down into bile and acid salts and eliminated. Studies have indicated that a low HDL (35 mg/dL) is a risk factor for coronary artery disease. Cigarette smoking lowers HDL, and exercise can raise it. Low-density lipoproteins (LDL) transport cholesterol to the peripheral cells. *(Braunwald, pp. 1161–1162; National Cholesterol Education Program, pp. 1–7)*

21. (E) When performing cardiopulmonary resuscitation in a small child, the heel of one hand should depress the sterum 1 to 1½ inches. The ratio of compression to breaths is 5:1 at a rate of 80 to 100 compression per minute. *(Effren, p. 33)*

22. (E) Beta-adrenergic blocking agents are used in the treatment of hypertension, coronary artery disease, and arrhythmias. The side effects are associated with the blockade of B_1 and B_2 receptors. Patients can complain of cold extremities and increased claudication, which is caused by peripheral vasospasm. Fatigue, insomnia, and hallucinations are direct effects of the beta blockers on the central nervous system. These side effects occur less often with lipid insoluble beta blockers (i.e., atenolol) that enter the brain in lower concentration. A beta-blocker can induce bronchospasm and is a relative contraindication in a patient with a history of asthma or bronchospasm. If a beta blocker is used in a patient with lung disease, a cardioselective agent should be considered. *(Kaplan, pp. 218–227)*

23. (A) Aortic dissection, myocardial infarction, and cerebral hemorrhage are all complications of hypertension. Aortic dissections in hypertensives may result from a combination of atherosclerosis and high pulsative wave stress. The major cause of stroke is hypertension and is directly related to the blood pressure elevation. *(Kaplan, pp. 136–143)*

24. (A) The majority of abdominal aortic aneurysms are asymptomatic and may be found on routine physical exam. If pain is present, it may be steady and located in the hypogastrium and lower back. Rupture of an aneurysm is associated with severe abdominal and/or back pain, hypotension, and shock. A normal aorta is 2 cm in diameter. Surgery is recommended, if possible, when the aortic aneurysm is 6 cm in diameter or wider. Fifty percent of aneurysms greater than 6 cm in diameter may rupture in 1 year. *(Braunwald, pp. 1548–1550)*

25. (E) Signs and symptoms of thoracic aneurysms are related to their size and location. Cough and deviation of the trachea occur with aneurysms of the descending thoracic aorta as a result of compression of the tracheobrachial tree and lung. Dysphagia occurs when there is compression of the esophagus and chest pain is related to compression of musculoskeletal structures. *(Braunwald, pp. 1551–1552)*

26. (E) Sudden cardiac death is defined as an unexpected natural death that is due to cardiac problems and associated with abrupt loss of consciousness. The most common cause of sudden cardiac death is coronary heart disease. Sudden cardiac disease in hypertrophic obstructive cardiomyopathy and aortic stenosis may be related to cardiac arrhythmias. Acute heart failure may cause sudden cardiac death as a result of arrhythmias or circulatory failure. *(Braunwald, pp. 742–749)*

27. (C) Serious complications of an acute myocardial infarction are rupture of the interventricular septum and rupture of a papillary muscle. A loud systolic murmur may be associated with both these complications. A differentiation can be made with a two-dimensional echocardiogram with Doppler. *(Braunwald, pp. 1283–1285)*

28. (A) Two major types of artificial valves are mechanical prostheses and bioprostheses (tissue valves). Mechanical valves have an excellent record of durability but are also associated with an increased risk of thromboembolism. With the hazard of thromboembolism, patients require anticoagulation therapy. Tissue valves were developed to decrease the risk of thromboembolism but are not as durable as mechanical valves. *(Braunwald pp. 1078–1081)*

29. (A) An atrial septal defect causes left-to-right shunt. The most common ASD is the ostium secundum type that is located in the region of the foramen ovale. An atrial septal defect is rarely diagnosed or causes symptoms in early life. Symptoms often develop in adults and include dyspnea, fatigue, supraventricular arrhythmias, and respiratory illness. *(Braunwald, pp. 915–916, 982)*

30. (D) One indication for cardiac pacing is symptomatic bradycardia. Medical therapy is usually not successful in speeding up the heart, so a pacemaker is indicated. Patients with asymptomatic bundle branch block and first degree AV block do not require cardiac pacing. Cardiac pacing is not indicated in asymptomatic sick sinus syndrome. If symptoms appear, however, a permanent pacemaker is indicated. (Braunwald, pp. 667, 717–718)

31. (E) Atrial fibrillation can occur in normal hearts or be associated with heart disease. Atrial fibrillation is associated with rheumatic heart disease, pulmonary emboli, coronary heart disease, hypertensive cardiovascular disease, cardiomyopathy, atrial septal defect, and following cardiac surgery. Thryotoxicosis can also be a precipitating cause of atrial fibrillation. (Braunwald, pp. 673)

32. (A) Headache, flushing, and hypotension are adverse reactions that are associated with nitroglycerin administration. The side effects are a result of the vasodilator properties of nitrates. (Braunwald, pp. 1327–1329)

33. (B) Mitral regurgitation can be associated with abnormalities of the mitral annulus, papillary muscles, chordae tendinae, and mitral leaflets. Disorders of the mitral annulus (i.e., rheumatic heart disease abscess), or dilation of left ventricle from heart disease result in dilation of mitral annulus. Papillary muscle dysfunction causes mitral regurgitation. This can be seen with an acute myocardial infarction or ischemia, because the papillary muscles are perfused by the coronary arteries. The cordae tendinae can rupture as a result of trauma, rheumatic fever, myxomatous degeneration, endocarditis, or a congenital abnormality. Abnormalities of the mitral leaflets are seen most frequently in rheumatic heart disease. (Braunwald, pp. 1034–1037)

34. (C) Angina, dyspnea on exertion, congestive heart failure, and syncope are indicators for valve replacement in aortic stenosis. Angina is due to the increased oxygen needs of the hypertrophied left ventricle and decreased oxygen delivery as a result of compression of the coronary arteries. Dyspnea on exertion and congestive heart failure are late symptoms and are caused by pulmonary venous hypertension. Syncope usually occurs during exertion as a result of a drop in cardiac output or a ventricular arrhythmia. (Braunwald, pp. 1057–1059)

35. (D) A loud S_1 is not present in aortic regurgitation. The murmur of aortic regurgitation is a high-pitched diastolic murmur. It begins immediately after A_2 and is best heard along the left sternal border, 3rd and 4th intercostal spaces. The systolic arterial pressure is elevated and the diastolic pressure is low resulting in a wide pulse pressure. The pulses are abrupt with a quick collapse and are often described as a waterhammer pulse. A bisferious pulse is present. (Braunwald, pp. 1064–1605)

36. (D) Dyspnea on exertion is usually the earliest symptom of left-sided heart failure. Patients with left ventricular disease develop high left ventricular filling pressures with exercise. This results in increased pulmonary capillary and pulmonary venous pressures causing shortness of breath with exertion. Orthopnea and paroxysmal nocturnal dyspnea usually develop at a later stage of left ventricular failure. Fatigue is often a complaint in patients with heart failure and low cardiac output. (Cohn, pp. 129–131)

37. (E) Liver disease is not a cause of acute pericarditis. Dressler's syndrome is characterized by acute pericarditis, fever, and pleuritis. It is an autoimmune syndrome that occurs weeks to months after an acute myocardial infarction. Chest trauma may result in the development of an acute pericarditis. Uremic pericarditis is a complication of chronic renal failure. The exact cause is unknown. Patients with malignant neoplasms may present with an acute pericarditis. Pericardial effusions can occur as a result of metastatic involvement of the pericardium. Primary tumors of the pericardium are rare. (Braunwald, p. 1488)

38. (D) Hypertrophic cardiomyopathy is a disease characterized by hypertrophy of the cardiac muscle without any identifiable cause. On physical exam, a systolic ejection murmur is best heard at the lower left sternal border and apex. Dyspnea is the most common symptom. Angina and syncope are also common complaints. Syncopal episodes are often related to arrhythmias. Ventricular arrhythmias are probably responsible for the majority of sudden death cases. The symptoms are increased with exertion. Syncope and sudden death have been associated with extreme exertion. Left ventricular hypertrophy is seen on the echocardiogram. (Braunwald, pp. 1422–1426)

39. (A) Captopril is an angiotension-converting enzyme inhibitor. It does not affect serum lipid levels. A thiazide diuretic can cause an elevation of low-density lipoproteins cholesterol, which is an atherogenic class of lipoproteins. Oral contraceptives, progestins, and anabolic steroids can also raise serum levels of lipoproteins. (Braunwald, pp. 515–516, 1167)

40. (E) Mitral valve prolapse syndrome is one of the most common valvular abnormalities. The majority of patients with MVP are asymptomatic. Symptomatic patients may complain of chest pain and palpitations. The chest pain is often atypical and is

not related to exertion and can be prolonged. Palpitations can be associated with atrial and ventricular premature contractions as well as supraventricular and ventricular tachyarrhythmias. The ausculatory findings associated with MVP syndrome are a midsystolic click and late systolic murmur. There is a great variability in physical findings. Patients may have both a click and a murmur or only one of the findings. The electrocardiogram can show nonspecific ST-T wave changes. (*Braunwald, pp. 1044–1049*)

41. **(C)** Patients with high LDL cholesterol (106 mg/dL) are at increased risk for developing coronary heart disease. LDL cholesterol transports cholesterol to peripheral cells. Elevated LDL will increase serum cholesterol levels. Very low-density lipoproteins (VLDL) are produced by the liver and small intestine. Triglycerides are very low-density lipoproteins. High levels of triglycerides can cause pancreatitis. Chylomicrons are large lipoprotein particles that consist of cholesterol and triglycerides. HDL cholesterol is inversely correlated with the risk of coronary heart disease. HDL cholesterol removes cholesterol from peripheral tissues and carries it back to the liver where it is eliminated. (*National Cholesterol Education Program, p. 17; Braunwald, pp. 1154–1162*)

42. **(E)** Contraindications to stress testing include unstable angina, congestive heart failure, severe hypertension, and severe aortic stenosis. Exercise can aggravate any of these clinical conditions. A patient with mild to moderate aortic stenosis may exercise safely but there is a risk of syncope or sudden death with aortic stenosis during vigorous exercise. A patient with premature ventricular contractions can safely do an exercise stress test. (*Braunwald, p. 238.*)

43. **(D)** Rheumatic fever is the major cause of mitral stenosis. Most patients do not develop symptoms of mitral stenosis for at least a decade after the onset of acute rheumatic fever. (*Braunwald, p. 1023*)

44. **(E)** Unstable angina is a serious condition and may be a warning of an impending myocardial infarction. The management of unstable angina includes bed rest, nitrates, beta-adrenergic blockers, and calcium channel blockers. Nitrates are the mainstay of therapy. They relieve pain and may improve global and left ventricular function. (*Braunwald, pp. 1353–1358*)

45. **(B)** Enzymes are released into the circulation by injured myocardial cells. Elevations of serum glutamic oxaloacetic transferase (SGOT), lactic dehydrogenase, and creatine kinase – MB (CK-MB) are used in the diagnosis of an acute myocardial infarction. There are three isoenzymes of creatine kinase – MM, BB, and MB. MM isoenzyme is present primarily in skeletal muscle. Brain and kidney contain BB isoenzyme and cardiac muscle contains MM isoenzyme and MB isoenzyme. Elevated CK–MB is usually the result of an acute myocardial infarction and is the most sensitive enzyme test for myocardial necrosis. (*Braunwald, pp. 1239–1241*)

46. **(B)** The major cause of cardiogenic shock is acute myocardial infarction. Cardiogenic shock occurs primarily with an anterior and anteroseptal myocardial infarction. The onset and severity of cardiogenic shock is related to the amount of functional myocardium that is lost. (*Braunwald, p. 572*)

47. **(D)** The present recommended antibiotic regimen for dental procedures and surgery of the upper respiratory tract is penicillin V 2.0 g orally 1 hour before the procedure then 1.0 g 6 hours later. Patients allergic to penicillin can take erythromycin 1.0 g orally 1 hour before and 50 mg 6 hours later. (*Shulman et al, pp. 1124A–1125B*)

48. **(C)** The ECG shows a true posterior myocardial infarction, indicating a prominent R wave in V_1–V_2. In the acute phase, there may be ST-segment depression with a tall, upright T wave in the right precordial leads as demonstrated in this ECG. (*Braunwald, p. 211*)

49. **(C)** This ECG shows a ventricular tachycardia at a rate of 150 beats per minute. Ventricular tachycardia is defined as three or more ventricular premature beats. The QRS complexes are widened and bizarre in appearance. (*Braunwald, pp. 694–695*)

50. **(A)** This ECG shows an acute anterior wall myocardial infarction with Q waves and loss of the R wave in leads V_1–V_4. There is ST-segment elevation in V_1–V_4, with T wave inversion in V_2–V_4. (*Scheidt, p. 19*)

51. **(E)** This ECG shows ventricular bigeminy. In ventricular bigeminy, there is pairing of a normal beat with a ventricular premature beat. In this ECG, ventricular premature beats have different contours and are multifocal. (*Braunwald, p. 693*)

52. **(B)** This ECG shows atrial flutter with 2:1 block. Regular sawtooth flutter waves are seen. The AV conduction rate remains constant with an atrial rate of 300 beats per minute and a ventricular rate of 150 beat per minute. In atrial fibrillation, the ventricular rhythm is grossly irregular with an atrial rate of 400 to 600 beats per minute. In sinus tachycardia, the atrial and ventricular rate is 100 to 180 beats per minute. Multifocal atrial tachycar-

dia is characterized by a marked variation in P-wave morphology and irregular P–P intervals. The atrial rate is 100 to 130 beats per minute. (Braunwald, pp. 660, 671–672, 675)

53. **(D)** Thrombolytic agents (i.e., streptokinase, tissue plasminogen activator (t-PA), have been used to lyse clots in an effort to limit myocardial infarctions. There is a possibility of bleeding complication with thrombolytic agents, so patients must be screened carefully. Absolute contraindications include a history of cerebrovascular disease, gastrointestinal bleeding, severe uncontrolled hypertension, bleeding diathesis, and recent severe trauma. (Braunwald, pp. 1253–1257)

54. **(A)** In PTCA, restenosis will occur within 6 months in approximately 20% of patients. Patients should be closely followed clinically and with exercise tests in the 6 months after PTCA. If restenosis develops, repeat catheterization with repeat PTCA, is often successful. (Braunwald, p. 1387)

55. **(C)** Vasovagal hypotension, which is the common faint, is the most common type of syncope. This is often precipitated by the sight of blood, a stressful or painful experience (i.e., venipuncture, trauma), crowding, and prolonged standing. The signs and symptoms associated with vasovagal syncope are pallor, weakness, nausea, and diaphoresis. The symptoms usually occur when the patient is in an upright position. It can usually be differentiated from other causes of syncope by the type of setting in which it happens, appearance of the patient and knowledge of the onset. (Braunwald, pp. 887–892)

56. **(A)** Bile acid sequestrants are used in the treatment of lipid disorders. They are often difficult to take because of the frequent gastrointestinal side effects, such as constipation, abdominal distension, nausea, vomiting, or diarrhea. Myositis and reversible liver damage are side effects associated with lovastatin. Flushing is a side effect of nicotinic acid. (Braunwald, p. 1169)

57. **(D)** The two major types of renovascular hypertension are caused by atherosclerotic disease and fibroplastic disease. Atherosclerotic disease is seen mostly in older men, whereas fibroplastic disease is seen more frequently in younger women. Renovascular disease should be suspected if the following clinical features are present: (1) abdominal bruit, particularly if lateral to midline; (2) severe, rapidly accelerating hypertension; (3) onset of hypertension before age 30, particularly in white women, as it may be due to fibroplastic disease; (4) onset after renal trauma; (5) rapidly deteriorating renal function. Headache, flushing, and palpita-

tions are associated with a pheochromocytoma. (Braunwald, pp. 842–843, 847)

58. **(E)** A number of events may precipitate heart failure in a previously compensated individual. The most common events are a reduction in therapy or dietary sodium excess. A patient may adjust his or her own medication as he/she begins to feel better or be more lenient with the sodium intake and precipitate heart failure. Tachyarrhythmias, bradycardia, atrial–ventricular dissociation, abnormal intraventricular conduction can all intensify heart failure. Systemic infections can increase the hemodynamic burden of the heart and precipitate heart failure. (Braunwald, pp. 474–475)

59. **(B)** Mitral regurgitation is a pansystolic murmur. It usually begins immediately after S1 and continues throughout systole. It is blowing, high pitched, and of constant intensity. Aortic stenosis is a crescendo decrescendo ejection murmur. It usually begins after the onset of S1 and ends before A2. (Braunwald, pp. 70, 1055–1057)

60. **(B)** The murmur of mitral regurgitation is best heard at the apex but can radiate to the axilla and occasionally the base of the heart. The murmur of aortic stenosis is best heard at the base of the heart but can radiate to the neck and apex. (Braunwald, pp. 1055–1057, 1040–1042)

61. **(A)** The normal aortic valve is tricuspid. Aortic stenosis can occur as a result of a congenital bicuspid valve. The bicuspid valve causes turbulent flow resulting in fibrosis and narrowing of the aortic valve. (Braunwald, pp. 1052–1054)

62. **(C)** With the valsalva maneuver, there is a decline in systemic venous return resulting in decreased filling of the right and left side of the heart. This results in a fall in stroke volume and arterial pressure that diminishes the murmurs of aortic stenosis and mitral regurgitation. (Braunwald, pp. 1040–1042, 1055–1057)

63. **(B)** Propranolol acts by decreasing heart rate, blood pressure, and contractility, thereby decreasing myocardial oxygen demand. (Braunwald, pp. 1330–1332)

64. **(C)** Diltiazem is a coronary vasodilator that will increase myocardial oxygen supply. Diltiazem will also lower blood pressure, which will decrease myocardial oxygen demand. (Braunwald, pp. 1332–1335)

65. **(C)** Nitroglycerin is a coronary vasodilator that increases myocardial oxygen supply. It is also a venodilator and reduces preload and can lower blood

pressure, which decreases mycardial oxygen demand. *(Braunwald, pp. 1328–1330)*

66. (B) Captopril is a potassium-sparing agent. It is an angiotensin-converting enzyme inhibitor and blocks the formation of angiotensin II, which stimulates aldosterone production. By decreasing aldosterone production, serum potassium levels may increase. Angiotensin-converting enzyme inhibitors should be used cautiously with potassium-sparing diuretics because of the potential for hyperkalemia. *(Braunwald, pp. 52, 877–878)*

67. (C) Hydrochlorothiazide is a diuretic and can cause an elevation of low-density lipoprotein cholesterol and a fall in serum potassium. Patients with hypokalemia may experience muscle weakness, polyuria, leg cramps, or increased ventricular ectopy. *(Braunwald, p. 516)*

68. (D) Diltiazem is a calcium channel blocker. It is used in the treatment of angina and hypertension. Calcium channel agents cause relaxation of the vascular smooth muscles in the coronary arteries and systemic arterial beds. Side effects include headache, dizziness, flushing, hypotension, leg edema, and gastrointestinal complaints. *(Braunwald, pp. 1667, 1332–1333)*

69. (D) Clonidine is an alpha-receptor agonist used in the treatment of hypertension. It does not affect serum potassium or serum lipid levels. Some of the side effects include dry mouth and drowsiness. *(Braunwald, pp. 873, 1167)*

70. (C); 71. (A); 72. (B); 73. (D) Enalapril is an angiotensin-converting enzyme inhibitor. It lowers blood pressure by blocking the action of angiotensin-converting enzyme, which is involved in converting angiotensin I to angiotensin II. Angiotensin II is a vasoconstrictor and stimulates aldosterone production.

Verapamil is a calcium channel blocker. It lowers blood pressure by decreasing systemic vascular resistance.

Metoprolol is a beta-adrenergic blocking agent. It lowers blood pressure by decreasing cardiac output, reducing renin activity and decreasing sympathetic discharge.

Prazosin is an alpha-adrenergic receptor blocker with its primary action as a postsynaptic alpha blocker. The antihypertensive effect of the drug is a result of blocking alpha-mediated vasoconstriction. *(Braunwald, pp. 873, 874, 877)*

74. (B); 75. (D); 76. (A); 77. (C) S_1 is a high-pitched sound caused by the closure of the mitral and tricuspid valves. S_2 is also high pitched and is the result of the closure of the pulmoinic and aortic valves. S_3 is a low-pitched heart sound and occurs as passive ventricular filling begins. An S_3 is heard with ventricular dysfunction or with marked left ventricular volume overload. An S_4 is a low-pitched heart sound and occurs with atrial contraction. S_4 is heard when there is increased left ventricular hypertrophy, and restricted diastolic filling. *(Braunwald, pp. 29–32)*

78. (B); 79. (C); 80. (A) Ventricular septal defect is the most common congenital malformation seen in children and infants. A ventricular septal defect can present anywhere in the interventricular septum and may vary in size. Symptoms are related to the size of the shunt and pulmonary vascular resistance. Coarctation of the aorta is narrowing of the thoracic aorta just distal to the insertion of the ligamentum arteriosum or just beyond origin of left subclavian artery. Features of coarctation include hypertension in arms and weak or absent femoral pulses. Coarctation is a cause of hypertension and is surgically correctable. A patient with an atrial septal defect may remain asymptomatic until the fourth or fifth decade. Symptoms of an atrial systal defect are dyspnea on exertion, fatigue, and palpitations secondary to supraventricular tachyarrhythmias. *(Braunwald, pp. 848, 982, 985)*

REFERENCES

Braunwald, E, ed. *Heart Disease: A Textbook of Cardiovascular Medicine, 3rd ed.* Philadelphia, PA: WB Saunders; 1988.

Cohn, JN. *Drug Treatment of Heart Failure,* 2nd ed. Secaucus, NJ: Advanced Therapeutics Communications International; 1988.

Effren, D. Cardiopulmonary Resuscitation, 3rd ed. Tulsa, OK. CPR Publishing, 1989.

Kaplan, NM. *Clinical Hypertension* 4th ed. Baltimore Md: Williams & Wilkins; 1986.

National Cholesterol Education Program. Highlights of the report of the expert panel on detection, evaluation, and treatment of high blood cholesterol in adults. NIH publication No. 88–2926. Washington, DC: Public Health Service; 1987.

Rautaharju, PM, Prince RJ, Eifler J, et al. Prognostic value of exercise ECG in men at high risk of future coronary heart disease: Multiple risk factor intervention trial experience. *J Am Coll Cardiol.* 1986; 8:1–10.

Scheidt, S. Basic electrocardiography. Abnormalities of electrocardiographic patterns. *CIBA Clin Symp.* 1984;36:1–32.

Shulman, ST, Amren DP, Bisro AL, et al. Prevention of bacterial endocarditis. A statement for health professionals by the committee on rheumatic fever and infective endocarditis of the council on cardiovascular disease in the young. *Circulation.* 1984; 70:1123–1127A.

Cardiology Subspecialty List:

Questions and Subspecialty
1. ECG findings
2. Cholesterol physiology
3. Cardiac arrhythmias
4. Mitral valve disease—complications
5. Cardiac arrhythmias
6. Cholesterol
7. Cardiac arrhythmias
8. Cholesterol
9. Congestive heart failure—treatment
10. Medication
11. Cardiac arrhythmias
12. Wolff–Parkinson–White syndrome—features
13. ECG findings
14. Angina—exacerbation
15. Hypertension—nonmedical treatment
16. ECG findings
17. Congestive heart failure—x-ray findings
18. Cardiac failure—causes of
19. Cardiopulmonary resuscitation
20. Cholesterol physiology
21. Cardiopulmonary resuscitation
22. Medications
23. Hypertension—complications
24. Aortic aneurysms characteristics
25. Thoracic aneurysms—clinical findings
26. Sudden cardiac death—causes
27. Murmurs
28. Prosthetic heart valves
29. Atrial septal defects
30. Cardiac pacemakers—indications
31. Atrial fibrillation—causes
32. Medications
33. Murmurs—causes
34. Murmurs—indications for treatment
35. Murmurs—physical findings
36. Heart failure—symptoms
37. Pericarditis—causes
38. Cardiomyopathy—characteristics
39. Medications
40. Mitral valve prolapse—characteristics
41. Coronary heart disease—risk factors
42. Stress testing—contraindications
43. Mitral stenosis—causes
44. Angina—treatment
45. Myocardial necrosis—laboratory evaluation
46. Cardiogenic shock—causes
47. Endocarditis—prophylaxis
48. ECG interpretation
49. ECG interpretation
50. ECG interpretation
51. ECG interpretation
52. ECG interpretation
53. Thrombolytic therapy—contraindications
54. Coronary angioplasty—results
55. Syncopes—causes
56. Medications
57. Renovascular hypertension—clinical findings
58. Heart failure—exacerbation
59. Murmurs
60. Murmurs
61. Murmurs
62. Murmurs
63. Medications
64. Medications
65. Medications
66. Medications
67. Medications
68. Medications
69. Medications
70. Medications
71. Medications
72. Medications
73. Medications
74. Heart sounds
75. Heart sounds
76. Heart sounds
77. Heart sounds
78. Congenital heart defects
79. Congenital heart defects
80. Congenital heart defects

Internal Medicine: Endocrinology

Peter Juergensen

Questions

DIRECTIONS (Questions 1 through 4): Each group of items in this section consists of lettered headings followed by a set of numbered words or phrases. For each numbered word or phrase, select

    A if the item is associated with (A) <u>only</u>,
    B if the item is associated with (B) <u>only</u>,
    C if the item is associated with <u>both</u> (A) <u>and</u> (B),
    D if the item is associated with <u>neither</u> (A) <u>nor</u> (B).

Questions 1 through 4

Match the following hormones with the site where they are produced.

    (A) posterior pituitary
    (B) anterior pituitary
    (C) both
    (D) neither

1. Leutinizing hormone and follicle stimulating hormone

2. Thyroid stimulating hormone and adrenocorticotrophic hormone

3. Antidiuretic hormone and thyroid stimulating hormone

4. Corticotropin releasing factor and melanocyte stimulating hormone

Questions 5 through 7

    (A) aldosterone
    (B) cortisol
    (C) both
    (D) neither

5. zona glomerulosa

6. zona reticularis

7. zona fasiculata

Questions 8 through 10

Match the following with its cause or symptom.

    (A) nephrogenic diabetes insipidus
    (B) neurogenic diabetes insipidus
    (C) both
    (D) neither

8. polyuria

9. psychogenic polydipsia

10. lithium

11. urinary tract obstruction

DIRECTIONS (Questions 12 through 38): For each of the items in this section, <u>ONE</u> or <u>MORE</u> of the numbered options is correct. Choose the answer

    A if only <u>1, 2, and 3</u> are correct,
    B if only <u>1 and 3</u> are correct,
    C if only <u>2 and 4</u> are correct,
    D if only <u>4</u> is correct,
    E if <u>all</u> are correct.

12. Myxedema may present with which of the following symptoms?
    (1) arthralgias
    (2) anovulation
    (3) hoarseness
    (4) diarrhea

13. NIDDM (noninsulin dependent diabetes mellitus) is characterized by a variety of metabolic defects including
    (1) deficient beta cell function
    (2) a reduction of insulin receptors
    (3) impaired transport of glucose into cells
    (4) postreceptor intracellular defects

SUMMARY OF DIRECTIONS				
A	**B**	**C**	**D**	**E**
1, 2, 3 only	1, 3 only	2, 4 only	4 only	All are correct

14. Prolactin secretion is enhanced by a variety of factors including

    (1) opiate narcotics
    (2) bromocryptine therapy
    (3) pregnancy
    (4) L-dopa therapy

15. Treatment of DKA (diabetic ketoacidosis) may result in

    (1) hypoglycemia
    (2) hypokalemia
    (3) hypophosphatemia
    (4) hypocalcemia

16. Causes of hyperthyroidism can include

    (1) subacute thyroiditis
    (2) painless thyroiditis
    (3) toxic multinodular goiter
    (4) struma ovarii

17. Hypothroidism may be caused by

    (1) Hashimoto's thyroiditis
    (2) iodine excess
    (3) iodine deficiency
    (4) chronic steroid therapy

18. Triiodothyronine (T_3) in the serum is derived from

    (1) secretion from the thyroid gland
    (2) iodination of tyrosine in the periphery
    (3) deiodination of T_4 in the periphery
    (4) oxidation of T_4 in the thyroid

19. T_4 is highly bound (more than 99%) in the plasma to

    (1) albumin
    (2) thyroid-binding globulin
    (3) thyroid-binding prealbumin
    (4) calmodulin-binding globulin

20. Fasting hypoglycemia may occur with

    (1) uremia
    (2) Addison's disease
    (3) insulin-producing islet cell tumors
    (4) acute hepatic necrosis

21. Clinical symptoms of acute adrenal insufficiency include

    (1) abdominal pain
    (2) hyponatremia
    (3) hypotension
    (4) hyperthermia

22. Endocrine causes for systolic and diastolic hypertension could include

    (1) primary aldosteronism
    (2) hyperthyroidism
    (3) hypercalcemia
    (4) Cushing's Syndrome

23. Hypercalciuria (excretion rate greater than 300 mg in males and greater than 250 mg in females in 24 hours) may be due to

    (1) primary hyperparathyroidism
    (2) sarcoidosis
    (3) vitamin D intoxication
    (4) thyrotoxicosis

24. Risk factors for nephrolithiasis include

    (1) hypercalciuria
    (2) hyperuricosuria
    (3) urine volume less than 1 L per day
    (4) high protein intake

25. Multiple endocrine neoplasia type I may include the following types of tumors

    (1) pituitary
    (2) parathyroid
    (3) pancreatic
    (4) medullary carcinoma of the thyroid

26. ACTH is stimulated by

    (1) TSH (thyroid stimulating hormone)
    (2) CRF (corticotropin releasing factor)
    (3) low cortisol
    (4) AVP (arginine vasopressin)

27. Aldosterone causes the kidney to

    (1) secrete potassium
    (2) absorb potassium
    (3) absorb sodium
    (4) secrete sodium

28. Short stature is a common endocrine problem seen in pediatric clinics. Differential diagnosis could include

    (1) familial
    (2) CNS tumors
    (3) hypothyroidism
    (4) growth hormone deficiency

29. Background diabetic retinopathy consists of

    (1) exudate
    (2) hemorrhages
    (3) microaneurysms
    (4) neovascularization

30. The Somogyi phenomenon is early morning hyperglycemia and ketonuria secondary to

    (1) excessive insulin administration
    (2) elevated epinephrine level
    (3) elevated growth hormone level
    (4) elevated cortisol level

31. First generation oral hypoglycemic agents include

    (1) tolbutamide
    (2) glipizide
    (3) acetohexamide
    (4) glyburide

32. SIADH (syndrome of inappropriate antidiuretic hormone release) can be caused by

    (1) narcotics
    (2) low serum osmolarity
    (3) adenocarcinoma of the lung
    (4) excessive H_2O drinking

33. Renal osteodystrophy refers to metabolic bone disease seen in end-stage renal disease. Possible bone lesions secondary to renal disease could include

    (1) osteomalacia
    (2) osteopetrosis
    (3) hyperparathyroid bone disease
    (4) fibrous dysplasia

34. Pheochromocytomas may be present in the

    (1) adrenals
    (2) organ of Zucherkandle
    (3) paravertebral sympathetic ganglion
    (4) kidney

35. Treatment for Cushing's disease can include

    (1) pituitary surgery
    (2) ketoconazole
    (3) op DDD
    (4) Dexamethasone

36. Osteomalacia is defined as excess unmineralized bone due to impaired bone mineralization. The possible etiologies include

    (1) vitamin D deficiency
    (2) hyperparathyroidism
    (3) hypophosphatemia
    (4) hyperthyroidism

37. A 21-hydroxylase deficiency in the newborn needs to be considered when there is

    (1) rapid weight gain
    (2) ambiguous genitalia
    (3) a breech delivery
    (4) the occurrence of shock or death

38. Complications of diabetes include

    (1) microangiopathy
    (2) gastroparesis
    (3) nocturnal diarrhea
    (4) segmental demyelinization

DIRECTIONS (Questions 39 through 63): Each of the numbered items or incomplete statements in this section is followed by answers or by completions of the statement. Select the <u>ONE</u> lettered answer or completion that is <u>BEST</u> in each case.

39. A patient has a nodule on palpation over the thyroid gland. Factors indicating possible carcinoma include

    (A) a scan with a hot nodule
    (B) a scan with a cold nodule
    (C) an echo with a clean cystic mass
    (D) biopsy with chronic lymphocytic infiltration
    (E) biopsy with a granulomatous lesion

40. ACTH (corticotropin) is a potent stimulatory for

    (A) estrogen release
    (B) testosterone release
    (C) cortisol production
    (D) ammonia generation
    (E) aldactone release

41. ACTH is inhibited by

    (A) high CRF
    (B) high cortisol
    (C) low cortisol
    (D) high estrogen
    (E) adrenalectomy

42. Adequacy of Levothyroxine replacement dose in primary hypothyroidism can be best determined by which of the following laboratory values?

    (A) T_3 RIA
    (B) reverse T_3
    (C) TBG
    (D) T_3 stimulation test
    (E) TSH

43. Klinefelter's syndrome is characterized by

    (A) a tall male
    (B) a short female
    (C) an abnormal XY chromosome
    (D) an XXY male
    (E) an XXY female

44. Infiltrative opthalmopathy secondary to thyroid is seen with

    (A) Graves' disease
    (B) Hashimoto's thyroiditis
    (C) toxic multinodular goiter
    (D) hypothyroidism
    (E) medullary carcinoma of the thyroid

45. The major clinical features of Turner's syndrome are

    (A) baldness with short stature
    (B) giantism alone
    (C) webbed neck, low hairline, and short stature
    (D) giantism with low hairline
    (E) short stature alone

46. Vitamin D is essential for normal calcium homeostasis and absorption. Of the following vitamin D sterols, which is the most important for calcium absorption?

    (A) $1, 25 - (OH)_2 D_3$
    (B) vitamin D_2
    (C) vitamin D_3
    (D) $24, 25 (OH)_2 D_3$
    (E) $25 - OHD_3$

47. Magnesium ammonium phosphate stones (struvite stones) are usually caused by

    (A) hyperparathyroidism
    (B) hyperthyroidism
    (C) renal tubular acidosis
    (D) infection
    (E) trauma

48. Parathyroid hormone can increase serum calcium

    (A) by directly stimulating the GI tract
    (B) by stimulating nephrogenic cyclic AMP
    (C) by decreasing bone turnover
    (D) by increasing serum $1, 25-(CO)_2 D_3$
    (E) by stimulating $25 - OHD_3$

49. Single-drug therapy for pheochromocytoma should **NOT** include

    (A) propranalol
    (B) prazosine
    (C) phenoxybenzanine
    (D) phentolamine
    (E) nitroprusside

50. The pituitary gland is located in the

    (A) glenoid fossa
    (B) sphenoid fossa
    (C) sella tursica
    (D) anterior skull
    (E) median eminence

51. Release of antidiuretic hormone (ADH) from the posterior pituitary is determined by the

    (A) serum osmolarity
    (B) serum viscosity
    (C) plasma ADH level
    (D) urine osmolarity
    (E) serum potassium level

52. Elevated VLDL with normal LDL is found to fit into which of the following Fredrickson classifications?

    (A) Type II a
    (B) Type II b
    (C) Type III
    (D) Type IV
    (E) Type V

53. The Dawn phenomenon is

    (A) hypoglycemia in the early AM
    (B) hypoglycemia in the late AM
    (C) hyperglycemia in early AM
    (D) ketoacidosis in the early AM
    (E) when NPH insulin peaks in patients

54. Oral hypoglycemic agents improve glucose control in diabetic patients by

    (A) improving insulin distribution
    (B) enhancing beta cell function
    (C) preventing gastric glucose absorption
    (D) enhancing glycogenolysis
    (E) preventing gluconeogenesis

55. The laboratory diagnosis of diabetes mellitus includes

    (A) a fasting glucose of < 140
    (B) a fasting glucose of < 100
    (C) a fasting glucose of > 140
    (D) a fasting glucose of > 100
    (E) 2-hour postprandial of > 100

56. The highly characteristic renal lesion of diabetes mellitus is called

    (A) membranous nephropathy
    (B) minimal change
    (C) Kimmelstiel–Wilson lesion
    (D) Pendred lesion
    (E) focal glomerular sclerosis

57. As a patient with diabetic ketoacidosis is being treated, the BP, pH, anion gap, and blood sugar improve except for the serum acetone level. With treatment, the level increases. The most likely etiology for this phenomenon is

    (A) laboratory error
    (B) lactate is being converted to acetone
    (C) glucose is being converted to acetone

(D) B-hydroxybutyrate is being converted to acetone

(E) glycogen is being converted to acetone

58. Appropriate laboratory work-up for adrenal insufficiency includes

(A) a TSH level
(B) an ACTH stimulation test
(C) a TRH stimulation test
(D) a CRF level
(E) a urine for ACTH level

59. TSH (thyrotropin) is stimulated by

(A) glucagon
(B) TRH (thyrotropin releasing hormone)
(C) prolactin
(D) ADH (antidiuretic hormone)
(E) ACTH (adrenocorticotrophic hormone)

60. Hyponatremia may be a presenting sign of

(A) ADH deficiency
(B) Grave's disease
(C) Cushing's syndrome
(D) hypothyroidism
(E) lithium therapy

61. Appropriate laboratory evaluation of Cushing's syndrome would include

(A) random ACTH level
(B) random cortisol level
(C) cortisol level at 4 PM
(D) 24-hour urine for cortisol
(E) cortisol level at 9 AM

62. Which of the following laboratory data would be most useful in the work-up of nephrolithiasis?

(A) urine culture
(B) urine phosphate level
(C) plasma to urine calcium ratio
(D) urine citric acid level
(E) 24-hour urine for osmolarity

63. A 25-year-old female on birth control pills is found to have an elevated T_4 of 17.2 μcg/dL (normal range 4.5 to 12.0 μcg/dL) on routine laboratory testing. The most likely etiology for the elevated T_4 would be

(A) decreased T_4 clearance
(B) an elevated TB_6 level
(C) daily levothyroxine intake of 0.025 μcg.
(D) an elevated TSH level
(E) decreased T_4 metabolism

Answers and Explanations

1. **(B)** LH (leuteinizing hormone) and FSH (follicle stimulating hormone) are secreted from the anterior pituitary.

2. **(B)** TSH (thyroid stimulating hormone) and ACTH (adrenocorticotrophic hormone) are secreted from the anterior pituitary.

3. **(C)** ADH (antidiuretic hormone) is secreted from the posterior pituitary and TSH (thyroid stimulating hormone) is secreted from the anterior pituitary.

4. **(D)** CRF (corticotropin releasing factor) is released by the hypothalamus and MSH (melanocyte stimulating hormone) is part of the ACTH molecule. *(Felig et al, pp. 249–259)*

5. **(A)** Layers of the adrenal gland are glomerulosa (outermost layer), fasiculata, and reticularis. The glomerulosa secretes only aldosterone.

6. **(B)** The reticularis secretes androgens, estrogens, and cortisol.

7. **(B)** The fasiculata makes up approximately 75% of the adrenal gland and secretes cortisol, androgens, and estrogen. *(Felig et al, pp. 514)*

8. **(C)** Nephrogenic diabetes insipidis and neurogenic diabetes insipidis by definition imply a polyuric state.

9. **(D)** Psychogenic polydipsia is seen with mental disorders and these patients drink an inordinate amount of fluid.

10. **(A)** Lithium will cause distal tubular injury, thus making these cells insensitive to ADH.

11. **(A)** Urinary tract obstruction will cause distal tubular injury, thus making those cells poorly responsive to ADH. *(Felig et al, pp. 361–364.*

12. **(A)** Symptoms of hypothyroidism can at times be difficult to detect, particularly if there is gradual progression of the disease or if another disease (i.e., CHF, sepsis) dominates. The severe form of hypothyroidism, called *myxedema,* may present with hoarseness, constipation, edema, arthralgias, anovulation, fatigue, and headaches. Diarrhea is not a symptom of myxedema, it can be seen with hyperthroidism. *(Federman, p. 16)*

13. **(E)** Noninsulin-dependent diabetes mellitus has a variety of etiologies. Beta cell function tends to decline over time in association with increased peripheral resistance to insulin. This resistance is composed of a reduction in insulin receptors, impaired cellular glucose uptake, and postreceptor defects. *(DeFronzo et al, pp. 52–81. Berger et al, p. 82)*

14. **(B)** Release of prolactin is accomplished by interrupting the normal inhibitory control mechanism that at present is felt to be dopamine. Bromocriptine (a dopaminergic agonist) and L-dopa will, therefore, inhibit dopamine release. Pregnancy with elevated estrogens directly stimulates prolactin. Opiates inhibit central dopamine release, thus increasing prolactin. *(Felig et al, pp. 272–273)*

15. **(A)** Treatment of DKA may cause hypoglycemia if vigorous insulin therapy is used. Incidence of hypoglycemia has been reduced with low-dose insulin regimens. Hypokalemia presents secondary to renal potassium wasting, poor intake and cellular shifts, and once acidosis improves and insulin therapy is initiated. Hypophosphatemia can be severe in DKA (rarely fatal), but is usually clinically silent. Hypocalcemia is not generally a condition associated with DKA. *(Kreisberg, pp. 681–695; Barrett et al, pp. 899–1104)*

16. **(E)** All options given can cause hyperthyroidism. Transient hyperthyroidism in subacute thyroiditis occurs in more than 50% of patients secondary to tissue injury to the gland and release of endogenous

T_4 stores. Painless thyroiditis may be the second most common cause of hypothyroidism due to lymphocytic infiltration of the gland. Autonomous hot nodules in the thyroid gland (toxic multinodular goiter) can cause marked hyperthyroidism. Struma ovarii (ovarian tumor) can cause ectopic thyroid production. *(Felig et al, p. 421)*

17. **(A)** Hashimoto's thyroiditis is an autoimmune thyroid disease that is the most common cause of hypothyroidism. Iodine excess will inhibit organification in large doses (Wolff–Chaikoff effect). Chronic iodine deficiency may result in goiter and hypothyroidism. Chronic steroid therapy does not cause hypothyroidism. *(Felig et al, pp. 445)*

18. **(B)** T_3 is directly secreted by the thyroid gland and by peripheral conversion of T_4 to T_3 (liver, muscles). Iodination of thyrosine in the periphery does not occur. Oxidation of T_4 does not occur. *(Felig et al, p. 392)*

19. **(A)** T_4 is approximately 80% bound to thyroid binding globulin (TBG), 15% to thyroid binding prealbumin (TBPA), and 5% to albumin. Calmodulin binding globulin does not exist. *(Felig et al, p. 396)*

20. **(E)** Insulin is broken down by the kidney; thus, more insulin can remain in circulation in patients with uremia. To maintain adequate glucose homeostasis, cortisol is one of the primary hormones necessary to prevent hypoglycemia. Islet cell tumors of the pancreas are classic for causing fasting hypoglycemia. With total liver necrosis, gluconeogensis will be absent, thus causing hypoglycemia. *(Felig et al, p. 1184)*

21. **(E)** Abdominal pain, even presenting as an acute abdomen, can be due to acute adrenal insufficiency. Hyponatremia with secondary increased ADH (antidiuretic hormone) and impaired free water clearance is common with Addison's disease. Both cortisol and mineralicorticoid are needed to maintain blood pressure. Fever can accompany adrenal crisis. *(Felig et al, p. 590)*

22. **(E)** Primary aldosteronism and Cushing's syndrome can increase blood pressure as the secretion of mineralicorticoid and the mineralicorticoid effect of cortisol cause sodium retention. Hypercalcemia by itself can increase blood pressure because it mediates the contractile elements of the vascular tree. Hyperthyroidism increase metabolic rate and cardiac output, thus increasing blood pressure. *(Felig et al, pp. 751–795, 713–714, 695)*

23. **(E)** Primary hyperparathyroidism can cause increased bone and gastrointestinal tract calcium ab-

sorption. Sarcoidosis and vitamin D intoxification cause GI calcium absorption. Thyrotoxicosis causes increased bone turnover with release of calcium. Hence, all can cause hypercalcuria. *(Felig et al, pp. 1531–1536)*

24. **(E)** Risk factors for kidney stone formation have been established (similar to the principle of coronary risk factors). Low–urine volume, high concentration of solute (calcium, urate, phosphate), pH (low for uric acid, high for infection or calcium phosphate) are all separate risk factors. High protein intake increases urate load and decreases pH. *(Felig et al, pp. 1500–1578)*

25. **(A)** Multiple endocrine neoplasia type I is usually made up of (the 3 Ps) pituitary, pancreatic, and parathyroid neoplasia. MEN type IIa has a medullary cancer of the thyroid (components of MEN type IIa are medullary carcinoma, pheochromocytoma, and hyperparathyroid). MEN type IIb consists of pheochromocytoma, medullary carcinoma, and marfanoid habitus. *(Felig et al, p. 1663)*

26. **(C)** Corticotropin releasing factor (CRF) and arginine vasopressin (AVP) both can stimulate ACTH (corticotropin or adrenocorticotropin). CRF and AVP are both produced in the hypothalamus, passed into the portal vessels of the anterior pituitary, and stimulate ACTH release. TSH stimulates the thyroid. Low cortisol by itself does not stimulate ACTH (it is through CRF or AVP, remember with the circadian rhythm, the afternoon cortisol level may be zero without causing release of ACTH). *(Felig et al, p. 523)*

27. **(B)** The effect of aldosterone at the renal tubule is potassium secretion and sodium retention. Retention of sodium, in turn, causes the kidney to retain fluid. *(Felig et al, p. 531)*

28. **(E)** Causes for short stature are quite extensive and are a common reason for pediatric visits to a pediatrician, especially in early adolescents. Etiology for short stature has been separated into congenital growth hormone deficiency (i.e. embryologic defects, inactive growth hormone) or acquired growth hormone deficiency (trauma, inflammatory disease, autoimmune) and CNS tumors that cause destruction of the pituitary. Hypothyroidism can also cause short stature. *(Felig et al, p. 1605)*

29. **(A)** Retinopathy is usually divided into background or proliferative. Background has evidence of retinal injury from diabetic vessel damage. Findings include hemorrhages, exudates, and microaneurysms. Laser therapy can be of great value. Neovascularization with vessels now growing into the vitreous is called proliferative retinopathy. *(Felig et al, p. 1116)*

30. **(E)** The underlying problem with Somogyi phenomenon is the excessive insulin doses resulting in hyperglycemia after counterregulatory hormones (epinephrine, growth hormone, and cortisol) are released. The overdosed patient will become hypoglycemic and the above events occur. It usually occurs in the early morning. *(Felig et al, p. 1137)*

31. **(B)** First-generation sulfonylureas are tolbutamide, chlorpropamide, acetohexamide, and tolazamide. Second-generation agents are glipizide and glyburide. *(Cahill et al, p. 14)*

32. **(B)** Inappropriate release of ADH has numerous etiologies including CNS lesion, adenocarcinoma of the lung, drugs (narcotics, phenothiazines), and pain. Low serum osmolarity or excessive H_2O drinking do not cause SIADH. *(Felig et al, pp. 368–374)*

33. **(B)** Renal osteodystrophy is a complicated disease process that may involve numerous etiologies and cause a variety of bone lesions. The most common lesions found are osteomalacia (from vitamin D deficiency or aluminum induction) and hyperparathyroid bone disease from secondary hyperparathyroidism. Less frequently, osteoporosis is seen. Osteopetrosis and fibrous dysplasia are not associated with renal failure. *(Felig et al, p. 1480)*

34. **(A)** Chromaffin cells are usually found in the adrenal glands and they can grow into pheochromocytomas. These cells are also found in the sympathetic nerve chain and on the organ of Zuckerkandl near the aortic bifurcation. They are not found in the kidney. *(Felig et al, p. 667)*

35. **(A)** Therapy of Cushing's disease can be quite difficult. If an ACTH producing tumor is present in the pituitary, it can be surgically resected. Ketoconazole and OP'DDD (mitotane) both can prevent adrenal cortisol production. Dexamethasone, a steroid, is used only in diagnosis, not treatment. *(Felig et al, pp. 615–617)*

36. **(B)** Both vitamin D deficiency and hypophosphatemia are the broad categories that head a long list of causes for osteomalacia. Hyperparathyroidism and hyperthyroidism do not cause osteomalacia. *(Felig et al, p. 1462)*

37. **(C)** A 21-hydroxylase block in the pathway of cortisol formation will result in low serum cortisol and aldosterone levels. Pathway is then shifted to the androgen excess. Clinical features include ambiguous genitalia in the male, severe salt washing, hypotension, shock, or death. It is important to determine this in a newborn as death can occur rapidly if undetected. Weight gain and type of delivery are not associated with a 21-hydroxylase block. *(Felig et al, p. 626)*

38. **(E)** Complications of diabetes are numerous, including accelerated atherosclerosis, diabetic neuropathy that may present with carpal tunnel, gastroparesis, GI motility disorders, deceased sensation, and nocturnal diarrhea. Segmental demyelination of the peripheral nerves and sorbitol deposition are the main causes of the neuropathy. *(Cahill et al, p. 17)*

39. **(B)** Thyroid tumors are classified into papillary, follicular, medullary, or undifferentiated. On scan they appear cold (they are usually nonfunctional). On echo they tend to be solid or have evidence of blood or fragments of tissue within the cyst. Chronic lymphocytic infiltration is seen with Hashimoto's thyroiditis. Granulomatous lesions are not seen with thyroid cancer. *(Felig et al, pp. 494–504)*

40. **(C)** ACTH is mainly responsible for stimulating cortisol. ACTH does help with the stimulation of cholesterol to pregnendone, which is the steroid needed for all subsequent steroid generation, including estrogen and testosterone, but it is not a stimulator of estrogen or testosterone release. Ammonia generation as well as aldosterone release are not under ACTH control. Aldactone is a drug that blocks aldosterone. *(Felig et al, pp. 513–518)*

41. **(B)** A high serum cortisol level will inhibit ACTH release. Also, high CRF or adrenolectomy will stimulate ACTH. High estrogen or low cortisol do not inhibit ACTH release. *(Felig et al, p. 530)*

42. **(E)** In primary hypothyroidism, when the TSH is elevated prior to replacement therapy, following the drop in TSH is the most sensitive assay. The goal is to achieve a normal TSH level (unless clinically contraindicated). T_3 RIA should normalize with T_4 therapy, but it is not sensitive enough. TBG is the binding protein that does not help. Reverse T_3 is presently a research tool. It may be of great value in diagnosis of sick euthryroid syndrome. T_3 stimulation test does not exist. *(Felig et al, p. 458)*

43. **(D)** Klinefelter's is usually caused by an extra chromosome, thus forming an XXY male with hypogonadism, usually associated with short stature and subnormal intelligence. Diagnosis needs to be entertained in a male with small firm testes, gynecomastia, and abnormal arm-to-body length. *(Felig et al, p. 1000)*

44. **(A)** Grave's opthalmopathy can be seen with hyperthyroid Grave's disease or with euthryroid Grave's. The etiology is unclear, but pathologically a lym-

phocytic and plasma cell infiltration occurs in the retroorbital space. Because the eye lies in the socket compartment, any additional mass added to the retroorbital space results in anterior displacement of the eye with resultant proptosis. *(Felig et al, p. 440)*

45. **(C)** Classic Turner's syndrome is a result of gonadal dysgenesis with streak gonads and they present with low hairline, low-set ears, webbed neck, broad chest, short stature, shortening of the fourth matacarpal, and commonly with renal abnormalities. They usually have a 45,X karyotype. *(Felig et al, p. 1006)*

46. **(A)** $1,25-(OH)_2D_3$ acts on the GI tract to cause calcium absorption and in concert with parathyroid hormone help maintain normal bone homeostasis. Vitamin D_2 and D_3 are metabolized to 25-OH D_3 in the liver and then hydroxylated to $1,25-(OH)2D_3$ or $24,25(OH)2D_3$ in the kidney. The true function of 24,25-(OH)2D3 is not clear at present, but it may be quite important in new bone formation. *(Felig et al, p. 1346)*

47. **(D)** Struvite (infection, triple phosphate) stones occur when the urine is supersaturated with magnesium, ammonium, and phosphate in the presence of urea-splitting bacteria. Proteus is the most common bacterium, although Klebsiella, Pseudomonas, Bacteriodes and Staphylococcus aureus also have been implicated. *(Felig et al, pp. 1521–1524)*

48. **(D)** Hypercalcemia of hyperparathyroidism is due to increased GI absorption of calcium mediated by $1,25-(OH)2D_3$. PTH stimulates increased $1,25-(OH)2D_3$ formation. Remember, this is in contrast to hypercalcemia of malignancy (either through bone metastasis or humoral causes) in which the hypercalcemia is due to bone calcium release, not increased GI absorption. PTH does not stimulate the GI tract directly, nor stimulate 25-OHD3. Nephrogenic cyclic AMP is a marker of PTH action at the kidney, but cyclic AMP does not cause hypercalcemia. *(Felig et al, pp. 1377–1384)*.

49. **(A)** Prazosine, phenoxybenzamine, phentolamine, or nitroprusside can be first-line drugs as they are all alpha-adrenergic antagonists. Propranolol, a beta-adrenergic antagonist, should never be used alone. By only blocking the vasodilator beta receptors with propranolol, there will then be unopposed alpha stimulation resulting in vasoconstriction and a rapid rise in blood pressure. *(Felig et al, p. 671)*

50. **(C)** The pituitary gland is located at the base of the skull in a saddle-shaped cavity termed the *sella tursica*. It is divided into anterior and posterior components. Along with the hypothalamus it provides the major components to a number of autoregulatory components of the endocrine system. *(Felig et al, p. 247)*

51. **(A)** Serum osmolarity is the most potent stimulus for ADH release. Serum osmolarity that is greater than 285 will cause a strong stimulus for ADH release. None of the other choices linked have any influence on ADH reflex. *(Felig et al, p. 341)*

52. **(E)** Fredrickson's classification is based on the following table:

Type	Lipoprotein abnormality
I	Chylomicrons markedly increased; VLDL & LDL are normal
IIa	LDL increased, VLDL normal
IIb	Both LDL and VLDL are increased
III	Abnormal cholesterol, normal VLDL and increased beta-VLDL
VI	VLDL increased and LDL normal
V	Chylomicrons markedly increased, VLDL increased, LDL normal

Type VI is also commonly seen in poorly controlled diabetics. *(Grundy, p. 2045)*

53. **(C)** Hyperglycemia in the early morning in those patients on insulin may be due to the dawn phenomenon. It is felt to be secondary to early morning rise in growth hormone secretion, which is a counterregulatory hormone and thus raises serum glucose. This is in contrast to the Somogyi effect, causing early morning hyperglycemia due to insulin overdose and release of all counterregulatory hormones. In patients with dawn phenomenon, the insulin dose is not excessive. *(Felig et al, p. 13)*

54. **(B)** Oral agents enhance beta cell function and thus increase insulin release. they also improve peripheral sensitivity to insulin. Both these actions tend to normalize blood sugar levels in the noninsulin dependent diabetic. *(Cahill et al, p. 13)*

55. **(C)** A fasting blood sugar of > 140 mg/dL on two occasions is diagnostic of diabetes mellitus. A ½ hour, 1 hour or 1 ½ hour blood sugar of > 200 mg can be diagnostic of diabetes during a glucose tolerance test. A 2-hour postprandial of > 200 is also diagnostic of diabetes. *(Cahill et al, p. 7)*

56. **(C)** Kimmelstiel–Wilson lesions include spherical nodular hyaline masses and sclerosis of the renal glomerulus. This is characteristic of diabetes mellitus. No other disease process is known to cause this lesion. *(Felig et al, pp. 1115–1116)*

57. (D) As diabetic ketoacidosis worsens, especially if there is concomitant lactic acidosis, B-hydroxybucerate is more likely to be formed. B-hydroxybucerate is not measured in the acetone assay. As DKA is treated, the B-hydroxybucerate will be converted to acetone, thus giving the paradoxical rise in serum acetone as the patient improves. *(Felig et al, p. 1150)*

58. (B) Appropriate tests would be a serum ACTH level and ACTH stimulation test to measure adrenal reserve. TSH level is to evaluate the thyroid, not adrenal. CRF is a research tool and is not needed, as ACTH level can be measured. Urine for ACTH cannot be done. *(Felig et al, p. 592)*

59. (B) TRH (thyrotropin releasing hormone) stimulates TSH (thyrotropin). Glucagon, prolactin, ADH, and ACTH do not stimulate TSH. T_4 and T_3 once slightly above normal suppress TSH. *(Felig et al, p. 400)*

60. (D) Hypothyroidism will cause an inability to secrete a water load secondary to elevated ADH level. Poor cardiac output and the renal tubule need thyroid hormone to excrete H_2O properly. ADH deficiency and lithium therapy cause hypernatremia. Grave's disease and Cushing's disease are usually not associated with inability to excrete a water load. *(Felig et al, pp. 453–454)*

61. (D) Glucocorticoid excess secondary to pituitary ACTH hypersecretion is labeled *Cushing's Disease.* Cushing's syndrome has numerous etiologies (iatrogenic, tumor, etc.). Laboratory work-up would include a 24-hour urine for cortisol (normal < 100 mg/24-hour). Random ACTH, random cortisol, and a 4 PM cortisol are of no diagnostic aid because they do not establish a cortisol excess state. ACTH has a wide daily fluctuation; cortisol is usually high in the early morning and low in the late afternoon (usual circadian rhythm). *(Felig et al, pp. 609–611)*

62. (A) The appropriate laboratory work-up for kidney stones should include a urine culture to rule out infection as the etiology for the stone disease. Stag-horn calculi in the renal pelvis are composed of struvite and are caused by infection. Urine phosphate and citric acid levels are nonexistent tests. A plasma-to-urine calcium ratio has no clinical relevance. The urine osmolarity only tells you if ADH is being secreted. *(Felig et al, pp. 1521–1524)*

63. (B) Isolated elevations of T_4 do not imply that the patient is hyperthyroid. The serum T_4 assay will measure both bound and free T_4. More than 99.95% of T_4 is bound; thus, if TB_6 is elevated, so too will the measurable T_4 in the serum. Increase in TB_6 can be seen with any elevated estrogen state (pregnancy, birth control pills), heredity and acute hepatitis. Elevated TSH level causing high T_4 is exceedingly rare. Decreased T_4 metabolism or clearance will not increase T_4. Levothyroxine dose of 0.025 mg. is miniscule (usual replacement close to 100 to 150 mg/day). *(Felig et al, pp. 395, 411, 458)*

REFERENCES

Felig P. Baster D. et al. eds. *Endocrinology and Metabolism.* New York: McGraw-Hill: 1987.

Federman D. Thyroid. S AM M. 1, May 1989.

DeFronzo RA, Ferrannin E, et al. New concepts in the pathogenesis and treatment of non-insulin dependent diabetes mellitus. *Am J Med.* 1983; 74(1a):52–81.

Berger M, Birchtold P. Insulin transport and action at target cells. *Joslin's Diabetes Mellitus*, 12th ed. Philadelphia, PA: Lea and Febiger; 1985.

Kreisberg A. Diabetic ketoacidosis: New concepts and trends in pathogenesis and treatment. *Ann Intern Med.* 1978;88:681–695.

Barrett E. DeFronzo, R. Diabetic ketoacidosis; Diagnosis and treatment. *Hosp Pract.* 1984; 19:89–104.

Cahill, F. Arky, A. et al. *VI Diabetes mellitus, Sci Am* January 1987.

Grundy M. Disorders of lipids and lipoproteins. In: Stein Jay H. et al. eds. *Internal Medicine*, 2nd ed. Boston, MA: Little, Brown; 1987.

Subspecialty List: Endocrinology

Internal Medicine: Neurology

Mary McClure

Questions

DIRECTIONS (Questions 1 through 16): Each of the numbered items or incomplete statements in this section is followed by answers or by completions of the statement. Select the ONE lettered answer or completion that is BEST in each case.

1. The most common source of low back pain is

   (A) vascular
   (B) nerve root compression
   (C) spondylogenic
   (D) visceral referred pain
   (E) psychogenic

2. Pupillary response to light in a person with a blind RIGHT eye, secondary to disease of the retina or optic nerve

   (A) will occur with light shining in the LEFT eye only
   (B) will occur with light shining in the RIGHT eye only
   (C) will occur with light shining in either eye
   (D) will not occur
   (E) will depend on the etiology of the lesion

3. Which of the following is **LEAST** likely to be informative in the diagnosis of multiple sclerosis?

   (A) CT scan
   (B) evoked responses
   (C) history and physical examination
   (D) MRI
   (E) CSF studies

4. The most common presenting symptom of Alzheimer's disease is

   (A) emotional lability
   (B) mild speech problems
   (C) memory deficits
   (D) agitation
   (E) handwriting changes

5. The best approach to the management of a mixed seizure disorder in a brain injured patient involves

   (A) the use of phenobarbital with caution
   (B) the use of phenytoin and ethosuximide only
   (C) the cautious use of two-drug therapy
   (D) referral to a neurologist or neurosurgeon
   (E) complete evaluation for potential metabolic etiology

6. The evaluation of new onset seizures in an adult includes all of the following **EXCEPT**

   (A) CT scan
   (B) chest x-ray
   (C) HIV testing
   (D) BUN electrolytes, creatinine
   (E) fasting blood sugar

7. A lesion of the right optic tract produces a

   (A) blind right eye
   (B) blind left eye
   (C) left homonymous hemianopsia
   (D) right homonymous hemianopsia
   (E) bitemporal hemianopsia

8. A patient's CT scan reveals multiple mass lesions. Which of the following is most likely to add diagnostic information?

   (A) chest x-ray
   (B) colonoscopy
   (C) amylase and lipase levels
   (D) abdominal ultrasound
   (E) head MRI

9. A patient with postconcussive syndrome is most likely to be helped by

   (A) referral for permanent disability
   (B) rest at home until symptoms have resolved
   (C) half-time work until symptoms have resolved
   (D) referral for inpatient rehabilitation
   (E) quick return to work

10. The most frequently encountered initial symptom(s) of botulism include(s)

(A) foot drop
(B) feeling of impending doom, dyspnea, and agitation
(C) tinnitus and vertigo
(D) blurred vision, diplopia, dysphonia
(E) cardiac dysrhythmias and blood pressure fluctuations

11. Which of the following is **NOT** in the differential diagnosis of Alzheimer's disease?

(A) depression
(B) bacterial meningitis
(C) vitamin B deficiency
(D) toxic encephalopathy
(E) brain tumors

12. Hyperalimentation without the addition of water soluable B vitamins can lead to

(A) Wernicke–Korsakoff's syndrome
(B) Tardive dyskenesia
(C) toxic myopathies
(D) scurvy
(E) transient global dementia

13. The most common symptom in a patient with spinal cord metatases is

(A) tingling
(B) pain
(C) numbness
(D) paresthesia
(E) focal weakness

14. Gower's maneuver is most indicative of

(A) cranial nerve dysfunction
(B) distal extremity weakness
(C) sensory impairment
(D) truncal ataxia
(E) proximal extremity weakness

15. Hemorrhagic CVA may be caused by all **BUT**

(A) arteriovenous malformation
(B) atrial fibrillation
(C) aplastic anemia
(D) anticoagulant therapy
(E) mycotic aneurysm

16. The most likely diagnosis in a patient whose CSF reveals

glucose, 20;

protein, 400;

WBC, 1200, 90% Polys is

(A) crypotococcal meningitis
(B) partially treated bacterial meningitis
(C) neoplastic meningitis
(D) aseptic meningitis
(E) acute bacterial meningitis

DIRECTIONS (Questions 17 through 25): For each of the items in this section, <u>ONE</u> or <u>MORE</u> of the numbered options is correct. Choose the answer

A if only <u>1, 2, and 3</u> are correct,
B if only <u>1 and 3</u> are correct,
C if only <u>2 and 4</u> are correct,
D if only <u>4</u> is correct,
E if <u>all</u> are correct.

17. Signs that are most helpful in distinguishing vertigo of peripheral vestibular origin from that of central origin include

(1) hearing loss
(2) diplopia
(3) tinnitus
(4) nausea and vomiting

18. Immediate diagnosis and treatment is required for which of the following headaches:

(1) migraine
(2) posttraumatic
(3) tension
(4) temporal arteritis

19. Parkinsonism is characterized by

(1) rigidity
(2) bradykinesias
(3) rhythmic tremor
(4) postural abnormalities

20. Argyll Robertson pupils

(1) react equally to light
(2) should suggest a serologic test for syphilis
(3) should suggest a fasting blood sugar determination
(4) react to near vision

21. Risk factors for cerebrovascular accident include

(1) alcohol consumption
(2) race
(3) hypertension
(4) asymptomatic bruit

22. Seizures occurring within 24 hours of a traumatic head injury

    (1) suggest serious brain injury
    (2) are associated with a 28% death rate
    (3) indicate a focal lesion
    (4) have no prognostic significance

23. Common triggers of cluster headaches include

    (1) histamine exposure
    (2) discontinuation of alcohol consumption
    (3) prolonged insomnia
    (4) daytime napping

DIRECTIONS (Questions 24 through 28): Each group of items in this section consists of lettered headings followed by a set of numbered words or phrases. For each numbered word or phrase, select the ONE lettered heading that is most closely associated with it. Each lettered heading may be selected once, more than once, or not at all.

For each anticonvulsant select the side effect(s) most likely to be attributed to its use.

(A) least likely to impair concentration, memory, and reaction time
(B) idiosyncratic fatal toxic hepatitis
(C) generalization of focal seizures during induction
(D) gingival hyperplasia, hirsutism
(E) benign liver tumors
(F) sedation, possible hyperactivity in children

24. phenobarbital

25. diphenylhydantoin (Dilantin)

26. valproic acid (Depakene)

27. carbamazepine (Tegretol)

28. ethosuximide (Zarontin)

DIRECTIONS (Questions 29 through 37): Each group of items in this section consists of lettered headings followed by a set of numbered words or phrases. For each numbered word or phrase, select

A if the item is associated with (A) only,
B if the item is associated with (B) only,
C if the item is associated with both (A) and (B),
D if the item is associated with neither (A) nor (B).

Questions 29 through 33

(A) generalized seizure
(B) partial seizure
(C) both
(D) neither

29. Petit Mal (absence)

30. psychomotor

31. presence of an aura

32. pseudoseizure

33. postictal period

Questions 34 through 37

(A) cluster headache
(B) migraine headache
(C) both
(D) neither

34. may be precipitated by frequent ergotamine use

35. may be relieved at menopause

36. associated with blue-hazel eyes, heavy smoking, alcohol use

37. generally unilateral, orbital, with ipsilateral lacrimation

Answers and Explanations

1. **(C)** Spondylogenic back pain involves sources in the bone, disc, joint, and soft tissues. Injuries, congenital conditions, and diseases are among the causes of spondylogenic back pain. Injuries or diseases involving nerve root compression are frequently more severe and produce greater pain that does not respond well to rest and NSAIDS. Visceral causes should always be considered and can be distinguished by location, radiation, type of pain, and associated symptoms. Certainly, the searing pain of a dissecting abdominal aortic aneurysm must be distinguished from benign back pain. Associated symptoms are also helpful in distinguishing urinary, pelvic, and pancreatic disease. Psychogenic back pain should remain a diagnosis of exclusion. *(Weiner and Goetz, pp. 260–265; Braunwald et al, pp. 34–41; Andreoli et al, pp. 712–713; Bates, p. 90)*

2. **(A)** The type of lesion is not significant, location is the determinant. In a lesion of the retina or optic nerve with the oculomotor nerve intact, a light stimulus in the blind eye will not be transmitted to the oculomotor nerve. However, a light stimulus in the normal eye will be transmitted and produce bilateral pupillary constriction. *(Weiner and Goetz, p. 304; Bates, pp. 150–151, 188, 193)*

3. **(A)** A thorough history and physical examination remain the cornerstone in the diagnosis of MS. The waxing and waning, often vague and variable symptoms suggest the clinical diagnosis. Evoked responses can be used to contribute information on latencies and CSF studies may reveal an elevated IGG disproportionate to the serum protein. An MRI is capable of demonstrating the white matter lesions and this confirms the clinical diagnosis. CT scanning may not reveal the lesions and does not add useful diagnostic information. *(Weiner and Goetz, pp. 814–815; Braunwald et al, pp. 1195–1999; Andreoli et al, pp. 100–106)*

4. **(C)** Alzheimer's patients present at various stages of their disease. A careful history reveals that although mood, personality, and handwriting changes may precipitate the evaluation, difficulty with memory has preceded the other symptoms, often in an insidious manner. *(Weiner and Goetz, pp. 198–200; Braunwald et al, pp. 131–133)*

5. **(D)** Many medications and combinations of drugs may be used in an attempt to control a mixed seizure disorder in a brain injured patient. The primary care provider cannot be expected to manage complex problems alone. Referral to a neurologist or neurosurgeon can offer the primary care provider as well as the patient with guidance in the most current therapeutic modalities. *(Weiner and Goetz, p. 224; Braunwald et al, pp. 1924–1925)*

6. **(C)** An adult with no history of a seizure disorder should be evaluated for all potential causes of seizures. A CT scan can rule out a mass lesion or lesions that may present with seizures. A primary lung cancer seen on chest x-ray may alter the treatment regimen of cerebral metastases. Severe hypoglycemia induces seizures and is readily treatable, as are other metabolic abnormalities. Seizures secondary to cerebral AIDS is rarely a presenting symptom. The CT reveals the mass lesions. HIV testing may add information but is not necessary for diagnosis of the space occupying lesion and, therefore, is not in the first line evaluation of new onset seizures. *(Warner and Goetz, pp. 86–90, Braunwald et al, pp. 1921–1926.*

7. **(C)** Because fibers originating in the nasal half of the retina cross at the chiasm and temporal fibers do not cross, a lesion in the RIGHT optic tract will block RIGHT temporal and LEFT nasal fibers. This produces a LEFT homonymous hemianopsia. (Remember that visual stimuli are transmitted to the retina reversed.) *(Weiner and Goetz, pp. 294–301; Wyngaard et al, pp. 73–74; Andreoli et al, pp. 717–719; Bates, p. 188)*

8. **(A)** A large percentage of cerebral tumors are metastatic with lung and breast the most likely sources. Colorectal cancer is much less likely to

metastasize to the central nervous system. Pancreatic enzymes are often normal in pancreatic cancer, which rarely metastasizes to the brain. Abdominal ultrasound may reveal tumors, but these are less likely to produce brain metastasis. If the CT scan is diagnostic, the expensive MRI is unnecessary. *(Weiner and Goetz, p. 30; Braunwald et al, pp. 1831, 1971–1972)*

9. **(E)** Postconcussive syndrome may follow mild to moderate head injury. Of itself it is not dangerous, nor does it imply serious sequelae. Symptoms are vague but headache is usual; most patients return to normal within 6 weeks. Those who do not should be encouraged to return to work as soon as possible, as patients who focus on symptoms may feel disabled for a longer time. *(Weiner and Goetz, pp. 224–225; Braunwald et al, p. 1965; Andreoli et al, pp. 783–784)*

10. **(D)** Botulism victims may develop a number of symptoms including respiratory, cardiac, and gastrointestinal complications. However, early symptoms very likely include blurred vision, diplopia, dysphagia, dysarthria, and dysphonia. It is important that the primary care provider remain alert to these early symptoms. Other symptoms may follow quickly with devastating results. *(Weiner and Goetz, p. 239; Andreoli et al, p. 761)*

11. **(B)** The patient with bacterial meningitis will present acutely with fever and neurological signs and symptoms. Alzheimer's has a more indolent early course. Fever is not expected unless concurrent infection exists. Depression may mimic Alzheimer's with limitations of functioning and memory. Lead poisoning can lead to encephalopathy. Memory loss, ataxia, and peripheral neuropathies can be seen in adults with lead poisoning. Some medications can produce toxic encephalopathies. Vitamin B deficiency may produce demyelination and axonal degeneration. Memory deficits can occur and may be mild or go on to dementia. Alzheimer's remains a diagnosis of exclusion at this time. *(Weiner and Goetz, pp. 198–205; Braunwald et al, pp. 852, 2012–2016; Andreoli et al, pp. 686–689)*

12. **(A)** Wernicke–Korsakoff's syndrome is a disease of thiamine deficiency. Most often seen in alcoholics who obtain many of their calories from alcohol rather than food, Wernicke–Korsakoff's syndrome can be seen in any setting where thiamine is deficient. Therefore, hyperalimentation should include this and other B vitamins. Tardive dyskinesia is a movement disorder caused by neuroleptic drugs. Toxic myopathies and transient dementias are not nutritional deficiency diseases. Scurvy is caused by vitamin C deficiency. *(Weiner and Goetz, pp. 151, 193–194; Braunwald et al, pp. 2001–2003; Andreoli et al, pp. 702–703)*

13. **(B)** Pain is the most common symptom of spinal cord metastases. The pain is frequently well-localized back pain but may be radicular. Pain may precede neurological symptoms by a few weeks and the goal is to begin treatment before this occurs. *(Weiner and Goetz, pp. 254–255; Braunwald et al, p. 2042)*

14. **(E)** Gower's maneuver is used to compensate for proximal muscle weakness. In the act of rising from the floor, patients use their hands to push off from the floor and again lean on their lower extremities to facilitate further straightening up. *(Weiner and Goetz, p. 228; Braunwald et al, p. 2073)*

15. **(B)** All the choices can lead to a CVA. However, atrial fibrillation is associated with embolic cardiovascular events. This will frequently occur in patients who fluctuate from atrial fibrillation to sinus rhythm. *(Weiner and Goetz, pp. 54–55; Braunwald et al, pp. 1933–1952; Andreoli et al, p. 770)*

16. **(E)** CSF glucose may be low in any of the meningitides listed. Protein as high as 400 is a good indication of acute bacterial meningitis, although it can be that high in cryptococcal or neoplastic meningitis. However, the WBC clearly identifies acute bacterial meningitis. Counts greater than 500 are rare in other diseases and 90% polys excludes the other diagnoses. *(Weiner and Goetz, p. 17; Braunwald et al, pp. 1982–1989; Andreoli et al, pp. 368–372)*

17. **(B)** The combination of hearing loss and tinnitus is very rare in central vertigo; nauseas and vomiting are common. The finding of hearing deficit and tinnitus in a patient with vertigo indicates a peripheral source. An additional distinguishing feature is Nystagmus, which is always present with peripheral lesions. *(Weiner and Goetz, p. 175; Braunwald et al, p. 78; Andreoli et al, p. 726)*

18. **(D)** Migraine headaches are chronic and most patients have a management regimen focused on pain relief. Posttraumatic headaches may persist for weeks following head trauma but, although annoying, are not serious and gradually subside. Tension headaches can be managed at home and involve avoidance of the triggers when possible and pain management. Temporal arteritis is an inflammatory process and may indicate a systemic vascular disorder. It is very responsive to steroid therapy, which should be initiated immediately as irreversible blindness can result. *(Weiner and Goetz, p. 1443; Andreoli et al, p. 656)*

19. **(E)** These symptoms are the hallmark of Parkinson's disease. Other disorders affecting the basal ganglia may demonstrate some of these findings. Encephalitis, particularly herpetic encephalitis often affects the basal ganglia, but history and viral

titres easily make the distinction. On the other hand, Parkinsonism is often associated with depression and later dementia. Careful examination of depressed and demented patients will rule out Parkinsonism. *(Weiner and Goetz, pp. 109–114; Braunwald et al, pp. 2017–2018; Andreoli et al, pp. 737–738)*

20. **(C)** Argyll Robertson pupils are bilaterally small, but may be irregular. They do not react to light, but do react to accommodation. They are characteristically seen in neurosyphilis. *(Weiner and Goetz, pp. 319–320; Braunwald et al, p. 643; Andreoli et al, pp. 719–720; Bates, p. 194)*

21. **(E)** All are among the many risk factors of stroke. In addition, atrial fibrillation and mitral valve prolapse, diabetes, obesity, hyperlipidemia, and hemolytic disorders are among risk factors for stroke. Congenital malformations such as aneurysms and arteriovenous malformations can lead to devastating sudden cerebrovascular events. *(Weiner and Goetz, p. 54; Braunwald et al, pp. 1933–1934, 1941; Andreoli et al, pp. 767–768)*

22. **(D)** Many factors may be involved early, including drug and alcohol abuse, which are common in traumatic injuries. Seizures may occur acutely with serious head injury and become chronic, but chronicity cannot be predicted accurately. Seizures within the first 24 hours may indicate focality, but also may result from generalized injury. Thus, the presence of a seizure or seizures in the immediate acute phase of head trauma is alone not prognostic. *(Weiner and Goetz, p. 224; Braunwald et al, pp. 1924–1925)*

23. **(D)** The trigger factors of cluster headaches are individual and variable. However, common triggers include alcohol use and sleep. During a period of frequent headaches, extra naps and heavy alcohol use should be avoided. During headache-free periods these may be benign. *(Weiner and Goetz, pp. 71, 72, 79; Braunwald et al, pp. 28, 29, 30)*

24. **(F); 25. (D); 26. (B); 27. (A); 28. (E)** Anticonvulsants share similar side effects. However, some are more common or more severe than others. Anticonvulsant therapy consists of minimizing the negative effects while obtaining optimal seizure control. Individualization is required. Many anticonvulsants produce some level of sedation. However, this is more common with phenobarbital, except in some young children where hyperactivity may be seen. Dilantin is less sedating but can promote gingival hyperplasia and hirsutism. Valproic acid is very useful for myoclonic and absence seizures but can occasionally produce fulminant hepatitis and death. This is more likely to occur in infancy and very early childhood. Carbamezepine should be in-

creased slowly, as gastrointestinal symptoms are common and often resolve in time. Bone marrow suppression is less likely but CBCs should be monitored. Nonetheless, a decrease in intellectual functioning, that is, memory and concentration, is not generally a problem with carbamezapine. Ethosuximide is effective in absence seizures but may cause gastrointestinal and bone marrow problems as well as difficulties in concentration. *(Weiner and Goetz, pp. 91–92; Braunwald et al, p. 1928; Barnhart, pp. 1599, 1600, 1539–1542, 511–514, 974–976)*

29. **(A); 30. (B); 31.(B); 32. (D); 33. (C)** An aura represents a focal manifestation of a seizure and aids in the distinction between partial complex and generalized seizures. A generalized seizure by definition does not present with an aura. Absence seizures are generalized seizures often beginning in childhood. The patient briefly (less than 30 seconds) loses contact with his/her environment. There is no postictal period. However, most other generalized seizures are followed by postictal periods, as are some partial seizures. Of interest, Jacksonian seizures may produce a postictal Todd's paralysis. —a pseudoseizure is not a neurologic event. *(Weiner and Goetz, p. 86; Braunwald et al, pp. 1921–1923; Andreoli et al, pp. 787–792)*

34. **(D); 35. (B); 36. (A); 37. (A)** Both migraine headaches and cluster headaches are vascular in origin. Cluster headaches are unilateral and orbital but also demonstrate ipsilateral lacrimation. Cluster headaches cluster, that is, occur frequently but give way to longer periods of freedom from them. They are more common in males, particularly those with blue or hazel eyes who smoke and use alcohol. During periods of attack, alcohol use is a common trigger and should be avoided. Cluster headaches are very severe and generally last 30 minutes to 2 hours and are not associated with nausea. Migraine headaches also tend to be ipsilateral, but nausea is common, and they are more likely to occur in females. They may decrease significantly with menopause. Migraines are often preceded by an aura and can last for a few hours or days. Ergotamine is useful for migraines, but if used frequently produces a dependency that in turn causes a migraine-like headache. *(Weiner and Goetz, pp. 71–72, 79, 68–70; Braunwald et al, pp. 28, 29, 30; Andreoli et al, pp. 708–710)*

REFERENCES

Andreoli T, Carpenter C, Plum F, Smith L, eds. *Cecil Essentials of Medicine*, 2nd Ed. Philadelphia, PA: W.B. Saunders; 1990.

Barnhart, E. *Physician's Desk Reference*, 43rd ed. Oradell, NJ: Medical Economics Co; 1989.

Bates, B. *A Guide to Physical Examination and History Taking,* 4th ed. Philadelphia, PA: J.B. Lippincott; 1987.

Braunwald, E., Isselbacher, KJ, Faucias, Petersdorf R, Wilson J, Martin J, eds. *Harrison's Principles of Internal Medicine,* 11th ed. New York, NY: McGraw-Hill; 1987.

Weiner W Jr, Goetz CG, eds. *Neurology for the Non-Neurologist,* 2nd ed. Philadelphia, PA: J.B. Lippincott; 1989.

Neurology Subspecialty List:

Questions Numbers and Subspecialty
1. Back pain
2. Ocular physiology
3. Multiple sclerosis
4. Alzheimer's
5. Seizure disorders
6. Seizure disorders
7. Ocular physiology
8. Cerebral metastases
9. Head trauma
10. Neurologic signs of botulism
11. Alzheimer's
12. Wernicke–Korsakoff Syndrome
13. Spinal cord metastases
14. Neurologic examination
15. Stroke
16. Meningitis
17. Vertigo
18. Headache
19. Parkinsonism
20. Argyll–Robertson pupils
21. Stroke
22. Head injury
23. Cluster headache
24–28. Anticonvulsant medication
29–33. Seizure disorders
34–37. Headaches

Internal Medicine: Rheumatology

Ricky D. Miller, William Reynolds

Questions

DIRECTIONS (Questions 1 through 11): For each of the items in this section, ONE or MORE of the numbered options is correct. Choose the answer

A if only 1, 2, and 3 are correct,
B if only 1 and 3 are correct,
C if only 2 and 4 are correct,
D if only 4 is correct,
E if all are correct.

1. Which of the following are frequently found in patients with osteoarthritis?

    (1) Heberden's nodes
    (2) swan-neck deformities of the fingers
    (3) rest usually decreases joint discomfort in early stages
    (4) morning stiffness

2. Which of the following laboratory findings suggests the diagnosis of osteoarthritis?

    (1) normal to slightly elevated sedimentation rate
    (2) clear synovial fluid on joint aspiration
    (3) normal white blood cell (WBC) count
    (4) elevated antinuclear antibody (ANA) test

3. Signs of bacterial septic arthritis include which of the following?

    (1) fever and chills
    (2) slow insidious onset
    (3) involves primarily large weight-bearing joints and the wrist
    (4) usually is polyarticular

4. Which of the following are characteristic of rheumatoid arthritis?

    (1) fatigue
    (2) weakness
    (3) morning stiffness
    (4) frequently affect the DIP joints of the hand

5. Which of the following would you consider important objectives in the treatment of rheumatoid disease?

    (1) relief of pain
    (2) suppression of inflammation
    (3) preservation of function
    (4) patient education

6. The most common neurologic problem seen in rheumatoid arthritis results from which of the following?

    (1) peripheral neuropathy
    (2) nerve root irritation
    (3) myelopathy secondary to vertebral involvement
    (4) cerebellar cortical degeneration

7. Which of the following lab findings are consistent with the diagnosis of rheumatoid arthritis?

    (1) mild normocytic anemia
    (2) elevated WBC count
    (3) elevated sedimentation rate
    (4) rheumatoid factor always present in high titers

8. Which of the following are potential side effects from the use of nonsteroidal, antiinflammatory medications?

    (1) gastrointestinal upset
    (2) rash
    (3) edema
    (4) elevated liver function test

9. Possible complications from the use of adrenocorticosteroid in patients with rheumatoid arthritis include

    (1) decrease hypoglycemic effects when used with insulin or oral hypoglycemics
    (2) osteoporosis
    (3) increased risk of digitalis toxicity in patients on digoxin
    (4) reactivate infectious processes

SUMMARY OF DIRECTIONS				
A	**B**	**C**	**D**	**E**
1, 2, 3 only	1, 3 only	2, 4 only	4 only	All are correct

10. Drug-related lupus-like syndrome can occur with which of the following drugs?

    (1) hydralazine
    (2) procainamide (Procan, Pronestyl)
    (3) phenytoin (Dilantin)
    (4) indomethacin (Indocin)

11. Which of the following are correct concerning rheumatoid arthritis?

    (1) occurs predominately in the second or third decade of life
    (2) is a highly predictable disease
    (3) the extent of articular involvement correlates well with the patient's complaints
    (4) affect women more often than men

DIRECTIONS (Questions 12 through 20): Each of the numbered items or incomplete statements in this section is followed by answers or by completions of the statement. Select the ONE lettered answer or completion that is BEST in each case.

12. Which of the following is considered the first drug of choice in the treatment of every new rheumatoid arthritis patient?

    (A) oral gold salts
    (B) aspirin
    (C) oral prednisone
    (D) indomethacin
    (E) intrarticular dexamethasone

13. In "rheumatoid disease" the majority of clinical and pathologic findings are a result of chronic inflammation of what structure?

    (A) synovial membranes
    (B) epiphyseal disc
    (C) articular cartilage
    (D) periosteal membrane
    (E) subchondrial bone

14. Which of the following tests is most useful in assessing the response in the treatment of rheumatoid arthritis?

    (A) Hgb and Hct (hemaglobin and hematacrit)
    (B) sedimentation rate
    (C) rheumatoid factor
    (D) synovial fluid exam
    (E) WBC count

15. The therapy for rheumatoid disease is based primarily on the use of modalities that perform what function?

    (A) stimulate phagocytosis
    (B) fight infection
    (C) reverse histamine reaction
    (D) inhibit prostaglandin production
    (E) suppress phagocytosis

16. All the following may be affected by SLE (systemic lupus erythematosus) **EXCEPT** the

    (A) heart
    (B) liver
    (C) joints
    (D) kidney
    (E) skin

17. Patients with rheumatoid arthritis can present with many types of deformities of the hand. Hyperextension of the PIP joint in conjunction with flexion at the DIP joint constitutes what deformity?

    (A) Dupturen's contracture
    (B) mallet finger
    (C) swan-neck deformity
    (D) boutonniere deformity
    (E) trigger finger

18. Ossification of the annulus, fibrosis of the intervertebral disc, and longitudinal ligament (Bamboo Spine) appearing on x-ray is classically associated with which of the following diseases?

    (A) systemic lupus erythematosus
    (B) osteoarthritis
    (C) degenerative disc disease
    (D) ankylosing spondylitis
    (E) posttraumatic changes from a compression fracture

19. A 52-year-old man presents with severe right ankle pain for 2 days and no other complaints. During the exam, the joint is erythematous, warm, and an effusion is noted. The patient is afebrile; WBC: 9000, with normal differential; BUN and creatinine are within normal limits. Uric acid level is 9.6 mg/dL (normal is 2.5 to 8 mg/dL). The most likely diagnosis is:

    (A) rheumatoid arthritis
    (B) osteoarthritis
    (C) pseudogout
    (D) gouty arthritis
    (E) bacterial septic arthritis

20. A 40-year-old female presents with a history of acute onset of right knee pain, chills, and sweats. Her temperature is 103.0° F. The right knee is erythematous, swollen with an effusion, and x-rays

reveal only soft tissue swelling. Arthrocentesis reveals 80,000/uL leukocytes with 90% polymorphonuclear cells. The patient's symptoms, physical, and laboratory findings are most consistent with which of the following?

(A) gouty arthritis
(B) osteoarthritis
(C) rheumatoid arthritis
(D) bacterial septic arthritis
(E) Lyme disease

DIRECTIONS (Questions 21 through 25): Each group of items in this section consists of lettered headings followed by a set of numbered words or phrases. For each numbered word or phrase, select the ONE lettered heading that is most closely associated with it. Each lettered heading may be selected once, more than once, or not at all.

Match the following diseases with the most appropriate description and physical findings:

(A) Multisystem disease characterized by persistent inflammatory synovitis, usually symmetrical and polyarticular with morning stiffness. PIP and MCP are joints frequently involved.

(B) Multisystem disorder characterized by fibrotic infiltration of the skin and various organ systems. Raynaud's phenomenon, fibrosis of the skin (scleroderma), and hypomotility of the esophagus is common.

(C) Earliest changes in this disease are frequently found in the sacroiliac joints of young men and is strongly associated with histocompatibility antigen HLA-B27.

(D) This may affect any joint, usually limited to one or few joints, and laboratory investigation is usually unremarkable.

(E) May involve virtually any organ system; common features include fatigue, fever, weight loss, and skin rashes (particularly malar rashes over both cheeks).

21. progressive systemic sclerosis (PSS)

22. rheumatoid arthritis (RA)

23. systemic lupus erythmatosus (SLE)

24. anklylosing spondylitis

25. osteoarthritis

Answers and Explanations

1. (B) Osteoarthritis is the most common disease of axial and peripheral diarthroidal joints. Progressive deterioration and loss of articular cartilage along with reactive changes at joint margins and subchondral bone are characteristic. Heberden's nodes are the formation of spurs at the dorsolateral and medial aspects of the distal interphalangeal (DIP) joints, usually developing slowly over months to years. The DIP joints are usually spared in rheumatoid arthritis. The clinical features of osteoarthritis are usually local; early in the disease, pain occurs after joint use and improves with rest. Later in the disease, pain occurs with minimal motion and even at rest. Morning stiffness and swan-neck deformities of the hands are more frequently found in rheumatoid arthritis. Morning stiffness is thought to be the result of synovial congestion and thickening along with joint effusion. Swan-neck deformity is the hyperextension of the PIP joint and flexion of the DIP joint. *(Rodman et al, pp. 40–41, 104–108)*

2. (A) The laboratory investigation in osteoarthritis (OA) is helpful in excluding other joint disease. There is no single diagnostic test for OA. Rheumatoid factors and antinuclear antibody (ANA) tests are negative, the erythrocyte sedimentation rate is usually normal to slightly elevated in patients with generalized or erosive OA. Synovial fluid exam reveals clear, straw-colored fluid with a low leukocyte count. The peripheral WBC count is usually normal. *(Rodman et al, p. 106)*

3. (B) Septic arthritis is a medical emergency. Failure to rapidly diagnosis this condition has the potential to cause permanent damage to the involved joint. Septic arthritis typically affects one joint or a few asymmetric joints. Patients with septic arthritis usually present with an acute onset of pain, fever, erythema, and swelling of the affected joint; systematic signs of infection are common. Weight-bearing joints (most commonly the knee) and the wrist are most commonly involved. *(Schwartz, pp. 1983–1984)*

4. (A) The onset of rheumatoid arthritis (RA) is frequently heralded by prodromal symptoms such as fatigue, anorexia, weight loss, weakness, generalized aching, and stiffness. Morning stiffness is frequent (see answer to question 1) in RA. The DIP joints can be involved in RA, but are usually spared and more consistently found in osteoarthritis. *(Rodman et al, pp. 40–41)*

5. (E) The treatment of rheumatoid diseases can be complex, with a wide varity of medications, surgical, and nonsurgical procedures available. The health care provider must be familiar with all treatment modalities; however, important general objectives must be kept in mind. The principal objectives of management must include: (1) relief of pain, (2) reduction or suppression of inflammation, (3) minimizing undesirable effects of the disease and treatment, (4) preservation of muscle and joint function, and (5) return to desirable and productive life. *(Rodman et al, pp. 46–47)*

6. (A) Neurologic involvement in RA usually involves peripheral nerve function secondary to chronic inflammation. Answers 1, 2, and 3 are all peripheral nerve problems seen in RA. Myelopathy due to vertebral involvement frequently occurs at the C1–C2 level. Approximately 50% of patients have mild perivascular infiltration of mononuclear cells in muscle and peripheral nerves. As the name implies, cerebellar cortical degeneration is a central nervous system disorder. The degeneration is due to chronic nutritional depletion commonly seen in alcoholics. *(Bennett and Claude, pp. 1998–2002)*

7. (B) The laboratory investigation in RA can be quite helpful, but the limitations of these tests must be understood by the health care practitioner. A normocytic anemia is common, occurring in approximately 40% of men and 60% of women affected. The erythrocyte sedimentation rate is usually elevated and the WBC count is usually normal. The rheumatoid factor is positive in approximately 70% of patients with RA and in 1% to 5% of normal patients. *(Rodman et al, pp. 44–46)*

8. **(E)** All the answers are correct. The side effects of nonsteroidal antiinflammatory medications need be known by all who treat inflammatory diseases. The side effects vary greatly with the individual drug types. Gastrointestinal problems occur in 1% to 10% of patients, rash occurs in 3% to 9% of patients, edema occurs in 1% to 3% of patients and may aggravate congestive heart failure. Elevation of liver function test can occur and should be followed at regular intervals. *(Geffner et al, pp. 1–47)*

9. **(E)** Regardless of the therapy, the frequency and severity of osteoporosis, a feature of RA, are increased by adrenocorticosteroid treatment. Compression fractures of the vertebral bodies are common. Decreased host resistance to acquired or reactivated infections is a well-documented feature of adrenocorticosteroid therapy. The use of these drugs aggravates latent or overt diabetes mellitus and the dose of insulin or oral hypoglycemics may need to be increased during therapy. Serum digoxin levels can be increased during therapy and rise to toxic levels; therefore, serum digoxin levels should be followed during therapy with adrenocorticosteroid medication. *(Fauci, pp. 132–133)*

10. **(A)** Drug-related lupus-like syndromes have been documented since 1953, with the use of hydralazine. There has been a steady accumulation of reports of lupus-like syndrome induced by various drugs. The syndrome occurs most commonly today with the use of procainamide (Procan, Pronestyl) and antiseizure medication such as phenytoin (Dilantin). Other medications that cause lupus-like syndromes are penicillamine, tetracycline, and isonazide. *(Rodman et al, p. 54)*

11. **(D)** RA affects women two to three times more often than men. Although, the disease can occur at any age, the peak incidence is in the fourth to the sixth decade of life. RA is not at all predictable. The disease can vary from intermittent and mild to unrelenting and eventually fatal. Because RA can involve periarticular structures, the extent of articular involvement does not correlate with the patients complaints. *(Rodman et al, pp. 38–41)*

12. **(B)** All the choices can be used in the treatment of RA, but aspirin is regarded as the drug of choice unless contraindicated. Aspirin is still the most tried, effective, and least expensive drug available for the treatment of RA. Between 3 to 6 g per day is usually required. *(Rodman et al, p. 46)*

13. **(A)** The classic presentation of RA is the result of chronic inflammation of synovial membranes. It is the formation of chronic granulation tissue (pannus) resulting from chronic synovitis that produces hydrolytic enzymes. These enzymes are capable of eroding articular cartilage, subchondral bone, ligaments, and tendons. *(Bennett and Claude, pp. 1999–2000)*

14. **(B)** The erythrocyte sedimentation rate (ESR) is diversely elevated in most patients and roughly parallels the disease activity, therefore, becoming a useful parameter for assessing response to therapy. WBC counts are most often normal, only 25% of patients are considered as having leukocytosis. Rheumatoid factor is not present in everyone with RA and does not change by the treatment of the disease. There is some correlation between the degree of anemia and the initial severity of the illness in RA, but anemia is present in only 40% of men and 60% of women, and does not correlate with the disease activity. *(Rodman et al, pp. 38–40)*

15. **(D)** The basis of therapy for RA is to suppress inflammation, because it is this process that leads to the destruction of skeletal and extraskeletal tissues. Prostaglandins are thought to act as mediators to stimulated inflammation. Inhibiting prostaglandin production is the major pharmacologic effect of aspirin, nonsteroidal antiinflammatory drugs, and corticosteroids. Gold-containing compounds, penicillamine, and antimalarials have a more specific antiinflammatory action and no inhibitory effects on the synthesis of prostaglandins. *(Rodman et al, pp. 16–19)*

16. **(B)** Systemic lupus erythematosus (SLE) affects many organ systems; however, no specific liver lesions are connected with the disease. In patients with SLE, 50% develop evidence of lupus nephritis and 25% have evidence of pericarditis, which can be transient and mild to massive pericardial effusion. Up to 85% of patients with SLE have skin, hair, or mucosal membrane changes (65% develop alopecia at some point) and 95% develop some type of arthritis or arthralgia. *(Rodman et al, pp. 52–53)*

17. **(C)** A hyperextension of the PIP joint in conjunction with flexion of the DIP joint describes a swanneck deformity. This deformity usually occurs in the index and middle fingers due to contraction of the interosseous and flexor muscles and tendons. Duptryen's contracture is caused by thickening and shortening of the palmar and sometimes the plantar fascia. A mallet finger deformity is usually the result of a traumatic injury in which the extensor tendon of the distal phalanx is ruptured. Boutonniere deformity is also common in RA, but is a flexion deformity of the PIP joint and extension of the DIP joint. A trigger finger refers to flexor tendon sheath inflammation in association with the development of a tendon nodule, giving rise to a "locking" of the digit in flexion. *(Rodman et al, pp. 164–167, 40–41)*

18. **(D)** "Bamboo spine" as described in the question is seen in patients with ankylosing spondylitis with the greatest frequency. SLE has no classical radiographic pattern; however, 15% of patients with SLE develop deforming arthritis and 5% to 8% develop aseptic necrosis. Osteoarthritis radiographically reveals joint space narrowing, subchrondral sclerosis, and osteophyte formation. Degenerative disc disease also shows joint space narrowing and osteophyte formation and spondylolisthesis may be present. Post traumatic changes from compression fractures usually involve anterior wedging of the vertebral body. *(Rodman et al, pp. 52–53, 178–180)*

19. **(D)** The patient presents with a monoarticular arthritis involving the ankle joint. The laboratory investigation reveals an elevated uric acid level and synovial fluid exam shows urate crystals classically seen in gouty arthritis. Bacterial septic arthritis is easily ruled out, as the patient has no fever, and one would expect a synovial white cell count in the range of 50,000 to 200,000. In rheumatoid arthritis, a monoarticular presentation is unlikely. Normal x-ray and urate crystals make the diagnosis of osteoarthritis remote. Pseudogout presents similarly, but crystal exam of the synovial fluid yields the rod-shaped crystals of calcium pyrophsophate. Also, one may find cartilaginous calcification on x-ray in pseudogout. Acute, gouty arthritis tends to affect the lower extremities, particularly the metatarsalphalangeal (MTP) joint (75% of patients), but is also frequently seen in the tarsal joints and ankle. The joints of the upper extremity can be affected, particularly the elbow, wrist, and metacarpalphalangeal joints. The shoulder, hips, and sacroiliac joint involvement is rare in pseudogout.

20. **(D)** This patient presents an acute onset of right knee pain, fever, and a swollen right knee. There are no x-ray findings consistent with bony pathology of intraarticular foreign body. There is an elevated synovial white count. These findings are most consistent with the diagnosis of bacterial septic arthritis. There are no urate crystals in the synovial fluid to accompany a diagnosis of gouty arthritis. Lyme disease is usually recognized clinically by an early, expanding, erythematous skin lesion (erythema chronicum migrans). One would not expect to find fever and a elevated synovial white count with osteoarthritis. *(Wyngaarden and Smith, pp. 1161–1168; Rodman, 116)*

21. **(B)** Progressive systemic sclerosis (PSS) is a multisystem disorder characterized by inflammation, fibrosis, and degeneration of the integument. These problems are associated with similar changes and prominent vascular lesions in the gastrointestinal tract, synovium, heart, lung, and kidneys. Raynauds phenomenon, fibrosis of the skin (scleroderma, and hypomotility of the esophagus are common) *(Wyngaarden and Smith, p. 623)*

22. **(A)** RA is a multisystem disease characterized by persistent inflammatory synovitis that is usually symmetrical and polyarticular associated with morning stiffness. RA is often associated with extraarticular involvement of other organ systems. Organs frequently affected include the skin, eye, cardiovascular system, respiratory system, spleen, and nervous system. *(Wyngaarden and Smith, p. 613)*

23. **(E)** SLE is an acute and chronic inflammatory process of unknown etiology that may involve virtually every organ system. The clinical presentation of SLE is highly variable and common features include fatigue, fever, weight loss, and the classic butterfly rash. Polyarthralgias and polyarthritis are the most common manifestations of SLE, occurring in 95% of patients. *(Wyngaarden and Smith, p. 617)*

24. **(C)** Anklylosing spondylitis (AS) usually presents during young adulthood in a male to female ratio of 3:1. The earliest changes in this disease are frequently found in the sacroiliac joints. There is an association with histocompatibility antigen HLA-B27. Inflammatory ocular disease, in particular, acute anterior uveitis, occurs in approximately one quarter of those patients with AS. *(Wyngaarden and Smith, p. 633)*

25. **(D)** Osteoarthritis is the most frequently encountered disorder of connective tissue affecting he joints in humans. It is a disease of both the articular cartilage and the subchondral bone. Osteoarthritis may affect any joint, but is usually limited to one or a few. There are no specific laboratory features of Osteoarthritis. *(Wyngaarden and Smith, p. 639)*

REFERENCES

Beeson, PB. In Wyngaarden JB, Smith, LH (eds.). *Cecil Textbook of Medicine*, 18th ed. Philadelphia: WB Saunders, 1988.

Bennett, Claude J. Rheumatoid arthritis. In Wyngaarden JB, Smith LH, (eds). *Cecil Textbook of Medicine*, 18th ed. Philadelphia: WB Saunders, 1988.

Fauci, A. Glucocorticosteroid therapy. In Wyngaarden JB, Smith LH, (eds). *Cecil Textbook of Medicine*, 18th ed. Philadelphia: WB Saunders, 1988.

Geffner, ES. *Compendium of Drug Therapy*. New York: McGraw-Hill, 1988.

Mercier LR, Pettid FJ. *Practical Orthopedics*. Chicago: Year Book Medical Publishing, 1984.

Rodman, GP, et al. *Primer on the Rheumatic Diseases*, 8th ed.

Schwartz, SI, et al. (eds). *Principles of Surgery*, 5th ed. New York: McGraw-Hill, 1989.

Rheumatology Subspecialty List:

Question Numbers and Subspecialty
1. Osteoarthritis—characteristics
2. Osteoarthritis—laboratory findings
3. Bacterial septic arthritis—characteristics
4. Rheumatoid arthritis—characteristics
5. Rheumatoid arthritis—treatment
6. Rheumatoid arthritis—complications
7. Rheumatoid arthritis—laboratory evaluation
8. Medications
9. Medications
10. Medications
11. Rheumatoid arthritis—characteristics
12. Medications
13. Rheumatoid arthritis—characteristics
14. Rheumatoid arthritis—laboratory evaluation
15. Rheumatoid arthritis—treatment
16. Systemic lupus erythematosus—clinical effects
17. Rheumatoid arthritis—clinical findings
18. Anklosing spondylitis—clinical findings
19. Gouty arthritis—diagnosis
20. Bacterial septic arthritis—diagnosis
21. Progressive systemic sclerosis—characteristics
22. Rheumatoid arthritis—characteristics
23. Systemic lupus erythematosus—characteristics
24. Ankylosing spondylitis—characteristics
25. Osteoarthritis—characteristics

Internal Medicine: Hematology/Oncology

Lynne P. Bolstad

Questions

DIRECTIONS (Questions 1 through 6): Each group of items in this section consists of lettered headings followed by a set of numbered words or phrases. For each numbered word or phrase, select the ONE lettered heading that is most closely associated with it. Each lettered heading may be selected once, more than once, or not at all.

Some side effects of chemotherapy may lead a patient to his/her oncologist when they are obviously related to the treatment regimen. However, when the connection is not clear to the patient, he/she may present to the primary care physician instead. Match the side effects listed below to the drugs with which they are most commonly associated.

    (A) methotrexate (MTX)
    (B) vincristine (VCR, Oncovin)
    (C) blenoxane (Bleomycin)
    (D) cyclophosphamide (Cytoxan)
    (E) nitrogen mustard (Mustargen)

1. peripheral neuropathy

2. fever/chills

3. stomatitis

4. hemorrhagic cystitis

5. constipation/paralytic ileus

6. dyspnea

DIRECTIONS (Questions 7 through 21): Each of the numbered items or incomplete statements in this section is followed by answers or by completions of the statement. Select the ONE lettered answer or completion that is BEST in each case.

7. Choosing appropriate blood components and quantities for transfusion requires adequate assessment of degree of volume of blood loss. In the first hour posthemorrhage, the most reliable measure of blood loss is

(A) patient description of symptoms
(B) hemoglobin/hematocrit
(C) pulse and postural blood pressures
(D) degree of peripheral edema
(E) degree of pallor

8. Initial therapy of idiopathic thrombocytopenic purpura (TIP) most commonly consists of

(A) splenectomy
(B) immunosuppressive agents
(C) B_{12} injections
(D) IV gamma globulin
(E) corticosteroids

9. All the following are common complications of Hemophilia A EXCEPT

(A) aseptic necrosis of the femoral head
(B) severe degenerative joint disease
(C) HIV infection
(D) compartment syndrome
(E) hepatitis

10. Transfusion of fresh frozen plasma (FFP) is the therapy of choice in controlling acute bleeding episodes in all the following coagulopathies EXCEPT

(A) hemophilia B
(B) factor XI deficiency
(C) vitamin K deficiency
(D) hemorrhagic diathesis of liver disease
(E) hemophilia A

11. A 55-year-old white female presents with nonspecific complaints of anorexia, fatigue, hair loss, and dry skin. Exam reveals a pale, fair-skinned woman with dry skin, mild vitiligo, and a beefy red tongue. Laboratory values reveal hypothyroidism and a macrocytic anemia. Which of the anemias listed below is most commonly associated with the findings above?

(A) anemia of chronic disease
(B) thalassemia minor
(C) folate deficiency

(D) pernicious anemia
(E) iron deficiency

12. A 14-year-old anemic patient has the following findings: gallstones, mild icterus, splenomegaly, elevated reticulocyte count, and decreased serum haptoglobin, yet feels reasonably well. These findings most strongly suggest

(A) autoimmune hemolytic anemia
(B) von Willebrand's disease
(C) idiopathic hemochromatosis
(D) B_{12} deficiency
(E) hereditary spherocytosis

13. All the health problems below are commonly associated with homozygous sickle cell anemia **EXCEPT**

(A) cholelithiasis
(B) CHF
(C) aseptic necrosis of the femoral head
(D) gout
(E) hepatic infarct

14. The primary pathological process in sickle cell anemia is that of

(A) diminished hemoglobin production
(B) splenic sequestration of RBCs
(C) increased RBC aggregation
(D) RBC membrane change upon deoxygenation
(E) hemoglobin polymerization upon deoxygenation

15. A 45-year old, generally healthy, white female comes in for an annual checkup. She feels fairly well, except for a gradual increase in fatigue and some occasional mild dysphagia. Her menses are becoming a bit irregular, and occasionally heavier. CBC shows WBC, 6400; H/H, 8.5/29; MCV, 68, MCH, 19.7, MCHC, 28.9: differential, WNL; poikilocytosis on smear. This presentation most strongly suggests

(A) folate deficiency
(B) pernicious anemia (PA)
(C) G6PD deficiency
(D) iron deficiency
(E) hereditary spherocytosis

16. All the following statements regarding polycythemia vera (PV) are true **EXCEPT**

(A) erythropoietin levels are increased in PV
(B) PV can progress to myelofibrosis
(C) PV can progress to other hematological neoplasms
(D) splenomegaly is commonly seen in PV
(E) pruritis and hyperuricemia are common findings in PV

17. A 50-year-old white male presents with complaints of increasing backache, fatigue, and weight loss of at least several weeks' duration, and acute onset 36 hours earlier of fever, loose cough, and dyspnea. Physical exam strongly suggests pneumonia (confirmed on x-ray), and also reveals pallor, petechiae on the face and legs, several recent bruises, mild hepatosplenomegaly, and several small palpable lymph nodes. The LEAST likely diagnosis is

(A) adult T-lymphocyte leukemia (ATL)
(B) aplastic anemia
(C) multiple myeloma
(D) acute myelogenous leukemia (AML)
(E) well-differentiated lymphocytic lymphoma

18. All the following statements are true of both acute lymphoblastic leukemia (ALL) patients and acute myelogenous leukemia (AML) patients **EXCEPT**

(A) a significant percentage of these children and young adults achieve a long-term remission and/or cure
(B) induction therapy should be initiated at a major medical or speciality cancer center
(C) both ALL and AML may present with signs and symptoms of bone marrow failure
(D) ALL and AML patients are at high risk for serious infection
(E) Leukostasis can develop and lead to hypoperfusion of vital tissues

19. All the following statements regarding chronic lymphocytic leukemia (CLL) are true **EXCEPT**

(A) CLL and diffuse well-differentiated lymphocytic lymphoma are both neoplasms of B-cell origin and are so similar that they follow essentially the same clinical course.
(B) CLL, which presents with massive splenomegaly, lymphadenopathy, and lymphocytosis has a median survival of 5 years
(C) Combination chemotherapy for CLL is routinely initiated at the time of diagnosis in an attempt to achieve decreased tumor load and possible remission as early in the disease process as possible.
(D) A Coombs + hemolytic anemia occurs in up to 20% of patients with CLL.
(E) Patients who demonstrate anemia and/or thrombocytopenia at the time of diagnosis of CLL have a 2-year median survival.

A 17-year-old white female presents with a 2-week history of right cervical adenopathy with no other symptoms. CBC is WNL, monospot is negative and CXR reveals slight mediastinal widening. Biopsy of the adenopathy reveals Sternberg–Reed cells, and final pathology report is one of Hodgkin's disease, nodular sclerosis type. PE (including indirect laryngoscopy) reveals no other lymphadenopathy or organomegaly; lymphograms and abdominal CT are WNL; chest CT reveals mildly enlarged mediastinal nodes.

20. This patient's disease is Stage

(A) $I_E A$
(B) II A
(C) III A
(D) III B
(E) IV A

21. Recommended therapy for this patient would consist of

(A) radiation therapy to the involved areas (involved field (IF) radiation therapy)
(B) single-agent chemotherapy, such as pulse therapy with high doses of an alkylating agent
(C) mantle field plus splenic irradiation (extended filed (EF) radiation therapy)
(D) combination chemotherapy, such as MOPP or ABVD
(E) bone marrow transplantation

DIRECTIONS (Questions 22 through 35): For each of the items in this section, ONE or MORE of the numbered options is correct. Choose the answer

A if only **1, 2, and 3** are correct,
B if only **1 and 3** are correct,
C if only **2 and 4** are correct,
D if only **4** is correct,
E if **all** are correct.

22. One of the mechanisms of thrombocytopenia is that of accelerated destruction of platelets. Common causes of this mechanism include

(1) prosthetic cardiac valves
(2) prosthetic joints
(3) idiopathic thrombocytopenic purpura (ITP)
(4) myeloproliferative disorders

23. Treatment of the underlying disease/precipitating factor is essential to successful management of disseminated intravascular coagulation (DIC). Common situations triggering this disorder include

(1) bacterial sepsis
(2) disseminated malignancy
(3) catastrophic obstetrical event
(4) massive trauma

24. Megaloblastic anemias are generally due to B_{12} or folate deficiency of some type. Which of the following are associated with folate deficiency?

(1) pregnancy
(2) tropical sprue

(3) dialysis
(4) alcohol abuse

25. Which of the following are associated with B_{12} deficiency?

(1) anticonvulsant therapy
(2) partial gastrectomy
(3) lead poisoning
(4) Crohn's disease

26. Von Willebrand's disease (vWD) is an autosomal dominant disorder involving diminished or defective synthesis of von Willebrand factor (vWF). This factor's role in the process of hemostasis includes

(1) conversion of factor IX to X
(2) facilitation of platelet adhesion
(3) activation of factor VII
(4) transport of factor VIII

27. A 40-year-old white female presents with easy bruising and significantly increased menstrual bleeding this month. CBC reveals WBC, 4400: H/H, 11.2/33; platelet count, 29,000. Differential diagnosis should include

(1) acute leukemia
(2) drug-induced thrombocytopenia
(3) SLE
(4) aplastic anemia

28. Causes of hereditary hemolytic anemia include

(1) hereditary spherocytosis
(2) G6PD deficiency
(3) thalassemia
(4) warm antibodies

29. Which of the following statements regarding thalassemia is/are true?

(1) The primary pathologic process in β-thalassemia major involves both defective erythropoiesis and hemolysis
(2) A common finding in undertransfused β-thalassemia major is splenomegaly
(3) Homozygous β-thalassemia results in hydrope fetalis
(4) HbH disease involves hemolysis

30. Work-up for iron deficiency (Fe def.) anemia should include

(1) UGI series
(2) stool for guaiac and O&P
(3) proctosigmoidoscopy and BE
(4) thyroid function studies

31. A patient has the following CBC: WBC, 4800; H/H, 8.6/26; MCV, 87; MCH, 29; MCHC, 33. Differential diagnosis should include

(1) myelopthisic anemia
(2) hereditary sideroblastic anemia
(3) anemia of chronic disorders
(4) thalassemia trait

32. Problems common to multiple myeloma include

(1) pathological fractures
(2) hypercalcemia
(3) spinal cord compression
(4) hyperviscosity syndrome

33. Which of the following statements about chronic myelogenous leukemia (CML) is/are true?

(1) combination chemotherapy is used to achieve remission in the chronic phase of CML
(2) presentation of CML commonly includes splenomegaly, leukocytosis, and symptoms of hypermetabolism
(3) the Philadelphia chromosome (Ph^1) is present in 20% to 30% of CML patients
(4) The majority of CML patients progress to a blastic phase that can be either myeloid or lymphoid.

34. Therapy and prognosis of lymphocytic ("non-Hodgkin's") lymphoma are determined more by histology than staging. High-grade, or aggressive, lymphomas include

(1) Burkitt's lymphoma
(2) diffuse lymphoblastic lymphoma
(3) diffuse bistiocytic (large cell immunoblastic) lymphoma
(4) diffuse well-differentiated lymphocytic lymphoma

35. In which of the following situations would it be unreasonable to consider bone marrow transplantation?

(1) a 6-year-old child with ALL in second remission
(2) a 36-year-old man with a non-Hodgkin's lymphoma in second relapse
(3) a 38-year-old woman in the chronic phase of CML
(4) a 68-year-old man with CML in blast crisis

Answers and Explanations

1. (B); 2. (C); 3. (A); 4. (D); 5. (B); 6. (C) Peripheral neuropathy is a common side effect of VCR: the patient can be reassured that this is not a new, bizarre manifestation of his/her disease. Fever often occurs 4 to 10 hours (occasionally sooner) after administration of Bleomycin, abating within 48 hours, and usually deceasing in severity with successive doses. When this does occur, one must always consider the possibility of infection and evaluate the patient appropriately. Acetaminophen and antihistamines may relieve symptoms of mild to moderate severity, and steroids may be effective when symptoms are severe. Stomatitis may occur with several chemotherapeutic agents, but particularly with MTX. One must always carefully evaluate for, and treat appropriately, herpes simplex and *Candida* infections that may also be involved. Hemmorrhagic cystitis can be seen with Cytoxan, and with the newer agent ifosfamide (Ifex), but one must also rule out a UTI when hematuria occurs. Constipation is common with use of VCR and, less commonly, with Velban. It should be treated early with multiple modalities (i.e., stool softeners, bulk agents, increased hydration). Paralytic ileus occurs less commonly and can, if not managed properly, in rare instances lead to bowel perforation. There is an 8% to 10% incidence of pulmonary fibrosis in patients receiving Bleomycin. Chest x-rays and pulmonary function studies with DLCO should be followed, and the drug should be discontinued if changes occur. In the patient presenting with dyspnea, this problem should be kept in mind while evaluating for other problems such as infection, pleural effusion, and pulmonary emboli. Nitrogen mustard does have side effects, the most common of which include severe nausea and vomiting, myelosuppression, thrombophlebitis, and tissue necrosis in the event of extravasation. *(Knobf et al, pp. 36–37, 46–47, 62–63, 78–81, 101–103)*

7. (C) The patient's description of symptoms is subjective and is affected by many other factors, such as pain, fear, and chronic health problems. Hematocrit/hemoglobin may be maintained at deceptively high levels for several hours after blood loss by compensatory vasoconstriction. Peripheral edema develops over a relatively long period of time, usually in the setting of chronic blood loss or anemia, as a result of some degree of high-output failure. Pallor has many causes in addition to blood loss, including hypoxemia, cold exposure, and fright. The earliest measurable parameters to change in response to blood loss are usually pulse, which rises, and blood pressure, which often demonstrates evidence of orthostatic hypotension fairly quickly after loss of blood volume large enough to require intervention. *(Braunwald et al, p. 1486)*

8. (E) A significant percentage of patients with ITP will normalize their platelet counts on high-dose prednisone, which is tapered after several weeks of therapy. If there is no response to this treatment regimen, or relapse occurs during or after tapering the steroids, splenectomy is usually considered. This is effective in significantly raising platelet counts in a high percentage of patients. Immunosuppressive agents (drugs such as cyclophosphamide, azathioprine, and vincristine) are generally considered only when both the above have failed, due to serious potential toxicities. IV gamma globulin is used for temporary phagocytic blockade in situations such as impending surgery or ITP in late pregnancy. Its value is limited because improvement is usually limited to approximately 4-weeks' duration. B_{12} is of no value in treating ITP. *(Braunwald et al, pp. 1472–1473)*

9. (A) There is no *specific* association of aseptic necrosis of the femoral head with hemophilia A. Severe degenerative joint disease follows multiple or chronic hemarthroses. The use of products such as cryoprecipitate and partially purified factor VIII concentrate has helped tremendously in decreasing the frequency and severity of this problem in recent years (although it is still seen commonly, particularly in older hemophiliacs who were born before these products were available). Hemophiliacs are at high risk for hepatitis and HIV infection due to their exposure to multiple blood products. Improved screening and a commercial heating process that inactivates HIV but not factor VIII have decreased, although not eliminated, this risk. Compartment syndromes occur due to extensive hemorrhage into soft tissue compartments and can result in muscle necrosis, ischemic nerve damage, and contractures if timely surgical intervention is not provided. *(Braunwald et al, pp. 1476–1477; Hoffbrand and Pettit, pp. 240–246)*

10. **(E)** The therapy of choice in hemophilia A (factor VIII deficiency) is infusion of partially purified factor VIII concentrate when available, or cryoprecipitate if it is not (this contains 50% of the factor VIII of FFP in 10% of the volume). Hemophilia B (factor IX deficiency) and factor XI deficiency must be differentiated from Hemophilia A, because cryoprecipitate and factor VIII concentrate do not supply these factors effectively, whereas FFP does. FFP, rather than vitamin K, is the therapy of choice for acute bleeding in vitamin K deficiency (as well as oral anticoagulant overdose) because it immediately supplies the diminished prothrombin factors (II, VII, IX, X, and proteins C and S) needed for hemostasis. Purified prothrombin complexes are avoided because these entail a high risk of thrombotic events. Administration of vitamin K (parenterally) requires 8 to 10 hours to permit normal factor synthesis. The hemorrhagic diathesis of liver disease involves vitamin K deficiency, decreased production of multiple coagulation factors, and increased production of coagulation inhibitors. Only FFP can immediately supply enough of the deficient factors to control acute hemorrhage although vitamin K administration may be helpful in long-term management). *(Braunwald et al, pp. 1476–1478; Hoffbrand and Pettit, pp. 240–249)*

11. **(D)** A high percentage of patients with PA are of Northern European descent and are fair haired and/or prematurely gray. Current thought is that this condition has an immunologic origin, probably an autoimmune response against gastric parietal cells. There is a strong association with other disorders of such origin, including thyroid disorders, Addison's disease, vitiligo, and hypoparathyroidism; 90% have antiparietal cell antibodies, 50% to 60% have antiintrinsic-factor antibodies. In PA, there is a loss of B_{12} absorption due to the absence of intrinsic factor in the stomach, and gastrin levels are often elevated. Findings may include pallor, slight icterus, smooth (sore) beefy red tongue, mild hepatosplenomegaly, and in more advanced cases, fast pulse, cardiomegaly, CHF, and CNS symptoms (neuropathy, ataxia, weakness, decreased finger coordination, decreased vibratory sense, positive Romberg, Babinski reflexes, and disturbed mentation). CBC and bone marrow demonstrate mega-

loblastic changes and serum B_{12} levels are low. These patients have a two-fold to three-fold increased incidence of gastric carcinoma, and so should be monitored accordingly. *(Braunwald et al, pp. 1499–1501; Hoffbrand and Pettit, pp. 56–57)*

12. **(E)** This presentation is consistent with a hemolytic anemia. The presence of gallstones in such a young person and the lack of specific symptoms strongly suggest chronic or congenital hemolysis, such as hereditary spherocytosis, rather than an acute acquired hemolytic process, such as autoimmune hemolytic (immunohemolytic) anemia (which generally occurs in adults, is often, although not always, acute in presentation, and has a positive direct Coombs' test). *(Braunwald et al, pp. 1506–1517)*

13. **(D)** Gout has no specific association with sickle cell anemia. Cholelithiasis is commonly associated with sickle cell anemia because of the icterus that occurs secondary to chronic hemolysis, and must always be kept in mind when evaluating the sickle cell patient with abdominal pain (i.e., one cannot automatically assume that such pain is due to sickle cell crisis). Chronic anemia and hypoxemia often lead to a chronic hyperdynamic cardiac state, and later to CHF. Skeletal infarction can readily lead to aseptic necrosis of the femoral head. Hepatic infarcts are common and can lead to significant hepatic parenchymal damage. *(Braunwald et al, pp. 1520–1522)*

14. **(E)** The Hb variant of sickle cell anemia, HbS, is a result of β chain abnormality. This abnormality causes extensive abnormal polymerization of Hb in the RBC upon deoxygenization of the blood. This in turn leads to deformation of the cell from its usual flexible biconcave shape to an elongated, rigid ("sickle") shape. The consequence is a significant increase in local hypoxia that then perpetuates the problem and can lead to infarcts of any organ/tissue. It also results in rapid RBC culling and destruction (hemolysis). Hb production is actually quite rapid, rather than diminished. Crises can occur due to marrow failure, caused by the stress of infection or folate deficiency, or due to vasoocclusive phenomena, precipitated by stresses such as vasoconstriction due to cold exposure, dehydration, or infection. The majority of people carrying this abnormal gene are of central African descent (heterozygotes may gain a small degree of protection against falciparum malaria). Heterozygotes (i.e., those with sickle cell trait) generally have minimal clinical disease, but homozygotes (i.e., those with sickle cell anemia) have a significantly diminished life expectancy; growth and development are retarded, and they are at significantly increased risk of infection. Chronic damage to multiple organs occurs due to infarcts. Treatment consists largely of trying to prevent crises from occurring and treating

the triggering condition when they do occur. Folate supplementation may be helpful, with only occasional need for transfusion. Genetic counseling should play an important role in preventing this disease. *(Braunwald et al, pp. 1518–1522; Hoffbrand and Pettit, pp. 93–98)*

15. (D) This is a hypochromic microcytic anemia. Folate deficiency and PA present a megaloblastic picture. Hereditary spherocytosis and G6PD deficiency would have become evident much earlier in life (this patient is also not in a high-risk group for G6PD deficiency). This CBC, including poikilocytosis on the smear, is typical for Fe deficiency anemia. Physical signs may include pallor, nail changes, angular cheilosis, atrophic glossitis, dysphagia (secondary to postcricoid web—most commonly seen in middle-aged women), and retinal hemorrhages when the anemia is severe and of rapid onset. Other typical lab findings include decreased serum Fe and ferritin levels, increased Fe-binding capacity (IBC), haptoglobin WNL, decreased FE stores on bone marrow aspiration, and reticulocyte count WNL or slightly elevated. Therapy consists of identifying and correcting the underlying cause of the deficiency, and supplementation. Up to 6 months of oral Fe 300 mg tid may be required to correct the anemia and replenish body stores. When oral absorption is poor, Fe-dextran complex can be given parenterally in several intramuscular injections (preferred route) or a single IV infusion, for a total of 1.5 to 2.0 g. Severe reactions can occur, particularly with the IV route; hence, a small test dose (50 mg) should be given. *(Braunwald et al, pp. 1495–1497; Hoffbrand and Pettit, pp. 34–40)*

16. (A) In *secondary* polycythemia, erythropoietin is increased in an effort to compensate for chronic hypoxia (as in chronic pulmonary diseases, high-altitude dwelling, congenital heart disease, Pickwickian syndrome, increased methemoglobin or sulfhemoglobin states), or due to conditions such as Cushing's syndrome and tumors (particularly renal). In PV, erythropoietin is *decreased* or absent, leukocyte alkaline phosphastase is increased, B_{12} is WNL or increased, and hyperuricemia, thrombocytosis, and leukocytosis are common. Clinical features, mostly due to increased blood viscosity, may include plethora, headaches, gout, fatigue/malaise, pruritis, edema, thrombotic or bleeding events, splenomegaly, and acne rosacea. Approximately 30% of patients with PV go on to develop myelofibrosis, and up to 15% may develop leukemias (or, less commonly, lymphomas). Intermittent phlebotomy is a safe mode of therapy. Myelosuppression is recommended in the advent of symptomatic thrombocytosis, rapidly enlarging spleen, or symptoms of hypermetabolism. This can be achieved with radioactive P^{32} every 3 months as

needed, or chemotherapeutic agents such as melphalan, busulfan, chlorambucil, or hydroxyurea. There is fear that myelosuppressive therapy may increase the risk of later leukemia or lymphoma, so phlebotomy alone is usually tried as initial therapy. *(Braunwald et al, pp. 147–148, 1529–1531; Hoffbrand and Pettit, pp. 214–217)*

17. (B) Thrombocytopenia may be seen in aplastic anemia, leukemias, myelomas, and lymphomas, and may present with petechiae, bruising, purpura, and/or unusual bleeding. All these conditions also cause an increased risk of infection, and an acute pneumonia (or other infection such as cellulitis or perirectal abscess) may well be the presenting complaint. Fever is very nonspecific symptom, and may be due to neoplastic activity or infection. All these conditions often present with anemia, which causes pallor and fatigue. Hepatosplenomegaly and/or lymphadenopathy are commonly seen in leukemias and lymphomas, and occasionally myelomas, but are generally not found in aplastic anemia. Bone pain may occur in leukemias due to the increasing activity of neoplastic cells in the marrow, and in myeloma due to skeletal destruction; retroperitoneal lymphadenopathy often causes back pain in lymphoma patients; bone pain is not a specific common finding in aplastic anemia. Weight loss is common in most neoplastic processes, but not in aplastic anemia. Initial work-up for this patient should include CBC, platelet count, ESR, chemical panel, U/A, protein electrophoresis, and bone marrow aspiration/biopsy, with further work-up to be based on these results (i.e., scans, lymph node biopsy, lumbar puncture, skeletal survey). *(Eiseman et al, pp. 193–228)*

18. (A) Both ALL and AML often do present with signs and symptoms of bone marrow failure, such as pancytopenia, bruising/petechiae/purpura, fatigue, and pallor due to anemia; but they may also present with significant leukocytosis. As the number of circulating blasts approaches and passes 100,000/mL, the risk of symptoms from leukostasis (due to interference with tissue perfusion) rises. In both ALL and AML, patients are immunocompromised, and sepsis and opportunistic infections are very common problems. Therapy aimed at long-term remission for any acute leukemia is intensive and complex, with many potential side effects and complications. A community hospital generally does not have the staff/materials/experience/equipment needed to support the critically ill leukemic undergoing induction therapy; thus, immediate transfer to a major treatment center upon diagnosis is essential. ALL is primarily a disease of children and young adults, with 50% of the children achieving long-term remission/possible cure (a lower percentage in adults and high-risk children). Successful therapy involves intensive multi-drug chemotherapy (VCR, prednisone, plus daunorubicin or L-asparaginase), prophylactic CNS radiation therapy, and maintenance chemotherapy for more than 1 year. AML is primarily a disease of adults and only 10% to 30% achieve a long-term remission, with very few cures. Induction therapy usually includes cytarabrine and daunorubicin (± 6 thioguanine); maintenance regimens are still being evaluated, and CNS relapse is rare (unlike ALL), so prophylactic RT is not employed. *(Braunwald et al, pp. 1541–1547)*

19. **(C)** Chronic lymphocytic leukemia is a disease that usually appears in the fourth or fifth decade of life, or later, and is characterized by increased mature appearing lymphocytes in the peripheral blood, associated with spleen, node, and bone marrow infiltration by a B-cell neoplasm. It is clinically indistinguishable from diffuse well-differentiated lymphocytic lymphoma. It is a relatively indolent disease that often presents with massive hepatosplenomegaly, peripheral lymphocytosis, and occasionally with lymphadenopathy, with surprisingly few symptoms—it is often picked up on routine exam or CBC. Stage A—lymphocytosis ± mild lymphadenopathy has a median survival of more than 7 years. Stage B—lymphocytosis, larger lymphadenopathy and hepatosplenomegaly—has a median survival of 5 years. Stage C—Stage B findings plus anemia and/or thrombocytopenia—has a 2 year median survival. No potentially curative therapy regime has been found. Single alkylating agents, such as low-dose daily or pulse high-dose chlorambucil, or pulse cyclophosphamide, are indicated to palliate hemolytic anemia, symptomatic organomegaly or lymphadenopathy, or systemic symptoms (such as fever, weight, loss, fatigue, night sweats). Steroid therapy may be of value in instances of hemolytic anemia, which occurs in about 20% of CLL patients, or autoimmune thrombocytopenia (differentiated from thrombocytopenia secondary to neoplastic marrow invasion by presence of antiplatelet antibodies and increased megakaryocytes in the marrow). Splenectomy may be helpful if such problems fail to respond to steroids, but is not otherwise indicated. Radiation therapy may control localized symptomatic disease; interferon is of no value. Hairy cell leukemia, another adult lymphoid leukemia (seen predominantly in males more than 40-years old) must be differentiated from CLL, as interferon *is* very effective in such patients with progressive disease, and alkylating agents are poorly tolerated. As in the other leukemias, infection is a major problem in patients with progressing disease; thus early diagnosis of infection and initiation of appropriate therapy is essential. *(Braunwald et al, pp. 1548–1550; Eiseman et al, pp. 196–200)*

20. **(B)** Staging is the same for all lymphomas and is especially vital in planning long-term management for Hodgkin's disease. The letter **B** denotes the presence of systemic symptoms: night sweats, recurrent fevers, more than 10% weight loss: **A** denotes the absence of these symptoms. In stage I, disease involves a single lymph node group (I) or is localized to a single extralymphatic organ or site (I_2). Stage II disease involves two or more node regions (II), or localized involvement of one extralymphatic organ or site plus one or more node regions (II_E) on the same side of the diaphragm. Stage III disease involves node regions on both sides of the diaphragm, and is designated III_s if spleen is involved, III_E if an extralymphatic organ is involved, and III_{SE} if both are involved. Stage III can be further defined as III_1—involving lymphatic structures in the upper abdomen: celiac, splenic, or hepatic portal nodes, or spleen, or IIIa—involving lower abdominal nodes: paraaortic, iliac, or mesenteric nodes (may be ± the upper abdominal nodes). Stage IV disease includes diffuse or disseminated involvement of one or more extralymphatic organs or tissues ± associated node involvement. *(Braunwald et al, pp. 1555–1558)*

21. **(C)** Radiation therapy is valuable in treating all the lymphomas, but especially Hodgkin's disease. If radiation therapy can achieve remission in 95% of patients with single-node disease in the neck, particularly if the pathology is of the lymphocyte-predominant type. EF is effective in achieving remission 90% of patients with Stage IA or IIA nodular sclerosing or mixed cellular Hodgkin's disease; if the spleen is normal sized, it can be included in the field and laparotomy/splenectomy avoided. In EF, a mantle field (cervical/axillary/mediastinal/preauricular/upper para-aortic nodes) is used for disease above the diaphragm, and an "inverted-Y" field (groin/retroperitoneal nodes) is used for disease below the diaphragm. Total axial lymph node irradiation (TANI), a combination of mantle plus "inverted-Y" fields plus a splenic port is effective in treating symptomatic localized disease (stages IB and IIB). Radiation therapy alone has achieved less than optimal results in Stage II disease with bulky mediastinal disease (more than one third the chest diameter on PA CXR), but combination chemotherapy plus radiation therapy can be effective in achieving remissions, and some cures. Stages III and IV are treated with combination chemotherapy such as MOPP (nitrogen mustard, vincristine [Oncovin], prednisone, procarbazine), and relapses are treated with a non–cross-resistant combination. ABVD (adriamycin, bleomycin, vinblastine, dacarbazine). Some centers are now using alternating cycles of MOPP and ABVD, or similar regimens, in an attempt to treat advanced disease more aggressively. Single-agent therapy is generally used only

in palliation of relapsed disease, rather than as primary therapy. Total body irradiation and high-dose chemotherapy in conjunction with autologous bone marrow transplantation is now being used in select (young, otherwise healthy) patients who have failed to benefit from chemotherapy. *(Braunwald et al, pp. 1559–1560)*

22. **(B)** Prosthetic cardiac valves cause damage to, and destruction of, platelets due to the mechanical action of the valves themselves and the turbulent flow patterns they create. ITP leads to destruction through an autoimmune process that involves the binding of antibodies or immune complexes to platelets, facilitating phagocytosis. Prosthetic joints cause neither damage to platelets nor any alteration of interactions with the immune system. Myeloproliferative disorders often do cause lowered platelet counts, but it is usually due to splenic sequestration and/or bone marrow infiltration by malignant cells. *(Braunwald et al, pp. 1471–1472)*

23. **(E)** Management of DIC has several components:

    1. Control of major symptoms. Administration of fresh frozen plasma, cyroprecipitate, and/or platelets to replace depleted blood components and prevent exsanguination, and heparin when thrombosis and/or incipient gangrene are evident.
    2. Treatment of the triggering disorder. Broad-spectrum antibiotic therapy after appropriate cultures are obtained in suspected sepsis, prompt delivery of fetus and placenta in the event of abruptio placenta, extraction of a retained dead fetus, surgical intervention after trauma, aggressive anti-tumor therapy (if possible) in the setting of malignancy, etc.
    3. Heparin prophylaxis where (2) is not rapidly manageable and chronic DIC is likely, for example, in acute promyelocytic leukemia, unresectable or disseminated malignancy, when surgical intervention must be postponed, and fat or amniotic fluid embolus. (Automatic initiation of heparin therapy, other than in the above situations, is controversial). *(Braunwald et al, pp. 1478–1479)*

24. **(E)** General causes of folate deficiency include: increased use, as in pregnancy, increased bone marrow turnover (e.g., hemolytic anemia), malignancy, inflammatory diseases, and growth spurts; malabsorption, as in inflammatory bowel disease, dermatitis herpetiformis/gluten-induced enteropathy, tropical sprue, and congenital malabsorption syndromes; excessive loss, as in CHF and dialysis; mixed mechanisms as in alcohol abuse or cirrhosis; inadequate diet (alcoholics, narcotic addicts, indigent, elderly); drug induced by such drugs as chemotherapeutic agents, anticonvulsants, barbiturates, triamterene, trimethoprim. Therapy consists of improving diet and supplemental folate 1 mg daily based on duration of the underlying cause. *(Braunwald et al, pp. 1500–1504; Hoffbrand and Pettit, pp. 48, 58–60)*

25. **(C)** General causes of B_{12} deficiency include: gastric malabsorption due to diminished or absent intrinsic factor post partial or total gastrectomy or in pernicious anemia; intestinal malabsorption as in Crohn's disease, blind loop syndrome, chronic pancreatitis, fish tapeworm, strict vegetarian diet (B_{12} is found only in animal products); and abnormal metabolism, which can be congenital or acquired (secondary to nitrous oxide exposure). Therapy consists of B_{12} intramuscularly (there are several dose/frequency regimens). Anticonvulsant therapy can cause a macrocytic anemia due to *folate* deficiency. Lead poisoning causes a hypochromic anemia by interfering with heme and globin synthesis, and some degree of hemolysis. *(Braunwald et al, pp. 1500–1504; Hoffbrand and Pettit, pp. 34, 48, 56–62)*

26. **(C)** Von Willebrand's disease is actually a heterogeneous disorder. In type 1, vWF synthesis is diminished; in type 2 (less common), it is defective in one of several ways. In types 1 and 2, the patient is heterozygous, and the degree of impairment of hemostasis is mild, with bleeding occurring only after surgery or trauma. In type 3 (a rare form: homozygous, or double heterozygous for two different defects), the patient has a more severe degree of impairment, with episodes of severe mucosal bleeding and hemarthrosis, vWF plays two roles in hemostasis: that of facilitation of platelet adhesion, and of transport of factor VIII. Therapy for vWD consists of prn transfusion of cryoprecipitate—1 unit often suffices for minor bleeding, with multiple units required over a period of time for trauma or surgery. *(Braunwald et al, p. 1473; Hoffbrand and Pettit, pp. 229, 238, 246)*

27. **(E)** All the problems above can initially present with simple thrombocytopenia. In this situation, WBC is borderline low, H/H are not unreasonably low for a menstruating female (who has had an abnormally heavy period). Bone marrow aspiration and biopsy are essential to evaluate the situation. Studies such as ANA and LE prep will help exclude SLE. History may suggest drug-induced thrombocytopenia, and in most instances, the platelet count will rise within a few days of terminating the causative medication. Other diagnoses to consider include ITP, hepatitis, CMV, HIV, Epstein–Barr virus, alcohol binging, and metastatic disease involving the bone marrow. *(Braunwald et al, pp. 1472–1473)*

28. **(A)** There are several groups of causes of hereditary hemolytic anemias. One is that of membrane

defects: hereditary spherocytosis, elliptocytosis, stomatocytosis, and acanthocytosis. Splenectomy is often helpful in these cases, and folate supplementation is sometimes of value. Another group is that of hemoglobin abnormalities (discussed later). The last is of red cell metabolic defects. The most common of these is G6PD deficiency (sex linked, seen most commonly in blacks, Eastern Mediterraneans, Sephardic Jews), in which symptoms are usually precipitated by environmental stress (infection, fava beans, metabolic acidosis, drugs such as sulfa, nitrofurantoin, and antimalarials). Treatment consists of prevention of acute crises and occasional transfusion. Others in this group are due to defects in the glycolytic pathway, such as glucose phosphate isomerase deficiency and pyruvate kinase deficiency. These are usually mild and may require no therapy, or folate supplementation and transfusions when hemolysis is severe, and occasionally splenectomy. Warm antibodies cause *acquired* auto-immune hemolytic anemia. (*Braunwald et al, pp. 1514–1518; Hoffbrand and Pettit, pp. 66–72*)

29. **(E)** Thalassemia is really a group of congenital defects in the synthesis of hemoglobin subunits. "Normal" adult hemoglobin (HbA) contains 2 α and 2 β subunits, production of which is controlled by two genes for α and one for β from each parent. The clinical presentation depends on the number of gene deletions (in α) or defects (in β) inherited. These are summarized below:

Gene Abnormality	Diagnosis	Laboratory Findings
α—αα	silent carrier	normal labs except ↑Hb A_z
α—α— or ——αα	α-thalassemia trait H&H.	↑MCV, nl or mild ↑Hb A_z
——α—	HbH disease	↓ MCV; HbH (β4); chemistries consistent with hemolysis; target cells
—/—	Hydrops fetalis	Hb Barts (γ4)
–/β	β–thalassemia minor (or "trait")	↓MCV; ↑Hb A_z mild ↓H/H nl or ↑HbF
–/–	β–thalassemia major (Cooley's anemia)	↓MCV, ↓MCH, ↑HbF, ↓or no HbA, ↓↓ H/H, bizarre shaped or nucleated RBCs; chemistries consistent with hemolysis; target cell

The thalassemias tend to be hypochromic and microcytic. α -thalassemia trait may cause varying degrees of anemia, usually asymptomatic. In HbH disease, both inadequate erythropoiesis and hemolysis occur. In hydrops fetalis, a Hb composed of four γ chains is produced, and is incompatible with life outside the uterus. β -thalassemias involve a variety of β chain defects and vary significantly in severity. In the minor form, the anemia is mild and generally does not require intervention. In the major form, the anemia is severe, puberty is delayed, significant skeletal abnormalities occur (including typical "chipmunk" facies due to expansion of the flat bones of the face and skull) consequent upon marrow expansion, and hepatosplenomegaly develops due to both extramedullary erythropoiesis and iron overload. Therapy generally consists of folate (due to rapid marrow turnover), splenectomy, multiple transfusions, starting in infancy, and administration of desferrioxamine to reduce iron overload. (*Braunwald et al, pp. 1525–1527; Hoffbrand and Pettit, pp. 82–93*)

30. **(A)** Thyroid function has no specific relationship to Fe deficiency. The most common cause of Fe deficiency is gastrointestinal (GI) blood loss, so thorough GI evaluation is essential. Common etiologies include hookworm infestations (common in underdeveloped nations), hiatus hernia, peptic ulcer disease, inflammatory bowel disease, neoplasms, chronic ASA ingestion, esophageal varices, telangiectasia, diverticular disease, angiodysplasia, and, occasionally, severe hemorrhoids. Other causes include pregnancy (due to Fe transfer to the fetus), uterine bleeding (menorrhagia, antepartum and postpartum bleeding), hemosiderinuria, malabsorption (seen in atrophic gastritis, celiac disease, post partial gastrectomy), dialysis, hematuria, and pulmonary hemosiderosis. (*Braunwald et al, pp. 1495–1497; Hoffbrand and Pettit, pp. 34–40*)

31. **(B)** Hereditary sideroblastic anemia is a disorder of ineffective erythropoiesis. Findings generally include hypochromic microcytic indices, with ringed sideroblasts and erythroid hyperplasia on bone marrow exam, and increased serum Pe and IBC. Hemochromatosis (Fe overload) is common due to increased intestinal Fe absorption and/or transfusions. β -thalassemia trait usually is also hypochromic/microcytic. This CBC demonstrates a normochromic normocytic anemia. This is commonly seen with a normal WBC and thrombocytopenia in a myelopthisic anemia due to infiltration of bone marrow by tumor, granuloma (usually in advanced TB), or fibrosis. The objective of therapy is the correction of the underlying disease process, which is often impossible, and then supportive measures. The anemia of chronic disorders also tends to present with normal indices, and has multiple eti-

ologies. These include chronic inflammatory states (such as RA, SLE, chronic infection, sarcoidosis, neoplasms, regional enteritis), renal failure, endocrine failure (as in Addison's disease, hypothyroidism, panhypopituitarism, hypogonadism), and liver disease (although this anemia may more commonly be megaloblastic). In all of these, Fe and IBC tend to both be reduced (if actual Fe deficiency is present, IBC may increase to normal). Treatment consists of optimal management of the underlying disease state; Fe supplementation is of little value, and transfusion is rarely needed. *(Braunwald et al, pp. 1497–1498, 1536, 1504–1506; Hoffbrand and Pettit, pp. 40, 90, 109–110)*

32. **(E)** Multiple myeloma is a malignant neoplasm of the plasma cell, usually producing a monoclonal immunoglobulin increase (seen on protein and/or urine electrophoresis). This disease tends to create multiple osteolytic lesions (best demonstrated on skeletal survey rather than bone scan), which are often very painful and can lead to pathological fractures, increased osteoporosis, hypercalcemia, and spinal cord compression. The excessive protein production can cause CNS symptoms due to hyperviscosity (confusion, paresthesias, somnolence, headache, and hemiplegia or coma when severe), amyloid deposition in (and failure of) multiple organs, and proteinuria/nephrotic syndrome. Tumor invasion of the bone marrow can cause depression of WBC, RBC, and/or platelets, hypogammaglobulinemia, and markedly increased susceptibility to infection. Cryoglobulin production and platelet dysfunction are common, and renal failure can occur as a result of amyloidosis, urate nephropathy, and other disorders. Radiation therapy may be of great value in controlling painful bone symptoms or impending cord compression. Chemotherapy is used to treat the systemic disease, usually consisting of pulse therapy with an alkylating agent (mephalan, cyclophosphamide, or chlorambucil) plus a steroid, and can achieve remission (although not cure). Allopurinol helps minimize hyperuricemia, and good hydration assists clearance of calcium and light protein chains. Plasmapheresis may be appropriate in severe hyperviscosity syndrome, and prompt assessment and treatment of infection is essential. *(Eiseman et al, pp. 225–228; Braunwald et al, pp. 1398–1400)*

33. **(C)** Chronic myelogenous leukemia (CML) is a neoplasm of the multipotent hematopoietic stem cell, which most commonly is found in middle-aged patients. The chronic phase is characterized by an elevated total WBC, predominantly granulocytic (but it is not uncommon to have increased eosinophil and/or basophil counts), with < 5% blasts in blood and marrow, low or absent leukocyte alkaline phosphatase (LAP), and presence of a specific chromosome marker called the Philadelphia (Ph[1]) chromosome (a translocation of chromosomes 22 and 9) in 80% to 95% of patients. These studies are valuable in differentiating CML from leukemoid reactions ($\uparrow \uparrow$ LAP, no Ph[1] chromosome), myelofibrosis ($\uparrow$ or normal LAP, no Ph[1] chromosome), and other myeloprofliferative disorders. Presentation often includes splenomegaly, leukocytosis with anemia (platelet counts are variable), hypermetabolism (weight loss, fever, hyperuricemia, sweating), and arthralgias; lymphoadenopathy may be present, and thrombohemorrhagic events may occur. Single-agent therapy (busulfan, cyclophosphamide, melphalan, or hydroxyurea) may be used to decrease the leukocytosis and symptomatology. It does not clear the Ph[1] chromosome abnormality from the marrow—it simply diminishes tumor load enough to remove the immature cells from the blood. It has not been demonstrated that conventional combination chemotherapy improves survival, although promising results are being achieved with intensive chemotherapy and radiation therapy followed by (HLA matched) bone marrow transplantation early in the chronic phase. Allopurinol decreases the hyperuricemia (which often otherwise increases on initiation of chemotherapy). Splenectomy is helpful only in relieving symptoms of hypersplenism, and does not change the overall course of the disease. Approximately 50% of patients will accelerate to a blastic phase or crisis, resembling acute leukemia within 3 to 4 years, with almost all patients ultimately continuing on to this state. Blastic crises may be myeloid in origin and two thirds of cases, and lymphoid in one third, consistent with the stem cell level of disease process. The blastic phase is usually very resistant to treatment, including bone marrow transplantation, and most patients die within 6 weeks of diagnosis of conversion to this phase (although the lymphoid cases may briefly respond). *(Braunwald et al, pp. 1527–1529; Eiseman et al, pp. 208–211)*

34. **(A)** Low-grade lymphomas are relatively indolent, high-grade more aggressive, and therapy varies accordingly. Low-grade includes small lymphocytic/plasmacytoid, consistent with CLL (diffuse well-differentiated lymphocytic); follicular small cleaved cell/diffuse areas, sclerosis (nodular poorly differentiated lymphocytic) and follicular mixed, small cleaved and large cell/diffuse areas sclerosis (nodular mixed lymphocytic histiocytic). Intermediate-grade includes follicular large cell/diffuse areas, sclerosis (nodular histiocytic); diffuse small cleaved cell (diffuse poorly differentiated lymphocytic); diffuse mixed, small and large cell/sclerosis, epithelioid cell component (diffuse mixed lymphocytic–histiocytic; and diffuse large cell/cleaved and noncleaved cell sclerosis (diffuse histiocytic). High grade includes large cell immunoblastic/plasma-

cytoid, clear cell, polymorphous, epithelioid component (diffuse histiocytic); lymphoblastic/convoluted
and nonconvoluted cell (diffuse lymphoblastic); and
small noncleaved cell/Burkitt's follicular areas (diffuse undifferentiated)—"Burkitt's" lymphoma. Although low-grade lymphomas are more indolent in
progression, the higher-grade lymphomas are actually more readily cured with intensive initial chemotherapy; the low-grade lymphomas have a relatively high relapse rate. Therefore, intensive
combination chemotherapy, ± radiation, is clearly
indicted in initial therapy of high-grade lymphomas. Therapy of low-grade lympohomas is more
controversial, with many electing to treat only as
needed to achieve local control of disease (regional
radiation therapy, less intensive chemotherapy).
Single-agent chemotherapy has fallen into disfavor,
except in diffuse well-differentiated lymphoma/
CLL. Intensive chemotherapy plus total body irradiation followed by autologous bone marrow transplantation is being investigated in patients who
have failed to benefit from chemotherapy (the bone
marrow is harvested after second remission is
achieved and purged of lymphoma cells with monoclonal antibodies, then reinfused after the patient
undergoes further intensive therapy). *(Braunwald et
al, pp. 1560–1565)*

35. **(D)** Bone marrow transplantation allows use of intensive total body irradiation (TBI) and/or chemotherapy at doses that would otherwise be lethal, in
attempting to achieve improved tumor cell kill and
higher chance of cure in treating several malignancies. The TBI/chemotherapy regimens are quite toxic, with many potential complications; moreover,
there is a 2- to 4- week period when a patient has
essentially no functioning marrow, until the donor
marrow begins to produce adequate mature blood
elements. Therefore transplantation must be performed at a major center, in order to provide the
necessary intensive support for such patients. Such
support includes effective isolation units, transfusion of HLA-matched platelets and irradiated pack-
ed red cells to inactivate lymphocytes that could
cause GVHD—(graft-versus-host-disease) long-
term central venous access (e.g., Hickman or Bro-
viac catheter), parenteral nutrition, constant infection surveillance with rapid intervention at any
sign of infection, etc. The tolerance/survival of marrow transplantation diminishes significantly with
age, and most centers refuse to consider patients

more than 45 to 50 years of age. Transplantation is
clearly acceptable in infants with severe combined
immune deficiency and young patients with severe
aplastic anemia, and is now being studied for use in
congenital defect such as sickle cell anemia and
thalassemia. It was initially used in end-stage relapsed leukemia patients with a low success rate,
due to the poor condition of the patients and high
tumor loads. It is now however, well-accepted for
children with ALL in second remission, as their risk
of relapse is large, but tolerance of transplantation
is fairly good and a significant number of long-term
remissions/? cures can be achieved. Still unresolved
is the question of transplantation in first remission
of ALL, due to the good numbers of long-term re-
mission/? cure. It may be reasonable in a patient in
good condition in first remission from AML, because these patients are at very high risk of relapse.
Studies are underway, with hopeful results, in
young, otherwise healthy patients with CML. CML
patients in blast crisis have not done so well (due to
high tumor load and its concomitant problems), particularly in the older patients, hence, these are patients in which transplantation is not commonly
considered. Work is being done with autologous
transplants in patients with relapsed lymphomas
and other malignancies, in which the patients' own
bone marrow seems clear of disease. In such a situation, the patients' own marrow is harvested, intensive therapy is given for the malignancy, and the
marrow is then given back to the patients. In appropriately selected patients, there is a good chance of
long-term remission of disease. *(Braunwald et al,
pp. 1536–1541)*

REFERENCES

Braunwald, E, Isselbacher KJ, Petersdorf, RG et al, ed.
Harrison's Principles of Internal Medicine, 11th ed. New
York: McGraw-Hill; 1987.

Eiseman B, Robinson, WA, Steele Jr G. *Follow-up of the
Cancer Patient.* New York: Thieme-Stratton; 1982.

Hoffbrand, AV, Pettit, JE. *Clinical Hematology,* London:
Gower Medical Publishing; 1988.

Knobf, MK, Lewis, KP, Fischer, DA, et al. *Cancer Chemotherapy Treatment and Care.* Boston, MA: G. K. Hall
Medical Publishers; 1981.

Subspecialty List: Hematology

Question Numbers and Subspecialty
1. Oncology: chemotherapy
2. Oncology: chemotherapy
3. Oncology: chemotherapy
4. Oncology: chemotherapy
5. Oncology: chemotherapy
6. Oncology: chemotherapy
7. Hematology: transfusion
8. Hematology: thrombocytopenia
9. Hematology: coagulopathy
10. Hematology: coagulopathy
11. Hematology: anemia
12. Hematology: anemia
13. Hematology: hemoglobinopathy
14. Hematology: hemoglobinopathy
15. Hematology: anemia
16. Hematology: Myeloproliferative disorders
17. Oncology: hematological neoplasms
18. Oncology: leukemia
19. Oncology: leukemia
20. Oncology: lymphoma
21. Oncology: lymphoma
22. Hematology: thrombocytopenia
23. Hematology: coagulopathy
24. Hematology: anemia
25. Hematology: anemia
26. Hematology: coagulopathy
27. Hematology: thrombocytopenia
28. Hematology: anemia
29. Hematology: hemoglobinopathy
30. Hematology: anemia
31. Hematology: anemia
32. Oncology: multiple myeloma
33. Oncology: leukemia
34. Oncology: lymphoma
35. Oncology: bone marrow transplantation

Pharmacology

Doris Rapp

Questions

DIRECTIONS (Questions 1 through 16): Each of the numbered items or incomplete statements in this section is followed by answers or by completions of the statement. Select the ONE lettered answer or completion that is BEST in each case.

1. Which of the following topical antifungal agents is contraindicated in infants?

    (A) undecylenic acid
    (B) clotrimazole
    (C) boric acid
    (D) tolnaftate
    (E) miconazole

2. The first-line drugs presently used against tuberculosis include

    (A) isoniazid and streptomycin
    (B) isoniazid, ethambutol, rifampin, and streptomycin
    (C) isoniazid, streptomycin, viomycin, and rifampin
    (D) isoniazid, ethambutol, and viomycin
    (E) isoniazid, viomycin, and cycloserine

3. Antihistamines are contraindicated in all the following medical conditions EXCEPT

    (A) glaucoma
    (B) hypertension
    (C) asthma
    (D) enlarged prostate
    (E) pregancy

4. The mainstay of therapy for all lipid disorders is

    (A) diet
    (B) Questran
    (C) Lopid
    (D) Mevacor
    (E) nyacin

5. When propranolol is to be used in the treatment of sinus tachycardia, the presence of another disease may be a relative contraindication or at least a precaution to its use. All the following are considered such precautions EXCEPT

    (A) congestive heart failure
    (B) asthma
    (C) hypertension
    (D) type I diabetes mellitus
    (E) A-V block

6. Which of the following micronutrients is considered to have the narrowest therapeutic index?

    (A) zinc
    (B) molybdenum
    (C) selenium
    (D) manganese
    (E) magnesium

7. All the following agents are used to manage asthmatics EXCEPT

    (A) theophylline
    (B) cromolyn sodium
    (C) nadolol
    (D) terbutaline
    (E) albuterol

8. All the following statements are true regarding the use of acyclovir in the treatment of herpes simplex EXCEPT

    (A) acyclovir ointment is used for the treatment of HSV-1 only
    (B) the infusion of IV acyclovir should be given slowly over 1 hour to prevent renal tubular damage.
    (C) headache and gastrointestinal discomfort are the most frequent adverse reactions to continuous acyclovir.
    (D) the dosage for chronic suppressive therapy is 200 mg three to five times per day.
    (E) absorption of oral acyclovir is unaffected by food

9. Mr. Brown has developed itching, crusted lesions in his beard area. New lesions develop each time he

shaves. A bacterial culture from a lesion showed *Staphylococcus aureus* (coagulase positive) and *Beta hemolytic Streptococcus*. Mr. Brown is allergic to penicillin. The appropriate course of therapy would be to start the patient on

(A) Burow's compresses and topical steroids
(B) topical antibiotics and wait for the report of antibiotic sensitivity
(C) Burow's compresses, topical steroids, and dicloxacillin 250 mg four times a day
(D) Burow's compresses, topical steroids, and erythromycin 250 mg four times a day
(E) Burow's compresses and wait for report of antibiotic sensitivity

10. Which of the following has the **LEAST** lipid solubility?

(A) atenolol and propranolol
(B) propranolol and labetalol
(C) pindolol and propranolol
(D) atenolol and nadolol
(E) metoperol and labetalol

11. Excessive doses of this vitamin may cause infantile idiopathic hypercalcemia.

(A) vitamin A
(B) vitamin B_{12}
(C) vitamin C
(D) vitamin D
(E) vitamin E

12. The antidepressant with the most sedative and anticholinergic effects associated with its use is

(A) amitriptyline
(B) nortriptyline
(C) imipramine
(D) desipramine
(E) amoxapine

13. Excessive amounts of which vitamin can cause ocular hemorrhage?

(A) vitamin A
(B) vitamin D
(C) vitamin E
(D) vitamin K
(E) vitamin C

14. Retrobulbar neuritis with typical central scotoma may be caused by pernicious anemia. This is associated with a deficiency of

(A) vitamin A
(B) vitamin B_{12}
(C) vitamin C
(D) vitamin E
(E) vitamin B_1

15. K.L. is a new patient referred to your office by her hometown pharmacist. K.L. has requested the refill of two prescriptions from out of state: digoxin 0.25 mg daily and furosemide 40 mg three times a day. You immediately recognize the potential for a problem which is

(A) hypovolemia; administer IV solution and terminate furosemide use
(B) hyperkalemia and digitoxicity; terminate both drugs until labs are ordered
(C) hypokalemia; order serum potassium and add supplements if value is low
(D) drug seeking behavior; alert the local authorities
(E) an impending MI; send to the emergency room

16. You have a 3-year old, 38-pound child with asthma who requires treatment with theophylline. What is the appropriate dose for him?

(A) 5 mg/kg/24 hours
(B) 5 mg/kg every 6 hours
(C) 10 mg/kg/24 hours
(D) 10 mg/kg every 6 hours
(E) 15mg/kg every 6 hours

DIRECTIONS (Questions 17 through 26): For each of the items in this section, ONE or MORE of the numbered options is correct. Choose the answer

A if only 1, 2, and 3 are correct,
B if only 1 and 3 are correct,
C if only 2 and 4 are correct,
D if only 4 is correct,
E if all are correct.

17. Phenobarbital and phenytoin are effective for generalized motor seizures. Which drugs are effective for absence seizures?

(1) ethosuximide
(2) phenobarbital
(3) valproic acid
(4) diazepam

18. A frightened mother phones you stating that her 5-year old has ingested about 20 of her synthroid 0.1 mg tablets. What is your advice to the mother?

(1) observe the child closely; should any symptoms occur, call back for instructions
(2) your child will go to sleep and sleep soundly for several hours; check on her periodically
(3) have the child eat some bread to "bind up" the drug particles and bring her to the emergency room
(4) induce emesis by using Syrup of Ipecac and bring her to the emergency room

19. The mother of the child in question 18 brings her daughter to the emergency room about 1 hour later, because the child has convulsed. You receive a call that the child is gravely ill. Your examination reveals her to be comatose. She has lost the gag reflex, has bibasilar rales and a temperature of 101°F. Labs revealed a serum glucose of 50 mg%. Which of the following procedures are considered correct medically for this patient?

   (1) begin an IV solution of D_5W
   (2) maintain ventilation—administer oxygen
   (3) administer digitalis glycosides and glucocorticoids
   (4) administer cholestyramine

20. Which of the following can interfere with interpretation of ovulation prediction kits?

   (1) phenytoin
   (2) amitriptyline
   (3) nitrofurantoin
   (4) oral contraceptives

21. Which of the following are useful in the treatment of migraine headaches?

   (1) tenormin
   (2) vicodin
   (3) midrin
   (4) sansert

22. Chronic vitamin A toxicity may cause damage to the

   (1) retina
   (2) pigment cells
   (3) neuroepithelium
   (4) vestibular chambers

23. A single, 25-year-old black woman was admitted to the hospital with classic symptoms of pelvic inflammatory disease (PID). The patient had been sexually active, using an I.U.D. for contraception. A laparoscopy with subsequent cultures grew *Hemophilus influenza*, *Chlamydia trachomatis*, and *Bacteroides oralis* from the endometrium, and *Trichomonas vaginalis* from the vagina. The most appropriate therapy would include

   (1) doxycycline
   (2) ampicillin
   (3) metronidazole
   (4) erythromycin

24. Self-blood glucose testing over urine glucose testing by the diabetic patient may offer the following advantage.

   (1) tests are more accurate; results are quantitative
   (2) detects glucose concentration at levels below the renal threshold value

   (3) provides immediate confirmation of hypoglycemic reactions
   (4) allows the clinician to alter treatment without the patient being hospitalized

25. Which of the following adverse reactions represents a contraindication to further administration of Pertussis-containing vaccines?

   (1) fever of 40.5°C or greater within 48 hours
   (2) hypotensive–hyporesponsive episode within 48 hours
   (3) persistent inconsolable crying lasting 3 or more hours
   (4) an unusual high-pitched cry occurring within 48 hours

26. The discomfort of oral ulcerations caused by HSV-1 may be relieved by

   (1) holding and swishing diphenhydramine elixir in the mouth for several minutes
   (2) holding and swishing diphenhydramine elixir mixed with an equal amount of Kaopectate concentrate in the mouth for several minutes
   (3) applying lidocaine hydrochloride 2% viscous to the lesions
   (4) swishing warm salt water in the mouth for several minutes

DIRECTIONS (Questions 27 through 34): Each group of items in this section consists of lettered headings followed by a set of numbered words or phrases. For each numbered word or phrase, select the ONE lettered heading that is most closely associated with it. Each lettered heading may be selected once, more than once, or not at all.

Questions 27 through 30

For each drug, select its most common usage.

   (A) fluphenazine (Prolixin)
   (B) oxybutynin (Ditropan)
   (C) tamoxifen (Nolvadex)
   (D) triazolam (Halcion)
   (E) astimazole (Hismanal)

27. allergic rhinitis

28. psychotic disorders

29. neurogenic bladder

30. insomnia

Questions 31 through 34

For each condition, select the drug most useful in its treatment

    (A) hypertension
    (B) peptic ulcer disease
    (C) muscle spasm
    (D) nausea
    (E) diabetes mellitus

C **31.** orphenadrine (Norflex)

D **32.** promethazine (Phenergan)

A **33.** enalapril (Vasotec)

B **34.** famotidine (Pepcid)

DIRECTIONS (Questions 35 through 50): Each group of items in this section consists of lettered headings followed by a set of numbered words or phrases. For each numbered word or phrase, select

    A if the item is associated with (A) <u>only,</u>
    B if the item is associated with (B) <u>only,</u>
    C if the item is associated with <u>both</u> (A) <u>and</u> (B),
    D if the item is associated with <u>neither</u> (A) <u>nor</u> (B).

Questions 35 through 38

    (A) diarrhea
    (B) constipation
    (C) both
    (D) neither

C **35.** EqualActin

B **36.** morphine

D **37.** Metamucil

A **38.** qunidine

Questions 39 through 42

    (A) sedation
    (B) excitation
    (C) both
    (D) neither

D **39.** terfenadine (Seldane)

A **40.** flurazepam (Dalmane)

A **41.** methyldopa (Aldomet)

A **42.** diphenhydramine (Benadryl)

Questions 43 through 46

    (A) bronchodilation
    (B) vasodilation
    (C) both
    (D) neither

D **43.** ranitidine (Zantac)

A **44.** theophylline (Theo Dur)

D **45.** trazodone (Desyrel)

B **46.** hydralazine (Apresoline)

Questions 47 through 50

    (A) angina
    (B) hypertension
    (C) both
    (D) neither

C **47.** diltiazem (Cardizem)

C **48.** propranolol (Inderal)

A **49.** nicardipine (Cardene)

B **50.** guanethidine (Ismelin)

Answers and Explanations

1. **(C)** It is possible that any agent may be absorbed through damaged skin. Some, however, are more readily absorbed than others. Boric acid is a weak fungistat and bacteriostat. Unfortunately, it is absorbed significantly through damaged skin, thus leading to possible systemic toxicity. Because of their underdeveloped drug metabolizing systems, infants may be especially sensitive to this agent. *(Swonger and Matejski, pp. 1066, 1975–1976)*

2. **(B)** Viomycin is considered a second-line drug. Its major side effects are auditory and nephrotoxicity. The first-line drugs are also potentially quite toxic. Isoniazid is associated with peripheral neuritis for which pyridoxine is often used prophylactically. It may also cause hepatitis. Ethambutol is associated with optic neuritis. Rifampin may affect liver function and negates the effect of oral contraceptives. Streptomycin, like other aminoglycosides, may damage the eighth cranial nerve and induce nephrotoxicity. All patients must be well monitored with appropriate laboratory tests. *(Goodman and Gilman, pp. 1199–1207; Mandell et al, pp. 1393–1395)*

3. **(B)** Antihistamines possess anticholinergic activity that may pose a potential hazard to patients with an enlarged prostate and those with acute narrow angle glaucoma. They may also be contraindicated in persons with asthma, but data supporting this potentially adverse effect for all asthmatics are not uniformly agreeable. *(Goodman and Gilman, pp. 605–624)*

4. **(A)** Treatment of hyperlipoproteinemia is indicated both for the relief of presenting symptoms and as part of the effort to decrease the risk of cardiac disease. Treatment begins with dietary restrictions. If triglycerides are elevated, weight reduction and alcohol eliminations are indicated and a low-fat diet is instituted. Other risk factors in cardiac disease such as stress, smoking, or lack of exercise may need to be addressed concurrently. Questran, lopid, and mevacor are lipid lowering agents that are added if diet alone is insufficient therapy. *(Goodman and Gilman, pp. 838–843)*

5. **(C)** Propranolol is a nonselective, beta-adrenergic receptor blocking agent. Blocking of beta receptors in the heart may worsen cardiac failure when sympathetic stimulation is often a vital component supporting circulatory function. Beta-receptor blockade in the lungs can lead to bronchoconstriction. Further, beta blockade may mask certain premonitory signs and symptoms (those that are adrenergically mediated) of acute hypoglycemia, thus making insulin dosage more difficult and predisposing the patient to the possibility of hypoglycemic attacks. *(Goodman and Gilman, pp. 192–203)*

6. **(C)** Clinical evidence of selenium deficiency includes the development of muscle tenderness, myalgia, and eventually a dilated cardiomyopathy. Twenty to forty micrograms daily of selenium as selenious acid is recommended for maintenance, and up to 100 µg/day for 4 weeks is needed for repletion. It is noted to be a toxic trace element. Suggested maintenance doses of the other trace elements are zinc, 15 mg/day; molybdenum, 20 to 120 µg/day; and manganese, 2.5 to 5.0 mg/day. *(Goodman and Gilman, pp. 1544–1550; Shils and Young, pp. 263–266)*

7. **(C)** Nadolol is a beta-adrenergic blocking agent and in blocking beta receptors in the lungs may cause bronchoconstriction. Theophylline and terbutaline cause bronchodilation, whereas cromolyn is used prophylactically in the treatment of asthma. Cromolyn inhibits both the immediate and nonimmediate bronchoconstrictive reactions to inhaled antigens. *(Goodman and Gilman, pp. 176–177, 589–600, 616–618; Briggs and Fink)*

8. **(A)** Acyclovir ointment appears to have some value in reducing healing time and duration of pain in HSV-1 and HSV-2 infections. *(Goodman and Gilman, pp. 1229–1231; Dorsky and Crumpacker, pp. 859–874)*

9. **(D)** *S aureus* (coagulase positive) and beta hemolytic *Streptococcus* organisms cause the majority of skin infections. These organisms may invade through breaks in the stratum corneum, through

the hair follicles, or through the bloodstream. Both organisms are sensitive to erythromycin, certain penicillins, and cephalosporin antibiotics. Systemic therapy is combined with topical therapy. Compresses with Burow's solution is used for impetigo. As long as systemic antibiotics are being used, topical steroids may be applied to reduce inflammation and speed restoration of the stratum corneum barrier. Solid clinical evidence shows that topical steroids enhance the rate of recovery and do not spread infection. Topical antibiotics are not needed when systemic antibiotics are employed. *(Goodman and Gilman, 1185; Mandell et al, pp. 1098–1099, 1168–1169)*

10. **(D)** Propranolol, labetalol, and pindolol are lipid soluble and this property accounts for their CNS side effects. *(Goodman and Gilman, pp. 192–203)*

11. **(D)** The absorption of calcium is influenced by vitamin D. Excessive doses of vitamin D are manifested as hypercalcemia with numerous clinical consequences, such as demineralization of bones, renal calculi, and metastatic calcifications in soft tissues. Additionally, hypercalcemia is associated with weakness, vomiting, diarrhea, and lack of muscle tone. Vitamins A, B_{12}, and C are not required for calcium absorption. *(Goodman and Gilman, pp. 1531–1540; Shils and Young, pp. 734–735)*

12. **(A)** See comparison. *(Swonger et al, pp. 418–422) Goodman and Gilman, pp. 413–422)*

Comparison for Answer 12

	Sedation	Anticholinergic effects
Amitryptiline	+ + +	+ + +
Nortryptiline	+ +	+ +
Imipramine	+ +	+ +
Desipramine	+	+/−
Amoxapine	+	+

13. **(C)** Although the information on this is sparce, recent literature has indicated that excessive vitamin E has been associated with ocular hemorrhage. Vitamin A toxicity in adults is associated with fatigue, weakness, anorexia, irritability, vomiting, loss of body hair, brittle nails, and skin disorders. It may also cause liver damage. Vitamin D excess may produce polyuria, polydipsia, nausea, vomiting, hypertension, and increased absorption of calcium. Vitamin K is produced primarily by gastrointestinal bacteria and is not associated with overt toxicity. *(Goodman and Gilman, pp. 1551–1592; Shils and Young, p. 353)*

14. **(B)** Vitamin B_{12} is released from food in the stomach and becomes attached to a glycoprotein called gastric intrinsic factor. This complex is absorbed with greater efficiency than B_{12} alone. The most common cause of B_{12} deficiency is inadequate production of intrinsic factor. This form of B_{12} deficiency anemia is called pernicious anemia. Severe B_{12} deficiency causes two principal symptom clusters: megaloblastic anemia and neuropathy. Retrobulbar neuritis is one form of neuropathy. Vitamins A, C, and E are absorbed independent of intrinsic factor. *(Goodman and Gilman, pp. 55–92; Shils and Young, p. 394)*

15. **(C)** The potential problem is hypokalemia caused by furosemide. A serum potassium level should be taken. Hypokalemia can lead to the potentiation of the digitalis glycosides and to digitalis toxicity. The preventive measure is to use potassium supplements along with the diuretic. If the measured potassium is not very low, recommending foods high in potassium including fresh fruits and vegetables may be useful in preventing hypokalemia and may obviate the need for potassium supplements. *(Goodman and Gilman, p. 741)*

16. **(B)** The recommended daily dose for a child of 19 kg is about 0.8 mg/kg/hr or 15 mg/hr. This times 24 hours equal 360 mg, which is almost identical to 5 mg/kg every 6 hours. The slight difference in calculation has to do with rounding off of kilograms to the nearest whole number. (Goodman and Gilman, p. 599; Silver et al, p. 819)

17. **(B)** Absence seizures, also known as petit mal epilepsy, differ considerably from generalized or grand mal seizures. They occur mostly in children; the attacks are of short duration and consist of syncope, or temporary cloudings of consciousness during which the individual may stare blankly or exhibit minor movements of the head and limbs. Ethosuximide and valproic acid are generally used to control absence seizures. Diazepam is used in status epilepticus. *(Goodman and Gilman, p. 461; Silver et al, p. 518)*

18. **(D)** Obviously, this could represent a huge overdose with a central nervous system stimulant. The child requires immediate medical attention. If problems arise, rapid treatment is necessary. Because thyroxin is a CNS stimulant, it is unlikely the child would go to sleep and sleep it off. She may become comatose, however, because of hypoglycemia, hyperpyrexia, and cardiac problems. *(Goodman and Gilman, pp. 1395–1397)*

19. **(E)** Because the child is comatose, ventilation needs to be maintained. She may have congestive heart failure as evidenced by the bibasilar rales. Therefore, digitalis glycosides are in order along with an IV solution. D_5W will provide glucose, which is needed to elevate her serum glucose back

to normal. Some patients have a rather flat response to glucose initially. Further, cholestyramine may be administered to interfere with thyroxine absorption. The addition of glucocorticoids will inhibit the peripheral conversion of T_4 to T_3. (*Goodman and Gilman, pp. 484–488*)

20. **(D)** Ovulation is the release of an egg from the ovary. This event is caused by a sudden surge in the level of luteinizing hormone (LH). Ovulation prediction tests try to determine this initial surge so that intercourse can follow to maximize the chances for fertilization. The progestin component of oral contraceptives produces feedback suppression of the hypothalamic–pituitary axis but primarily affects LH. This would inhibit growth of the expelled follicle, but in most cases the follicle is not released because of the action of the estrogen component. Dilantin, elavil, and macrodantin do not interfere with ovulation. (*Goodman and Gilman, pp. 554–557*)

21. **(E)** The exact mechanism of antimigraine action of beta blockers has not been proven, but abundant evidence supports their beneficial effects. Vicodin is a combination of hydrocodone and acetaminophen, both analgesics whose effects are additive. Hydrocodone, a narcotic, suppresses the affective component of pain. Midrin is also a combination product containing acetaminophen plus a sympathomimetic amine that acts by constricting dilated cranial and cerebral arterioles. Sansert is methylsergide, which inhibits the effects of serotonin, a substance that may be involved in the mechanism of vascular headaches. (*Stein, pp. 2183–2184*)

22. **(A)** Vitamin A has long been associated with good vision, especially good night vision. With slow chronic toxicity, visual problems can ensue subsequent to deposition of carotenoid products. (*Goodman and Gilman, pp. 192–203*)

23. **(B)** Sexually transmissible agents of importance in PID are *Neisseria gonorrhea* and *C trachomatis*. Treatment of nongonococcal PID requires an antibiotic directed at the agents of nongonococcal urethritis, combined with an antianaerobic agent such as a combination of doxycycline and metronidazole. Doxycycline will cover *Chlamydia*. Metronidazole will cover the *Trichomonas* and bacteroides. If there is a treatment failure, a broad spectrum penicillin or cephalosporin may have to be added to cover the *H influenza*. (*Mandell et al, pp. 743–744, 1079*)

24. **(E)** All these statements are true. Home glucose monitoring allows the patient to maintain records that facilitate better insulin management. This will lessen the likelihood of developing diabetic complications. (*Paulshock and Johnson*)

25. **(E)** Pertussis is a bacterial infection that presents with the clinical features of whooping cough. The primary problem associated with the vaccine is central nervous system irritation, which is indicated by all four choices in this question. (*Silver et al, p. 139*)

26. **(A)** Diphenhydramine elixir, alone or mixed with an equal amount of water, or Kaopectate concentrate held and swished around the mouth for several minutes often relieves the discomfort of oral ulcerations. Lidocaine viscous is also effective as this is a topical anesthetic. Using warm salt water would irritate the vesicles even more and increase the discomfort. (*Scott et al, pp. 23–26*)

27. **(E)** Astimazole is a new once-a-day antihistamine released in 1989. It has shown good effects in the treatment of allergic rhinitis. (*Goodman and Gilman, p. 978*)

28. **(A)** Fluphenazine (Prolixin) is a phenothiazine that has activity at all levels of the central nervous system as well as on multiple organ systems. It has been used extensively in the management of manifestations of psychotic disorders. (*Goodman and Gilman, p. 403*)

29. **(B)** Oxybutynin (Ditropan) exerts direct antispasmodic effect on smooth muscle and inhibits the muscarinic action of acetylcholine on smooth muscle. As such, it has wide usage in managing patients with voiding difficulties. (*Swonger and Matejski, pp. 770–771*)

30. **(D)** Triazolam (Halcion) is a type of benzodiazepine. It is a hypnotic with a short duration of action. It increases the duration of sleep and decreases the frequency of nocturnal awakenings. It is recommended for short-term management of insomnia characterized by difficulty in falling asleep, frequent nocturnal awakenings, and/or early morning awakenings. (*Goodman and Gilman, p. 352*)

31. **(C)** Orphenadrine (Norflex) is indicated as an adjunct to rest, physical therapy, and other measures for the relief of discomfort associated with acute painful musculoskeletal conditions. Its mechanism of action has not been completely elucidated, but probably relates to its analgesic properties. (*Goodman and Gilman, p. 489*)

32. **(D)** Promethazine (Phenergan) is a phenothiazine derivative that has many uses, some of which include treatment of allergic rhinitis, urticaria, nausea, and as a preoperative sedative. (*Goodman and Gilman, p. 412*)

33. **(A)** Enalapril (Vasotec) is an antihypertensive agent belonging to the category of ACE inhibitors.

It will control the majority of blood pressures with once-a-day dosing. *(Goodman and Gilman, p. 799)*

34. **(B)** Famotidine (Pepcid) is classified as an H_2 receptor antagonist. It as well as cimetidine and ranatidine are useful in the treatment of peptic ulcer disease. *(Pollonia et al, pp. 139–142)*

35. **(C)** As the name implies, Equal-Actin is equally effective in the treatment of diarrhea and constipation. It decreases the number of bowel movements and improves the consistency of the fecal content to equalize the bowel water balance. It is helpful in treating patients with the irritable bowel syndrome. *(Goodman and Gilman, p. 949)*

36. **(B)** Morphine and other narcotics are associated with a number of gastrointestinal side effects, including anorexia, constipation, biliary tract spasm, and intestinal cramps. *(Goodman and Gilman, p. 502)*

37. **(B)** Metamucil is a bulk-forming laxative consisting of psyllium mucilloid. It increases the water content of the feces and thereby the mass of the stool is increased as well, offering a physical stimulus to peristalsis. Transit time through the colon is hastened and a "natural type" of bowel movement occurs. *(Goodman and Gilman, p. 997)*

38. **(A)** Quinidine is an antiarrhythmic agent of natural source, that is, it comes from the bark of a Peruvian tree, *Cinchona officinatis*. Many patients cannot tolerate it due to its side effect of diarrhea. *(Swonger and Matejski, pp. 623–624)*

39. **(D)** Terfenadine (Seldane) is a relatively new antihistamine that is chemically and pharmacologically distinct from other antihistamines. It is very well tolerated and causes little if any sedation. This has been a point in favor of this drug over conventional antihistamines. *(Goodman and Gilman, p. 622)*

40. **(A)** Flurazepam (Dalmane) is a sedative hypnotic of the benzodiazepine group. It has its major use as a sleeping aid. *(Goodman and Gilman, p. 352)*

41. **(A)** Methyldopa (Aldomet) is an antihypertensive agent belonging to the centrally acting sympatholytic group of drugs. Its major side effect is drowsiness. *(Goodman and Gilman, p. 798)*

42. **(A)** Diphenhydramine (Benadryl) is an antihistamine belonging to the ethanolamine group associated with the highest incidence of drowsiness as a side effect. In fact, Benadryl is often used as a hypnotic, especially in hospitalized patients. *(Goodman and Gilman, p. 623)*

43. **(D)** Ranitidine (Zantac) is an H_2 receptor blocker used in the treatment of peptic disorders. *(Goodman and Gilman, pp. 624–627)*

44. **(A)** Theophylline competitively inhibits phosphodiesterase, the enzyme that degrades cyclic AMP, thus elevating cyclic AMP levels. In bronchial smooth muscle cells, cyclic AMP produces relaxation of muscle fibers. *(Goodman and Gilman, pp. 590–598)*

45. **(D)** Trazadone (Desyrel) is an antidepressant. *(Goodman and Gilman, p. 419)*

46. **(B)** Hydralazine (Apresoline) is an antihypertensive that lowers blood pressure by exerting a peripheral vasodilating effect through a direct relaxation of vascular smooth muscle. *(Goodman and Gilman, p. 795)*

47. **(C)** Diltiazem is a calcium antagonist that is most effective in angina due to coronary artery spasm. It is also used to treat elevated blood pressure. *(Goodman and Gilman, pp. 798, 820)*

48. **(C)** Propranolol has long been used to treat both angina and hypertensive. It also has many other uses, such as the treatment of cardiac arrhythmias and migraine headaches to mention only two. It is a beta-adrenergic blocking agent. *(Goodman and Gilman, p. 793)*

49. **(A)** Nicardipine is a new calcium channel blocker currently approved for treatment of angina. It most likely will receive other approved uses; especially in management of hypertension. *(Lessem et al, pp. 146–153)*

50. **(B)** Guanethidine is an older drug not used often any longer, partly because of the way it is metabolized, but primarily because of side effects—the most notable of which is orthostatic hypotension and impotency in males. It remains an effective blood pressure lowering agent. *(Goodman and Gilman, p. 795)*

REFERENCES

Briggs D, Fink J. Rational use of theophylline in treating the asthmatic patient. University of Alabama at Birmingham. Division of C.M.E.; 1988.

Dorsky DI, Crumpacker CS. Drugs five years later: Acyclovir. *Ann Intern Med.* 1987; 107(6):859–874.

Goodman LS, Gilman AG. *The Pharmacological Basis of Therapeutics*, 7th ed. New York: Macmillan; 1985.

Lessem JN, Barone EJ, Berl T, et al. *Am J. Hypertens.* 1989; 2(3):146–153.

Mandell GL, Douglas RG Jr, Bennett JE. *Principles and Practice of Infectious Disease*, 2nd ed. New York: John Wiley; 1985.

Paulshock BZ, Johnson LH. Monitoring techniques in non-insulin dependent diabetes mellitus. *Primary Care.* 1988; 15(2).

Pollonia A, Marchis, Greco A, et al. *Int J Clin Pharmacol Res.* 1988; 8(2): 139–142.

Scott TF, McNair P, Lawrence C, Witkowski JA. Herpes simplex virus infections, Part 2. Diagnosis and treatment. *Selected Readings.* 1986; 12(2); 23–26.

Shils E, Young R. *Modern Nutrition in Health and Disease*, 7th ed. 1988. Philadelphia, PA: Lea and Febiger; pp. 263–266.

Silver HK, Kempe CH, Bruyn HB, Fulginiti VA. *Handbook of Pediatrics*, 15th ed. E. Norwalk, CT: Appleton & Lange; 1987.

Swonger AK, Matejski MP. *Nursing Pharmacology*, 1st. ed. Glenview, IL: Scott, Foresman and Co; 1988.

Subspecialty List: Pharmacology

CHAPTER 8

Psychiatry

Janet Stayer Kozel

Questions

DIRECTIONS (Questions 1 through 23): For each of the items in this section, ONE or MORE of the numbered options is correct. Choose the answer

A if only 1, 2, and 3 are correct,
B if only 1 and 3 are correct,
C if only 2 and 4 are correct,
D if only 4 is correct,
E if all are correct.

1. The schizophrenic premorbid personality is often noticeable in childhood and adolesence and is distinguished by
   (1) deficiency of social skills with development of small social network
   (2) impaired self-confidence in relationships with the opposite sex
   (3) episodes of neurotic-like illness such as anxiety, obsessions, and phobias
   (4) a tendency to confine close relationships to family members

2. An acute manic episode is characterized by a mood that is elevated, expansive, or irritable. Associated symptoms include
   (1) hyperactivity, reduced need for sleep, and poor concentration
   (2) religious preoccupation, spending sprees, and the playing of word games
   (3) increased self-esteem (grandiosity), pressure of speech, and poor social judgement
   (4) increased productivity, elevated frustration tolerance, and good humor

3. A major depressive episode is usually associated with which symptoms in addition to depressed mood?
   (1) reduced ability to feel pleasure
   (2) decreased interest in activities
   (3) diminished energy
   (4) insomnia, appetite changes, and feelings of guilt

4. The following are true about insomnia
   (1) when found it is always indicative of an underlying disorder
   (2) its significance is dependent upon its timing in the usual pattern of sleep
   (3) it is unaffected by times of going to bed, waking, working, and exercise
   (4) it can be associated with the use of alcohol or other drugs

5. Recommended sleep hygiene methods for patients complaining of insomnia include
   (1) avoiding caffeine, nicotine, and alcohol
   (2) avoiding prolonged naps
   (3) establishing a set wake-up time
   (4) establishing a set time of going to sleep

6. Which of the following are characteristics included in the criteria for diagnosing attention-deficit hyperactivity disorder in children
   (1) an inability to remain seated in the classroom
   (2) difficulty following instructions or completing tasks
   (3) intrusiveness and frequent interruptions into conversations or activities of others
   (4) marked distress over minor changes in environment or schedule

7. Identify which of the following are commonly abused prescription drugs
   (1) methamphetamine (Dexidrine), alprazolam (Xanax)
   (2) imipramine (Tofranil), carbamazepine (Tegretol)
   (3) chlordiazepoxide (Librium), meperidine (Demerol)
   (4) bethanechol (Urecholine), buspirone (BuSpar)

8. Which of the following are true of alcohol withdrawal syndrome?

    (1) it causes elevated blood pressure with orthostatic drop
    (2) patients are in serious danger of seizures
    (3) it can cause hallucinations and delirium
    (4) it is not a frequent cause of mortality

9. Withdrawal from sedative/hypnotic types of drugs

    (1) resembles alcohol withdrawal syndrome
    (2) resembles opiate withdrawal syndrome
    (3) can produce seizures
    (4) resembles cocaine withdrawal syndrome

10. Which of the following are true regarding opiate withdrawal syndrome?

    (1) it carries a risk of status epilepticus
    (2) patients have observable piloerection, dilated pupils, and diarrhea
    (3) it causes auditory hallucinations
    (4) patients usually complain of physical discomfort such as joint pain and muscle cramping

11. The DSMIII-R criteria for the diagnosis of schizophrenia include

    (1) the presence of psychosis persisting at least 1 week
    (2) impairment in the level of functioning in general lifestyle areas
    (3) persisting signs of illness for at least 6 months
    (4) pervasive signs of a mood disorder persisting throughout the illness

12. Psychosis is a symptom of an underlying disorder. When an acutely psychotic patient is encountered, the differential diagnosis should include

    (1) acute drug reaction
    (2) bipolar (manic/depressive) disorder
    (3) major depression
    (4) schizophrenia

13. Simple phobias must be distinguished from panic disorder and

    (1) often cause panic attacks in public places
    (2) consist of a persistent fear of a specific object

    (3) generally result in marked impairment in functioning
    (4) are very common in the general population

14. Somatiform disorders are characterized by

    (1) symptoms that suggest a physical ailment
    (2) negative physical and laboratory findings
    (3) a concomitant physical ailment
    (4) intentional patient malingering

15. Reversible causes of dementia in the elderly include

    (1) a major depressive episode
    (2) vitamin deficiency
    (3) prescription medication effects
    (4) hydrocephalus

16. Common causes of irreversible chronic, progressive dementia include

    (1) Alzheimer's disease
    (2) Parkinson's disease
    (3) multiple small strokes
    (4) alcoholism

17. A work-up of the patient presenting with dementia should include, in addition to a complete history, physical, and neurologic examination,

    (1) laboratory studies including thyroid function and serum B_{12} and folate determination
    (2) abdominal x-rays and complete genitourinary evaluation
    (3) CT scan and electroencephalograph
    (4) lumbar puncture and cerebrospinal fluid examination

18. Imipramine (Tofranil) is a tricyclic antidepressant that commonly causes side effects including

    (1) orthostatic hypotension
    (2) dry mouth
    (3) blurred vision
    (4) diarrhea

19. Lithium carbonate, a salt commonly used to treat bipolar affective (manic/depressive) illness, can cause

    (1) dry mouth
    (2) tremor
    (3) constipation
    (4) diarrhea

20. Caution must be used in prescribing benzodiazepines, such as alprazolam (Xanax), because of

    (1) jitteriness
    (2) drowsiness
    (3) abnormal motor movements
    (4) impaired motor control

21. Antipsychotic medication, such as haloperidol (Haldol), can cause neurologic side effects, for example,

    (1) acute dystonia
    (2) abnormal motor movements
    (3) motor agitation
    (4) parkinsonism

22. The borderline personality is characterized by

    (1) manipulative behavior including suicidal threats
    (2) tempestuous interpersonal relationships
    (3) impulsivity and frequent mood shifts
    (4) persistent psychotic thinking

23. Personality disorders are

    (1) caused by biological factors exclusively
    (2) often occur with a patient meeting criteria for more than one disorder
    (3) often associated only with discrete episodes of mental illness
    (4) maladaptive traits that cause impairment or emotional distress

DIRECTIONS (Questions 24 through 27): Each group of items in this section consists of lettered headings followed by a set of numbered words or phrases. For each numbered word or phrase, select the ONE lettered heading that is most closely associated with it. Each lettered heading may be selected once, more than once, or not at all.

    (A) anxiolytic
    (B) tricyclic antidepressant
    (C) sedative/hypnotic
    (D) antipsychotic
    (E) MAO inhibitor

24. amitriptyline (Elavil)

25. lorazepam (Ativan)

26. flurazepam (Dalmane)

27. thioridazine (Mellaril)

DIRECTIONS (Questions 28 through 32): Each group of items in this section consists of lettered headings followed by a set of numbered words or phrases. For each numbered word or phrase, select

    A if the item is associated with (A) only,
    B if the item is associated with (B) only,
    C if the item is associated with both (A) and (B),
    D if the item is associated with neither (A) nor (B).

Questions 28 through 30

    (A) generalized anxiety disorder
    (B) panic disorder
    (C) both
    (D) neither

28. discrete spontaneous episodes

29. sustained state of tension and irritability

30. depression

Questions 31 and 32

    (A) preoccupation with body size and weight
    (B) binge eating accompanied by some extreme measure to prevent weight gain
    (C) both
    (D) neither

31. anorexia nervosa

32. bulimia nervosa

DIRECTIONS (Questions 33 through 50): Each of the numbered items or incomplete statements in this section is followed by answers or by completions of the statement. Select the ONE lettered answer or completion that is BEST in each case.

33. The prevalence of schizophrenia, which has been relatively constant across cultural boundaries, is approximately

    (A) 1%
    (B) 5%
    (C) 0.25%
    (D) 8%
    (E) 10%

34. When lithium is used to treat bipolar affective illness, which lab tests are used in routine monitoring of the patient for side effects?

    (A) uric acid, WBC
    (B) CBC, liver enzymes
    (C) T3 uptake, liver enzymes
    (D) TSH, creatinine
    (E) electrolytes, glucose

35. Hallmark features of narcolepsy include

    (A) daytime "sleep attacks"
    (B) cataplexy
    (C) sleep paralysis
    (D) hypnogogic hallucinations
    (E) all of the above

36. What diagnosis should be strongly suspected in an overweight, hypertensive, middle-aged male, who complains of sleepiness and whose wife complains that he snores

    (A) coronary artery disease
    (B) chronic obstructive pulmonary disease
    (C) obstructive sleep apnea syndrome
    (D) major depression
    (E) narcolepsy

37. Many of the most common side-effect complaints of tricyclic antidepressants are related to their anti-cholinergic effects and include

    (A) blurred vision
    (B) urinary retention
    (C) constipation
    (D) dry mouth
    (E) all of the above

38. Which of the following medications is frequently used in the treatment of children with attention-deficit hyperactivity?

    (A) amitriptyline (Elavil)
    (B) phenelzine (Nardil)
    (C) methylphenidate (Ritalin)
    (D) carbamazepine (Tegretol)
    (E) lorazepam (Ativan)

39. Cocaine is a stimulant drug that has become a common drug of abuse. A prominent feature of cocaine withdrawal is

    (A) somnolence
    (B) depression
    (C) psychosis
    (D) muscle cramping
    (E) abdominal pain

40. Psychotropic drug use in the elderly

    (A) is contraindicated
    (B) must be closely monitored for side effects
    (C) should always be in low doses
    (D) should not be a first-line approach to treatment
    (E) none of the above

41. Individuals with antisocial personality disorder are

    (A) responsive to rehabilitation measures and psychotherapy
    (B) generally males with a lifelong pattern of irresponsible and often criminal behavior
    (C) not likely to risk their own safety when engaging in antisocial behavior
    (D) often improved in their behavior when forced to take responsibility, as in becoming a parent
    (E) rarely dangerous to others in their behavior

42. The Minnesota Multiphasic Personality Inventory (MMPI)

    (A) is used in place of a lengthy psychiatric interview to assess patients
    (B) is an old test of personality function that is rarely used today
    (C) can be used as a measure of "intelligence"
    (D) is a self-report test used to assess symptoms of mental illness and personality dysfunction
    (E) can easily be manipulated by an intelligent patient wishing to present a positive picture

43. A neurotransmitter that has been implicated as a causative factor in depression is

    (A) epinephrine
    (B) serotonin
    (C) amphetamine
    (D) tryamine
    (E) phenylalanine

44. A personality pattern characterized by excessive inflexibility and perfectionistic views is called

    (A) narcissistic personality disorder
    (B) an unclassified personality problem
    (C) oppositional defiant disorder
    (D) passive-aggressive personality disorder
    (E) obsessive-compulsive personality disorder

45. A number of medical disorders can cause alteration in mood and can mimic a major depressive episode including

    (A) hypothyroidism
    (B) hyperthyroidism
    (C) systemic lupus erythematosus
    (D) brain tumor
    (E) all the above

46. Initial management of the acutely suicidal patient should include

    (A) psychotherapy
    (B) antidepressant medication
    (C) hospitalization and close observation
    (D) antianxiety medication
    (E) electroconvulsive therapy (ECT)

47. Mental retardation is classified in four levels: mild, moderate, severe, and profound and is caused by

    (A) congenital abnormalities
    (B) genetic abnormalities
    (C) trauma
    (D) nonorganic etiology
    (E) all the above

48. A patient is determined to be "incompetent" if he/she

    (A) is psychotic
    (B) is disoriented
    (C) is dangerous to himself/herself and others
    (D) is unable to make decisions in his/her own best interest
    (E) is unable to determine right from wrong

49. Closed head injury can cause a variety of psychiatric syndromes, both temporary and permanent, including

    (A) personality changes
    (B) psychosis
    (C) depression
    (D) disruption of sleep patterns
    (E) all the above

50. Chronic heavy metal poisoning is an often overlooked syndrome that can cause symptoms resembling

    (A) schizophrenia
    (B) depression
    (C) Parkinson's disease
    (D) panic disorder
    (E) all the above

Answers and Explanations

1. **(E)** It has long been recognized that schizophrenia occurs in association with many personality types. However, the socially withdrawn type of personality is more strongly represented in schizophrenics and their first-degree relatives. The reason for this is unknown, but it can be a valuable piece of historical information when forming a differential diagnosis. *(Kendell, p. 7)*

2. **(A)** The manic does have an elevated mood, increased energy, and rapid thought processes, with a reduced need for sleep. However, his/her energies are poorly focused and his/her judgment impaired to such a degree that activities are often disorganized and counterproductive. He/she generally has little tolerance for interference, and while such a person can be in an expansive mood when things go well, can abruptly become hostile and even violent. *(Dunner, p. 2)*

3. **(E)** The presence of melancholia (the loss of pleasure in activities) associated with at least three of the following: sleep disturbance, eating disturbance or weight change, reduced energy, inappropriate guilt, loss of libido, reduced concentration, morbid or nihilistic thoughts, or psychomotor changes, fulfill the criteria for diagnosis of major depression. *(Dunner, p. 3)*

4. **(C)** Insomnia is a symptom, a subjective complaint requiring evaluation and carries a broad differential diagnosis. It can be the result of bad habits: for example, no exercise, alcohol, tobacco, or caffeine use, or working and worrying right up until bedtime. A careful history must be obtained, including whether the sleeplessness includes difficulty falling asleep, waking during the night, or waking in the early morning hours. Fragmented sleep can be a symptom of depression, alcohol abuse, or medication effect, among other things. Major primary sleep disorders must be ruled out. All-night polysomnography in a sleep lab is sometimes needed for a definitive diagnosis. *(Aldrich, p. 314)*

5. **(A)** When bad habits are affecting a patient's sleep, he/she needs to be encouraged to keep a more structured schedule. Getting up at the same time each morning tends toward becoming sleepy at the same time each night. Getting up at the same time is easier to achieve than controlling falling asleep. Habits that interfere with efficient sleep, namely daytime naps, drug and alcohol use, should be discouraged. *(Zarcone, pp. 490–493)*

6. **(A)** Children with Attention Deficit Hyperactivity Disorder (ADHD) often tend to move excessively, are intrusive in their behavior, and are unable to focus their attention on tasks. Rigidity of behavior is more indicitive of Pervasive Development Disorder or in its extreme, Autistic Disorder. *(APA, pp. 50–53)*

7. **(B)** Alprazolam and chlordiazepoxide are benzodiazepines, which are the most commonly prescribed class of psychoactive medications. They can cause tolerance, intoxication, and withdrawal. Meperidine, a synthetic opioid with morphinelike action, is a frequently abused pain reliever. Methamphetamine is a stimulant and is commonly abused for weight control or to combat fatigue. The other agents do not produce tolerance, intoxication, withdrawal symptoms or the maladaptive behavior symptoms associated with substance abuse. *(APA, pp. 165, 175–176, 182–183, 184–185)*

8. **(A)** Elevated blood pressure with an orthostatic drop is an easily observable sign of alcohol withdrawal syndrome. Seizures, and even status epileptiform, are dangerous and potentially fatal complications of withdrawal from alcohol. Hallucinations and delirium are additional complications and complete the picture of delirium tremens of the "DTs". *(Ellinwood et al, pp. 6–11)*

9. **(B)** Drugs, including benzodiazepines (Valium, Librium, Dalmane, etc.) and barbiturates are cross-tolerant with alcohol and produce the same with-

drawal syndrome. It should be kept in mind that some of the longer acting agents, such as diazepam (Valium), can cause a delayed syndrome several days after discontinuation of the drug. It is important to recognize and promptly treat withdrawal before it progresses with an appropriate cross-tolerant agent such as pentobarbital or chloridiazepoxide. *(Ellinwood et al, pp. 6–11)*

10. **(C)** Gooseflesh, markedly dilated pupils in diffuse light, and diarrhea are easily observable signs of acute opiate withdrawal. Opiate withdrawal can cause severe discomfort, but is not life-threatening as is sedative/hypnotic/alcohol withdrawal. The necessity of using objective signs in the treatment of opiate addiction is obvious, due to the tendancy of these patients toward drug-seeking behavior. *(Ellinwood et al, pp. 3, 7, 12)*

11. **(A)** By definition, symptoms of illness existing for less than 6 months cannot be called schizophrenia, and are diagnosed as schizophreniform disorders. The total time of mood disturbance must be less than that of thinking disturbances, or another diagnosis such as schizoaffective or major depression with psychotic features should be made. *(APA, pp. 187–195)*

12. **(E)** Psychosis is an indication of a brain chemical malfunction. Many different causes must be entertained. The first step in narrowing a differential diagnosis is to take a careful history, including the duration of symptoms and the patient's premorbid level of functioning. One must of course, rule out nonpsychiatric causes of brain dysfunction. *(Davidson, pp. 1–14)*

13. **(C)** Panic disorder causes discrete episodes of panic that occur spontaneously and often become psychologically linked with the circumstances in which they occur. A phobia is the fear of a single distinct object, such as cats. As opposed to panic disorder, simple phobias are common, result in little debilitation, and do not, in themselves, cause patients to seek treatment. *(APA, pp. 243–245)*

14. **(A)** Somatiform disorders present in many forms. Symptoms occur in many body systems, commonly gastrointestinal, cardiovascular, or genitourinary. Often, pain is experienced that cannot be correlated with the anatomic distribution of the nervous system. Occasionally, they occur concurrently with or subsequent to a genuine physical ailment or trauma. The patient is not conscious of the production of his/her symptoms. To him/her they are felt as "real." *(APA, pp. 263–267)*

15. **(E)** Although Alzheimer's disease and multiinfarct disease are the leading causes of dementia in the elderly, there are numerous causes that can be treatable. Careful evaluation must be undertaken to rule out metabolic causes, including drug interactions, overmedication, vitamin deficiencies, and thyroid disease. Primary psychiatric disease can cause reversible dementia. In the condition of normal-pressure hydrocephalus, shunting can alleviate symptoms. *(Jenike, pp. 117–121)*

16. **(E)** The cause of progressive dementia must be carefully evaluated. Although it may be irreversible, the course can sometimes be modified by treatment, enabling the patient continued function at a certain level and perhaps remaining longer at home. Psychotropic medications used judiciously, and treatment of the underlying disorder, can be helpful. *(Jenike, pp. 117–121, 126–136)*

17. **(B)** Complete and careful evaluation of the patient with dementia should be undertaken with the goal of discovering possible treatable etiology. In the absence of gastrointestinal or genitourinary symptoms, work-up of these systems is not indicated. Lumbar puncture is not routinely indicated and should not be a part of the initial examination. *(Jenike, pp. 117–121)*

18. **(A)** Imipramine is a tricyclic antidepressant that, in addition to the usual anticholinergic side effects, can produce a significant drop in standing blood pressure. This may require discontinuation of the drug and use of another antidepressant. It must be used with particular care in the elderly, because of the hazard of falls. *(Baldessarini, pp. 178–179, 182–183)*

19. **(C)** Diarrhea and tremor are common side effects of lithium treatment. They can occur at therapeutic or toxic levels. When they occur, a serum lithium level should be obtained, as the symptoms can precede more dangerous consequences of lithium toxicity. *(Baldessarini, pp. 117–118)*

20. **(C)** Alprazolam (Xanax), a commonly prescribed anxiolytic, has a side-effect profile typical of the benzodiazepines. Care must be taken to caution patients in its use while operating heavy machinery or a motor vehicle, as it can markedly slow motor speed as well as cause drowsiness. *(Baldessarini, pp. 256–257)*

21. **(E)** Neuroleptically induced neurologic side effects are common. They usually occur in the first weeks of treatment and may not be dose-related. Anti-

cholinergic medication or amantadine (Symmetrel) may relieve symptoms. The offering agent may have to be discontinued and an alternate treatment chosen. Of particular importance are the movement disorders indicative of tardive dyskinesia, which may be irreversible. *(Baldessarini, pp. 68–80)*

22. **(A)** A borderline personality is distinguished by a great deal of character dysfunction. Their lives are generally marked by one crisis after another, which they respond to in impulsive ways. They do have periods when reality testing is impaired, but this generally is limited to times of crisis. *(APA, pp. 346–347)*

23. **(C)** Personality disorders are characterological flaws that impair a person's ability to function in society. A patient may exhibit traits of more than one described disorder. It has been believed by some that environment plays a part in shaping the personality. *(APA, p. 335)*

24. **(B)** The general term *tricyclic* antidepressants has been used for the group of antidepressant agents having a three-ring type structure. These agents have similar properties and side effects and are distinguished from the monoamine oxidase inhibitor type. Imipramine (Tofranil) was the first tricyclic antidepressant to be used. There are now several agents that do not fit into either of these catagories and sometimes are referred to as "atypical" antidepressants. *(Baldessarini, pp. 131–135)*

25. **(A)** Lorazepam is a relatively short-acting benzodiazepine. Its lack of active metabolites and low tissue accumulation make it a favored drug for anxiety treatment. *(Baldessarini, p. 250)*

26. **(C)** Flurazepam is also a benzodiazepine. It has relatively greater sedating effects and thus more commonly is used to induce sleep rather than to treat daytime anxiety. *(Baldessarini, pp. 250–251)*

27. **(D)** Thioridazine is a relatively low-potency antipsychotic agent. It has high sedative effects and a low tendency to cause extrapyramidal side effects. The choice of an antipsychotic agent must be individualized to the patient. *(Baldessarini, pp. 22, 25)*

28. **(B)** Panic disorder is characterized by sudden onset of pounding heart, shortness of breath, dizziness, and extreme anxiety. Patients often feel as though they are about to die. The initial attack often occurs in young adulthood. In severe forms, it can progress to development of phobias associated with situations in which panic attacks have previously occurred. *(Gorman and Liebowitz, pp. 1–4)*

29. **(A)** Generalized anxiety disorder is characterized by the development over time of chronic feelings of tension, anxiety, and restlessness. Discrete episodes of frank panic do not occur. Abuse of alcohol or sedatives often occurs in an attempt to self-medicate. *(Gorman and Liebowitz, pp. 32, 4, 10–11)*

30. **(C)** The difference between major depression disorder, generalized anxiety disorder, and panic disorder can often be quite blurred. In all three disorders, depressed mood and anxiety can coexist. In anxiety and panic disorders, the onset of tension or panic attacks often precede the onset of depressed mood by a significant period of time. *(Gorman and Liebowitz, pp. 4, 10–11)*

31. **(A)** Anorexia nervosa is a disorder characterized by a refusal to maintain a normal body weight. The person has a distorted body image and sees herself/himself as fat even when severely undernourished. Such persons are preoccupied with body size and shape. *(APA, pp. 65–67)*

32. **(C)** Bulimics have a disorder characterized by binge eating during which they feel a lack of control over their eating behavior. Bulimics, like anorexics, have a preoccupation with their weight and body features. They engage in means to prevent weight gain such as self-induced vomiting, abuse of laxatives, fasting between binges, or overly strenuous exercise. *(APA, pp. 67–69)*

33. **(A)** Various studies conducted by researchers in numerous developed and developing countries have shown rates approximating 1% or 10 per 1000 population. There have been some inconsistencies in uniformity and diagnostic criteria and data collection, but it is obvious that the disorder occurs in all populations and has a historical basis. *(Helzer, pp. 4–5)*

34. **(D)** Lithium is excreted by the kidneys; thus, blood levels are dependant upon renal function. Lithium can also have long-term effects on renal and thyroid function. Lithium-induced hypothyroidism can be a side effect of lithium treatment and is treated with thyroid replacement. Thus, in addition to routine lithium blood levels, renal and thyroid function should be monitored. *(Baldessarini, pp. 115, 119–121)*

35. **(E)** Narcolepsy is a disorder involving more than just excessive daytime sleepiness. Hypersomnolence is more commonly caused by other disorders or poor habits. The diagnosis of true narcolepsy, which is relatively rare, can be made only in the presence of at least one of the other symptoms. Sleep attacks plus cataplexy, is considered pathonemonic of narcolepsy. An all-night polysomno-

graph and daytime sleep latency testing is confirmatory. *(Guilleminault, pp. 338–341)*

36. **(C)** Obstructive sleep apnea is a common cause of excessive daytime somnolence. Snoring is a common observable sign of upper airway obstruction. This is not a benign condition. In addition to sleepiness being quite debilitating and potentially dangerous, lowered PO_2 during sleep and other physiologic changes can lead to hypertension and potentially fatal cardiac arrythmias. *(Lugaresi et al, p. 498)*

37. **(E)** Tricyclic antidepressants vary in their potency of anticholinergic effects. The patient's underlying medical status must be taken into account in choosing an antidepressant. Conditions such as benign prostatic hypertrophy can worsen markedly. *(Baldessarini, p. 183)*

38. **(C)** Methylphenidate (Ritalin), along with methamphetamine (Dexidrine), and pemoline (Cylert) are stimulants commonly used to treat children with attention-deficit hyperactivity disorder. Amitriptyline and phenelzine are antidepressants. Carbamazepine is an anticonvulsant with several psychiatric uses. *(Baldessarini, pp. 126–219)*

39. **(B)** The most common symptom of acute cocaine withdrawal after heavy use is depression. This can also be accompanied by anxiety and irritability. Often, cocaine abusers also abuse sedative medications or alcohol in an attempt to self-medicate these feelings. Cocaine does not produce a physical withdrawal syndrome as do opiates, sedative/hypnotics or alcohol. *(APA, pp. 142–143, 177–179)*

40. **(B)** When psychoactive drugs are used in the elderly, care must be taken to closely monitor response to the drug. Impaired gastrointestinal, liver, and/or renal function can alter absorption and elimination patterns. Interactions with other prescribed or over-the-counter medications can occur. Psychotropic drugs can be effectively and safely used in the elderly when precautions are taken, and can enhance and even prolong life. *(Jenike, pp. 6–7, 9–14)*

41. **(B)** Antisocial personalities do not respond well to treatment. They do not learn from their mistakes and tend to blame others for their misfortunes. Statistically, they are predominantly males, and are well represented in prison populations. *(APA, pp. 342–346)*

42. **(D)** The MMPI is a well-standardized test that has been used extensively for more than 40 years. It does not take the place of a careful psychiatric examination, but augments it. It includes sophisticated internal validation factors that point out certain patterns of manipulation on the part of the patient. *(Clarkin and Sweeney, p. 5)*

43. **(B)** Some of the new antidepressants have potent serotonin uptake blocking effects. Amphetamine was once used as an antidepressant, with limited results. Phenylalanine and tyrosine are amino acid precursors of centrally active catecholamines. *(Baldessarini, pp. 151–155)*

44. **(E)** A tendency towards perfectionism and minute attention to detail can be desirable in certain occupations. The obsessive compulsive is, however, impaired in his/her ability to discriminate what is important. Taken to the extreme, the patient is so preoccupied with details, he/she cannot complete the task at hand. *(APA, pp. 354–356)*

45. **(E)** It is very important to rule out nonpsychiatric causes of a psychiatric appearing presentation. Many metabolic dysfunctions may cause brain dysfunction and mimic symptoms of psychiatric illness. At times, there may be an underlying life-threatening situation that is potentially correctable. *(Dunner, p. 12)*

46. **(C)** A statement of suicidal intent by a patient must be taken very seriously. An actively suicidal patient is not a candidate for outpatient treatment because of the potential lethality of an overdose of many psychiatric medications. Initiation of treatment and stabilization is best accomplished in an inpatient setting and can generally be done in 1 week to 10 days. *(Baldessarini, pp. 195–197)*

47. **(E)** Mental retardation varies widely in cause and degree of impairment. Causes can include genetic, such as Down's syndrome; congenital, as in fetal alcohol syndrome; traumatic, as a result of childhood head injury; or have no readily identifiable cause. *(APA, pp. 28–33)*

48. **(D)** Competency is a legal term used to define the ability of a person to make decisions based on his/her own best interest. It is further broken down to pertain to the specific task at hand, such as competency to draw up a will, make a contract, or participate in a legal defence. A person may be deemed competent to perform some tasks and not others. *(Baldessarini, p. 280)*

49. **(E)** A closed head injury causes trauma to the brain by creating shear forces and contusions within the skull. Depending upon the force of the blow and the movements of the brain within the skull, many different brain functions may be impaired. Healing and accommodation of the remaining intact brain can bring about the return of some functions within about 2 years of injury. *(APA, pp. 4–8)*

50. **(B)** Lead, cadmium, and mercury are commonly encountered potential poisons. They each can have neurobehavioral effects with chronic exposure that can mimic psychiatric illness. The complaints are usually subtle and include tremor, fatigue, memory loss, mood changes, insomnia, and others. Once again, when encountering a depressed patient, rule out other medical causes first. *(Molinaro, pp. 261–269)*

REFERENCES

Aldrich, MS. Cardinal manifestations of sleep disorders. In: Kryger, Roth, Dement, (eds.). *Principles and Practice of Sleep Medicine.* Philadelphia, PA: WB Saunders; 1989.

American Psychiatric Association. *Diagnostic and Statistical Manual of Mental Disorders,* 3rd ed. Washington, DC: American Psychiatric Association; 1987.

Baldessarini, RJ. *Chemotherapy in Psychiatry,* 2nd ed. Cambridge, MA: Harvard University Press; 1985.

Clarkin J, Sweeney J. Psychological assessment. In: Michels R, (ed). *Psychiatry,* Vol. I. Philadelphia, PA: JB Lippincott; 1988.

Davidson K. Symptomatic psychoses. In: Michels R (ed). *Psychiatry,* Vol. I. Philadelphia, PA: JB Lippincott; 1988.

Dunner DL. Affective disorder: Clinical features. In: Michels R (ed). *Psychiatry.* Vol. I. Philadelphia, PA: JB Lippincott; 1988.

Ellinwood E, Woody G, Krichnan R. Treatment for drug abuse. In: Michels R (ed). *Psychiatry.* Vol. II. Philadelphia, PA: JB Lippincott; 1988.

Gorman J, Liebowitz M. Panic and anxiety disorders. In: Michels R (ed). *Psychiatry.* Vol. I. Philadelphia, PA: JB Lippincott; 1988.

Guilleminault, C. Narcolepsy syndrome. In: Kryger, Roth, Dement (eds). *Principles and Practice of Sleep Medicine.* Philadelphia, PA: WB Saunders; 1989.

Helzer, JE. Schizophrenia: Epidemiology. In: Michels R (ed). *Psychiatry.* Vol. I. Philadelphia, PA: JB Lippincott; 1988.

Jenike M. *Handbook of Geriatric Psychopharmacology.* Littleton, MA: PSG Publishing Co; 1985.

Kendell E. Schizophrenia: Clinical features. In: Michels R (ed). *Psychiatry.* Vol. I. Philadelphia, PA: JB Lippincott; 1988.

Lugaresi E, Cirignotta F, Montagna P. Snoring: Pathogenic, clinical, and therapeutic aspects. In: Kryger, Roth, Dement (eds). *Principles and Practice of Sleep Medicine.* Philadelphia, PA: WB Saunders; 1989.

Molinaro J. *A Primary Care Approach to Heavy Metal Poisoning.* JAAPA. Jul/Aug 1989.

Zarcone, P. Sleep hygiene. In: Kryger, Roth, Dement, (eds). *Principals and Practice of Sleep Medicine.* Philadelphia, PA: WB Saunders; 1989.

Subspecialty Listing: Psychiatry

Question Numbers and Subspecialty
1. General psychiatry
2. General psychiatry
3. General psychiatry
4. Sleep disorders medicine
5. Sleep disorders medicine
6. Child psychiatry
7. Substance abuse
8. Substance abuse
9. Substance abuse
10. Substance abuse
11. General psychiatry
12. General psychiatry
13. General psychiatry
14. General psychiatry
15. Geriatric psychiatry
16. Geriatric psychiatry
17. Geriatric psychiatry
18. General psychiatry
19. General psychiatry
20. General psychiatry
21. General psychiatry
22. General psychiatry
23. General psychiatry
24. General psychiatry
25. General psychiatry
26. General psychiatry
27. General psychiatry
28. General psychiatry
29. General psychiatry
30. General psychiatry
31. Eating disorders
32. Eating disorders
33. General psychiatry
34. General psychiatry
35. Sleep disorders medicine
36. Sleep disorders medicine
37. General psychiatry
38. Child psychiatry
39. Substance abuse
40. General psychiatry
41. General psychiatry
42. General psychiatry
43. General psychiatry
44. General psychiatry
45. General psychiatry
46. General psychiatry
47. Child psychiatry
48. Forensic psychiatry
49. General psychiatry
50. General psychiatry

CHAPTER 9

Obstetrics and Gynecology

Denyse Mahoney

Questions

DIRECTIONS (Questions 1 through 21): For each of the items in this section, ONE or MORE of the numbered options is correct. Choose the answer

- A if only 1, 2, and 3 are correct,
- B if only 1 and 3 are correct,
- C if only 2 and 4 are correct,
- D if only 4 is correct,
- E if all are correct.

1. Which of the following mothers' offspring would require treatment with hepatitis B immune globulin and hepatitis B vaccine at birth?

    (1) mother with active hepatitis B in last month of pregnancy
    (2) mother with active hepatitis A
    (3) mother who is HBsAG positive
    (4) mother with convalescent titers for hepatitis A

2. Endomyometritis commonly occurs after cesarean section (less common after vaginal delivery); factors involved in the pathogenesis of endomyometritis are:

    (1) history of previous episode of pelvic inflammatory disease
    (2) presence of normal cervical and vaginal flora that become pathogenic in the upper genital track
    (3) the presence of anemia or other chronic diseases prior to delivery
    (4) the ideal medium of the postpartum endometrial cavity for proliferation of bacteria

3. A patient was delivered by forceps and is presently 2 days postpartum. She is found to have a swollen, erythematous right leg with a positive Homan's sign. Which of the following contributed to her present postpartum complications?

    (1) decreased blood flow from her lower extremities during the last weeks of pregnancy
    (2) hypercoagulable state of pregnancy

    (3) decreased activity secondary to postpartum state
    (4) use of oxytocin to stimulate labor

4. A patient develops mastitis postpartum. Which of the following would be signs and symptoms?

    (1) chills and fever
    (2) engorgement of breast within 48 hours after onset of lactation
    (3) areas of inflammation, redness, and induration of one breast
    (4) green discoloration of breast milk

5. A woman presents in labor at 5 cm dilated in breech presentation. Which of the following causes a higher incidence of breech presentation?

    (1) fetal anomalies
    (2) uterine anatomic abnormalities
    (3) premature onset of labor
    (4) grandmultipartity

6. Breech presentation is associated with a higher incidence of cord prolapse. What other malpresentations are also associated with this obstetric emergency?

    (1) transverse lie
    (2) brow presentation
    (3) compound presentation
    (4) face presentation

7. A 25-year-old patient has undergone a rapid, spontaneous vaginal delivery followed by a prolonged third stage of labor, and an eventual manual removal of the placenta. She continues to bleed heavily after placental removal, with an estimated blood loss of greater than 1000 ml. What are the subsequent steps to control the hemorrhage?

    (1) exploration of the uterus for retained products
    (2) administration of methyergonovine (methergine)
    (3) vigorous fundal massage
    (4) packing of the uterus

SUMMARY OF DIRECTIONS				
A	**B**	**C**	**D**	**E**
1, 2, 3 only	1, 3 only	2, 4 only	4 only	All are correct

8. Which are indications for a low vertical or classical uterine incision at the time of cesarean section?

   (1) transverse lie of the fetus
   (2) an estimated fetal weight of 4500 g.
   (3) premature baby
   (4) frank breech presentation

9. A 35-year-old patient presents to labor and delivery at 18 weeks' gestation, complaining of fullness in her vagina. On pelvic exam, the cervix is 6 cm with ballooning of the membranes into the vagina. Additional information you might obtain from the patient that would explain her present condition would be

   (1) history of previous septic abortion
   (2) previous second trimester abortion that was without contractions
   (3) a known balanced chromosomal abnormality in the patient
   (4) history of patient's mother receiving DES during her pregnancy

10. A woman has undergone a suction curettage for a hydatidiform mole. What subsequent steps should be done to ensure she does not develop choriocarcinoma?

    (1) serial serum beta HCG levels should be obtained every 1 to 2 weeks until negative
    (2) prophylatic chemotherapy should be administered
    (3) the patient should be advised not to become pregnant for at least 1 year
    (4) patient should undergo a radical hysterectomy and bilateral salpingo-oophorectomy

11. At 34-weeks' gestation, a patient's fundal height measures 40 cm. The sonogram at that time reveals polyhydramnios. What else may be found on ultrasound at this time?

    (1) large ovarian cyst
    (2) calcification of the placenta
    (3) placenta previa
    (4) fetal congenital anomalies

12. Preterm labor occurs more frequently in twin gestations. What other antenatal complications occur at a greater frequency in twin gestations?

    (1) fetal anomalies
    (2) preeclampsia
    (3) intrauterine growth retardation
    (4) gestational diabetes

13. Respiratory depression is a known side effect of magnesium sulfate (a medication commonly used in pregnant woman). Which of the following are a means of monitoring the amount of magnesium administered and preventing this complication?

    (1) observing changes in the fetal heart rate
    (2) checking maternal deep tendon reflexes
    (3) monitoring blood pressure
    (4) serum magnesium

14. A 32-year-old patient presents to labor and delivery at 37-weeks' gestation with a complaint of vaginal bleeding. Her history includes two previous cesarean sections. A sonogram performed showed the following (See Figure 9–1)

Which of the following procedures should not be performed on this patient?

    (1) bimanual pelvic exam
    (2) bed rest with IV fluids
    (3) attempted vaginal delivery
    (4) repeat cesarean section

15. At 36 weeks, a 28-year-old patient presents with a complaint of leaking fluid from her vagina on the fetal monitor. How would you determine whether this was amniotic fluid?

    (1) obtain a specimen of fluid and send it for L/S ratio
    (2) place some fluid on a glass slide and check for "ferning" under the microscope
    (3) estimate amniotic fluid volume on ultrasound
    (4) test fluid with nitrazine paper

16. A patient has documented spontaneous rupture of membranes at 32 weeks' gestation. It has been decided to manage the patient conservatively with bed rest, monitoring white blood cell count and maternal temperature. What are the major risks to the mother and fetus when conservative management is followed?

    (1) prolapsed cord
    (2) development of late decelerations on nonstress testing
    (3) onset of chorioamnionitis
    (4) onset of vaginal bleeding secondary to placenta previa

Figure 9–1. A 32-year-old patient at 37-week's gestation. AF, amniotic fluid; B, maternal bladder; Cx, cervix; P, placenta.

17. Which of the following medications are commonly used to arrest preterm labor?

(1) magnesium sulfate
(2) indomethicin
(3) ritodrine
(4) ethanol

18. Pregnancy complicated by insulin dependent diabetes prior to gestation has the following additional complications

(1) increase in fetal congenital anomalies
(2) increased cesarean section rate
(3) increased incidence of preeclampsia/eclampsia
(4) increase in fetal respiratory distress syndrome

19. In caring for a mother with diabetes, which of the following are important means of fetal surveillance?

(1) accurate dating of pregnancy
(2) fasting serum glucose at 100 mg/dL
(3) biweekly NSTs after 34 weeks
(4) maternal 24-hour urinary estriol excretion

20. A 32-year-old woman has been followed by her gynecologist for secondary infertility, her last pregnancy having been 8 years earlier. Her preliminary infertility work-up reveals she is ovulating and her husband's fertility work-up is within normal limits. Her history reveals a past use of an intrauterine device (IUD) that was removed 2 years previously because of an episode of PID. She undergoes a laparoscopy. What would be the expected findings at the time of surgery?

(1) pelvic endometriosis
(2) pertubular adhesions
(3) ovarian cysts
(4) bilateral hydrosalpinx

21. A 35-year-old woman undergoes a dilation and curettage for irregular menstrual bleeding. The endometrial curettings are consistent with the secondary phase of the menstrual cycle. With this information, which of the following is a correct statement about this patient?

(1) the patient is entering premature menopause
(2) the endometrium is under predominantly estrogen stimulation
(3) the patient is taking oral contraceptives
(4) the patient has ovulated

DIRECTIONS (Questions 22 through 44): Each of the numbered items or incomplete statements in this section is followed by answers or by completions of the statement. Select the ONE lettered answer or completion that is BEST in each case.

22. When reviewing the events of a patient's labor, what is the most predictive factor in determining whether she will develop a postop infection after cesarean section?

(A) history of previous cesarean section
(B) whether cesarean section was an emergency
(C) duration of labor prior to cesarean
(D) presence of medical complications, such as preeclampsia or diabetes
(E) malpresentation of fetus such as breech or transverse lie

23. On postop day number 5, a patient has persistent spiking temperature despite triple antibiotic for 48 hours. She is also found to be tachypneic and tachycardic. What is the most important postop complication to rule out?

(A) pneumonia
(B) tuboovarian abscess
(C) endomyometritis
(D) sepsis
(E) pulmonary embolus

24. A 36-year-old woman, with two previous full-term pregnancies presents for her first prenatal visit at 12 weeks' gestation. What tests must she be advised to undergo?

(A) immediate high resolution ultrasound
(B) genetic amniocentesis
(C) maternal serum alphafetoprotein at present visit
(D) amniocentesis for chromosomal abnormalities at 24 weeks
(E) chromosomal analysis of herself and of the father of the baby

25. A 27-year-old black female with chronic hypertension is being monitored during the active phase of labor. Late decelerations are noted on the monitor. What can be summarized from such fetal heart rate pattern?

    (A) the patient has developed superimposed preeclampsia
    (B) the patient has placenta previa
    (C) the decelerations are secondary to head compression and are of no significance
    (D) the patient probably has intrauterine growth retardation and therefore uteroplacental insufficency
    (E) the patient should undergo a pelvic exam to rule out cord prolapse

26. The tracing shown in Figure 9–2 was obtained on a 23-year-old woman at 41½ weeks during antepartum testing. The tracing can be described as

    (A) suspicious for fetal compromise
    (B) as a reactive nonstress test
    (C) as a negative oxytocin challenge test
    (D) a fetal heart pattern consistent with a cord pattern
    (E) as an indication that the patient must be wrong on her dates of conception

27. A patient is admitted to labor and delivery with contractions every 4 minutes, lasting 45 seconds. On admission, her pelvic exam revealed a 4 cm dilated cervix. One hour later, her exam was 5 cm dilated. Which of the following is an accurate statement about her labor pattern?

    (A) the fetal presentation should be determined because breech presentation progresses rapidly

    (B) an intrauterine pressure catheter should be placed to determine intensity of uterine contractions
    (C) if this is a first pregnancy, she is making good progress
    (D) this is adequate progress for the latent phase of labor
    (E) she had entered her second stage of labor

28. A gestational diabetic at 40 weeks has an estimated fetal weight of 4300g by sonogram. What major complication of vaginal delivery would warrant doing a preliminary cesarean section without a trial of labor.

    (A) a higher incidence of placental insufficency in gestational diabetes
    (B) a higher incidence of infection postop in gestational diabetes
    (C) a higher incidence of breech presentation in pregnancies complicated by diabetes
    (D) a higher incidence of shoulder dystocia in pregnancies complicated by diabetes
    (E) a higher incidence in diabetes of the uterine atony following delivery of a large baby

29. A large baby, 9½ pounds, is delivered with midforceps to a 32-year-old patient. The placenta delivered spontaneously without difficulty. The uterus appears to be well contracted with pitocin, but the patient continues to bleed vaginally, presenting bright, red blood. What is the most likely cause of this persistent bleeding?

    (A) retained placental products
    (B) lacerations of the cervix or vagina
    (C) previously undiagnosed coagulopathy

Figure 9–2. A 23-year-old woman at 41½ weeks.

(D) bleeding is from a rectal tear, secondary to the forceps

(E) uterine atony

30. A 27-year-old woman presents in labor at term with a history of a previous cesarean section for cephalopelvic disproportion. What is the most important historical information needed prior to attempting vaginal delivery after a cesarean?

(A) birthweight of previous baby
(B) length of labor in previous pregnancy
(C) strength of contractions in present labor
(D) uterine incision in previous cesarean section
(E) the number of previous cesarean sections

31. At 11 weeks of pregnancy, a patient presents to the Emergency Room with a complaint of vaginal bleeding and lower abdominal cramping. On pelvic exam, there is a large amount of blood in the vagina and placental tissue present in the os. This describes which kind of spontaneous abortion?

(A) inevitable
(B) septic
(C) missed
(D) incomplete
(E) induced

32. A 17-year-old female presented at the GYN clinic, requesting an abortion. She is presently 10 weeks pregnant. What would be the safest, most efficient means of abortion at this time?

(A) intraamniotic saline injection
(B) suction curettage after cervical dilation with prostaglandin suppository
(C) hysterotomy
(D) dilation and curettage
(E) administration of IV oxytocin

33. At 16-weeks' gestation, a patient presents with a complaint of vaginal bleeding. Her quantitative beta HCG is higher than expected at 16 weeks' gestation and her fundal height is approximately 16 to 18-week size. Although she denies a past history of hypertension, her blood pressure is 140/90. No fetal heart sounds can be heard on doptone and there is no sign of a fetus on ultrasound. What would be her most likely diagnosis?

(A) threatened abortion
(B) incomplete abortion
(C) hydatidiform mole
(D) fetal demise at 16 weeks
(E) twin gestation

34. A 28-year-old patient presents to labor and delivery at 38 weeks with a history of sudden onset of sharp pain in her lower abdomen and back, which has since subsided. On evaluation, her blood pressure is 150/100 and there is no detectable fetal heart movement on ultrasound. She also complains of profuse vaginal bleeding. On the fetal monitor, she is having frequent contractions. What is the most likely cause of fetal demise?

(A) placenta previa
(B) chronic hypertension
(C) diseminated intravascular coagulopathy
(D) placental abruption
(E) chronic renal failure

35. A woman at 20-weeks' gestation is diagnosed with fetal demise. She has elected to await the onset of spontaneous labor. What blood test should be drawn at this time to avoid a major complication of intrauterine fetal demise?

(A) beta HCG
(B) PT and PTT and fibrinogen
(C) liver function test
(D) CBC
(E) prolactin level

36. At 42-weeks' gestation, a patient's labor is induced. At 5 cm dilated, she undergoes an artificial rupture of membranes with very little fluid present. What other characteristic of postdate pregnancy might be present at the time of rupture of membranes?

(A) chorioamnionitis
(B) blood tinged fluid
(C) vernix present in fluid
(D) meconium stained fluid
(E) hyperstimulation of uterine contractions

37. In prenatal clinic, a 32-year-old patient presents at 24 weeks' gestation. On history, you find her first child weighed 9½ pounds. Her second child was stillborn. What screening test would you order at 28 weeks?

(A) alpha fetoprotein
(B) VDRL
(C) blood type and Rh
(D) 50 g glucose challenge
(E) toxoplasmosis titers

38. A 29-year-old patient presents to the Emergency Room at 17 weeks' gestation with a complaint of right upper quadrant and right lower quadrant pain of 6 hours duration. The pain is associated with nausea and vomiting. On exam, she has diffuse abdominal tenderness and decreased bowel sounds and her fundal height is consistent with dates and is nontender. She has no CVA tenderness. Her temperature is 102.4°F and the WBC count on

CBC is 18,000. Her urinalysis shows no WBCs or proteinuria. What is the most likely diagnosis?

(A) hyperemesis graviderm
(B) acute appendicitis
(C) pylonephritis
(D) unilateral PID
(E) degenerating myomata

39. Complications secondary to anesthesia are one of the most common causes of maternal mortality. The most life-threatening complication of general anesthesia in the pregnant woman is?

(A) hypotension
(B) atelectis
(C) aspiration
(D) uterine atony
(E) eclampsia

40. A 24-year-old patient presents to a GYN clinic for a routine exam. Her OB/GYN history is significant for having her first child at age 16 and her second at age 18. Since separation from her husband at age 19, she has had several sexual partners. On pelvic exam, she has condylomata acuminata on her labia. What gynecologic neoplasm is this woman at risk for?

(A) ovarian cancer
(B) AIDS
(C) endometrial cancer
(D) cervical cancer
(E) cancer of the labia

41. A 23-year-old patient presents to planned parenthood, requesting birth control. Her GYN history is significant for several sexual partners, a recent episode of PID secondary to *Chlamydia*, and one induced abortion. Which of the following forms of birth control would you be least likely to recommend for her use?

(A) contraceptive sponges
(B) intrauterine device
(C) oral contraceptives
(D) diaphram
(E) condoms

42. A 30-year-old patient complains of progressively worse dysmenorrhea. Her pain begins 2 to 4 days prior to onset of bleeding and is associated with spotting. Additionally, she complains of pain on intercourse (dysparunia). You think the patient may have endometriosis. What is the best way to make the diagnosis?

(A) a 6-month course of danazol (danocrine) to see whether the symptoms subside
(B) pelvic ultrasound
(C) treatment with prostaglandin synthetase inhibitors to see if the symptoms abate

(D) diagnostic laparoscopy
(E) diagnostic hysteroscopy

43. Which menstrual irregularity would most likely occur in a woman suffering from anorexia nervosa or in a woman who is a marathon runner?

(A) menorrhagia
(B) amenorrhea
(C) oligomenorrhea
(D) polymenorrhea
(E) metrorrhagia

44. A 25-year-old woman presents with a history of prolonged episodes of amenorrhea followed by prolonged bleeding. She has been sexually active for 6 years and has never conceived. On physical exam, she is obese and somewhat hirsute. On pelvic exam, her ovaries are enlarged bilaterally. The most likely diagnosis is?

(A) progesterone secreting tumor on the ovaries
(B) hyperprolactinemia syndrome
(C) congenital adrenal hyperplasia
(D) polycystic ovary syndrome
(E) hypothyroidism

DIRECTIONS (Questions 45 through 48): Each group of items in this section consists of lettered headings followed by a set of numbered words or phrases. For each numbered word or phrase, select the ONE lettered heading that is most closely associated with it. Each lettered heading may be selected once, more than once, or not at all.

Question Range 45 through 48

For the number of weeks of gestation, match the events of pregnancy that occur at the time of pregnancy.

(A) 6 weeks
(B) 28 weeks
(C) 20 weeks
(D) 16 to 20 weeks
(E) 14 weeks

45. fundal height at umbilicus

46. fetal movements first perceived by mother

47. gestational sac first seen on sonogram (abdominal)

48. optimal time to draw maternal serum alpha fetoprotein

Question Range 49 through 52

The following are a list of drugs. Match the known side effects if ingested by a pregnant woman.

(A) alcohol
(B) nitrofuratoin
(C) coumarin

(D) cocaine

(E) phenytoin

49. anomalies are caused by the drug's effect on the fetal clotting factors

50. higher incidence of stillborns secondary to placental abruption when this drug is used during second and third trimesters

51. taken in large amounts causes definitive syndrome in the fetus, but unsure if occasional use causes fetal harm

52. the maternal benefits of this drug outweigh the known fetal effects

DIRECTIONS (Questions 53 through 73): For each of the items in this section, ONE or MORE of the numbered options is correct. Choose the answer

A if only 1, 2, and 3 are correct,
B if only 1 and 3 are correct,
C if only 2 and 4 are correct,
D if only 4 is correct,
E if all are correct.

53. A 62-year-old female who is 12 years postmenopausal complains of urinary urgency, frequency, and occasional incontinence. On pelvic exam, she has a urethral carbuncle and her vaginal mucosa appears atrophic: shiny, pale pink with white patches, and bleeds slightly to touch. Her urinalysis and urine cultures are negative. How would you best treat this patient?

(1) antibiotic by mouth
(2) testosterone cream to be applied to affected areas
(3) vaginal suppositories containing sulfa antibiotics
(4) estrogen-containing cream per vagina

54. A 26-year-old female who is G2P2 and whose LMP was 8 weeks earlier presents to the Emergency Room with a complaint of lower abdominal pain and vaginal bleeding described as spotting. Her vital signs are stable and on abdominal exam she has good bowel sounds and no tenderness. On pelvic exam, she has mild cervical motion tenderness and a 6 to 8 week size uterus. Her serum beta HCG is positive and her hematocrit is 39. You suspect a threatened abortion but want to rule out ectopic pregnancy. What would be the next appropriate step?

(1) pelvic ultrasound, with vaginal probe if available
(2) diagnostic laparoscopy
(3) serial quantative beta HCG
(4) exploratory laparotomy

55. A 31-year-old female G1P1 presents to the Emergency Room with lower abdominal pain, vaginal bleeding, and a 6-week history of amenorrhea. Her GYN history is significant for history of oral contraceptive use in the past and having undergone an uncompleted induced abortion. Additionally, she has had an episode of PID and subsequent secondary infertility. Eight months prior to admission, she underwent a laparotomy for microsurgery on her fallopian tubes in an attempt to correct her infertility. A culdocentesis performed in the emergency room was positive for blood and exploratory laparotomy revealed an ectopic pregnancy. What risk factors did this patient have for developing an ectopic pregnancy?

(1) a history of an induced abortion
(2) a history of PID
(3) a history of oral contraceptive use
(4) a history of tubal surgery

56. A 19-year-old G0P0. female presents to the Emergency Room with a complaint of lower abdominal pain, vomiting, and fever of 2-days duration. Her last period was normal and ended 3 days prior to the onset of pain. On physical exam, her temperature was 103°F, and she had decreased bowel sounds and bilateral lower abdominal tenderness with rebound tenderness. On pelvic exam, she had marked cervical motion tenderness and bilateral adnexal tenderness. The diagnosis of PID was made and the patient was admitted for IV antibiotic therapy. Which of the following organisms could be responsible for the infection?

(1) *Neisseria gonorrhea*
(2) anaerobic bacteria such as *Bacteroid's*
(3) *C trachomatis*
(4) *Clostridum difficile*

57. A 22-year-old G2P2, presents to the GYN clinic with a history that her boyfriend had a positive culture for gonorrhea. She complains only of a vaginal discharge. On abdominal exam, she has mild bilateral lower abdominal tenderness and on pelvic exam, a mucopurulent discharge from the cervix and mild cervical motion tenderness. She appears to have mild PID and because she could tolerate medication by mouth, she is treated on an outpatient basis. Which of the following regimens are adequate treatment for outpatient PID?

(1) vibramycin, 100 mg b.i.d orally
(2) 2.4 million U procaine penicillin intramuscularly with probenicid and erythromycin 25 mg orally for 7 days
(3) trimethoprim-sulfamethoxazole, 2 tabs orally, b.i.d. for 7 days
(4) ceftriaxone, 250 mg, intramuscularly for one dose and doxycycline 100 mg orally, b.i.d. for 10 days

58. A 29-year-old G3P1Ab2 female is seen in the Emergency Room with a 24-hour history of bilateral lower abdominal pain, right greater than left. She complains of slight nausea and has had one episode of vomiting. She is sexually active and uses only condoms for birth control. Her last period was lighter than normal. Her past gynecologic history is significant for one previous episode of PID. Her abdominal exam reveals slightly decreased bowel sounds and mild bilateral tenderness without rebound tenderness. On pelvic exam, she has moderate cervical motion tenderness and fullness in her right adnexa. Her temperature is 38.2°C, and WBC on CBC is 14,000. She is admitted with a diagnosis of PID, but which of the following should also be considered in this patient?

    (1) acute appendicitis
    (2) adenexal torsion
    (3) ectopic pregnancy
    (4) ruptured tubal ovarian abscess

59. A 24-year-old female presents with a complaint of labial bumps that are painful when she urinates. On questioning the patient, she reveals she has felt feverish and has had generalized malaise. On pelvic exam, she has several vesicular lesions on the labia and a few ulcerative lesions. The lesions are painful to touch. Which of the following could be the cause of this patient's symptoms?

    (1) condylomata acuminata
    (2) secondary syphilis
    (3) lymphogranuloma venereum
    (4) herpes

60. A 42-year-old G2P2 female has a known history of uterine myomata that are approximately 14-week size. Within the past year, her periods have become progressively heavier and longer. A dilation and curettage performed 6 months earlier showed normal pathology and failed to decrease the bleeding. Which of the following are acceptable indications for hysterectomy in the patient?

    (1) heavy uterine bleeding causing anemia
    (2) the possibility of myomatas developing into cancer
    (3) inability to adequately evaluate the size of the ovaries
    (4) prevention of the development of pelvic adhesions

61. Endometrial hyperplasia is a pathology found in women with irregular menstrual bleeding. It is characterized by excessive growth of the endometrium, which is usually a result of a persistently high level of estrogen that is unopposed by progesterone. Which of the following women are likely to have endometrial hyperplasia?

    (1) a young woman suffering from anorexia nervosa
    (2) a 35-year-old woman with a long history of anovulatory cycles
    (3) a woman with a 10-year history of oral contraceptive use
    (4) an obese woman who has postmenopausal bleeding

62. On a routine pelvic examination, a 5-cm cystic mass is palpated on the left side of a 22-year-old female. Her last menstrual period was approximately 13 days prior to the exam. It is decided to give her birth control pills in an attempt to suppress ovarian function. Six weeks later, she is reexamined and the cyst is 8-cm in size. Which of the following would be the next step in treating this patient?

    (1) continue birth control pills and reexamine the patient in 8 weeks
    (2) perform laparoscopy to determine whether the cyst is functional versus neoplastic
    (3) obtain ultrasound to rule out endometrioma
    (4) perform exploratory laparotomy in order to remove cysts

63. A 19-year-old female who is sexually active and uses no form of birth control presents to the Emergency Room with a complaint of severe abdominal pain. Her last menstrual period (LMP) was approximately 6 weeks before the onset of the pain. She has a history significant for irregular periods. On abdominal exam, she has decreased bowel sounds and rebound tenderness. On pelvic exam, she has a small amount of dark red blood in her vagina and marked tenderness to cervical motion. Prior to bringing the patient to the operating room for an exploratory laparotomy, which tests below would be helpful in differentiating whether this patient has a ruptured corpus luteal cyst versus ectopic pregnancy?

    (1) hemoglobin and hematocrit
    (2) urinary pregnancy test sensitive to 25 mIU beta HCG
    (3) white blood cell count on CBC
    (4) serum pregnancy test

64. A 63-year-old female whose status is post-four spontaneous deliveries and a total abdominal hysterectomy for fibroids 15 years earlier presents with a complaint of fullness in her vagina. Additionally, she has noted loss of urine with coughing or sneezing, which is getting progressively worse. On pelvic exam, she has a second-degree cystocele and when asked to valsalva, loses small amounts of urine. Which of the following would be adequate therapy for this patient?

    (1) Marshall–Marchetti–Kranz
    (2) placement of a vaginal pessary

(3) anterior vaginal repair

(4) repair of vesicovaginal fistula

65. A 40-year-old G3P3 woman goes to her gynecologist for a routine GYN exam. On physical exam, which of the following are part of a routine gynecologic exam?

(1) bimanual pelvic exam

(2) breast exam

(3) speculum exam of the cervix and vagina

(4) abdominal exam

66. When performing a pelvic exam, it is important to

(1) adequately drape the patient to avoid excessive exposure

(2) insist that family members including the patient's husband leave the examining room

(3) explain to the patient each step of the procedure

(4) refrain from informing the patient that a particular part of the exam will be painful

67. When performing a pelvic exam, which cervical changes would be indicative of pregnancy?

(1) a multiparous cervix

(2) softening of the cervix

(3) presence of Nabothian cysts on the cervix

(4) blueish discoloration of the cervix

68. When obtaining a menstrual history, which of the following are important questions to ask?

(1) duration and amount of menstrual flow

(2) age of onset and frequency of menses

(3) date of last menstrual period and whether it was normal

(4) presence of intermenstrual bleeding

69. A 42-year-old female with a known history of uterine myomata presents with a complaint of increased bleeding during menses and spotting 4 to 5 days prior to onset of period. On pelvic exam, she has a 14-week size irregular uterus, consistent with fibroids. On speculum exam, there is a small polyp that can be seen in the endocervical canal. Which of the following would be an appropriate procedure for this patient to undergo next?

(1) endometrial biopsy with endocervical curettage

(2) ultrasound of the pelvis

(3) fractional dilation and curettage

(4) CAT scan of the pelvis

70. A 23-year-old crack abuser presents to the Emergency Room with a complaint of vaginal spotting and no period for 6 weeks. A pregnancy test is positive and her pelvis is consistent with a 6-week gestation. She is discharged with the diagnosis of threatened abortion. Two days later, she returns and miscarries. A VDRL drawn at the time of the initial visit is found to be positive. Upon questioning, the patient then remembers having a bump on her vulva approximately 4 weeks earlier. If the patient failed to get treatment at this time, which of the following symptoms would she then develop?

(1) maculopapular skin rash, often on the palms of the hands and soles of the feet

(2) generalized malaise, headaches, and anorexia

(3) condylomata lata on the vulva, thighs, and buttocks

(4) signs of PID

71. A 27-year-old G2P1Ab1 at 32 weeks' gestation presents to her obstetrician with a complaint of not feeling the baby move for 24 hours. On ultrasound, intrauterine fetal demise is confirmed. There is no sign of fetal movement and there is no fetal cardiac motion. The patient is induced and delivers spontaneously approximately 12 hours later. Which of the following are appropriate means of helping parents deal with the loss of the child?

(1) allow the parents to hold and examine the stillborn child if they choose

Figure 9–3. A 32-year-old G3P2Ab1 female at 40-week's gestation.

(2) heavily medicate the mother during labor and particularly the delivery, so she will have no recollection of the delivery

(3) photographs of the child should be taken and either given to the parents or kept on file for future viewing

(4) discourage the father (or other support person) from being present during labor and delivery to spare him the pain

72. A 32-year-old G3P2Ab1 female at 40-weeks gestation is being monitored in labor and develops the fetal heart rate depicted in Figure 9–3. Which of the following is true about this patient's tracing?

(1) these are late decelerations
(2) it is indicative of a cord compression pattern
(3) it shows fetal tachycardia
(4) these are variable decelerations

73. A 16-year-old female is seen in the emergency room as a rape victim. She undergoes a physical and pelvic exam. Prior to being discharged from the Emergency Room, she should be offered which of the following?

(1) follow-up visit in order to be tested for pregnancy and obtain a repeat VDRL
(2) information on how to contact a rape crisis counselor
(3) treatment for gonorrhea and *Chlamydia*
(4) medication to prevent pregnancy

Answers and Explanations

1. (B) Babies born to mothers with active hepatitis B and babies born to mothers who are chronic carriers (chronic HBsAG positive) have a high incidence of developing acute and chronic hepatitis, hepatoma, and cirrhosis. Treatment of these neonates is, therefore, necessary. Treatment consists of hyperimmune serum globulin (HBIG) and the hepatitis B vaccine (HBvac). These are both given at birth and the HBvac is given in two more doses, beginning at 1 month of age. *(Burrow and Ferris, p. 332)*

2. (C) Organisms that normally colonize the cervix and vagina act as pathogens in the upper genital tract postpartum or postop cesarean section. These organisms gain entrance to the upper tract during labor because of prolonged ruptured membranes and repetitive pelvic exams. The upper genital tract, primarily the endometrial cavity, is dark, vascular, and has necrotic decidua. It becomes, therefore, the ideal media for bacterial growth. *(Burrow and Ferris, p. 350)*

3. (A) The patient's symptoms are describing a deep vein thombosis (DVT), a known complication in the pregnant and postpartum patient. The factors that increase the risk of DVT in a pregnant or recently pregnant woman are the hypercoaguable state of pregnancy. A number of blood coagulation factors rise during pregnancy. These include fibrinogen, factor VIII, factor VII, and other vitamin-K dependant clotting factors. During pregnancy, depression of the systemic fibrinolytic activity occurs which returns to normal after delivery of the patient. In the puerperium, however, there are secondary rises of fibrinogen and circulatory platelets. Answers 2 and 3 are anatomical/mechanical reasons for increased chance of DVT. Decreased blood flow from the lower extremities occurs secondary to the enlarged uterus and because of decreased patient mobility, secondary to an operative delivery such as forceps or cesarean section. *(Cunningham et al, p. 478; Niswander, p. 174)*

4. (B) Chills and fever occur with mastitis, as does the localization of an area of redness, hardening, and induration on the breast. Mastitis typically occurs during the third and fourth week postpartum. Postpartum breasts do become engorged within 24 to 48 hours, but it is bilateral without localized induration or erythemia. Postpartum engorgement resolves spontaneously with support and application of ice packs. Mastitis does not cause breast milk to change color but the offending organism, *Staphlococcus aureus*, can be cultured from the breast milk. Treatment consists of an oral (or if necessary parenteral) penicillinase-resistant antibiotic for 10 days. If an abcess has formed, incision and drainage may be necessary. *(Cunningham et al, 485)*

5. (E) As term approaches, the fetus assumes the longitudinal lie in the vertex presentation. The reason for vertex predominance is the piriform shape of the uterus. Although the fetal head is larger at term than the podalic pole, the breech and flexed extremities are bulkier and, therefore, adapt to the fundus better. Congenital anomalies, particularly anencephalic and hydrocephalic babies, will present more commonly as breech. Presumably, this is because the piriform-shaped uterus accommodates these anomalies more efficiently. Uterine anomalies such as bicornate and septate uterus predispose to breech presentation. Prior to 32 weeks, the amniotic cavity is larger and the amount of amniotic fluid is greater; therefore, more fetuses are in the breech presentation. Breech presentation is more common in grandmultiparous women because of relaxed uterine musculature. *(Cunningham et al, pp. 178–180, 349)*

6. (B) Transverse lie occurs when the long access of the fetus is perpendicular to that of the mother. Transverse lie can either be back up or back down and, once in labor, the chance of cord prolapsing is greater due to inadequate filling of the pelvis by the presenting part. The only means of delivering a transverse lie is cesarean section. In a compound presentation, an extremity comes into the pelvis alongside the presenting part. Excluding the presence of a cord prolapse or other signs of fetal distress, a vaginal delivery can be attempted. Brow and face presentations adequately fill the birth canal and, therefore, prevent a higher incidence of cord prolapse. *(Cunningham et al, pp. 360–362)*

7. **(A)** There are several things the practitioner should do once it appears that the patient is bleeding heavily postdelivery. The first is to examine the patient for retained products by exploring the uterus manually and then examining the cervix and vagina for lacerations. Once lacerations have been ruled out, the practitioner should then attempt manually to contract the uterus and to administer medication that will cause uterine contractions. Oxytocin is usually given first and if the uterus does not respond, ergonovine or methylergonovine should be administered. The ergotrates cause sustained uterine contractions and are, therefore, more efficacious but can cause hypertension and hence are contraindicated in some cases. A prostaglandin derivative, prostaglandin F_2 alpha, has recently been used intramuscularly (or intrauterine) and has been found to be efficacious once oxytocin and ergotrates have failed. Packing of the uterus had been used as a means of controlling postpartum hemorrhage but was found to be ineffective and dangerous because of concealed hemorrhage. As with any situation when there is the potential for shock to develop, the patient's cardiovascular status should be monitored. At least one, if not two, large gauge IV catheters should be placed and specimens for blood crossmatch should be obtained. *(Cunningham et al, 417–419)*

8. **(B)** In general, a low vertical or classical uterine incision is done when it is anticipated that delivery through a low transverse incision would lacerate or tear laterally into the large branches of the uterine artery and vein. Because delivery of a transverse lie requires intrauterine manipulation, a low vertical incision provides greater room. The lower uterine segment is not adequately developed in the preterm baby, and particularly in the absence of labor, delivery is usually by low, vertical incision. A large baby in the vertex position is not an indication for a low, vertical incision, nor is a breech presentation. Additional indications for a low, vertical (or classical) incision are a myomata that occupies the lower segment anteriorly, in some cases of placenta previa, and patients with invasive carcinoma of the cervix. *(Cunningham et al, pp. 362,453; Niswander, p. 380)*

9. **(C)** The patient's condition is describing an incompetent cervix. Patients with an incompetent cervix typically present in the second trimester with the complaint of spotting and a bulging feeling in their vagina. They do not complain of painful contractions. On pelvic exam, there is cervical dilation with the membranes bulging through the os in an hourglass configuration. Although the exact cause of incompetent cervix is not known, it has been associated with previous cervical trauma, including dilation and curettage, conization, and cautery of the cervix. Abnormal cervical development has been noted as one of the genital tract abnormalities that occur in women whose mothers were exposed to diethylstilbestrol (DES). Incompetent cervix is known to occur in these women. A previous first trimester abortion is not associated with a higher incidence of incompetent cervix. Babies born to women with incompetent cervix do not have a chromosomal abnormality. *(Cunningham, pp. 498–499)*

10. **(B)** Gestational trophoblastic neoplasia consists of benign GTN, most often hydatidiform mole, and malignant GTN, which includes nonmetastatic and metastatic GTN. Approximately 20% of women who have a hydatidiform mole will go on to develop some form of malignant GTN, one of which is choriocarcinoma. To best detect these patients, serum beta HCG tests are drawn every 1 to 2 weeks until they are negative. Additionally, a women who has had a mole should not become pregnant for 1 year, as pregnancy would interfere with the means of following the trophoblastic disease. Oral contraceptives are a safe and most efficient means of preventing pregnancy. Once beta HCG levels are negative, the patient needs to be followed monthly for 6 months and then every 2 months for 1 year. Should the level of HCG plateau or begin to rise, the patient should undergo further work-up and eventually receive chemotherapy. In nonmetastatic GTN, single-agent chemotherapy is effective with either methotrezate or actinomycin D. Prophalatic chemotherapy was considered a possibility in some centers, but morbidity and mortality associated with therapy did not outweigh the benefits. A radical hysterectomy is not indicated for any stage of GTN, but hysterectomy at the time of diagnosis of a hydatidiform mole is acceptable for a woman who has finished childbearing. It is not necessary to remove the adnexa but it is still necessary to follow beta HCG levels to detect possible metastatic trophoblastic tissue. *(Cunningham et al, pp. 540–553; Neshein, pp. 1–7)*

11. **(D)** Polyhydramnios or hydramnios is excessive amniotic fluid. In most cases of mild polyhydramnios, there is no etiology, but moderate to severe hydramnios is usually associated with fetal anomalies. The anomalies are primarily those of the central nervous system, which includes anencephaly, and gastrointestinal anomalies such as esophageal atresia. These anomalies are easily diagnosed on ultrasound. Other conditions in which hydramnios occurs are diabetes, immune and nonimmune hydrops, and in one twin of a twin gestation. A large ovarian cyst may be found in a woman with a great-

er than expected fundal height, but would not be found concurrently with polyhydramnios. Calcification of the placenta occurs with postdate pregnancy or in intrauterine growth retardation, both of which are usually associated with oligohydramnios. *(Cunningham et al, pp. 554–556)*

12. **(A)** It is more likely that preeclampsia will develop in twin gestations. In fact, twin gestation is one of two instances in which preeclampsia will occur prior to 20 weeks, hydatidiform mole being the other. Congenital anomalies of one or both twins is more common in multiple as compared to single gestations. Frequently, hydramnios accompanies the anomalous twin. Intrauterine growth retardation occurs secondary to intrauterine crowding and subsequent placental insufficiency. The growth retardation can be in both twins or one alone. When there is a significant difference in the growth of a twin it is called discordancy. Because of the higher perinatal mortality rate in discordant twins, nonstress testing and frequent ultrasound examinations are performed in order to detect discordant growth at an early stage. Other complications of twin gestation are a higher incidence of cesarean section secondary to malpresentation, postpartum hemorrhage secondary to uterine atony, maternal anemia, and a higher incidence of spontaneous abortion. *(Cunningham et al, pp. 629–647; Niswander, pp. 371–372)*

13. **(C)** Magnesium plasma levels of 4 to 7 mEq/L are known to prevent eclamptic seizures. When the levels are above 10 mEq/L, respiratory depression develops. It is, therefore, advantageous to follow plasma levels periodically, approximately every 8 hours to prevent toxicity. A clinical means of monitoring magnesium levels is to follow the intensity of patellar deep tendon reflexes. Preeclampsia tends to be a hyperstimulatory state; thus, the deep tendon reflexes tend to be hyperreflexic. Magnesium sulfate has a depressive effect upon this hyperreflexia; it therefore becomes a good bedside means of monitoring magnesium levels. If patellar reflexes return to normal, it can be presumed that the magnesium levels are within the therapeutic but not toxic level. Loss of patellar reflexes is associated with plasma levels of greater than 10 mEq/L and impending respiratory depression. Although administration of $MgSO_4$ will cause decreased fetal heart rate variability, this is not an adequate or consistent means of monitoring plasma levels. Because $MgSO_4$ has only a minimal affect on lowering blood pressure, it is not a good means of monitoring levels. *(Cunningham et al, pp. 681–682)*

14. **(A)** The figure in the sonogram is showing a complete placenta previa. The sonogram is the most definitive means of diagnosing a placenta previa. A bimanual exam would be completely contraindicated, as it would result in severe hemorrhage secondary to digital disruption of the placental site. A sterile speculum exam can be performed if done in an environment where emergency cesarean section is readily available. Because the patient is 37 weeks, there would be no reason to treat the patient conservatively with IV fluids and bed rest. If the patient is preterm and active bleeding has subsided, it is possible to treat conservatively. The patient would then remain on strict bed rest and avoid use of tampons and douching and refrain from sexual intercourse. If the previa is partial or low lying and the patient is preterm, conservative treatment may result in avoiding cesarean section; as gestation progresses, the placenta may move away from the cervical os. A vaginal delivery would be completely contraindicated in the instance presented in the question because it is a complete previa at 37 weeks and there is no chance that the placenta would migrate upwards. A repeat cesarean section would be the only reasonable course of action in this case. The patient's history of previous cesarean is the probable etiology of the placenta previa. Previas are more common in women who have undergone previous cesarean sections, multiparous patients, and in advanced maternal age. *(Cunningham et al, pp. 712–714)*

15. **(C)** The accurate diagnosis of spontaneous rupture of membranes is important to ascertain if the patient has not yet begun labor (premature rupture of membranes) or if the patient is in premature gestation, prior to 37 weeks (preterm rupture of membranes). In order to evaluate a patient for spontaneous rupture of membranes, the patient must be in the dorsal lithotomy position. A sterile speculum examination is performed. Evidence of rupture of membranes would be clear or blood-tinged fluid in the posterior fornix of the vagina, or "pooling," and escape of clear fluid from the cervical os when the patient coughs. The fluid is then checked with nitrazine paper. Because amniotic fluid is basic with a pH of approximately 7.0 to 7.5 and vaginal secretions are 4.5 to 5.5, it can be surmised that if fluid obtained from the vagina turns nitazine paper blue (indicative of a higher pH) it is amniotic fluid. Ferning is also a phenomenon of the basic amniotic fluid in the acidic vagina. A ferning pattern is seen on the glass slide when placed under the light microscope. Although in preterm rupture of membranes, it is important to obtain amniotic fluid from the vaginal fornix for lecithin/sphingomyelin (L/S) ration, L/S is an indication of fetal lung maturity, not a test for the presence of or the absence of ruptured membranes. Ultrasound determination of amniotic fluid volume is an important means of evaluating premature and preterm rupture of membranes, but it is not a means of diagnosing rupture of mem-

branes (for instance, postdate pregnancy, intrauterine growth retardation, and fetal congenital anomalies). *(Cunningham et al, pp. 309, 557–558; Niswander, p. 323)*

16. **(B)** The major risk involved in conservative management of preterm rupture of membranes is the onset of chorioamnionitis, which increases both maternal and fetal morbidity and mortality. Babies born after the onset of chorioamnionitis have a higher rate of incidence of respiratory distress, sepsis, and intraventricular hemorrhage. The maternal complications are endomyometritis and sepsis. Vaginal delivery is the preferred route of delivery, but because of malpresentation of the preterm fetus, there is usually a higher incidence of cesarean section. The diagnosis of chorioamnionitis is difficult. Usually by the time the mother has developed a fever greater than 38°C, the infection is already well established. An increase in the maternal white blood cell count on CBC is also used to predict on the onset of chorioamnionitis, but has not been found to be a consistent indicator of the development of infection. Because of the variable lie (i.e., breech, transverse) of the preterm infant and the ruptured amniotic sac, the incidence of prolapsed cord is much greater in preterm rupture of membranes. Patients with preterm rupture of membranes should undergo nonstress testing to determine reactivity and fetal heart rate (sustained fetal tachycardia is another indication of the onset of chorioamnionitis). A cord pattern or variable decelerations, not late decelerations, would be a more likely finding on NST. The cord pattern would be secondary to decreased amniotic fluid and possibly occult prolapse. Spontaneous rupture of membranes is not possible with a complete previa as the os is covered with placenta. *(Cunningham et al, p. 751)*

17. **(B)** Magnesium sulfate and ritodrine are the most commonly used tocolytic agents. The presumed affect of magnesium is that it works as an antagonist to calcium at the myometrial level. $MgSO_4$ is given in the same dose for preterm labor as in preeclampsia: a 4-g loading dose followed by 2 g/hr. Obviously, it also has the same side effects, primarily respiratory depression. Ritodrine is a β_2 adrenergic agonist. Its effect is on the adrenergic receptors of the smooth muscle of the myometrium to decrease its contractile potential. Ritodrine also has some β one activity; it therefore can cause maternal tachycardia and subsequent chest pain, and EKG changes consistent with ischemia. It can also cause pulmonary edema and hyperglycemia. The ability to actually stop preterm labor with these tocolytic agents has been questioned. Some studies have shown no significant difference in preterm delivery when use of tocolytic agents is compared to conservative therapy of bed rest and hydration. Because

prostaglandins are involved in the initiation of myometrial contractions and, therefore, of labor, the use of prostaglandin synthetase inhibitor drugs (such as indomethacin) to arrest labor seemed logical. Unfortunately, they were found to cause premature closure of the fetal ductus arteriosus. Ethanol was once used intravenously to arrest labor; but its effect of intoxication, lethargy, and respiratory depression in the mother and fetus have since discourage its use. *(Cunningham et al, pp. 756–758)*

18. **(E)** Congenital anomalies are increased threefold in fetuses born to women who are diabetic prior to pregnancy. Clinicians feel that this rate is greatly decreased if the mother is in excellent diabetic control prior to conception. Congenital heart defects are the most common anomalies, followed by neural tube defects. Women with diabetes have a higher incidence of cesarean section delivery. A primary reason is because of the higher incidence of macrosomia and subsequent cephalopelvic disproportion and the possibility of shoulder dystocia. There is general disagreement about the timing of delivery of a diabetic women. Many centers feel women should be delivered prior to 40 weeks because of the higher incidence of intrauterine fetal demise after 36 weeks. Elective induction, especially with an unfavorable cervix, often leads to cesarean section. The cesarean section rate for diabetic women (gestational and pregestational) is approximately 50%. There is a fourfold increase in preeclampsia/eclampsia in women with overt diabetes and gestational diabetics with fasting hyperglycemia. Because the lungs of babies born to diabetic mothers mature at a later gestational age, they have an approximately five times greater a chance of having respiratory distress syndrome. This makes elective delivery prior to 38 weeks a very difficult decision. Amniocentesis for long maturity is often performed prior to elective delivery. An L/S ratio of greater than 2 has been found to be inaccurate in predicting fetal lung maturity in diabetic mothers. If present, phosphatidyl glycerol (PG) is the best indicator of fetal lung maturity in diabetics. *(Cunningham et al, pp. 816–822; Niswander, pp. 92–98)*

19. **(B)** Accurate dating of a pregnancy is very important in both gestational and overt diabetes. This is because of the need to begin fetal surveillance in the third trimester, the incidence of fetal macrosomia, the higher incidence of fetal respiratory distress syndrome, and the greater possibility of elective induction. An accurate LMP, pelvic exam in the first trimester and an early sonogram for dating purposes are helpful in accurately assessing gestational age. Because of the higher incidence of stillbirths, prenatal surveillance is begun as early as 28 weeks in diabetic mothers. This testing is usually in the form of nonstress test (NST), followed by an

oxytocin challenge test if the NST is nonreactive. NST in diabetic pregnancy is found to be predictive of fetal well-being for only approximately 4 to 5 days and, therefore, after 32 to 34 weeks should be done on a biweekly basis. There is controversy over which means of fetal surveillance is most accurate in diabetics: some centers advocate OCTs or biweekly biophysical profiles instead of NSTs. A fasting glucose of 100 mg/dL is too high for a diabetic mother. A fasting glucose should be between 60 to 90 mg/dL in order to maintain good control. In a gestational diabetic controlled on diet alone, a fasting glucose of greater than 110 is an indication for initiating insulin therapy. The 1-hour postprandial glucose should be below 120 to 140. Twenty-four-hour urinary estriol determinations were previously used to monitor fetal well-being antenatally. It has been subsequently found an inaccurate and costly means of fetal surveillance. *(Cunningham et al, pp. 816–822; Niswander, pp. 93–98)*

20. **(C)** Laparoscopy is one of the final steps in a fertility work-up. Although tubal occlusion secondary to PID can be diagnosed on hysterosalpingogram, additional infertility-causing problems can be diagnosed on laparoscopy, particularly when dye (usually methylene blue or indigo carmine) is injected at the time of surgery. IUDs may cause peritubular adhesions that are responsible for decreased tubal functioning and, therefore, infertility. These adhesions can be seen only on laparoscopy. Because of this, patient's history of PID, it is very likely that bilateral hydrosalpinx is the cause of secondary infertility diagnosed at laparoscopy. Pelvic endometriosis can definitely only be diagnosed on laparoscopy and does not cause peritubular adhesions and tubal occlusion. However, this patient's past history of PID makes endometriosis a less likely cause of infertility. Simple ovarian cyst seldom causes infertility. *(Jones et al, pp. 293–294)*

21. **(D)** In the normal menstrual cycle, the endometrium undergoes hormonal stimulation in preparation for implantation of the fertilized ovum. During the first half of the cycle, the endometrium is under the influence of estrogen, which is secreted from the developing follicle. This estrogen causes cellular proliferation of the endometrium, termed *the proliferative phase*. After ovulation, progesterone is secreted from the corpus luteum and the effect of this hormone on the endometrium is to cause secretion of glycogen and mucus from the glandular cells. This phase is termed the *secretory phase* and is dependent upon the occurrence of ovulation with the subsequent development of a corpus luteum. This patient could not be going through premature menopause because she has ovulated. Because a secretory endometrium is secondary to progesterone stimulation, this patient's endo-

metrium could not be under estrogen stimulation. The second choice is therefore incorrect. The third choice is also incorrect because oral contraceptives prevent ovulation and therefore the development of the corpus luteum and secretion of progesterone. *(Hacker, et al, pp. 400–401; Jones et al, pp. 68–78)*

22. **(C)** Duration of labor prior to cesarean section is the most predictive factor in whether a patient develops a postoperative infection. It was previously believed that the number of pelvic exams while in labor and duration of rupture of membranes was equally predictive but controlled studies showed that it was the length of labor that determined the number of pelvic exams and the possibility of ascending infection secondary to rupture of membranes. Although diabetes and other medical complications do affect incidence of postoperative infection, they are not the most causative. *(Burrow and Ferris, p. 350)*

23. **(E)** The diagnosis of pulmonary embolus is very difficult to make. The most common sign present is tachypnea. Pulmonary embolus is the most dangerous complication of DVT. It occurs approximately 5 to 7 times more frequently in women who have undergone cesarean section. The most definitive means of diagnosing PE is angiography. A ventilation–perfusion scan can also be used, but it is not as accurate. An arterial blood gas is helpful in making the diagnosis. Answer A would be a good possibility except that the patient with pneumonia should be responding to triple antibiotics. Tuboovarian abcesses are infrequent as a complication of cesarean section. It is more commonly seen in PID that failed to respond to triple antibiotics after 48 hours, as should sepsis. *(Cunningham et al, pp. 479–480; Niswander, pp. 1177–1178)*

24. **(B)** Age 35 has been arbitrarily designated as the age at which a mother must be advised to undergo genetic amniocentesis to rule out Down's syndrome. The risk of an offspring with Down's syndrome at age 30 is 1 in 885, whereas at age 35, it is 1 in 365; at age 40, it is 1 in 100, and at age 45, it is 1 in 35. Although a woman may decide against amniocentecis, it is the practitioner's responsibility to advise her of the incidence of Down's syndrome in her age group and to refer her to available genetic counseling. *(Cunningham et al, pp. 516–518)*

25. **(D)** Late decelerations are a result of uteroplacental insufficiency. A late deceleration occurs when the fetal heart rate begins to slow after the onset of the contraction and returns to baseline after the contraction is completed. Late decelerations by definition must occur with every contraction, and are often the consequent of fetal hypoxia and subsequent acidosis. Many maternal factors cause uter-

oplacental insufficiency and, therefore, intrauterine growth retardation. Some of these factors are severe preeclampsia, chronic hypertension, chronic renal disease, severe diabetes with vascular involvement, and heavy maternal smoking. Although it is very likely that a patient with chronic hypertension with superimposed preeclampsia might develop late decelerations, the diagnosis of superimposed preeclampsia cannot be made solely on a fetal heartrate pattern. The diagnosis would instead be made if the patient developed hyperflexia, proteinuria, and generalized edema in addition to her chronic hypertension. A patient with placenta previa would more than likely develop vaginal bleeding and fetal bradycardia. Decelerations that are secondary to head compression are early decelerations and if they are not severe are of no consequence. A prolapsed cord would typically show a cord pattern (variable deceleration) or bradycardia on fetal monitoring. (Cunningham et al, pp. 291, 298, 764–765)

26. **(B)** A nonstress test is called reactive if there are two fetal heartrate accelerations accompanying a fetal movement within a 20-minute period. The fetal heartrate accelerations should be 15 beats per minute above the baseline, lasting for 15 seconds. A reactive nonstress test is a means of assuring fetal well-being in the antepartum period in a high-risk pregnancy. Indications for conducting antepartum testing are gestational or insulin-dependent diabetes, postdate pregnancy (starting at 41 weeks), intrauterine growth retardation, preeclampsia, chronic hypertension, history of previous preterm delivery or stillbirth, and multiple gestations (i.e., twins, triplets). Because this above pattern is reactive, it is, therefore, not suspicious for fetal compromise. An oxytocin challenge test entails administration of oxytocin in order to cause contractions. There are no contractions on this tracing. A positive oxytocin challenge test is one in which late decelerations occur with each contraction and is indicative of some degree of fetal compromise. A negative OCT is one in which late decelerations do not occur consistently. Oxytocin challenge tests are performed when the NST is nonreactive or if on NST there are spontaneous contractions with late or suspicious decelerations. There is no way on fetal heartrate tracings to determine fetal age. A cord pattern would show variable decelerations, which do not appear on the above tracing. (Cunningham et al, pp. 1291–1292)

27. **(C)** A woman in labor with her first pregnancy should dilate 1.2 cm per hour once she has entered the active phase of labor. The active phase of labor is defined as the onset of rapid change in cervical dilation and usually occurs after reaching 4 cm dilation. A multiparous patient usually dilates 1.5 cm in the active phase. The latent patient precedes the active phase and is defined as the onset of regular uterine contractions, but slow dilation of the cervix. In a nulliparous patient, the latent phase should last no longer than 20 hours; in multiparous women, approximately 14 hours. Answer A is incorrect because it implies the situation is describing more rapid progress than normal, which is not true. Answer B implies that progress is inadequate and therefore necessitating an intrauterine pressure catheter. Answer D is also incorrect because the question does not describe the latent phase. E is incorrect because the second stage of labor is determined from full dilation until delivery of the baby. (Burke, p. 31)

28. **(D)** Shoulder dystocia, or the inability to deliver the anterior shoulder after delivery of the head, is a complication of a macrosomic baby. Pregnancies complicated by gestational and insulin-dependant diabetes tend to make larger babies. These babies typically have a larger transthoracic diameter, particularly when compared to babies of nondiabetic mothers. The incidence of shoulder dystocia is, therefore, higher in diabetic mothers. In a study done by Acker and colleagues, on the risk factors for shoulder dystocia, 73.3% of diabetics with a fetal weight greater than 4000 g developed shoulder dystocia when compared to 52.4% in nondiabetics. It was suggested in this article that if the estimated fetal weight on ultrasound was greater than 4000 g in a diabetic woman, then elective cesarean section should be performed. Other factors contributing to a higher chance of shoulder dystocia are maternal obesity, postdate pregnancy, prolonged second stage of labor, and midforceps or vacuum extraction. Although there is placental dysfunction in diabetic pregnancies, this would not warrant primary cesarean without a trial of labor. A higher incidence of infection does occur with diabetics postoperatively; therefore, vaginal delivery would be preferred over operative. Breech presentation does not occur in diabetics at a greater frequency. Uterine atony will occur with overdistension subsequent to a large fetus, but maternal diabetes itself would not make this entity more common. (Cunningham et al, pp. 366–368; Acker et al, p. 767)

29. **(B)** The information in the question gives numerous reasons for postpartum bleeding. They are uterine overdistension secondary to a large baby, midforceps delivery and therefore the possibility of cervical tears, and multiparity, which predisposes to a less contractive uterus. The information given states, however, that the uterus is well contracted; thus uterine atony would be an incorrect answer, as would retained products, because the placenta delivered spontaneously. Midforceps delivery is associated with a higher incidence of cervical and vagi-

nal lacerations; therefore, careful inspection of the cervix and vagina should follow such a delivery. In the above incident lacerations would be the most likely answer. Causes of excessive postpartum bleeding (postpartum hemorrhage) are overdistension of the uterus secondary to a large infant, polyhydramnios or multiple gestation, midforceps and rotation forcep delivery, delivery through an incompletely dilated cervix, the use of halothane anesthetics, which cause uterine relaxation, and finally, women who had very rapid or very slow dilation. Retained placenta and abnormally adherent placenta such as placenta accreta, increta, or percrete are also causes of postpartum hemorrhage. Because the question states that the placenta delivered spontaneously, accreta could not be a likely cause. Previously undiagnosed coagulopathy might be a cause for postpartum hemorrhage, but in the above case, not the most likely. Rectal tears or fourth-degree lacerations are more common with forceps delivery, but are usually easily repairable, and, therefore, do not cause much bleeding. (*Cunningham et al, pp. 405–406, 415–418, 436*)

30. **(D)** Knowledge of the uterine scar is the most important factor in determining whether a patient is a candidate for vaginal delivery after a cesarean section. The safest and most commonly used incision is the lower segment transverse incision. A classical incision on the uterus is known to easily rupture during labor. The low transverse incision ruptures less than 2% of the time. Therefore, VDAC (vaginal delivery after cesarean) is contraindicated in patients who have a classical incision. It is questionable whether patients with a low vertical incision on the uterus should undergo a trial of labor. The incidence of spontaneous rupture is minimal, but greater than low transverse. Studies show there are no increased complications in women who undergo VDAC after more than one previous cesarean section. The indication for the primary cesarean section should not be a deterrant because the success rate of VDAC in patients with a recurrent indication such as cephalopelvic disproportion or failure to progress is approximately 60%. Length of labor and intensity of present contractions have no effect on the decision to allow a patient a trial of labor. (*Cunningham et al, pp. 408, 446*)

31. **(D)** Incomplete abortions are characterized by heavy vaginal bleeding and placental tissue present in a dilated cervical os. The bleeding is heavy because there has been incomplete separation of the placenta and, therefore, inadequate myometrial contraction of the blood vessels. Bleeding from an incomplete abortion can be severe enough to cause marked hypovolemia and shock. Inevitable abortion occurs when a patient has crampy abdominal pain and spotting, and upon pelvic exam, the cervi-

cal os is open and there is evidence of spontaneous rupture of membranes. Leaking membranes may be seen from the cervical os or the vaginal vault. Septic abortion occurs when the signs and symptoms of spontaneous abortion are accompanied by a temperature elevation of greater than 38°C. This diagnosis is made only after other sources of fever have been excluded, such as UTI. A missed abortion is one in which the fetus dies but the products of conception are retained for 4 to 8 weeks. A patient typically notes loss of pregnancy signs such as nausea, vomiting, and breast tenderness. On sequential pelvic exams, the uterus fails to enlarge, and in fact will decrease in size. On ultrasound, there is no evidence of fetal viability and it is often used to verify the diagnosis. Induced abortion is one in which the mother elects to terminate the pregnancy. (*Cunningham et al, p. 497; Niswander, pp. 215–218*)

32. **(B)** Suction curettage is the safest means of elective abortion in the first trimester. It is more efficient if preceded by a preliminary means of dilating the cervix. This can be accomplished with prostaglandin suppository in the vagina or with laminaria tents inserted into the cervix. Intraamniotic saline injection is infrequently used and only during the second trimester. Hysterotomy, dilation and extraction, and the use of oxytocin are reserved for the second trimester abortions. (*Cunningham et al, pp. 502–505; Hacker and Moore, pp. 591–595*)

33. **(C)** Hydatidaform mole is one component of gestational trophoblastic neoplasm (GTN). Moles occur in a gestation in which there is a proliferation of trophoblastic tissue. It can be a complete mole, in which there is no sign of a fetus, or a partial mole, in which the fetus may be viable, or there are findings consistent with a nonviable fetus. The most common symptom of hydatidiform mole is several episodes of vaginal bleeding. A size-to-dates dicrepancy is also common. Approximately one half of the patients are larger than dates and one-fourth are smaller. The trophoblast is responsible for production of human chorionic goadotrophin (HCG); therefore, the levels of beta HCG in the serum are often greater than expected for the weeks of gestation. The occurrence of preeclampsia prior to 20 weeks is highly suggestive of hydatidiform mole. On ultrasound, there are very characteristic findings and it is the best means of diagnosing a mole. Answer A is incorrect because with a threatened abortion at 18 weeks, there should be fetal heart tones. An incomplete abortion usually occurs prior to 12 to 14 weeks and would more than likely have a decreasing beta HCG level. A fetal demise at 16 weeks would also have decreasing beta HCG levels and would not be associated with hypertension. Although in twin gestation, hypertension/preeclampsia may occur before 20 weeks, there would

be a higher level of beta HCG level and a larger fundal height. Fetal heart tones should be obtainable at 16 weeks. *(Cunningham et al, pp. 541–545; Acker et al, pp. 2–4)*

34. **(D)** Placental abruption is the separation of the placenta before delivery of the fetus. Separation can occur in various degrees, and it can be partial or complete. Abruption can be associated with vaginal bleeding or the bleeding may remain hidden within the uterus. If the separation is of a significant degree, the blood loss will be extensive because the uterus cannot contract down upon the torn vessels that supply the placenta. The baby's blood supply is subsequently disrupted and fetal death occurs. The mother is also severely affected. She will develop shock secondary to blood loss and also has a high chance of developing a consumptive coagulopathy. The coagulopathy is most often hypofibrinogenemia with elevation of fibrinogen-fibrin degradation products. Pregnancy-induced and chronic hypertension are often associated with placental abruption. It is also seen in trauma, short umbilical cord, sudden decompensation of the uterus, and uterine anomaly. Placenta previa does not present at term with vaginal bleeding, but infrequently with fetal demise, and is not typically associated with hypertension. Chronic hypertension does not cause abruptio placenta, but in the above cases, the separation of the placenta is the cause of fetal demise. Disseminated intravascular coagulopathy is a known complication of preeclampsia and abruption, but would probably not cause fetal demise without some other precipitating event such as abruption. Chronic renal failure is associated with a higher incidence of fetal wastage but the case presented is more consistent with an acute occurrence. *(Cunningham et al, pp. 701–712)*

35. **(B)** A consumptive coagulopathy, primarily hypofibrinogemia, occurs within 4 to 6 weeks of intrauterine fetal demise. It is felt to be secondary to the release of thromboplastin from the dead fetus. Because the products of conception tend to shrink postdemise and labor is more effective if initiated on its own, a woman is allowed to await spontaneous labor is she so chooses. She must be monitored for the possibility of coagulopathy with weekly PT and PTT, plus fibrinogen and platelet counts. The use of postaglandin E$_2$ vaginal suppository has increased the number of women who have elected immediate termination because it has greatly increased coagulation factors and, therefore, there should be no change in liver function tests. The hemoglobin and hematocrit levels would fall if the patient went into DIC, but that would occur significantly after the change in coagulation factors. Prolactin levels would have no effect upon the incidence of DIC postfetal demise. *(Cunningham et al, pp. 716–719)*

36. **(D)** A pregnancy that progresses past 42 weeks is associated with increased fetal morbidity and mortality. One reason for the increased fetal risk is decreased amniotic fluid with subsequent cord compression. Cord compression may result in fetal distress, which in turn causes fetal defecation in utero and subsequently meconium-stained fluid. Because postdate pregnancies are associated with these complications and an increased risk of intrauterine demise, patients are monitored from 40½ weeks. This monitoring can be one or more of the following: nonstress testing, biophysical profile, or oxytocin challenge test. These tests have all been associated with high false-positive and false-negative results. In many cases, induction is performed at 42 weeks regardless of antepartum test results. Babies born after 42 weeks' gestation can either be large for dates, which increases the risk for failed induction, cephalopelvic dysproportion, and shoulder dystocia, or these babies can be growth retarded. A growth-retarded fetus has a greater chance for stress during labor and, when born, appears as if it has lost weight, particularly muscle mass and subcutaneous fat. Chorioamnionitis does not occur more commonly with postdate pregnancy. In fact, it is more common with preterm delivery. Blood-tinged fluid is sometimes associated with partial placental abruption but is not a common finding in postdate pregnancy. The presence of vernix would indicate a preterm or term fetus. Ruptures of membranes either spontaneous or artificial are usually followed by a greater intensity of contractions, but usually hyperstimulation. *(Cunningham et al, pp. 759–763)*

37. **(D)** The optimal time to screen for gestational diabetes is 28 weeks. In some patients, pregnancy is a diabetogenic state. Human placental lactogen is a hormone secreted by the placenta with levels increasing during the latter half of pregnancy. This hormone has an antiinsulin effect in the mother and in predisposed patients will cause glucose intolerance. The glucose challenge test (also called the 50-g glucola or O'Sullivan) is the most commonly employed screening test. It consists of taking 50 g of glucola in a nonfasting state, and having a plasma glucose drawn 1 hour later. If the plasma glucose is 135 to 140 mg/dL, the patient then has to undergo a 3-hour glucose tolerance test. Most centers now feel that all pregnant women should undergo routine screening for gestational diabetes at 28 weeks. Others feel only those women with a significant obstetric or family history need be screened. Criteria for this screening are maternal age greater than 30, a family history of diabetes, a prior macrosomic baby, a baby with a congenital anomaly, or a stillborn. Women who are hypertensive or obese also have a higher incidence of gestational diabetes. Alpha fetoprotein screening is only accurate between 15 to 20 weeks. Although women infected with syphilis

have a high incidence of stillborns, hopefully they have undergone treatment after the first obstetric loss. Additionally, babies infected with syphilis are usually growth retarded, not macrosomic. Rh negative women should receive rhogam at 28 weeks but their blood type and Rh should be drawn at the first prenatal visit. Babies that have congenital toxoplasmosis are generally smaller for gestational age, have microcephaly or hydrocephaly. *(Cunningham et al, pp. 617–619, 812–816)*

38. **(B)** Acute appendicitis is the most important surgical diagnosis to rule out during pregnancy. It is also one of the most difficult diagnoses because the enlarging uterus displaces the appendix and, therefore, the location of pain. Additionally, many of the presenting complaints of appendicitis are common complaints of pregnancy such as nausea, anorexia, and vomiting. A mild leukocytosis is also common in pregnancy, particularly during the third trimester. If the diagnosis of appendicitis is a serious consideration, the patient should undergo exploratory laparotomy. To delay would increase the occurrence of severe peritonitis, gangrene, spontaneous abortion, preterm labor, and increased maternal morbidity. Another possible surgical complication of pregnancy that could be present in the above patient is acute cholecystitis. Hyperemesis gravidarum would be an unlikely diagnosis because it is primarily a first trimester phenomenon and is not associated with a fever or markedly elevated WBC count. If this patient had pyelonephritis, she would probably have costal vertebral angle (CVA) tenderness, and WBCs in the urine. If PID occurs at all during pregnancy, it is extremely rare and only before 12 weeks. Degeneration of uterine myomata does cause pain, mild leukocytosis, and slightly elevated temperature. Usually, however, it is not associated with decreased bowel sounds, nausea, and vomiting, and ordinarily there is some uterine tenderness and a palpable myomata. *(Cunningham et al, pp. 831–832)*

39. **(C)** The aspiration of acidic gastric contents or undigested food particles will cause severe respiratory distress and possibly death. In order to prevent this complication, the mother should be fasting for 6 to 12 hours prior to general anesthesia, and medication to reverse gastric acidity should be administered immediately prior to intubation. Additionally, intubation should be performed with pressure on the cricoid cartilage to occlude the esophogus, and extubation should be performed with the mother awake and on her side. A true fasting state with minimal gastric contents is extremely difficult to achieve in obstetric patients. A woman seldom knows when she will begin labor and, more importantly, gastric emptying and peristalsis are delayed or inhibited at the onset of labor. Subse-

quently, all pregnant women should be treated as if they have a full stomach. In the fasting state, the stomach continues to secrete gastric juices that have a very low pH. To neutralize this pH, antacids are administered within 45 minutes of intubation. Maternal hypotension does not accompany general anesthesia, but is the major side effect of spinal and epidural anesthesia. Atelectasis frequently occurs within the first 24 hours after general anesthesia, but is not life threatening. If left untreated, in some instances atelectasis will progress to pneumonia. Three of the inhalation anesthetics used in obstetrics do cause uterine relaxation and in some cases uterine atony. These agents are halothane, enflurane, and isoflurane. They are used in conjunction with nitrous oxide and given in the smallest possible amounts to avoid this complication. Although uterine atony is associated with lower hematocrit postdelivery and greater chance of blood transfusion, these complications are not as life threatening as aspiration. Eclampsia probably does not occur more with general anesthesia and, in fact, in severe preeclampsia/eclampsia, general anesthesia is the preferred means of anesthesia. *(Cunningham et al, pp. 329–339)*

40. **(D)** Cervical cancer and its precursor, cervical intraepithelial neoplasia (dyplasia), occur more often in women who are sexually active at an early age (before age 20) and who have multiple sexual partners. Originally, women who were married young and had children at a young age were considered at risk, but it is now felt that cervical cancer is due to sexual intercourse at an early age and multiple sexual partners. Women who smoke are also at a higher risk of developing cervical cancer. Infection has been considered a possible etiology of CIN. The most commonly implicated agent is the human papillomavirus (HPV), the same virus that causes condylomata accumulata. HPV types 6 and 11 are usually associated with benign lesions such as condylomata, whereas types 16 and 18 are associated with severe dysplasia and carcinoma in situ (CIN III). Although evidence is strong in suggesting HPV as having either a causative or exacerbative effect on neoplastic changes in the cervix, many women with CIN or invasive carcinoma have no evidence of the virus. Early sexual relationships and multiple partners have not been a historical finding in women who develop ovarian or endometrial cancer. In fact, endometrial cancer is more common in nulliparous women. Labial cancer occurs at a much later age than the above gynecologic neoplasms. AIDS is not considered a cancer. *(Jones et al, pp. 643–654: pp. 58–64)*

41. **(B)** The patient described would not be a good candidate for an IUD for several reasons. She has a

history of PID and intrauterine devices have been associated with a higher risk of developing PID. This risk is particularly high in a patient with multiple sexual partners, a recent episode of PID, and women under the age of 25. The patient is also nulliparous: IUDs are more difficult to tolerate in women who have never had an intrauterine pregnancy. Additionally, since the patient has a greater risk of developing PID, her future fertility should be a factor in the decision. There may also be a higher chance of having an ectopic pregnancy with an IUD in place; the patient in this instance already has one risk factor for an ectopic pregnancy, PID; she does not need a second factor. As long as she was a nonsmoker and had no other contraindications, oral contraceptives could be recommended to this patient. Oral contraceptives have also been found to have a protective effect against the development of pelvic inflammmatory disease. If the patient is well motivated a diaphram could be suggested. Because it is a barrier device, it also has a protective effect against the aquisition of sexually transmitted diseases. The diaphragm also has minimal medical complications and therefore few contraindications. The contraceptive sponge has been associated with a slightly higher risk of developing toxic shock syndrome, but it is an acceptable form of birth control. Condoms are a good means of preventing the spread of sexually transmitted diseases, are readily available, and are without significant medical contraindications. Condoms and the contraceptive sponge are not as effective against pregnancy prevention as the pill and the IUD. (*Hacker et al, pp. 358–368; Jones et al, pp. 225–231*)

42. **(D)** Endometriosis is endometrial-like tissues found outside the uterus that respond to cyclic hormonal stimulation. Because this ectopic tissue can be found in various locations, most commonly on the ovaries, tubes, uterosacral ligaments, and posterior cul de sac, symptoms of the disease vary greatly. Progressively worse dysmenorrhea, unresponsive to PG synthetase inhibitors, is a common presenting complaint. Infertility occurs in approximately 20% to 40% of women with endometriosis and is often the reason a woman undergoes a workup. Frequently, women with endometriosis also complain of dysparunia. This is considered to be secondary to endometrial implants in the uterosacral ligament. Because of the various ways that endometriosis presents, laparoscopic visualization is the only means of definitively formulating the diagnosis. Endometrial implants are not visualized on ultrasound. However, endometriomas, cysts formed on the ovary secondary to excessive bleeding from endometrial tissue, can be seen on sonography. There is, however, no way of differentiating an endometrioma from a simple ovarian cyst, a dermoid, or other pelvic pathology. Laparoscopic diag-

nosis should be made prior to the administration of any medical therapy such as danazol is given. The absence of response to PG synthetase inhibitors may be a means of making the preliminary diagnosis of endometriosis but not the conclusive diagnosis. Hysteroscopy would be of no help in making the diagnosis, as endometriosis is extrauterine. (*Jones et al, pp. 303–326*)

43. **(B)** Women who lose 25% of their ideal body weight secondary to anorexia nervosa and women who engage in vigorous or stressful exercise often have secondary amenorrhea. This is probably due to hypothalamic dysfunction. These women typically have low gonadotropin levels and low estrogen levels. Due to their lack of estrogen, findings on physical exam may include decreased breast size, an atrophic vaginal mucosa, and possibly absent cervical mucus. In general, these patients are anovulatory. Weight gain and decreased exercise will often restore normal hypothalamic functioning. Oligomenorrhea or episodic menstrual bleeding occurring at greater than 35-day intervals is due to anovulatory cycles. It is seen in women who engage in moderate exercise but not anorexia, in which complete cessation of menses is more common. Menorrhagia is cyclic menstrual bleeding that is excessive in amount or duration. Polymenorrhagia, which is often due to anovulatory cycles, is episodic bleeding occuring at less than 21-day cycles. Metorrhagia is uterine bleeding between periods and is usually due to uterine polyps or carcinoma, but can be due to estrogen withdrawal or anovulation. (*Hacker and Moore, pp. 424–427; Jones et al, pp. 351–375*)

44. **(D)** The signs and symptoms of polycystic ovarian syndrome (PCO) are due to hyperandrogenism, which is a result of overproduction of androgen by both the ovaries and adrenal gland. Clinically, patients with the syndrome are hirsute, have menstrual irregularity, and are infertile. Approximately 50% of these women are obese, most have acne, and 15% are virilized. The ovaries have multiple follicular cysts, which are arrested in development. The ovarian stroma consists of luteinized thecal cells that produce androgens. This excess androgen plus that produced by the adrenal gland stimulate LH secretions, which in turn continue stimulation of the ovaries and more androgen secretion. The excess androgen is converted peripherally into estrogen. Because women with PCO are anovulatory, this estrogen is unopposed by progesterone. The unopposed estrogen effect on the endometrium places these women at greater risk for development of adenomatous hyperplasia and possibly endometrial carcinoma. The high levels of estrogen also causes the amenorrhea and at other times, excessive bleeding. Congenital adrenal hyperplasia also presents with hirsutism and virilism

but these patients usually have a male body type and do not have enlarged ovaries. Excess androgen production prevents the secretion of progesterone; therefore, this patient's symptoms would not be due to a progesterone secreting tumor. Patients with hyperprolactemia are usually amenorrheic but usually have galactorrhea and are not hirsute. Hypothyroidism also causes amenorrhea, but not hirsutism. *(Hacker and Moore, pp. 430–435; Jones et al, pp. 169–174, 351–375)*

45. **(C)** A fundal height at the umbilicus roughly corresponds to 20 weeks' gestation. On physical examination, there are several ways of determining fundal height and, therefore, gestational age. A fundus palpable to the pubic symphysis is 12 weeks; at the umbilicus, 20 weeks. Those weeks between these two landmarks are approximated. After 20 weeks, and before 32 weeks, fundal height is measured with a tape measure in centimeters. Weeks' gestation correspond ($\pm$/-1 cm) to the measured centimeters from the top of the symphysis to the top of the fundus. *(Cunningham et al, pp. 1260; Medical Letter)*

46. **(D)** Women who have previously been pregnant will first feel fetal movement between 16 and 18 weeks. With a first pregnancy, women will usually feel movement between 18 and 20 weeks. Gestational age can be approximated to when fetal movement is first perceived. *(Cunningham et al, pp. 218)*

47. **(A)** At 6 weeks' gestation, a gestational sac can be seen on abdominal ultrasound. After 8 weeks, the embryo can be seen and measurements of crown–rump length can be made. A fetal heart can be visualized at 7 weeks. *(Cunningham et al, p. 284, Niswander, p. 29)*

48. **(D)** Maternal serum alpha fetoprotein is a screening test to detect the presence of numerous fetal abnormalities, the most common of which are neural tube defects. The major protein secreted by the early fetus is alpha fetoprotein. This protein is secreted into the amniotic fluid and crosses the fetal membranes into the maternal circulation. The level of alpha fetoprotein is elevated in the amniotic fluid of an abnormal fetus and, therefore, in the maternal serum. This elevation is best detected between 16 and 20 weeks. In addition to open neural tube defects, other abnormalities detected include congenital nephrosis, esophageal and duodenal atresia, exophalos, Turner and Potter's syndromes, fetal death or fetal blood in amniotic fluid. *(Cunningham et al, p. 277)*

49. **(C)** Coumarin is a small molecule that easily crosses the placenta and is taken up by the fetus. The anomalies it causes are a result of hemorrhage secondary to its anticoagulant effect. Exposure dur-ing the first trimester causes anomalies that are collectively termed *fetal warfarin syndrome*. Use of coumarin during the second and third trimesters causes optic atrophy, cataracts, microcephaly, microphthalmia, blindness, and mental retardation. Heparin is a large molecule that does not cross the placenta and is, therefore, the drug of choice for anticoagulation. *(Cunningham et al, pp. 565–566)*

50. **(D)** The use of cocaine during pregnancy causes an increased chance of placental abruption that is most likely secondary to its vasoconstrictive effects. Because of the placental abruption, there is a higher incidence of stillborn fetuses. Use of cocaine is also felt to cause an increase in preterm delivery and intrauterine growth retardation. *(Cunningham et al, p. 568)*

51. **(A)** Women who are considered alcoholics, who ingest large amounts of alcohol frequently, will very often produce a child with fetal alcohol syndrome. Children born with the syndrome have characteristic cardiovascular, limb, and craniofacial defects. Additionally, they are found to be growth retarded, have impaired fine and gross motor function, and lower IQs. The effects on a fetus of a small amount of alcohol ingested during pregnancy is still uncertain. It is best to abstain entirely. *(Cunningham et al, p. 567–568)*

52. **(E)** Phenytoin (Dilantin) is one of the most commonly used anticonvulsant medications. It is considered a cause of minor craniofacial and digital anomalies but is not definitive if these are secondary to drug, versus a genetic disposition found in women who have a seizure disorder. Nonetheless, the adverse effects of terminating the medication, consequent seizures, and potentially causing maternal and fetal hypoxia outweigh the chance of developing the anomalies. If a patient is already pregnant and is well controlled by Dilantin, she should remain on the medication. *(Cunningham et al, p. 566)*

53. **(D)** The patient's symptoms are describing postmenopausal atrophic changes affecting the vagina, bladder, and urethra. The patient may also complain of vaginal discharge, itching, burning, and dyspareunia. These symptoms are all due to estrogen depletion and, therefore, are treated best with estrogen replacement. Replacement can be either in the form of systemic estrogen or local application in the form of vaginal creams or suppositories. Estrogen is well absorbed through the vaginal mucosa; thus, a relatively small dose can be used with minimal systemic effects. Because some estrogen is systemically absorbed, local therapy is still associated with the known complications of estrogen replacement. Oral estrogen with progesterone is effective treatment for atrophic vaginitis/cystitis and has the advantage of also treating osteoporosis. Antibiotics, orally or locally, would not be indicated in the above patient, as the urine culture was negative. Testosterone is not indicated for the treatment of atrophic vaginitis. *(Hacker and More, pp. 438–443; Jones et al, pp. 416–420)*

54. **(B)** On ultrasound, (abdominal) a gestational sac is visible at 7-weeks' gestation and at 8 weeks, a fetal pole can be seen. Both can be seen more clearly and somewhat earlier on vaginal probe sonography. The presence of a fetal pole and gestational sac within the endometrial cavity would rule out an ectopic pregnancy. Sonographic findings in the presence of an ectopic pregnancy are generally nonspecific. There may be a sonolucency in the endometrial cavity, suggestive of a gestational sac called a pseudogestational sac. The adnexa may contain a mass with a mixed echogenic pattern and there may be fluid in the posterior cul de sac. A gestational sac may be seen in the adnexa and in advanced gestations, an actual fetal pole with visible fetal heart motion is noted. Quantitative levels of beta human chorionic gonadotrophin (beta HCG) are known to double within 48 hours in a viable pregnancy. In an ectopic pregnancy, the trophoblastic tissue that produces beta HCG does not function as adequately as in a normal pregnancy, and therefore this doubling time will not occur. Instead it will either maintain a plateau or rise only a small degree. Although an ectopic pregnancy must always be suspected when a pregnant woman presents with abdominal pain and bleeding, the above patient's physical findings are not significant enough to subject the patient to either laparotomy or laparoscopy. If ultrasound failed to show an intrauterine gestation and beta HCG levels sequentially did not double, then laparoscopy would be indicated. If the patient had rebound tenderness or more severe tenderness on pelvic exam, a culdocentesis would be an appropriate diagnostic procedure. If the patient arrived in the Emergency Room hypotensive and tachycardic, with a history of amenorrhea or known pregnancy, immediate exploratory laparotomy would be indicated. *(Cunningham, pp. 520–522; Niswander, p. 29; Hacker and Moore, pp. 341–348, 485–489)*

55. **(C)** Ectopic pregnancy is responsible for the greatest number of maternal deaths in the first trimester. The incidence of ectopic pregnancy is increasing in the United States. The increase in sexually transmitted diseases and subsequent tubal damage and pelvic adhesions are primarily responsible for the rise in ectopic pregnancy. A woman who has had PID has a sevenfold increase in her chance of developing a tubal pregnancy. Women who undergo tubal surgery to correct infertility have a 30% to 50% chance of developing a subsequent ectopic pregnancy. The improvement in microsurgical tech-

nique and increase in women requiring tubal surgery secondary to PID has increased the number of women undergoing this procedure and has subsequently added to the increased rate of ectopics. Additional factors in the increased prevalence of tubal pregnancy is conservative surgery at the time of ectopic incident, which results in an 11% chance of developing a second ectopic pregnancy, and the increased number of women requesting a reversal of a bilateral tubal ligation. An induced abortion uncomplicated by PID does not predispose a patient to the development of an ectopic pregnancy. Birth control pills change the cervical mucosa and make it less permeable to the gonorrhea bacteria. Women on the pill are, therefore, somewhat protected against the development of PID. *(Jones et al, p. 480)*

56. **(A)** The patient in the questions has many of the classic presenting signs and symptoms of acute PID. Because of her age, the severity of her presenting symptoms, and most importantly, her parity, she is a good candidate for in-hospital treatment. *Gonorrhea* and *Chlamydia* are the most commonly implicated organisms in PID. Gonococcal PID typically presents with symptoms of fever, lower abdominal pain, and tenderness. Chlamydial PID on the other hand is more indolent: symptoms are usually mild tenderness and low-grade temperature. Unfortunately, *Chlamydia* causes as much, if not more, tubal damage as gonorrhea, and is, therefore, as likely to cause infertility. Anaerobic bacteria are typically the etiologic agent in a second episode of PID, but can occur in a first episode particularly when gonorrhea or *Chlamydia* has rendered the environment anaerobic. If a patient has been symptomatic for several days, it is probable that she has developed an anaerobic infection and the choice of antibiotic therapy should address both these bacteria. Two strains of mycoplasma have also been implicated in the etiology of PID: these are *Mycoplasma hominis* and *Ureaplasma urealyticum*. *C difficile* is the organism responsible for pseudomembranous enterocolitis, a side effect of antibiotic administration, usually with ampicillin and clindamycin. *(Hacker and Moore, pp. 304–308; Jones et al, pp. 511–522)*

57. **(D)** Forty-five percent of women who culture positive for gonorrhea will have concurrent *Chlamydia*. Antibiotic therapy must, therefore, treat both these organisms. Because of the increasing prevalence of penicillin-resistant strains of *Neisseria gonorrhea*, ceftriaxone, which is highly effective against even resistant strains, is presently the drug of choice for gonorrhea. Doxycycline or any of the tetracyclines is the drug of choice for *Chlamydia*, but there are some strains of gonococcus that are resistant to tetracycline. Combined therapy with ceftriaxone and doxycycline is, therefore, the best outpatient

treatment for PID. Cefoxitin, 2 g intramuscularly, with probenecid 1 g orally and a tetracycline is an acceptable alternative to ceftriaxone. If a patient is allergic to penicillin and the practitioner is not willing to risk the cross reactivity with cephalosporins, spectinomycin, 2 g intramuscularly, can replace the ceftriaxone. Trimethoprim-sulfamithoxazole is effective against both gonorrhea and *Chlamydia*, but resistant strains of both organisms have developed against the drug. If a patient fails to improve within 48 hours on an outpatient basis, she should be admitted for IV therapy. In-hospital therapy should include coverage for gonorrhea, *Chlamydia*, and anaerobic bacteria. No single drug is adequate; the following combinations are all possible choices: cefoxitin or cefotetan with doxycycline; gentamycin and clindamycin (clindamycin does cover some strains of *Chlamydia*) or ampicillin, gentamycin, and metronidazol (Flagyl) with the addition of doxycycline. *(Hacker and Moore, pp. 305–309; Jones et al, pp. 518–520; Medical Letter, p. 5–8)*

58. **(A)** This patient's past history of a previous episode of PID and generally mild symptoms are highly suggestive of recurrent salpingitis. Nevertheless, the other possibilities should be considered and an attempt should be made to rule them out. A serum or urine pregnancy test would be indicated, particularly if there is a history of amenorrhea or abnormal menses. If the pregnancy test were negative, an ectopic condition would not be a possibility. Acute appendicitis usually presents with a higher fever and a higher WBC count, but in its earlier stages, can present as did the above patient, particularly because her pain is right sided and her history includes symptoms of nausea and vomiting. Careful observation, surgical consultation, and possible laparotomy may be required to completely rule out appendicitis. An adnexal mass, usually ovarian cyst, can twist and will present as unilateral lower abdominal pain with only mild leukocytosis and fever. These symptoms are secondary to necrosis due to the torsion and possible rupture of the cyst. Sonogram would be helpful in identifying a pelvic mass, but to definitively diagnose a twisted adnexal mass, laparoscopy/laparotomy would be necessary. Clinically, the pain associated with twisted adnexa is usually colicky in nature. A patient with a ruptured tuboovarian abscess is ordinarily acutely ill and can present in septic shock. Typically, these patients have high fever, greater than 30°C, high WBC counts, and on abdominal exam, have marked tenderness, rebound, and rigidity. On pelvic exam, severe cervical motion tenderness and possibly a palpable mass is noted. *(Hacker and Moore, pp. 309–310)*

59. **(D)** Herpes genitalis is a venereal disease caused by the herpes simplex virus. 90% of the time, it is caused by the herpes simplex type II virus and 10% of the time by the herpes simplex type I virus. The initial episode is usually the most severe, although some patients are asymptomatic. The virus can migrate up the nerve fiber and remain dormant; therefore, the patient can develop recurrent episodes. The first episode can be associated with a generalized viremia and the patient may present with generalized malaise and low-grade fever. Recurrent episodes are usually precipitated by stress, menstruation, and upper respiratory infection. The principal way in which to differentiate this lesion from other labial lesions is that it is painful to touch. The definitive diagnosis is made on culture. Secondary syphilitic lesions are condyloma latum; they are raised, round, plateau-like lesions of various sizes that often occur in clusters. The lesions are extremely infectious and occur on the labia vulva, the surrounding perineum, and inner thigh and buttocks. These lesions are not painful to touch and neither is the chancre lesion that is characteristic of primary syphilis. Condylomata acuminata is caused by the human papilloma virus and is a sexually transmitted disease. These lesions can occur on the vulva, vagina, perineum, or cervix. They are white, verrucous growths that when large and multiple are described as cauliflower-like. The lesion of lymphogranuloma venerum is a painless vulvovaginal ulcer progressing to adenitis, usually to the nodes of the anus and rectum. *Chlamydia* is the causative agent. *(Hacker and Moore, pp. 299–303; Jones et al, pp. 578–584)*

60. **(B)** Fibroids, or more correctly, leiomyomata are abnormal but benign growths of the myometrium. The major indications to perform a hysterectomy for myomata are bleeding severe enough to cause anemia, severe pelvic pain, or secondary dysmenorrhea, and urinary tract symptoms of frequency or urinary retention. Probably the most important reason to remove fibroids is the inability to adequately access the adnexa. When the myomata is greater than 12-weeks size, it prevents adequate palpation of the ovaries on bimanual exam. An ovarian cancer may then be missed or the malignant ovary may be mistaken for the known uterine myomata. Additional reasons for hysterectomy would be growth of the myomata following menopause and rapid increase in size in premenopausal women. Leiomyomata develop into malignant lesions (sarcomas) only less than 1% of the time; prophylactic removal of a myomata to prevent cancer is, therefore, not an indication for hysterectomy except in the above-stated conditions of rapid growth and postmenopausal growth. Even with these conditions, malignant leiomyosarcoma are rare. Pelvic adhesions may form on myomata, but in general, they form only after surgical intervention, PID, or endometriosis. *(Hacker and Moore, pp. 272–275, 473)*

61. (C) Endometrial hyperplasia is found on pathologic specimen usually on dilation and curettage or on an endometrial biopsy performed in the office. It is considered a premalignant lesion and in some instances will progress to endometrial cancer. It is found in women who experience abnormal uterine bleeding secondary to overstimulation of the endometrium by estrogen unopposed by progesterone. Premenopausally, endometrial hyperplasia occurs in women who are anovulatory; women who fail to ovulate do not form a corpus luteum and, therefore, do not produce progesterone. These women usually have a less severe form of hyperplasia called simple hyperplasia or cystic glandular hyperplasia. Postmenopausal women with endometrial hyperplasia also have excessive estrogen stimulation of the endometrium without the protective effect of progesterone. This is often seen in women receiving estrogen replacement without progesterone added to the regimen. It is also seen in women who are not taking exogenous estrogen; the source of estrogen in these women appears to be the peripheral conversion of androsteredione (from the adrenal gland) to estrone. This conversion takes place in adipose tissue and consequently occurs at a greater rate in obese women. Adenomatous hyperplasia is a more severe form of endometrial hyperplasia and is more often found in postmenopausal women. Compared with simple hyperplasia, it is more likely to progress to endometrial carcinoma. In its most severe form, it is called carcinoma in situ. Anorexic women have low levels of both estrogen and progesterone secondary to minimal secretion of FSH and LH. Women on oral contraceptives are anovulatory but the progesterone component and relatively low level of estrogen prevent hyperplasia. *(Hacker and Moore, pp. 276–278, 716–723)*

62. (D) If a patient is less than 40 years of age and an adnexal/ovarian cyst is less than 6 cm in size, the patient can be placed on birth control pills and observed for 6 weeks. A large percentage of patients, 60% to 70%, will respond to such a regimen and no adnexal mass will be palpable at the next examination. In the case presented, the cyst not only did not respond to hormonal treatment, it grew larger. Exploratory laparotomy is the preferred means of treatment for both diagnostic and therapeutic reasons. Although a simple or uniloculated cyst can be differentiated on ultrasound from a multiloculated cyst, differentiating a benign multilocular cyst from a malignant one is impossible on ultrasound. In order to adequately diagnose the etiology of an adnexal mass, removal and pathologic diagnosis is necessary. Laparoscopy is again not adequate means of distinguishing whether an adnexal mass is a functional cyst or malignant lesion. Functional cysts such as corpus luteum or follicular, greater than 6 cm in size should be removed in

order to prevent torsion or rupture that can present as a surgical emergency. *(Hacker and Moore, pp. 279–288)*

63. (C) This patient requires exploratory laparotomy for either ruptured ectopic pregnancy or ruptured hemorrhagic corpus luteum. Because hemoperitoneum causes an elevation of the WBC count, this test would not help in deciding the origin of the peritoneal irritation. A low hemaglobin and hematocrit (Hbg and Hct) would also be expected in both cases. As the presence of a corpus luteal cyst frequently causes prolonged amenorrhea with irregular or nominal bleeding, the only way to determine whether this patient's amenorrhea is secondary to pregnancy is to obtain a pregnancy test. Urinary pregnancy tests that are sensitive to 25 mIU/mL of urinary human chorionic gonadotrophin are positive in more than 95% of ectopic pregnancies. Most serum pregnancy tests are sensitive to 10 mIU/mL and are, therefore, very accurate in diagnosing pregnancy. *(Hacker and Moore, pp. 280; Jones et al, pp. 488)*

64. (A) The patient's clinical symptoms of stress incontinence, physical findings of cystocele, and reproduction of incontinence with stress are all indicative of urinary stress incontinence (USI). This type of incontinence occurs when the proximal urethra drops below the pelvic floor secondary to pelvic relaxation. An increase of intraabdominal pressure such as coughing is, therefore, not transmitted equally to the bladder and proximal urethra. This unequal pressure results in greater bladder pressure that overrides urethral resistance and causes incontinence of urine. Stress incontinence can be diagnosed clinically on good history and with the stress test as mentioned in the question and with the Q-Tip test. Additional means of diagnosing urinary stress incontinence are cystometrogram, cystouretheroscopy, and uroflowmetry. Cystoceles occur when the bladder descends into the upper vaginal wall, and are commonly found in women with USI. Kegel exercise, pelvic diaphram exercises, and placement of a pessary are nonsurgical means of correcting stress incontinence. The Kegel exercises are successful only in women with minimal symptoms and few anatomic defects. Pessaries are usually only used in women who are unfit for surgery. An anterior repair or anterior colporrphaphy is done through the vagina and involves plication of the pubocervical fascia to support the bladder and urethra. A Marshall–Marchetti–Kranz is done through a retropubic approach and involves elevating the vesicourethral junction via sutures to the symphisis pubis. An additional surgical procedure, the modified Pereyra method, is a combined abdominal–vaginal approach to correction of the problem. All surgical procedures attempt to return the proximal urethra to its normal position: above the pelvic floor, thus correcting the incontinence. *(Hacker and Moore, pp. 314–320; Jones et al, 460–478)*

65. (E) A large percentage of women see only their gynecologist routinely. The general health care of women then falls into the hands of the practitioner who does routine GYN exams. Obviously, a bimanual exam of the pelvic organs: uterus, ovaries, tubes, and bladder is part of the gynecologic exam, as is inspection of the cervix and vagina on speculum exam. A breast exam and an explanation of self-examination are important. Breast cancer is the most common malignant neoplasm in women. Early detection via routine exam, self-exam and screening mammography allows for greater cure rates. Screening mammograms should be done first at age 35 to 40 for a base line and then repeated at physician-determined intervals between ages 40 to 50. After 50, it is suggested women undergo annual mammography. Woman at increased risk for breast cancer should have their baseline mammogram at age 35 and their subsequent mammograms at closer intervals. *(Jones et al, pp. 6–13)*

66. (B) The ability of a practitioner to adequately perform a pelvic exam depends on the patient's preparation for the examination. Communication prior to and throughout the exam is extremely important. Patients tolerate such exams much better when they are informed of what the practitioner is doing or about to do. Preparation by adequately draping the patient is a good means of keeping the patient comfortable and somewhat lessens the sense of self-consciousness and loss of control many women experience during a pelvic examination. Although it may make the examiner uncomfortable, allowing one family member to remain in the examination room may help the patient tolerate the procedure better. When the patient is an adolescent, allowing a mother or sister in the room may greatly decrease her anxieties. Some patients will actually feel more uncomfortable with the husband or a family member remaining in the room. Again, good communication with the patient will alert the practitioner to this possibility. The patient should be informed when a part of the exam may be painful. To avoid doing so may prevent the completion of the exam secondary to the patients' mistrust of the examiner and general discomfort. When informing the patient of impending pain, stress that the discomfort will be far reduced if the patient can relax and not tighten up in response to the anticipated pain. *(Jones et al, pp. 3–7)*

67. (C) Generalized engorgement of pelvic organs causes cyanosis and the discoloration of the cervix called *Chadwick's sign*. The uterus, both the corpus (body) and cervix undergoes softening during pregnancy; this is termed *Hegar's sign*. A multiparous cervix is one in which the os is slit-like when compared to a circular os, which is found in a nulliparous woman. A multiparous os is only indicative of a previous pregnancy, not a present one. Because a nulliparous woman is one who has never completed a pregnancy, she in fact could be pregnant. Nabothian cysts can either accompany or follow a chronic cervicitis and have no connection to pregnancy. They appear as translucent nodules on the ectocervix. *(Bates, p. 391)*

68. (E) Whether a patient is being interviewed during a routine exam or being seen for a gynecologic emergency, a thorough menstrual history is important. First, the date of the last menstrual period (LMP) should be obtained and whether the LMP was normal in amount, duration, and interval. The patient should also be asked about her two previous periods and whether they were normal. Next, the patient should be asked about her menstrual cycle: is it regular in interval, and what is the interval? A normal menstrual cycle is 28 to 30 days. A history of irregular cycles is indicative of anovulatory cycles or other endocrine abnormalities. Duration of menstrual flow, presence of clots, and amount of bleeding and associated pain are additional information that should be obtained. Age of menarche and onset of menopause and perimenopausal symptoms are also important in menstrual history. Intermenstrual bleeding can be spotting just prior to menses or at time of ovulation. It can also be indicative of uterine cancer and should always be investigated. Finally, a history of premenstrual syndrome should be elicited. The symptoms are extremely variable and including bloating, painful breast swelling, fatigue, depression, anxiety, irritability, and hostility. It may also include a craving for sweets and binge eating. *(Hacker and Moore, pp. 14, 263; Jones et al, pp. 5–6)*

69. (B) An endometrial biopsy can be performed in an office or clinic with either local anesthesia in the form of paracervical block or just premedication with analgesics. The endometrium is sampled with an extremely small suction-type curette in several, usually 4 to 6, different sites. In the case of this patient, as in any woman suspected of having cancer, an endocervical curetting should be performed prior to obtaining endometrial samples. In the case where polyps are visualized in the endocervical canal, they can be either of endocervical origin or endometrial. The polyps can often be removed in office if they are small, but if they are of considerable size, should be removed in an operating room. Endometrial polyps are seldom malignant in premenopausal women, but in menopausal or postmenopausal women, they should be removed in the operating room. This will allow adequate dilation of the cervix in order to remove all the polyps for pathologic diagnosis. A traditional dilation and curettage (D&C) would not only provide the above patient with endometrial sampling and removal of the polyp (which was probably causing the intermenstrual bleeding), it may also be therapeutic. The patient's increased menstrual bleeding is probably secondary to her known myomata. Submucosal myomata will often cause excessive bleeding; curettage will decrease this bleeding; it thus becomes not only a diagnostic but also therapeutic procedure. Endometrial sampling, whether by D&C or endometrial biopsy, is indicated in any woman (40 years of age) who has intermenstrual bleeding or a marked change in her bleeding pattern. A sonogram would adequately identify myomata but would not be helpful in determining whether there has been malignant endometrial changes. CAT scan provides greater imaging when compared to ultrasound, particularly if pelvic or periaortic nodes are suspected, but it still does not provide the necessary pathologic diagnosis for this patient. (*Hacker and Moore, p. 278; Jones et al, pp. 19-25, 723–726*)

70. **(A)** Syphilis, particularly in people who use IV drugs and crack or cocaine, is greatly increasing in frequency. It is theorized that many women are exchanging sex for drugs and that is why it is increasing in this population. Primary syphilis is characterized by a chancre that is a nontender ulcerative lesion usually found on the vulva, but can be also found in the vagina or on the cervix. It will appear between 10 and 60 days from the time of inoculation and spontaneously regress after 4 to 6 weeks. It is usually associated with tender, inguinal nodes. Because serologic tests are usually negative at this time, the primary means of making the diagnosis is by obtaining a specimen from the lesion. The spirochete can be seen on dark-field microscopy. Secondary syphilis that is characterized by the symptoms mentioned in the question occurs anywhere from 3 to 6 weeks after the appearance of the chancre. The condylomata, late lesions, are extremely infectious and again the spirochete can be seen under the dark-field microscope. The VDRL is positive at this time and there is also inguinal adenopathy present. Benzathine penicillin G, 2.4 million U in a one-time dose is the treatment for primary, secondary, or latent syphilis (less than 1 year's duration). Tertiary syphilis, which may affect any organ system of the body, particularly the central nervous system, is treated with three doses of benzathine penicillin G at weekly intervals. For patients allergic to penicillin, tetracycline 500 mg, orally, for 15 days is given for primary, secondary, and latent; 500 mg, orally, for 30 days for tertiary syphilis. There are no signs of PID with syphilis. (*Hacker and Moore, p. 301; Jones et al, pp. 577–579; Medical Letter, pp. 5–8*)

71. **(B)** One of the best means of antepartum fetal surveillance is the mother's perception of fetal movement. Whenever a woman complains of decreased fetal movement, she should immediately undergo fetal monitoring to obtain a reactive tracing and ultrasound to document fetal well-being. Intrauterine demise or neonatal death is not only a medical problem, it is also a psychosocial problem. The practitioner who deals with pregnant women must learn how to deal with women who have suffered a stillborn or neonatal loss. Couples should be allowed to see their child and hold or examine the baby. Often the child has undergone maceration or has a disfiguring anomaly. Wrapping the child to conceal or lessen these changes will help reduce the parents' shock. Although mothers and fathers often will not opt to view their dead child, it has been shown that to do so will help the parents accept the death and grieve appropriately. Taking pictures has also been found to help the parents in accepting the child's death. Additionally, many parents who originally could not deal with the demise can later return to view the pictures. Mothers should be appropriately medicated for pain and should not be "snowed." Being knocked out with good amounts of amnesiacs and analgesics will take away the realization that the child was actually born dead. Often, these women will not accept that their babies were stillborn but in fact believe that something was done to kill the child. Again, an awareness of the stillbirth enhances the mothers ability to appropriately grieve. Allowing the father to remain with the mother during the labor and delivery will allow him to better accept the reality of the child's death. It will also allow the couple to provide each other with support and encouragement. Often in our attempt to help the mother with the pain of labor and delivery of a stillborn, we forget that the father too has lost a child. (*Capitulo and Maffia, pp. 81–86*)

72. **(C)** Variable deceleration is caused by umbilical cord compression. The onset of the decelerations varies according to its relationship to the contraction and the shape of the deceleration varies when compared to the other decelerations. Variable decelerations occur when the cord is around the babies' neck or a limb and also occurs when there is oligohyramnios. Changing the mother's position from the right side to left side, or placing her in Trendelenburg or knee-chest position may relieve the pressure on the cord. The variable deceleration then may resolve with position change. Severe variable decelerations, those lasting greater than 60 seconds, often occur during the second stage of labor, as the patient starts to push. Late decelerations begin after the onset of the contractions and occur consistently at the same time of each contraction and appear similar in form. Late decelerations usually are indicative of some kind of uteroplacen-

tal insufficiency such as chronic hypertension, pregnancy-induced hypertension, sudden and severe maternal hypotention (as seen with some epidural anesthesia). Placing the patient on her left side will cause maximum blood flow to the placenta and often alleviates the late decelerations. The baseline fetal heart rate in this tracing is 150 bpm, the normal fetal heartrate is anywhere between 120 to 160. A rate above 160 bpm is considered fetal tachycardia. *(Hacker and Moore, pp. 190–194; Freeman and Garite, p. 75)*

73. **(E)** Rape makes up about 7% of all violent crime in this country. Approximately 3 to 10 times as many rapes are committed than are reported. Practitioners who care for women at some time in their career must deal with a woman who has been raped. Practitioners are called upon to obtain evidence and treat the patient both medically and psychologically. The patient should be treated for both gonorrhea and *Chlamydia* at the time she is initially seen. A baseline VDRL and pregnancy test should also be drawn and the patient should be seen again in 6 weeks in order to repeat these tests and to repeat GC and *Chlamydial* cultures. The patient must be informed about the possibility of pregnancy. A certain percentage of women are protected against pregnancy with a preexisting form of birth control such as birth control pills, IUD, bilateral tubal ligation, or hysterectomy *(Cunningham et al, pp. 621–624)*

REFERENCES

Acker DB, Sachs BP, Friedman EA. Risk factors for shoulder dystocia. *Obstetrics and Gynecology*, 1985; 66 (6):762–767.

Bates Barbara. *A Guide to Physical Examination*, 4th ed. Philadelphia, PA: Lippincott; 1987.

Burke, L. The use of the Friedman curve in labor management. *Cinc J Med.* 1975; 56:29–36.

Burrow and Ferris. *Medical Complications During Pregnancy.* Philadelphia, PA: WB Saunders; 1988.

Capitulo KL, Maffia A. *The Perinatal Bereavement Team: Development and Function, Women and Loss.* New York: Praeger Publishers, 1985.

Cunningham FG, MacDonald PC, Gant NF. *Williams Obstetrics*, 18th ed. Norwalk, CT: Appelton and Lange; 1989.

Freeman RK, Garite TJ. *Fetal Heart Rate Monitoring.* Baltimore, MD: Williams and Wilkins; 1981.

Hacker NF, Moore JG. *Essential of Obstetrics and Gynecology*, 1st ed. Philadelphia, PA: W.B. Saunders; 1986.

Jones HW, Wentz AC, Burnett LS. *Novak's Textbook of Gynecology*, 11th ed. Baltimore, MD: Williams and Wilkins; 1988.

Neshein BI. Induced abortion by the suction method. *Acta Ob Gynecol. Scand.* 1984; 63:591–595.

Niswander KR. *Manual of Obstetrics, Diagnosis and Therapy.* 3rd ed. Boston, MA: Little, Brown; 1987.

Treatment of sexually transmitted diseases. *The Medical Letter, on Drugs and Therapeutics.* Rochelle, NY: The Medical Letter; 1988.

Obstetrics and Gynecology Subspecialty List:

Question Number and Subspecialty

1. OB—Hepatitis B vaccine—indications
2. OB—Endomyometritis—pathogenesis
3. OB—Deep vein thrombosis—causes
4. OB—Mastitis—characteristics
5. OB—Breech presentation—causes
6. OB—Cord prolapse—association with malpresentations
7. OB—Postpartum bleeding—management
8. OB—Cesarean section—indications
9. OB—Incompetent cervix—history
10. OB—Gestational trophoblastic neoplasia—characteristics
11. OB—Polyhydramnios—characteristics
12. OB—Twin gestations—complications
13. OB—Magnesium—effects in pregnancy
14. OB—Placenta previa—management
15. OB—Spontaneous rupture of membranes—diagnosis
16. OB—Spontaneous rupture of membranes—complications
17. OB—Medications
18. OB—Diabetes in pregnancy—complications
19. OB—Diabetes in pregnancy—monitoring
20. GYN—Infertility—characteristics
21. GYN—Menstrual cycle—characteristics
22. OB—Caesarean section—postop complications
23. OB—Pulmonary embolism
24. OB—Genetic amniocentesis—indications
25. OB—Fetal monitoring
26. OB—Fetal monitoring
27. OB—Labor patterns
28. OB—Complications of vaginal delivery
29. OB—Postpartum bleeding—causes
30. OB—Vaginal delivery—contraindications
31. OB—Incomplete spontaneous abortion—characteristics
32. OB—Elective abortions—types
33. OB—Hydatidiform mole—characteristics
34. OB—Placenta abruption—characteristics
35. OB—Intrauterine fetal demise—complications
36. OB—Postdate pregnancy—characteristics
37. OB—Gestational diabetes—screening indications
38. OB—Acute appendicitis in pregnancy
39. OB—General anesthesia in pregnancy—complications
40. GYN—Condylomata acuminata—complications
41. GYN—Birth control—indications
42. GYN—Endometriosis—diagnosis
43. GYN—Menstrual irregularites—characteristics
44. GYN—Polycystic ovary syndrome—characteristics
45. OB—Events of pregnancy
46. OB—Events of pregnancy
47. OB—Events of pregnancy
48. OB—Events of pregnancy
49. OB—Medication
50. OB—Drugs in pregnancy
51. OB—Drugs in pregnancy
52. OB—Medication
53. GYN—Postmenopausal atrophic changes—treatment
54. OB—Ectopic pregnancy—laboratory evaluation
55. OB—Ectopic pregnancy—risk factors
56. GYN—Pelvic inflammatory disease—causes
57. GYN—Pelvic inflammatory disease—treatment
58. GYN—Right lower quadrant pain—differential diagnosis
59. GYN—Herpes genitalis—characteristics
60. GYN—Hysterectomy—indications
61. GYN—Endometrial hyperplasia—characteristics
62. GYN—Adnexal/ovarian cysts—management
63. GYN—Corpus luteal cyst vs. ectopic pregnancy—differential
64. GYN—Stress incontinence—management
65. GYN—Routine examination
66. GYN—Pelvic examination—procedure
67. GYN—Pelvic examination—findings
68. GYN—Menstrual history—considerations
69. GYN—Endometrial biopsy—indications
70. OB—Syphilis—characteristics
71. OB—Intrauterine fetal demise—management
72. OB—Fetal monitoring
73. GYN—Rape—management

CHAPTER 10

Practice Test
Questions

DIRECTIONS (Questions 1 through 7): For each of the items in this section, ONE or MORE of the numbered options is correct. Choose the answer

A if only 1, 2, and 3 are correct,
B if only 1 and 3 are correct,
C if only 2 and 4 are correct,
D if only 4 is correct,
E if all are correct.

1. Hypercalcemia may be caused by

   (1) primary hyperparathyroidism
   (2) thyrotoxicosis
   (3) humoral hypercalcemia of malignancy
   (4) thiazide diuretics

2. Treatment of hyperthyroidism can include

   (1) steroids
   (2) lithium
   (3) propylthiouracil
   (4) methimazole

3. Complications of iatrogenic Cushing's syndrome include

   (1) cataracts
   (2) osteoporosis
   (3) myopathy
   (4) growth spurt

4. Osteoporosis, a disease in total bone mass, may be caused by

   (1) menopause
   (2) hyperthyroidism
   (3) Cushing's syndrome
   (4) alcoholism

5. Diabetes mellitus may present with

   (1) polyuria
   (2) polydipsia
   (3) ketosis
   (4) blurry vision

6. The appropriate laboratory work-up for a pheochromocytoma would include

   (1) serum for metanephrins
   (2) serum for VMA
   (3) 24-hour urine for prostaglandins
   (4) 24-hour urine for fractionated catecholamines

7. Clinical signs of hypocalcemia include

   (1) positive Chovstek's sign
   (2) cramps and tingling
   (3) tetany
   (4) negative Trousseau's sign

DIRECTIONS (Questions 8 through 17): Each of the numbered items or incomplete statements in this section is followed by answers or by completions of the statement. Select the ONE lettered answer or completion that is BEST in each case.

8. Hypercalcemia should be suspected if a patient has a serum calcium level of

   (A) 8.0 mg/dL with albumin of 3.0 g/dL
   (B) 9.0 mg/dL with albumin of 3.0 g/dL
   (C) 10.0 mg/dL with albumin of 4.0 g/dL
   (D) 10.0 mg/dL with albumin of 2.0 g/dL
   (E) 9.5 mg/dL with albumin of 3.8 g/dL

9. Dexamethasone suppression test is used to aid in the diagnosis of

   (A) Graves' disease
   (B) Addison's disease
   (C) Cushing's disease
   (D) Reidel's disease
   (E) rheumatoid arthritis

10. Kidney stones can have a variety of mineral components. Which of the following is NOT a cause for stones

    (A) cystine
    (B) oxalate
    (C) magnesium
    (D) purine
    (E) phosphate

11. Clinical features of Cushing's syndrome include

(A) thick skin
(B) hirsutism
(C) improving strength
(D) hair loss
(E) abdominal pain

12. High-density lipoprotein is associated with

(A) decreased cardiac mortality
(B) increased cardiac mortality
(C) diabetes
(D) hypertension
(E) high saturated fat intake

13. A patient presents with osteolytic lesions on x-ray; bone pain, deformity, bone scan with numerous hot lesions and bone biopsy demonstrate intense osteoblastic bone resorption and large numbers of osteoclasts. The most likely bone lesion would be

(A) hyperthyroid bone disease
(B) hyperparathyroid bone disease
(C) Paget's disease
(D) metastatic breast cancer
(E) osteoporosis

14. NPH insulin usually has its peak activity at

(A) 4 to 6 hours
(B) 18 to 24 hours
(C) 10 hours
(D) 6 to 14 hours
(E) 16 hours

15. Monitoring adequate blood sugar control in the diabetic would include which of the following tests?

(A) 12 MN blood sugar
(B) glycohemoglobin level
(C) 24-hour urine for glucose
(D) 6 PM blood sugar
(E) 8 AM insulin level

16. Antihistamines are contraindicated in all the following medical conditions EXCEPT

(A) glaucoma
(B) hypertension
(C) asthma
(D) prostatic hypertrophy
(E) pregnancy

17. All the following are used in the management of asthma EXCEPT

(A) theophylline
(B) cromolyn sodium
(C) nadolol
(D) terbutaline
(E) albuterol

DIRECTIONS (Questions 18 and 19): For each of the items in this section, ONE or MORE of the numbered options is correct. Choose the answer

A if only 1, 2, and 3 are correct,
B if only 1 and 3 are correct,
C if only 2 and 4 are correct,
D if only 4 is correct,
E if all are correct.

18. Phenobarbital and phenytoin are effective in the management of generalized motor seizures. Which drug(s) is/are effective in petit mal or absence seizures?

(1) ethosuximide
(2) phenobarbital
(3) valproic acid
(4) diazepam

19. Which of the following are useful in the treatment of migraine headache?

(1) tenormin
(2) vicodin
(3) midrin
(4) sansert

DIRECTIONS (Questions 20 and 21): Each of the numbered items or incomplete statements in this section is followed by answers or by completions of the statement. Select the ONE lettered answer or completion that is BEST in each case.

20. The evaluation of new onset seizures in an adult should include all the following EXCEPT

(A) CT Scan
(B) chest radiograph
(C) HIV testing
(D) BUN, electrolytes, and creatinine
(E) fasting blood sugar

21. The most common symptom of a patient with a spinal cord metastases is

(A) paraparesis
(B) pain
(C) numbness
(D) paresthesia
(E) focal weakness

DIRECTIONS (Questions 22 through 24): For each of the items in this section, ONE or MORE of the numbered options is correct. Choose the answer

    A if only 1, 2, and 3 are correct,
    B if only 1 and 3 are correct,
    C if only 2 and 4 are correct,
    D if only 4 is correct,
    E if all are correct.

22. Seizures occurring within 24 hours of a traumatic head injury

    (1) suggest serious brain injury
    (2) are associated with a 28% mortality
    (3) indicate a focal lesion
    (4) have no prognostic significance

23. Hematuria

    (1) is not painful except when there is passage of large clots in the ureter or urethra
    (2) occurs in sepsis and other systemic disorders
    (3) occurs in acute interstitial nephritis
    (4) occurs in cystic and inflammatory diseases

24. In the patient with hyperchloremic acidosis you will find

    (1) decreased serum bicarbonate
    (2) sulfate and phosphate excreted normally
    (3) increased reabsorption of chloride ions
    (4) renal excretion of acid is reduced

DIRECTIONS (Question 25): Each of the numbered items or incomplete statements in this section is followed by answers or by completions of the statement. Select the ONE lettered answer or completion that is BEST in each case.

25. Which of the following symptoms are least likely to be seen in acute pyelonephritis?

    (A) nausea and vomiting
    (B) leukocytosis
    (C) CVA tenderness or pain on deep abdominal palpation
    (D) cystitis
    (E) fever and chills

DIRECTIONS (Questions 26 through 39): For each of the items in this section, ONE or MORE of the numbered options is correct. Choose the answer

    A if only 1, 2, and 3 are correct,
    B if only 1 and 3 are correct,
    C if only 2 and 4 are correct,
    D if only 4 is correct,
    E if all are correct.

26. Proper care of an amputated digit includes

    (1) placing the amputated part in a bath of lactated Ringer's solution
    (2) perfusing exposed arteries with iced saline solution
    (3) placing the amputated part, protected in a bag of crystalloid solution, on ice
    (4) avoiding the use of ice and keeping the amputated part at room temperature

27. Hemorrhage in the acute setting is best controlled by

    (1) manual compression of vessels proximal to the bleeding site
    (2) the use of vascular clamps
    (3) tourniquets
    (4) direct pressure to the bleeding site

28. Principles of fluid resuscitation in the acute management of hypovolemic shock includes

    (1) insertion of large-bore peripheral IVs
    (2) rapidly infusing 2 L of lactated Ringer's solution
    (3) type-specific blood is preferred for life-threatening shock
    (4) immediate insertion of central venous catheters

29. Signs and symptoms of small bowel obstruction include

    (1) intermittent, crampy abdominal pain
    (2) vomiting
    (3) abdominal distention
    (4) diarrhea

30. Radiologic studies that are helpful in the diagnosis of acute cholecystitis include

    (1) plain KUB
    (2) RUQ ultrasound
    (3) technetium 99m scans (HIDA)
    (4) oral cholecystogram

SUMMARY OF DIRECTIONS				
A	**B**	**C**	**D**	**E**
1, 2, 3 only	1, 3 only	2, 4 only	4 only	All are correct

31. Which of the following are common characteristics of acute mesenteric ischemia?

    (1) it is typically a disease of the elderly and infirm
    (2) often follows a period of hemodynamic instability
    (3) often due to embolic or thrombotic events
    (4) patients complain of pain that is disproportionate to a relatively benign physical exam

32. The hallmarks of acute arterial occlusion include

    (1) pain
    (2) pallor
    (3) pulselessness
    (4) paralysis and paresthesia

33. Certain high-risk patients may require antibiotics in addition to incision and drainage for the treatment of soft tissue abscesses. These include

    (1) patients manifesting systemic toxicity
    (2) diabetic patients
    (3) patients with valvular heart disease
    (4) patients with cirrhosis

34. Which of the following statements are characteristic of perirectal abscesses?

    (1) if mistreated could lead to life-threatening sepsis
    (2) form fistulas-in-ano when they drain spontaneously
    (3) require general anesthesia for proper drainage
    (4) occur with greater frequency in the immunocompromised patient

35. Clinical findings often seen with mandibular fractures include

    (1) malocclusion
    (2) rhinorrhea
    (3) deviation of the jaw on opening
    (4) raccoon eye

36. When closing lacerations in the Emergency Room setting it is important to relieve tension on the wound edges to achieve an optimal result. Techniques to reduce wound tension include

    (1) undermining soft tissues
    (2) splinting the affected part

    (3) closing the wound in layers
    (4) application of adhesive strips

37. Characteristics of full-thickness burn wounds include

    (1) blister formation
    (2) white or charred appearance
    (3) sensitive to pin prick
    (4) will not heal spontaneously

38. Indications that a cast is too tight include

    (1) increasing pain
    (2) poor capillary refill
    (3) paresthesias
    (4) pain on passive extension of the digits

39. Diagnostic peritoneal lavage is extremely useful in determining which trauma patients require urgent exploratory laparotomy. Indication for peritoneal lavage in multisystem trauma include

    (1) patients with altered mental status from head injury or intoxication
    (2) situations in which the patient will have lengthy nonabdominal surgery
    (3) unexplained hypotension
    (4) situations in which CT scanning is not available

DIRECTIONS (Questions 40 through 44): Each of the numbered items or incomplete statements in this section is followed by answers or by completions of the statement. Select the ONE lettered answer or completion that is BEST in each case.

40. The primary pathologic effect of acetaminophen poisoning is

    (A) bronchospasm
    (B) bone marrow suppression
    (C) reversible mental status changes
    (D) hepatic dysfunction
    (E) cardiac dysfunction

41. The major toxic effect of carbon monoxide is

    (A) hypoxia
    (B) inhibition of surfactant
    (C) primary myocardial depression
    (D) bronchospasm
    (E) hemolysis

42. The proper rate and sequence of ventilation and chest compression in two-person CPR is

    (A) one ventilation after five compressions at a rate of 80 to 100 compressions per minute
    (B) two ventilations after ten compressions at a rate of 80 to 100 compressions per minute

(C) one ventilation after ten compressions at a rate of 80 to 100 compressions per minute

(D) two ventilations after three compressions at a rate of 80 to 100 compressions per minute

(E) three ventilations after three compressions at a rate of 80 to 100 compressions per minute

43. The leading cause of mortality in the first four decades of life is

(A) congenital defects
(B) cancer
(C) infectious disease
(D) multisystem trauma
(E) bronchospastic diseases

44. A positive anterior drawer sign is indicative of

(A) medial collateral ligament tear
(B) lateral collateral ligament tear
(C) anterior cruciate ligament tear
(D) medial meniscus tear
(E) lateral meniscus tear

DIRECTIONS (Question 45): For each of the items in this section, ONE or MORE of the numbered options is correct. Choose the answer

A if only 1, 2, and 3 are correct,
B if only 1 and 3 are correct,
C if only 2 and 4 are correct,
D if only 4 is correct,
E if all are correct.

45. Which of the following statements regarding pelvic fractures are correct?

(1) mortality in patients with pelvic fractures can reach as high as 20%
(2) a displaced fracture of the pelvic ring indicates that there is at least one other fracture
(3) anterior pelvic fractures are commonly associated with uretheral injuries
(4) few patients with pelvic fractures sustain hemorrhage sufficient to require transfusion

DIRECTIONS (Questions 46 through 52): Each of the numbered items or incomplete statements in this section is followed by answers or by completions of the statement. Select the ONE lettered answer or completion that is BEST in each case.

46. Malignant neoplasms of the musculoskeletal system

(A) generally have a good prognosis
(B) include osteoblastomas and giant cell tumors
(C) rarely require surgical excision
(D) are usually painful
(E) rarely metastasize

47. Statistically, the most common type of childhood maltreatment seen by health care practitioners is

(A) nonorganic failure to thrive
(B) physical abuse
(C) sexual abuse
(D) emotional/verbal abuse
(E) neglect

48. The most common bacterial pathogen for otitis media at all ages is

(A) Group A beta hemolytic strep
(B) *E coli*
(C) *S pneumoniae*
(D) *S aureus*
(E) *B catarrhalis*

49. Asthmatic children

(A) rarely present before 5 years of age
(B) have a generally poor prognosis
(C) rarely require pharmacologic therapy
(D) present with hyperreactivity of the airways to a variety of stimuli and a high degree of reversibility of the obstructive process
(E) demonstrate rales as the diagnostic feature on physical exam

50. Which of the following is the most important first step in treating a child who is unresponsive after suspected cardiopulmonary arrest?

(A) applying cardiac monitor
(B) initiating closed chest cardiac massage
(C) determining if patient is having respiratory difficulty and establishing a patent airway
(D) assessing whether circulatory problems exist by checking brachial, femoral, or carotid pulses
(E) establishing an IV line

51. The most common type of burn seen in children is

(A) scald burns
(B) flame burns
(C) electrical burns
(D) flash burns (exploding flammable materials)
(E) George Burns

52. A patient has a type III epiphyseal fracture (Salter fracture). This type of fracture is described as

(A) the epiphyseal plate has slipped from its origin and there is a fracture through the metaphysis producing a triangular metaphyseal fragment
(B) a crushing injury damaging the epiphyseal plate usually producing growth arrest
(C) the epiphyseal plate has slipped with a fracture involving the epiphysis

(D) an intraarticular fracture extending through the epiphysis, epiphyseal plate, and metaphysis

(E) the epiphyseal plate separates from the metaphysis without displacement or injury to the growth plate

DIRECTIONS (Questions 53 through 64): For each of the items in this section, ONE or MORE of the numbered options is correct. Choose the answer

A if only 1, 2, and 3 are correct,
B if only 1 and 3 are correct,
C if only 2 and 4 are correct,
D if only 4 is correct,
E if all are correct.

53. Painless rectal bleeding in children may be caused by

(1) Meckel's diverticulum
(2) rectal fissures
(3) juvenile polyps
(4) intussusception

54. Status epilepticus is when a patient has continuous seizures for 20 minutes, or more than two seizures without a lucid period. Which of the following is/are true regarding the cause, management, and outcome of this condition?

(1) may be caused by poor compliance in the use of seizure medication
(2) appropriate laboratory studies include determination of blood glucose level, arterial blood gasses, electrolytes, and blood level of anticonvulsant medication
(3) treatment includes: establishing airway, giving oxygen, intravenous glucose, and consideration of giving naloxone, thiamine, and correction of metabolic abnormalities; use of an anticonvulsant like phenobarbital
(4) complications include death from anoxia, aspiration, or trauma. Encephalopathy from anoxia, acute renal failure due to myoglobinuria, and rhabdomyolysis and respiratory arrest caused by medications

55. Treatment for an avulsed secondary tooth includes

(1) cleaning the tooth thoroughly by scrubbing all dirt and foreign matter from the tooth
(2) inserting the tooth into the open socket or placing the tooth under the patient's tongue until a dentist is seen
(3) wrapping the tooth in gauze until a dentist is seen
(4) seeing a dentist as soon as possible

56. A 5-year-old female presents with a single swollen, firm, nontender anterior cervical node. The child has been entirely healthy for the last several months. There has been no known exposure. Your differential diagnosis includes which of the following?

(1) Beta streptococcus adenitis
(2) malignancies
(3) cat scratch fever
(4) atypical mycobacterium

57. Acetaminophen is a common ingestion in the pediatric population. Which of the following is/are true for an ingestion of this type in a child older than 1 year of age?

(1) the local or national poison control number should be called. They are likely to suggest that Syrup of Ipecac be given to this alert child at the dose of 10 mL
(2) the child has vomited from the Syrup of Ipecac. You should wait 30 minutes until vomiting has ceased and then administer activated charcoal
(3) serum acetaminophen levels should be drawn at 2 hours postingestion
(4) the antidote for acetaminophen is N-acetylcysteine (Mucomyst)

58. Factor(s) tending to increase the suspicion that a physical injury to a child has a nonaccidental etiology include

(1) a history that does not explain the extent or characteristics of the injury
(2) an explanation of his/her involvement in the traumatic incident that is not compatible with the child's developmental level
(3) a long delay in seeking medical help
(4) parents who seem overly anxious and distraught

59. Adverse reactions to DTP vaccine that occur in more than 5% of vaccine recipients include

(1) pain or swelling at the site
(2) fever greater than 38°C
(3) anorexia or vomiting
(4) febrile convulsion

60. *Haemophilus influenzae* type b (HIB) frequently causes the following infections in children

(1) meningitis
(2) otitis media
(3) epiglottitis
(4) urinary tract infection

61. Incidence studies of acute otitis media show that

   (1) the peak incidence is in the second 6 months of life
   (2) in the first year of life, 60% of children will have at least one episode of otitis media
   (3) by age 3, 80% of children will have experienced otitis media
   (4) the incidence of otitis media decreases after the first year of life

62. Abnormal sexual development is manifested by

   (1) no sign of puberty in a girl of 15
   (2) onset of puberty in a girl age 9
   (3) bilateral/unilateral breast development in a girl prior to age 8
   (4) no sign of puberty in a boy of 13

63. Human breast milk offers which of the following advantages to neonates?

   (1) secretory IGA
   (2) a high vitamin D content
   (3) epidermal growth factor
   (4) higher iron content than formula

64. The Denver Developmental Screening Test (DDST)

   (1) is a screening instrument designed to determine whether a particular child's development falls within the normal range
   (2) is an intelligence test for children
   (3) consists of a progressive sequence of developmental tasks that test personal–social, fine motor/adaptive, language, and gross motor skills
   (4) requires extensive testing material and is difficult and time consuming to administer

65. A newborn infant in the delivery room is commonly evaluated by the Apgar score. The following is/are true statements

   (1) a score is given at 1 and at 5 minutes
   (2) the 1-minute score is most predictive of neurologic residual and long-term outcome
   (3) signs including heartrate, muscle tone, and color are given a score
   (4) a total score of 5 indicates an infant in the best possible condition

66. Innocent murmurs are characterized by which of the following?

   (1) present in 50% of children
   (2) may have an abnormality of 2nd heart sound
   (3) are systolic in timing
   (4) frequently have an associated click

DIRECTIONS (Questions 67 through 70): Each group of items in this section consists of lettered headings followed by a set of numbered words or phrases. For each numbered word or phrase, select the ONE lettered heading that is most closely associated with it. Each lettered heading may be selected once, more than once, or not at all.

For each description of a skin lesion, select the disease with which it is associated

   (A) lichen sclerosis et atrophicus
   (B) psoriasis
   (C) eczema
   (D) tuberous sclerosis
   (E) pityriasis rosea

67. herald patch

68. hourglass distribution in anogenital area

69. adenoma sebaceum

70. lichenification

DIRECTIONS (Questions 71 through 76): For each of the items in this section, ONE or MORE of the numbered options is correct. Choose the answer

   A if only 1, 2, and 3 are correct,
   B if only 1 and 3 are correct,
   C if only 2 and 4 are correct,
   D if only 4 is correct,
   E if all are correct.

71. The thick ascending limb of the loop of Henle, absorbs sodium chloride rapidly and causes

   (1) a decreased osmolality and tubular fluid concentration of sodium chloride to drop to 30 mmol/L
   (2) the voltage across the lumen to become positive
   (3) the tubular fluid to become dilute
   (4) concentration of fluid in the distal loop when it passes through this region

72. The statement/statements most accurately associated with scleroderma (progressive systemic sclerosis) in renal tissue would be

   (1) renal failure is associated with 40% to 50% of all deaths
   (2) renal involvement is rarely the presenting symptom
   (3) closely resembles accelerated nephrosclerosis
   (4) petechial hemorrhages and wedge-shaped cortical infarcts

SUMMARY OF DIRECTIONS				
A	**B**	**C**	**D**	**E**
1, 2, 3 only	1, 3 only	2, 4 only	4 only	All are correct

73. In adult polycystic kidney disease, you would find

(1) cortical and medullary cysts
(2) renal failure as a newborn
(3) hepatic cysts and intracranial aneurysms
(4) reduced bicarbonate absorption

74. The normal range of serum osmolality is 285 to 295 mOsm/L and is calculated: (1 mOsm glucose = 180 mg/L; 1 mOsm BUN = 28 mg/L)

(1) $2(Na^+ mmol/L) + glucose\ mmol/L + BUN\ mmol/L$

(2) $2(Na^+ mOsm/L) + \dfrac{glucose\ mOsm/L}{1.8\ mmol} + \dfrac{BUN\ mOsm/L}{28\ mmol}$

(3) $2(Na^+ meq/L) + \dfrac{glucose\ mg/dL}{18} + \dfrac{BUN\ mg/dL}{2.8}$

(4) $2(Na^+ meq/L) + glucose\ mEq/L + BUN\ mEq/L$

75. 50% to 70% of body weight is composed of water that is

(1) two thirds intracellular fluid
(2) one third extracellular fluid
(3) regulated by the amount of solvent in each compartment
(4) not dependent on the amount of adipose tissue

76. The concentration of urine depends largely on

(1) the loop of Henle
(2) large osmotic pressure gradient between the papilla and cortex
(3) the countercurrent system
(4) nephrons

DIRECTIONS (Questions 77 through 85): Each of the numbered items or incomplete statements in this section is followed by answers or by completions of the statement. Select the ONE lettered answer or completion that is BEST in each case.

77. In Rheumatoid Disease the majority of clinical and pathological findings are a result of chronic inflammation of what structure?

(A) synovial membranes
(B) epiphyseal disc
(C) articular cartilage
(D) periosteal membrane
(E) subchondrial bone

78. A 52-year-old man presents with severe right ankle pain for 2 days and no other complaints. During the exam, the joint is erythematous, warm, and an effusion is noted. The patient is afebrile, WBC: 9000, with normal differential, BUN and creatinine are within normal limits. Uric acid level is 9.6 mg/dL (normal is 2.5 to 8 mg/dL). The most likely diagnosis is

(A) rheumatoid arthritis
(B) osteoarthritis
(C) pseudogout
(D) gouty arthritis
(E) bacterial septic arthritis

79. Which of the following signs and symptoms are most commonly found in a pregnant woman with pyelonephritis?

(A) lower abdominal pain, fever, and chills
(B) premature onset of contractions
(C) fever and chills, nausea and vomiting, and flank pain
(D) urinary frequency, urgency, and dysuria
(E) a brownish discoloration of urine

80. At 10-weeks gestation a 23-year-old G1 P0 breaks out in a rash that begins first on her face and then spreads downward. One week earlier, she suffered fever, malaise, and myalgias. Which test should be obtained immediately to determine whether her fetus will be affected by an infection resulting in severe congenital abnormalities?

(A) VDRL
(B) cervical cultures for gonorrhea
(C) chlamydial cultures
(D) rubella titers
(E) group B beta strep cultures

81. At 32 weeks, a 16-year-old G 1 P0 presents to the obstetric clinic complaining of headache; her blood pressure is 140/85. According to her prenatal chart, her first trimester blood pressures were 100/70. At this time she has 2+ protein in her urine and she is hyperreflexic. What is the most likely diagnosis?

(A) chronic hypertension
(B) migraine headache
(C) eclampsia
(D) chronic renal disease
(E) preeclampsia

82. The above patient is admitted to the hospital and placed on bed rest. Instead of improving, her blood pressure increases to 160/100, the proteinuria remains at 2+ to 3+, and she remains hyperreflexic. A decision to deliver her baby is made, what medication must be started at this time?

(A) hydrochlorothiazide
(B) hydralazine

(C) magnesium sulfate
(D) diazepam
(E) furosemide

83. When performing a Pap smear you are attempting to obtain cells from the area that undergoes dysplastic changes. This area is called the

(A) endocervix
(B) squamocolumnar junction
(C) posterior vaginal fornix
(D) exocervix
(E) internal os

84. The primary means by which oral contraceptives prevent pregnancy is

(A) inhibition of endometrial implantation of the embryo
(B) inhibition of the release of prolactin and, therefore, prevention of ovulation
(C) inhibition of the release of estrogen from the follicle and, therefore, ovulation
(D) inhibition of spermatozoa by pill-induced changes in the cervical mucus
(E) inhibition of the midcycle gonadotrophin surge and, therefore, ovulation

85. A 15-year-old patient presents with a complaint of severe menstrual cramps that prevent her from attending school and maintaining her normal daily activity. The pain usually occurs on the first day of her menses and has gotten progressively worse since the onset of menarche at age 13. Pelvic exam is without significant findings. You make the diagnosis of primary dysmenorrhea and decide to treat her in the following manner

(A) tylenol with codeine
(B) oral contraceptives
(C) prostaglandin synthetase inhibitors
(D) diagnostic laparscopy
(E) tocolytic agents

DIRECTIONS (Questions 86 through 93): Each group of items in this section consists of lettered headings followed by a set of numbered words or phrases. For each numbered word or phrase, select the ONE lettered heading that is most closely associated with it. Each lettered heading may be selected once, more than once, or not at all.

Questions 86 through 89

Match the following vaginal infections with the appropriate description.

(A) *Trichomonas*
(B) atrophic vaginitis
(C) gonorrhea

(D) candidiasis
(E) *Gardnerella vaginalis*

86. thick white discharge with vaginal itching and burning, marked erythemia of vulvovaginal mucous membranes

87. vaginal itching and burning, thin blood-tinged discharge; thin friable vulvar and vaginal epithelium

88. soreness with vaginal itching and burning; frothy yellow–green discharge, diffusely reddened mucous membranes.

89. musty, malodorous discharge, thin and greyish in color

Questions 90 through 93

For the number weeks of gestation match the events of pregnancy that occur at the time

(A) 6 weeks
(B) 28 weeks
(C) 20 weeks
(D) 16 to 20 weeks
(E) 14 weeks

90. fundal height at umbilicus

91. fetal movements first perceived by mother

92. gestational sac first seen on sonogram (abdominal)

93. optimal time to draw maternal serum alpha fetoprotein

DIRECTIONS (Questions 94 through 96): Each of the numbered items or incomplete statements in this section is followed by answers or by completions of the statement. Select the ONE lettered answer or completion that is BEST in each case.

94. The test of choice for diagnosis of a pericardial effusion is

(A) chest x-ray
(B) CT scan of chest
(C) MUGA
(D) Echocardiogram
(E) right heart catheterization

95. All the following physical findings may be associated with mitral stenosis EXCEPT

(A) diastolic apical rumble
(B) Graham–Steele diastolic murmur
(C) opening snap
(D) S₃ gallop
(E) loud S₁

Figure 10–1.

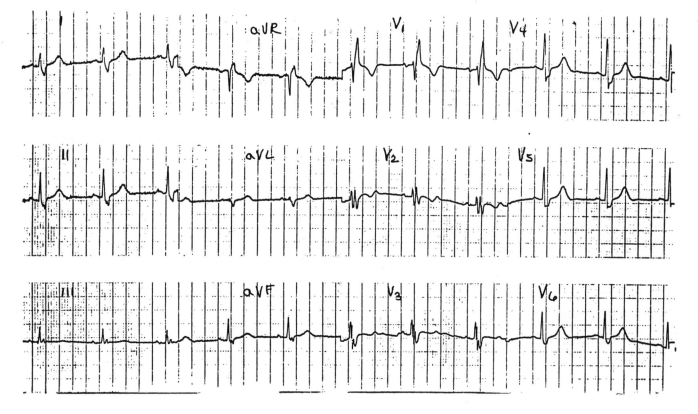

Figure 10–2.

96. All the following are causes of left ventricular hypertrophy **EXCEPT**

    (A) mitral stenosis
    (B) systemic arterial hypertension
    (C) hypertrophic obstructive cardiomyopathy
    (D) aortic insufficiency
    (E) aortic stenosis

97. Electrocardiogram Figure 10–1 demonstrates

    (A) inferior wall myocardial infarction
    (B) left ventricular hypertrophy
    (C) anterolateral ischemia
    (D) right bundle branch block
    (E) left atrial enlargement

98. Electrocardiogram Figure 10–2 demonstrates

    (A) paced rhythm
    (B) left bundle branch block
    (C) right bundle branch block
    (D) idiopathic subaortic stenosis
    (E) posterior wall myocardial infarction

DIRECTIONS (Questions 99 through 110): For each of the items in this section, <u>ONE</u> or <u>MORE</u> of the numbered options is correct. Choose the answer

    A if only <u>1, 2, and 3</u> are correct,
    B if only <u>1 and 3</u> are correct,
    C if only <u>2 and 4</u> are correct,
    D if only <u>4</u> is correct,
    E if <u>all</u> are correct.

99. Electrocardiographic findings in cardiac tamponade include

    (1) diffuse low voltage
    (2) prolonged QT interval
    (3) electrical alternans
    (4) left bundle branch block

100. Risk factors for developing coronary artery disease are

    (1) caffeine intake
    (2) tobacco smoking
    (3) alcohol consumption
    (4) high blood pressure

101. Which of the following arrhythmias can cause syncope?

    (1) severe bradycardia
    (2) premature ventricular contractions
    (3) asystole
    (4) premature atrial contractions

102. The following findings are associated with acute pericarditis

    (1) ST elevation
    (2) pericardial friction rub
    (3) dyspnea
    (4) chest pain often aggravated by leaning forward

103. Secondary causes of hypertension include

    (1) pheochromocytoma
    (2) renal parenchymal disease
    (3) use of estrogen-containing oral contraceptive pills
    (4) primary aldosteronism

104. The first heart sound (S_1)

    (1) is caused by the closure of the mitral and tricuspid valves
    (2) precedes the palpable upstroke in carotid pulse
    (3) is a high-pitched sound
    (4) is best heard at the 2nd or 3rd intercostal spaces

105. Physical findings associated with heart failure are

    (1) pulmonary rales
    (2) congestive hepatomegaly
    (3) S_3 gallop
    (4) S_4

106. Causes of ST segment elevation are

    (1) Prinzmetal's angina
    (2) acute pericarditis
    (3) acute myocardial injury
    (4) early repolarization

107. Manifestations of digitalis intoxication include

    (1) prolonged QT interval
    (2) anorexia
    (3) urinary retention
    (4) arrhythmias

108. Endocarditis prophylaxis is recommended for

    (1) cystoscopy
    (2) colonoscopy
    (3) gallbladder surgery
    (4) dental procedures

109. Factors associated with a poor prognosis after an acute myocardial infarction are

(1) congestive heart failure
(2) positive stress test after a myocardial infarction
(3) poor left ventricular systolic function
(4) ventricular arrhythmias during first 24 hours

110. What are the guidelines for the classification of blood pressure?

(1) mild hypertension is a diastolic pressure of 90 to 104 mm Hg
(2) normal systolic blood pressure is < 160 mm Hg
(3) severe hypertension is a diastolic pressure > 115 mm Hg
(4) isolated systolic hypertension is systolic pressure > 180 mm Hg with diastolic < 90 mm Hg

DIRECTIONS (Questions 111 through 119): Each of the numbered items or incomplete statements in this section is followed by answers or by completions of the statement. Select the ONE lettered answer or completion that is BEST in each case.

111. When lithium is used to treat bipolar affective illness, which lab tests are used in routine monitoring of the patient for side effects?

(A) uric acid, WBC
(B) CBC, liver enzymes
(C) T3 uptake, liver enzymes
(D) TSH, creatinine
(E) electrolytes, glucose

112. Hallmark features of narcolepsy include

(A) daytime "sleep attacks"
(B) cataplexy
(C) sleep paralysis
(D) hypnogogic hallucinations
(E) all the above

113. What diagnosis should be strongly suspected in an overweight, hypertensive, middle-aged male, who complains of sleepiness and whose wife complains that he snores:

(A) coronary artery disease
(B) chronic obstructive pulmonary disease
(C) obstructive sleep apnea syndrome
(D) major depression
(E) narcolepsy

114. Initial management of the acutely suicidal patient should include

(A) psychotherapy
(B) antidepressant medication
(C) hospitalization and close observation
(D) antianxiety medication
(E) electroconvulsive therapy (ECT)

115. All the following are true in cases of Lyme disease EXCEPT

(A) there is an expanding erythematous annular lesion
(B) the treatment of choice is trimethoprim/sulfamethoxazole
(C) it is the most commonly reported tick-borne disease in the United States
(D) it is a disease of stages if left untreated
(E) if arthritis develops, it primarily affects the knee joint

116. Two consecutive tuberculin skin tests are read in the same individual as negative and positive, respectively. He is considered a "true" converter. The following are true of a converter EXCEPT

(A) the tests were given within 2 years of each other
(B) the first test was 7 mm induration and the second test was 14 mm induration
(C) the person in considered newly infected
(D) chemoprophylaxis is not necessary if he is less than 25-years old and has a negative chest x-ray
(E) he should receive treatment prophylactically if he is a child less than 3 years old

117. Of all hepatitis infections, hepatitis B (HBV) has the "alphabet soup" of lab values. All the following are true regarding these values EXCEPT

(A) the surface antibody indicates past infection and is considered protective
(B) the core antibody IgG indicates infection even if the surface antigen is negative
(C) the E antigen in the presence of the surface antigen can indicate a greater likelihood for chronic disease
(D) the surface antigen is the first evidence of acute infection
(E) the core antigen is usually not detected in the serum by conventional lab methods

DIRECTIONS (Questions 118 and 119): Each group of items in this section consists of lettered headings followed by a set of numbered words or phrases. For each numbered word or phrase, select

A if the item is associated with (A) <u>only</u>,
B if the item is associated with (B) <u>only</u>,
C if the item is associated with <u>both</u> (A) <u>and</u> (B),
D if the item is associated with <u>neither</u> (A) <u>nor</u> (B).

(A) preoccupation with body size and weight
(B) binge eating accompanied by some extreme measure to prevent weight gain
(C) both
(D) neither

118. anorexia nervosa

119. bulemia nervosa

DIRECTIONS (Questions 120 through 129): For each of the items in this section, <u>ONE</u> or <u>MORE</u> of the numbered options is correct. Choose the answer

A if only <u>1, 2, and 3</u> are correct,
B if only <u>1 and 3</u> are correct,
C if only <u>2 and 4</u> are correct,
D if only <u>4</u> is correct,
E if <u>all</u> are correct.

120. Which of the following are frequently found in patients with osteoarthritis?

(1) Heberden's nodes
(2) swan-neck deformities of the fingers
(3) rest usually decreases joint discomfort in early stages
(4) morning stiffness

121. Signs of bacterial septic arthritis include which of the following?

(1) fever and chills
(2) slow insidious onset
(3) involves primarily large weight-bearing joints and the wrist
(4) usually is polyarticular

122. Which of the following are characteristic of rheumatoid arthritis?

(1) fatigue
(2) weakness
(3) morning stiffness
(4) frequently affects the DIP joints of the hand

123. Somatiform disorders are characterized by

(1) symptoms that suggest a physical ailment
(2) negative physical and laboratory findings
(3) a concomitant physical ailment
(4) intentional patient malingering

124. A major depressive episode is usually associated with which symptom(s) in addition to depressed mood?

(1) reduced ability to feel pleasure
(2) decreased interest in activities
(3) diminished energy
(4) insomnia, appetite changes, and feelings of guilt

125. The schizophrenic premorbid personality is often noticeable in childhood and adolescence and is distinguished by

(1) deficiency of social skills with development of small social network
(2) impaired self-confidence in relationships with the opposite sex
(3) episodes of neurotic-like illness such as anxiety, obsessions, and phobias
(4) a tendency to confine close relationships to family members

126. Psychosis is a symptom of an underlying disorder. When an acutely psychotic patient is encountered, the differential diagnosis should include

(1) acute drug reaction
(2) bipolar (manic/depressive) disorder
(3) major depression
(4) schizophrenia

127. Simple phobias must be distinguished from panic disorder and

(1) often cause panic attacks in public places
(2) consist of a persistent fear of a specific object
(3) generally result in marked impairment in functioning
(4) are very common in the general population

128. Imipramine (Tofranil) is a tricyclic antidepressant that commonly causes side effects including

(1) orthostatic hypotension
(2) dry mouth
(3) blurred vision
(4) diarrhea

129. The borderline personality is characterized by

(1) manipulative behavior including suicidal threats
(2) tempestuous interpersonal relationships
(3) impulsivity and frequent mood shifts
(4) persistent psychotic thinking

DIRECTIONS (Questions 130 through 142): Each of the numbered items or incomplete statements in this section is followed by answers or by completions of the statement. Select the ONE lettered answer or completion that is BEST in each case.

130. All the health problems listed below are commonly associated with homozygous sickle cell anemia EXCEPT

(A) cholelithiasis
(B) CHF
(C) aseptic necrosis of the femoral head
(D) gout

131. A 14-year-old anemic patient has the following findings: gallstones, mild icterus, splenomegaly, elevated reticulocyte count, and decreased serum haptoglobin, yet feels reasonably well. These findings most strongly suggest

(A) autoimmune hemolytic anemia
(B) von Willebrand's disease
(C) idiopathic hemochromatosis
(D) B_{12} deficiency
(E) hereditary spherocytosis

132. All the following statements regarding chronic lymphocytic leukemia (CLL) are true EXCEPT

(A) CLL and diffuse well-differentiated lymphocytic lymphoma are both neoplasms of B-cell origin and are so similar that they follow essentially the same clinical course
(B) CLL, which presents with massive splenomegaly, lymphadenopathy, and lymphocytosis has a median survival of 5 years
(C) combination chemotherapy for CLL is routinely initiated at the time of diagnosis in an attempt to achieve decreased tumor load and possible remission as early in the disease process as possible
(D) A Coombs ± hemolytic anemia occurs in up to 20% of patients with CLL
(E) patients who demonstrate anemia and/or thrombocytopenia at the time of diagnosis of CLL have a 2-year median survival.

133. A 55-year-old white female presents with non-specific complaints of anorexia, fatigue, hair loss, and dry skin. Physical exam reveals a pale, fair-skinned woman with dry skin, mild vertigo, and a beefy red tongue. Laboratory values reveal hypothyroidism and macrocytic anemia. Which of the anemias listed below is the most commonly associated with the findings above?

(A) anemia of chronic disease
(B) thalassemia minor

(C) folate deficiency
(D) pernicious anemia
(E) iron deficiency

134. A 50-year-old white male presents with complaints of increasing backache, fatigue, and weight loss of at least several weeks' duration, and acute onset 36 hours earlier of fever, loose cough, and dyspnea. Physical exam strongly suggests pneumonia (confirmed on x-ray), and also reveals pallor, petechiae on the face and legs, several recent bruises, mild hepatosplenomegaly, and several small palpable lymph nodes. The LEAST likely diagnosis is

(A) adult T-lymphocyte leukemia (ATL)
(B) aplastic anemia
(C) multiple myeloma
(D) acute myelogenous leukemia (AML)
(E) well-differentiated lymphocytic lymphoma

135. Target lesions are pathognomonic of

(A) erythema marginatum
(B) erythema multiforme
(C) erythema annulare
(D) erythema nodosum
(E) erythema gyratum repens

136. The most common skin cancer is

(A) squamous cell carcinoma (SCC)
(B) primary melanoma
(C) actinic keratosis (AK)
(D) keratoacanthoma
(E) basal cell carcinoma (BCC)

137. All the following are considered elevated lesions EXCEPT

(A) plaques
(B) macules
(C) wheals
(D) pustules
(E) scales

138. The drug of choice in treating uncomplicated erysipelas is

(A) tetracycline
(B) cephalothin
(C) vancomycin
(D) penicillin
(E) nafcillin

139. The LEAST likely symptom associated with acute pyelonephritis would be

(A) nausea and vomiting
(B) leukocytosis

(C) CVA tenderness or pain on deep abdominal palpation
(D) cystitis
(E) fever and chills

DIRECTIONS (Questions 140 through 142): Each group of items in this section consists of lettered headings followed by a set of numbered words or phrases. For each numbered word or phrase, select

A **if the item is associated with (A) only,**
B **if the item is associated with (B) only,**
C **if the item is associated with both (A) and (B),**
D **if the item is associated with neither (A) nor (B).**

(A) Lyme disease
(B) Rocky Mountain spotted fever

140. Bell's palsy is a neurological complication

141. tetracycline is the treatment of choice

142. vesicular lesions may develop as the disease progresses

DIRECTIONS (Questions 143 through 156): For each of the items in this section, ONE or MORE of the numbered options is correct. Choose the answer

A **if only 1, 2, and 3 are correct,**
B **if only 1 and 3 are correct,**
C **if only 2 and 4 are correct,**
D **if only 4 is correct,**
E **if all are correct.**

143. Which of the following are part of the treatment regimen for an acute episode of cystitis in pregnancy?

(1) repeat culture and sensitivity several days after therapy is complete
(2) ten-day course of antibiotic therapy
(3) repeat urine cultures periodically during remainder of prenatal course
(4) chronic suppressive therapy

144. Which of the following anatomical changes during pregnancy are responsible for a higher incidence of pyelonephritis in pregnant women?

(1) women with at least one previous pregnancy
(2) incomplete bladder emptying that predisposes to vesicoureteral reflux
(3) increased vascular supply to the bladder and ureters
(4) dilation of upper urinary tract; namely, hydronephrosis

145. After delivery of an RH positive baby to an RH negative mother, the mother is given a rhogam shot. When is rhogam also indicated in an Rh-negative mother?

(1) after an ectopic pregnancy
(2) following amniocentesis
(3) routinely at 28 weeks
(4) following spontaneous or induced abortion

146. A 21-year-old G 3 P 1011 female reveals at the time of her first prenatal visit that the father of her baby is an IV drug user. You advise her to be tested for acquired immune deficiency disease (AIDS) and the test results are positive. She is presently 10 weeks pregnant; what additional counselling/testing should you now perform?

(1) the patient should be advised to undergo immediate abortion because of the detrimental affects of pregnancy on AIDS
(2) she should be counselled about the likely possibility that she will transmit the AIDS virus to her baby
(3) she should be given antibiotic prophalaxis for *Pneumocystis carnii* pneumonia
(4) the patient should be tested for hepatitis B, gonorrhea, and *Chlamydia*

147. A patient is day 3 postoperative following a cesarean section. On two separate occasions her temperature has spiked to greater than 101°F. If the presumptive diagnosis is endomyometritis, which of the following are acceptable antibiotic therapies?

(1) ampicillin, gentamicin, and clindamycin
(2) penicillin and gentamicin
(3) a second or third generation cephalosporin
(4) ampicillin and doxycycline

148. A 34-year-old female has a Pap test result that showed CIN II or moderate dysplasia. Which of the following procedures could be performed next to further evaluate the abnormal Pap?

(1) simple hysterectomy
(2) cone biopsy
(3) antibiotic treatment for cervicitis
(4) colposcopic examination

149. A 35-year-old woman requests birth control pills. Before prescribing a combination estrogen/progesterone pill you must obtain a negative history of which of the following?

(1) previous deep vein thrombosis
(2) smoking
(3) ischemic heart disease
(4) migraine headache

SUMMARY OF DIRECTIONS				
(A)	**(B)**	**(C)**	**(D)**	**(E)**
1, 2, 3	**1, 3**	**2, 4**	**4**	**All are**
only	**only**	**only**	**only**	**correct**

150. A patient is considering permanent sterilization by tubal ligation. What important aspects of the procedure and complications should be explained during presurgical counselling?

   (1) the permanent nature of the procedure and poor outcome of reversal
   (2) the possibility of development of PID secondary to the procedure
   (3) the possibility of pregnancy after the procedure with a higher incidence of ectopic pregnancy
   (4) the possibility that menstrual irregularities may occur after the procedure

151. A couple comes to your office with a complaint of being unable to get pregnant. They have been attempting to conceive for greater than 1 year. Your history reveals that the woman has had an irregular menstrual cycle for many years and has had no previous pregnancy. Her husband denies having previously sired any children. After a thorough physical and pelvic exam, what would be the next steps in evaluating this couple's infertility?

   (1) the woman should be instructed to do a basal body temperature chart
   (2) the woman should undergo a hysterosalpingogram
   (3) the man should have a semen analysis performed
   (4) the woman should have a serum estriol drawn at approximately day 14 of her cycle

152. Varicella (chickenpox)

   (1) has an average incubation period of 14 days
   (2) cannot be transmitted through blood transfusions
   (3) is usually treated symptomatically
   (4) occurs only in children and young adults

153. Bullae on lower extremities include the following diagnosis

   (1) pemphigus vulgaris
   (2) epidermolysis bullosa aquisita (EBA)
   (3) bullous diabeticorum
   (4) bullous pemphigoid

154. Viral disease(s) occurring in children

   (1) rubella
   (2) rubeola
   (3) Kawasaki
   (4) scarlet fever

155. The risk of HIV transmission to health care workers

   (1) is greatly reduced when universal precautions are implemented
   (2) is lower than the risk of hepatitis B virus (HBV) transmission
   (3) is approximately 0.5% following a single needlestick exposure to blood from an HIV-infected patient
   (4) has been documented from exposure to body fluids other than blood, such as feces, sputum, urine, or vomitus

156. AIDS-associated Kaposi's sarcoma

   (1) may present in the lung as nodular infiltrates
   (2) is seen primarily in IV drug users
   (3) may respond to alpha-interferon administration
   (4) when treated with radiotherapy is associated with a high response rate and an improved prognosis

DIRECTIONS (Questions 157 through 169): Each of the numbered items or incomplete statements in this section is followed by answers or by completions of the statement. Select the ONE lettered answer or completion that is BEST in each case.

157. Which of the following tests is used initially to evaluate the presence of HIV infection in a patient?

   (A) HIV antibody status by ELISA
   (B) HIV serum p24 antigen status
   (C) HIV antibody status by Western Blot
   (D) T-lymphocyte subset studies
   (E) In vitro culture of HIV from patient's blood

158. All the following statements about patterns of HIV infection in the United States are true **EXCEPT**

   (A) the cumulative incidence of AIDS cases is disproportionately higher in blacks and Hispanics than in whites
   (B) the highest risk of HIV infection in pediatric patients occurs in children born to women who themselves are at risk of HIV infection
   (C) the percentage of reported AIDS cases in New York and San Francisco compared to the total United States population has gradually increased over time

(D) it is estimated that as of December 1988, 1.0 to 1.5 million people have been infected with HIV

(E) Estimates predict 365,000 AIDS cases by 1992 in the United States alone

159. All the following statements regarding PCP are true **EXCEPT**

(A) the definitive diagnosis is made by obtaining pneumocysts on silver stain of sputum, bronchial washings, or lung tissue
(B) it is the leading cause of death in AIDS patients
(C) it occurs in 80% to 90% of all AIDS patients
(D) treatment failure is defined as lack of clinical improvement after 3 days
(E) most AIDS patients will survive their first episode of PCP

160. Which of the following is the most sensitive indicator of bleeding tendency in a preoperative patient?

(A) prothrombin time (PT)
(B) partial thromboplastin time (PTT)
(C) platelet count
(D) fibrinogen
(E) history and physical

161. Ulcerative colitis most frequently involves the

(A) cecum
(B) ileum
(C) left colon
(D) right colon
(E) rectum

162. Chovstek and Trousseau signs can be seen in patients with

(A) hypercalcemia
(B) hypomagnesemia
(C) hypocalcemia
(D) hypermagnesemia
(E) hypophosphatemia

163. Which of the following is **NOT** associated with pancreatitis?

(A) alcohol
(B) gallstones
(C) hyperlipidemia
(D) carcinoma
(E) hyperparathyroidism

164. "Apple Core" lesions on barium enema are pathognomic for

(A) diverticulitis
(B) sigmoid volvulus
(C) Gardner's syndrome
(D) carcinoma of the colon
(E) villous adenoma

165. Name the correct sequence of events in thyroid hormone secretion.

(A) TSH—TRH—T_4—T_3
(B) TRH—TSH—T_3—T_4
(C) TRH—TSH—T_4—T_3
(D) TSH—TRH—T_3—T_4
(E) TRH—T_4—TSH—T_3

166. Pneumaturia is diagnostic of

(A) rectovaginal fistula
(B) colovesicular fistula
(C) diverticulitis
(D) carcinoma
(E) urinary tract infection

167. Which of the following operations for duodenal ulcer has the best morbidity and mortality?

(A) proximal gastric vagotomy
(B) partial gastrectomy
(C) truncal vagotomy and pyloroplasty
(D) truncal vagotomy and ontrectomy
(E) truncal vagotomy and gastrojejunostomy

168. What substance is secreted by the chief cells of the stomach?

(A) gastrin
(B) pepsin
(C) pepsinogen
(D) gastric acid
(E) glucagon

169. Hemorrhage complicating duodenal ulcer

(A) usually is massive secondary to penetration into the gastroduodenal artery
(B) is a more frequent complication than either obstruction or perforation
(C) requires gastric resection for its control
(D) can be controlled by endoscopic techniques with decreased mortality
(E) can be controlled with simple ligation without the risk of recurrent hemorrhage

DIRECTIONS (Questions 170 through 173): Each group of items in this section consists of lettered headings followed by a set of numbered words or phrases. For each numbered word or phrase, select the ONE lettered heading that is most closely associated with it. Each lettered heading may be selected once, more than once, or not at all.

(A) esophageal webbing
(B) traumatic esophageal rupture
(C) linear tearing of the gastroesophageal junction
(D) esophageal spasm
(E) associated with long-standing gastroesophageal reflux

170. Barrett's esophagus

171. Boerhaave's syndrome

172. Mallory–Weiss syndrome

173. Plummer–Vinson syndrome

DIRECTIONS (Questions 174 through 185): For each of the items in this section, <u>ONE</u> or <u>MORE</u> of the numbered options is correct. Choose the answer

    A if only <u>1, 2, and 3</u> are correct,
    B if only <u>1 and 3</u> are correct,
    C if only <u>2 and 4</u> are correct,
    D if only <u>4</u> is correct,
    E if <u>all</u> are correct.

174. Which of the following characteristics of gastric ulcers indicate the need for surgery?

(1) associated with a duodenal ulcer
(2) reappearance after a period of healing
(3) large size
(4) less than 30% healing after 3 weeks of medical therapy

175. What are the most common causes of large bowel obstruction?

(1) carcinoma
(2) volvulus
(3) diverticulitis
(4) ulcerative colitis

176. Parathyroid physiology is responsible for the metabolic regulation of

(1) calcium
(2) magnesium
(3) phosphorous
(4) chloride

177. Which of the following play(s) a prominent role in development of diverticulitis?

(1) sex
(2) diet
(3) familial history
(4) age

178. Which of the following regarding bilirubin is/are correct?

(1) bilirubin is formed mostly from the breakdown of hemoglobin
(2) once formed, bilirubin joins with albumin to form a stable protein pigment complex
(3) conjugated bilirubin is acted upon by bacteria in the intestine to produce urobilinogen and urobilin

(4) the hepatic parenchymal cell is a site of bilirubin conjugation with *glucoronic* acid

179. Which of the following physical findings is most likely to be associated with bowel obstruction?

(1) distention
(2) tenderness
(3) auscultatory "rushes"
(4) tympany upon percussion

180. When examining a patient suspected of sustaining vascular injury, the following should be of concern

(1) shock
(2) type of trauma
(3) fracture
(4) color of blood

181. Symptoms in classic stroke from unilateral carotid artery disease may include

(1) ipsilateral hemiplegia
(2) contralateral hemiplegia
(3) contralateral blindness
(4) ipsilateral blindness

182. A fusiform aneurysm

(1) is usually secondary to trauma
(2) is usually secondary to atherosclerosis
(3) can be caused by infection
(4) involves the entire circumference of the artery

183. For which of the disorders listed below is a pacemaker indicated?

(1) acquired heart block
(2) sick sinus syndrome
(3) Stokes–Adams attacks
(4) A–V disassociation

184. Which of the following tests are best used to differentiate between restrictive and obstructive pulmonary disease?

(1) total lung capacity
(2) ventilation–perfusion scanning
(3) forced expiratory volume in 1 second divided by the forced vital capacity
(4) chest x-ray

185. Which of the following are physical findings consistent with a consolidated pneumonia?

(1) rales
(2) increased vocal fremitus
(3) dullness with percussion
(4) decreased whispered pectoriloquy

DIRECTIONS (Questions 186 through 200): Each of the numbered items or incomplete statements in this section is followed by answers or by completions of the statement. Select the ONE lettered answer or completion that is BEST in each case.

186. Which of the following is in the correct order for frequency of occurrence in bronchogenic carcinoma starting with the most frequent and progressing to the least frequent cell type?

(A) adenocarcinoma, small cell anaplastic carcinoma, large cell carcinoma, epidermoid carcinoma
(B) epidermoid carcinoma, adenocarcinoma, large cell carcinoma, small cell anaplastic carcinoma
(C) small cell anaplastic carcinoma, large cell carcinoma, epidermoid carcinoma, adenocarcinoma
(D) small cell anaplastic carcinoma, adenocarcinoma, large cell carcinoma, epidermoid carcinoma
(E) large cell carcinoma, small cell carcinoma, adenocarcinoma, epidermoid carcinoma

187. Deep regular respirations with periods of apnea best describe which of the following?

(A) Cheyne–Stokes respiration
(B) Biots breathing
(C) Kussmaul respiration
(D) stridulous breathing
(E) apnea

188. A fifty-year-old male presents with a history of persistent cough, hemoptysis, and weight loss, and states he had "several lung infections" over the past 3 to 4 months. The patient is a 30-pack-year smoker and also complains of right shoulder and chest pain. The patient is afebrile, pale, and dyspneic with exertion. The chest x-ray suggests mediastinial widening and perihilar adenopathy.
Which of the following diagnosis is most consistent with the given history?

(A) bronchiectasis
(B) chronic obstructive pulmonary disease (COPD)
(C) chronic bronchitis
(D) asthma
(E) bronchogenic carcinoma

189. A 19-year-old female is involved in an automobile accident; she is hospitalized with a fractured femur, her past medical history is unremarkable. The patient suddenly develops dyspnea, cough, anxiety with retrosternal lateralized chest pain. Vital signs are pulse: 120, respiration: 32, blood pressure: 120/80, Temperature: 100.1°F. Chest x-ray shows

mild bilateral atelectasis and the EKG is normal. The most likely diagnosis is which of the following?

(A) pneumonia
(B) myocardial infarction
(C) pulmonary embolism
(D) costochondritis with hyperventilation
(E) unrecognized pneumothorax

190. Which agent provides the most rapid effect and best therapeutic index in the treatment of asthma?

(A) inhaled beta-adrenergic agonist medication
(B) subcutaneous epinephrine
(C) IV aminophyllin
(D) hydrocortisone
(E) oral aminophyllin

191. Of the following, which is the best of all clinical respiratory measurements for assessing the progress of various types of pulmonary fibrotic diseases?

(A) arterial blood gases
(B) vital capacity
(C) inspiratory reserve volume
(D) total lung capacity
(E) tidal volume

192. The most reliable physical finding in acute appendicitis is

(A) hyperesthesia of the skin overlying the right lower quadrant
(B) localized right lower quadrant tenderness
(C) tenderness on rectal examination
(D) psoas sign
(E) all the above are equally reliable

193. Which study is most accurate in confirming the diagnosis of venous thrombosis and the extent of involvement?

(A) impedance plethysmography
(B) ultrasound
(C) ultrasound and real-time B-mode imaging
(D) radiolabeled fibrinogen
(E) venography

194. Bilateral nonpitting edema is associated with

(A) cardiac disease
(B) lymphedema
(C) renal disease
(D) cirrhosis
(E) venous disease

195. Which arteriosclerotic aneurysm is most common?

(A) abdominal aortic aneurysm
(B) carotid artery aneurysm
(C) popliteal aneurysm
(D) femoral aneurysm
(E) subclavian artery aneurysm

196. Frequent causes of cardiac arrest or fibrillation include all the following **EXCEPT**

    (A) acute myocardial infarction
    (B) a serum potassium of 5.0 mEq/L
    (C) anoxia
    (D) a serum potassium of 7.0 mEq/L
    (E) drugs

197. Which of the following statements regarding bladder cancer is true?

    (A) its most common histology is adenocarcinoma
    (B) its most common presenting symptom is painless hematuria
    (C) early pulmonary metastases are characteristic
    (D) its most common presenting symptom is urinary retention
    (E) surgery is the only effective treatment

198. All the following statements about intermittent claudication are correct **EXCEPT**

    (A) it is the most common complaint produced by limb ischemia
    (B) the onset of pain occurs at rest
    (C) the onset of pain occurs during exertion
    (D) the cessation of pain occurs after rest
    (E) the symptoms may remain stable for years or improve

199. What is the site of the most common form of extracranial vascular disease?

    (A) external carotid artery
    (B) common carotid artery
    (C) internal carotid artery
    (D) subclavian artery
    (E) vertebral artery

200. Which congenital defect is most often recognized at birth or on the first day of life and is lethal if not corrected?

    (A) tetralogy of Fallot
    (B) transposition of the great vessels
    (C) patent ductus arteriosus
    (D) atrial septal defect
    (E) ventricular septal defect

Answers and Explanations

1. **(E)** Hypercalcemia may have numerous etiologies. Primary hyperparathyroidism, a common cause for hypercalcemia, stimulates 1,25 90H$_2$ D3 generation (which increases gastrointestinal (GI) tract calcium absorption), enhances renal calcium reabsorption, and helps mobilize calcium from bone. Approximately 20% of patients with thyrotoxicosis will have hypercalcemia secondary to direct thyroid hormone-induced bone turnover and resorption. Humoral hypercalcemia of malignancy releases a humoral substance from the malignant cells (usually squamous cancer) that enhances bone resorption. Thiazide-induced hypercalcemia may be due to increased GI calcium absorption, enhanced renal calcium recovery, stimulation of parathyroid hyperplasia, and increased bone resorption. *(Felig et al, pp. 1376–1413)*

2. **(E)** A variety of treatments are available for hyperthyroidism. Steroids can decrease TSH production and acutely decrease T$_4$ release and are of value in thyroid storm. Lithium can inhibit T$_4$ release from the gland but is rarely used as an antithyroid drug. Propylthiouracil (PTU) causes iodination defects and prevents T$_4$ to T$_3$ conversion in the periphery. Methimazole (Tapazole) causes decreased secretion of T$_4$ and organification defects of the thyroid gland, but lacks the peripheral effects of PTU. PTU and methimazole are the two most common antithyroid drugs. *(Felig et al, p. 416)*

3. **(A)** Myopathy commonly ensues after long-term steroid therapy. Cataract and osteoporosis (especially that of trabecular bone) are common side effects of steroid therapy. Steroids cause growth retardation, not growth spurts. *(Felig et al, p. 793)*

4. **(E)** The list for etiologic causes for osteoporosis is quite lengthy and includes all the listed answers. Low estrogen levels accelerate bone loss as well as thyrotoxicosis. Elevated steroid levels seen with Cushing's inhibits calcium absorption and directly affect bone formation. Alcohol is toxic to the bone and marrow. *(Felig et al, p. 1471)*

5. **(E)** Polyuria occurs with uncontrolled diabetes mellitus, as glucose acts as an osmotic agent. Polydipsia is due to dehydration and hyperosmolarity. Ketosis is due to the absence of insulin and fat breakdown. Blurry vision is a manifestation of corneal fluid shifts with changing serum glucose levels, especially with high glucose levels. *(Cahill et al, p. 7)*

6. **(D)** Twenty-four hour collection for catecholamines (fractionated for epinephrine or nonepinephrine totals) would help in the diagnosis towards pheochromocytoma. The laboratory diagnosis can at times be quite difficult. Urine collections for 24 hours for metanephrines or VMA can be used, serum levels cannot. Assay for prostaglandins would not be of benefit. *(Felig et al, pp. 668–671)*

7. **(A)** Hypocalcemia will present with a variety of clinical manifestations including cramps, tingling, overt tetany, seizures, irritability, poor concentration, learning disability, psychosis, and occasionally extrapyramidal symptoms. On physical exam, the Chovstek's sign (twitching of lips produced by tapping the facial nerve) and Trousseau's sign (hand tetany or carpopedal spasm, induced by inflating a blood pressure cuff 20 mm Hg above systolic BP for 3 minutes) are positive. *(Felig et al, p. 1422)*

8. **(D)** Normal serum calcium level is usually 8.5 to 10.5 mg/dL (can change to mmd/L by dividing by 4.0). Approximately 40% of serum calcium is bound to protein and 50% is free or ionized. Serum calcium level needs to be corrected for the low albumin. Thus, for each drop in albumin of 1.0, the calcium level should be corrected upward by 0.8 mg/dL. The simplest calculation, total serum calcium minus albumin, is equal to the corrected total serum calcium. Thus, for answer D it would be $(10 - 2) + 4 = 12$ mg/dL, which is hypercalcemic. *(Felig et al, p. 1363)*

9. **(C)** Low- or high-dose dexamethasone suppression test can be used to help in the diagnosis of Cushing's disease. One milligram of dexamethasone is given at 11 AM and a 6 AM serum cortisol should be <5.0 because the circadian rhythm will have been blocked by the dexamethasone. The absence of ACTH release will then prevent the early morning rise of cortisol. A serum cortisol level of >5.0 implies absence of the blockade; ACTH is then released even in the presence of dexamethasone and that is suggestive of Cushing's disease. The test has no useful purpose for Addison's, Graves, or rheumatoid arthritis. Reidel's disease does not exist, although there is a Reidel's thyroiditis. *(Felig et al, p. 575)*

10. **(D)** Cystine, oxalate (as calcium oxalate) magnesium (as magnesium ammonia phosphate) and calcium phosphate are components of renal stones. Purine is not a urinary stone component. Purine is a nucleic acid that has uric acid as a metabolic end product. *(Felig et al, p. 1506)*

11. **(B)** Hirsutism occurs with increased adrenal androgen production. Cushing's syndrome will result in excess androgen formation. Other symptoms include myopathy with weakness, obesity, thin skin with easy bruising, and large striae. *(Felig et al, p. 607)*

12. **(A)** High density lipoprotein is associated with decreased atherosclerosis and is thus felt to be protection against heart disease. It helps remove LDL (low density lipoproteins) from the circulation. Elevated HDLs are usually not seen in patients who consume diets high in saturated fats. *(Felig et al, pp. 1274, 1280–1282)*

13. **(C)** Paget's disease is an active bone lesion in which large amounts of bone are broken down by osteoclasts and new unorganized weaker bone is layed down. Treatment with calcitonin or diphosphonates can be quite helpful to patients with Paget's. *(Felig et al, pp. 1487–1491)*

14. **(D)** The peak action of NPH insulin is between 6 to 14 hours. Regular insulin will peak within 2 to 4 hours. The combination of these agents can provide for uniformly stable glucose levels. *(Felig et al, p. 1132)*

15. **(B)** Glycohemoglobin (HbA1c) is an assay that allows for measurement of diabetic control over longer periods of time. Glucose can alter the hemoglobin molecule in a nonenzymatic fashion, thus, constant high glucose will increase the HbA1c level and suggest hyperglycemic episodes. Improving glucose control will gradually decrease the HbA1c level over 1 to 2 weeks. *(Felig et al, p. 1112)*

16. **(B)** Antihistamines possess anticholinergic activity that may be harmful to patients with enlarged prostate and those with acute narrow-angle glaucoma. They may also be contraindicated in patients with asthma. Data supporting this are not uniformly agreed upon. *(Goodman and Gilman, pp. 605–624)*

17. **(C)** Nadolol is a beta-adrenergic blocking agent, and in blocking beta receptors in the lungs, bronchoconstriction results. Theophylline, albuterol and terbutaline cause brochodilation, whereas cromolyn is used prophylactically in the treatment of asthma. Cromolyn inhibits both the immediate and nonimmediate bronchoconstrictive reactions to inhaled antigens. *(Goodman and Gilman, pp. 589–600, 616–618, 176–177)*

18. **(B)** Absence or petit mal seizures differ considerably from generalized or grand mal seizures. They occur most frequently in children; the attacks are of short duration and consist of syncope or temporary clouding of consciousness during which the individual may stare blankly or exhibit minor movement of the head and limbs. Ethosuximide and valproic acid are generally used to control absence seizures. Diazepam is used in controlling acute grand mal seizures. *(Goodman and Gilman, p. 461; Silver et al, p. 139)*

19. **(E)** The exact mechanism of antimigraine action of beta blockers has not been proven, although abundant evidence supports their beneficial effects. Vicodin is a combination of hydrocodone and acetaminophen, both analgesics with additive effects. Hydrocodone, a narcotic, suppresses the affective component of pain. Midrin is also a combination product containing acetaminophen plus a sympathomimetic amine that acts by constricting dilated cranial and cerebral arterioles. Sansert is methylsergide that inhibits the effects of serotonin, a substance possibly involved in the mechanism of vascular headaches. *(Stein, pp. 2183–2184)*

20. **(C)** An adult with no history of seizure disorder should be evaluated for all potential causes of seizures. A CT scan can rule out a mass lesion or lesions that may present with seizure. A primary lung cancer seen on chest radiograph may alter the treatment regimen of cerebral metastases. Severe hypoglycemia induces seizures and is readily treatable, as are other metabolic abnormalities. Seizures secondary to cerebral lesions of AIDS are rarely a presenting symptom. The CT scan will detect the lesions. HIV testing may add information but is not necessary for diagnosis of the space occupying lesion. *(Weiner and Goetz, pp. 86–90; Braunwald et al, pp. 1921–1926)*

21. **(B)** Pain is the most common symptom of spinal cord metastases. The pain is frequently well localized but may be radicular in nature. Pain may precede the onset of neurologic symptoms by several weeks. The goal is to formulate the diagnosis and begin treatment prior to neurologic deficit. *(Weiner and Goetz, pp. 254–255; Braunwald et al, p. 2042)*

22. **(D)** Many factors may be involved early, including drug and alcohol abuse, which are common in traumatic injuries. Seizures may occur acutely with serious head injury and become chronic, but chronicity cannot be predicted accurately. Seizures within the first 24 hours may indicate focality but also may result from generalized injury. Thus, the presence or absence of a seizure or seizures in the immediate acute phase of head trauma is not, in and of itself, prognostic. *(Weiner and Goetz, p. 224; Braunwald et al, p. 1924–1925)*

23. **(E)** Hematuria, presence of blood in the urine, may be occult or gross. It may result from trauma, bleeding disorders, infections, stones, glomerular disease, or neoplasm. It generally denotes structural genitourinary disease. Its relationship to voiding, onset, and red blood cell morphology may indicate location and type of lesion. It is usually not painful except when large clots are produced. *(Andreoli et al, p. 484)*

24. **(E)** Hyperchloremic acidosis results from impaired renal excretion of acid and decreased serum bicarbonate. Sulfate and phosphate are excreted normally and there is also increased reabsorption of chloride ions. This form of metabolic acidosis is due to renal insufficiency and results in an increase in the normal anion gap. *(Cox and Kathpolia, p. 1208)*

25. **(D)** Acute pyelonephritis is associated with nausea, vomiting, fever, chills, flank pain, leukocytosis, costovertebral angle tenderness, or pain on deep palpation of the abdomen. The patient may or may not have the classic symptoms of cystitis such as frequency and dysuria. Acute pyelonephritis frequently requires hospital admission and IV antibiotics. *(Stamm and Turck, pp. 1191–1192)*

26. **(B)** Cooling an amputated part will extend the time to successful replantation from 6 to 12 hours. The amputated part should not be placed directly on ice. Attempts to cannulate or ligate exposed vessels may cause serious initimal damage. The amputated part should be placed in a bag of lactated Ringer's solution, then placed on ice. *(Urbaniak, pp. 1653–1654)*

27. **(D)** Direct pressure to the bleeding site is the most effective method of controlling hemorrhage in the acute setting. Tourniquets can cause distal ischemia. The use of clamps in the acute setting is discouraged, as damage may be done to associated neural structures. *(Committee on Trauma, ACS; p. 15)*

28. **(A)** Hypovolemic shock is best treated by rapid infusion of 2 L of lactated Ringer's solution delivered via large-bore peripheral IVs. The bolus of lactated Ringer's solution serves as both a treatment as well as diagnostic movement to access the patient's response. Large-bore peripheral catheters are easy to insert and have flow characteristics sufficient to deliver large volumes of fluid. Central venous lines are time consuming to insert, carry with them some morbidity, and do not allow for rapid fluid delivery. Type-specific blood is the preferred form of urgent blood replacement. *(Committee on Trauma, ACS; p. 5)*

29. **(A)** Peristaltic abdominal pain, nausea, and vomiting as well as abdominal distention are all closely associated with small bowel obstruction. These patients may also report an *absence* of flatus and bowel movements. *(Beal, p. 891)*

30. **(A)** Cholecystitis is obstruction of the cystic duct or ampulla of the gallbladder usually due to an impacted stone. This leads to ischemia, edema, and necrosis of the gallbladder wall. Plain films will show only a small percentage of radiopaque gallstones, but may help rule out other processes. Ultrasonography will detect the presence of gallstones, but gives only suggestive evidence as to the presence of obstruction. HIDA scans have a high degree of accuracy in demonstrating the presence or absence of flow through the gallbladder, cystic duct, and into the duodenum. HIDA scans should be considered the gold standard in the diagnosis of this entity. Oral cholecystograms are a poor choice in this setting as the nausea and vomiting that accompany this condition prevent absorption of the contrast material. *(Beal, p. 885)*

31. **(E)** Acute mesenteric ischemia often follows periods of hypotension from myocardial infarctions, arrhythmias, major trauma, sepsis, etc. There is often a discrepancy between a relatively benign physical exam and complaints of severe pain. This is due to the fact that initial colon damage is limited to the mucosa with peritoneal signs developing only after progression to transmural bowel infarction. *(Williams, p. 474)*

32. **(E)** These symptoms are often referred to as the "5P's." Pallor is the result of peripheral vasconstriction. Paresthesias and paralysis are due to severe nerve and muscle ischemia. Pulselessness may be an acute event or a chronic manifestation of peripheral vascular disease. Pain is often continuous and severe, its onset accurately marking the time of the occlusion. *(Simmerman and Fogarty, pp. 698–699)*

33. **(E)** Any patient who is immunosuppressed or exhibits signs of systemic toxicity requires oral broad-spectrum antibiotics. These patients will require close observation. If erythema and swelling increase, admission for IV antibiotics should be considered. *(Warren, p. 983)*

34. **(E)** Perirectal abscesses are formed by communication with the rectosigmoid colon. When these abscesses drain spontaneously they form fistulas-in-ano. These abscesses should be explored under general anesthesia, as they can be quite extensive and require adequate drainage. *(Warren, p. 992)*

35. **(A)** Mandibular fractures will often produce malocclusion and pain upon opening of the mouth. Broken teeth are often seen. "Raccoon's eyes" and rhinorrhea are indicative of severe midface injury as is often seen in maxillary or nasoethmoid fractures. *(Georgiade and Manstein, pp. 411–412)*

36. **(B)** Splinting of the body part involved and the use of adhesive strips do little to reduce wound edge tension. The most effective measures are undermining soft tissues to gain length and closure of the wound in layers. *(Lammers, pp. 478–530)*

37. **(C)** Burn wounds are characterized by the depth of tissue penetration achieved by the thermal force (Fig. 5–1). Wounds are classified as partial thickness superficial, partial thickness deep, and full thickness. Partial-thickness superficial wounds occur when only the epidermis and superficial dermal elements are involved. Partial-thickness deep wounds penetrate through the epidermis and into the middermis. These wounds are characterized by blister formation and intense pain. These wounds will heal spontaneously. Full-thickness wounds occur with destruction of all epidermal and dermal cells. These wounds have a dry, pearly white, or charred black appearance. They are insensitive to pin prick. They will not heal spontaneously, but will require skin grafting. *(Zawacki, pp. 26–27)*

38. **(E)** Circumferential casts that are too tight produce increasing pain, swelling, coolness, decreasing capillary refill, and pain on passive extension of the digits. In this case, the cast should be split, including the cast padding, and wrapped with an elastic bandage. This maintains immobility of the involved extremity while restoring circulation. *(Simon, pp. 13–14)*

39. **(A)** The important issue this question raises is the role of abdominal CT scanning in multisystem trauma. The issue in question for the ER personnel is whether or not the multiply injured patient has significant bleeding, (thus requiring exploration), not the specific organ involved. CT scanning of the abdomen and pelvis should be reserved for the stable patient with unisystem injury. Multiinjured patients should have peritoneal lavage performed as a quick, specific screening test for hemoperitoneum. *(Committee on Trauma, ACS; pp. 117–118)*

40. **(D)** Acetaminophen toxicity can be divided into four stages:

    Stage I—mild, easily dismissed symptoms lasting up to 24 hours
    Stage II—RUQ pain and tenderness, elevation of LFTs, oliguria lasting 24 to 48 hours
    Stage III—Peak liver function abnormalities, occasional complete liver failure with hepatorenal syndrome, anorexia, nausea, and/or vomiting lasting 72 to 96 hours
    Stage IV—Resolution of hepatic insufficiency 4 days to 2 weeks

    A high arylating mebatolite of acetaminophen is formed during its metabolism that binds to hepatocytes and causes hepatic necrosis. The minimum dose capable of causing hepatic toxicity is estimated to be 140 mg/kg in children and 7.5 g in adults. *(Linden and Romack, p. 721)*

41. **(A)** Hypoxemia is the primary pathophysiologic event in carbon monoxide (CO) poisoning. CO acts as a competitive inhibitor of oxygen binding by coupling with hemoglobin. The affinity of CO for hemoglobin is 240 times greater than that of oxygen. Myocardial depression is seen in CO poisoning as a function of hypoxemia. Bronchospasm and surfactant inhibition are not characteristics of this disorder. *(Reisdoff and Wiegenstein, pp. 809–810)*

42. **(A)** The proper sequence of two-person CPR is one ventilation per 5 compressions. A brief pause is made in compressions to allow for adequate ventilation. All PAs should be familiar with current American Heart Association CPR recommendations. *(Standards and Guidelines, JAMA, pp. 2905–2984)*

43. **(D)** Multisystem trauma accounts for more deaths in persons aged 1 to 33 years than all other diseases *combined*. Trauma is the leading cause of death for all persons aged 1 to 44 years. *(Baker et al, p. 313)*

44. **(C)** The anterior cruciate ligaments are intracapsular structures that prevent anterior/posterior dislocation of the tibia upon the femur. These ligaments insert onto the inner sides of the femoral condyles. Backward movement of the tibia upon the femur is indicative of posterior cruciate ligament tears. Medial collateral ligament tears would best be demonstrated by valgus stress, lateral ligaments by varus stress. *(Hoppenfeld, pp. 186–187)*

45. (A) Pelvic fractures are exceeded only by skull fractures in terms of associated complications and mortality. Pubic rami and pubic bone fractures account for 70% of all pelvic fractures and are often associated with genitourinary trauma. All patients with pelvic fractures should be assumed to have a urethral or bladder laceration until proven otherwise. Displaced fractures that disrupt the pelvic ring always should be assumed to have associated fractures and fracture dislocations. Up to 50% of patients have a transfusion requirement in association with pelvic injuries. *(Simon, pp. 196–197)*

46. (D) Neoplastic diseases of the musculoskeletal system constitute a serious problem because of the generally poor prognosis of malignant neoplasms in these areas, thus making A an incorrect choice. Those listed under B, osteoblastomas and giant cell tumors, are examples of benign neoplasms and as so are not an appropriate response when discussing the general topic of malignant neoplasms. C is false because these malignant neoplasms frequently require surgical excision and E is incorrect because these tumors commonly metastasize. The only correct choice is D, in that malignant neoplasms commonly include pain as a prominent clinical feature. *(Kempe et al, pp. 624–625)*

47. (B) The most common types of child abuse and neglect seen by physicians are approximately 70%, physical abuse; 25%, sexual abuse; and 5%, failure to thrive due to underfeeding. Emotional abuse and neglect may actually be more common, but children are rarely brought to health care providers with symptoms of these diagnoses as a chief complaint. *(Behrman et al, p. 79)*

48. (C) *S pneumoniae* accounts for 30% of organisms cultured from effusions. Group A beta strep and *S aureus* occur in 5%. *E coli* occurs in neonates along with other gram-negative bacilli in about 20% of effusions. *S aureus* occurs 5% of the time and *B catarrhalis*, 20%. *(Behrman et al, p. 880)*

49. (D) The correct response to this question is D because asthmatic children do present with these listed findings. A is false because 80% to 90% of asthmatic children have their first symptoms before age 4 to 5 years. B is false because, generally, asthmatic children have a favorable prognosis and respond to treatment. C is false because pharmacologic therapy is the mainstay of treatment for asthma. There are numerous pharmacologic agents used alone or in combination for effectively relieving the signs and symptoms of asthma. E is false because a wheeze is the hallmark sign on physical exam that is associated with asthma; rales is more typical of pneumonia. *(Behrman et al, pp. 495–500)*

50. (C) Cardiopulmonary arrest in the pediatric patient is primarily a result of respiratory difficulties resulting from obstruction and hypoxia. Patency of airway should be the first priority of treatment once it is established that the patient is unresponsive or having respiratory difficulty. Airways may be established by the head tilt and chin lift method or by gently lifting the occiput of the head off the bed or surface by a towel or hand under the occiput and placing the patient in the "sniffing position." Breathing and circulation should then be evaluated and cardiac monitors and IVs should be initiated if initial attempts at CPR are ineffective. *(Barkin, pp. 10–19)*

51. (A) Scald burns are the most common burn in children. Flame burns are more common in older children who play with matches or flammable material. *(Barkin, p. 237)*

52. (C) A type I epiphyseal fracture is a separation of the epiphysis from the metaphysis without displacement or damage to the growth plate. A type II involves slippage of the growth plate with a fracture into the metaphysis of the bone. Type III fracture involves a slippage of the growth plate with a fracture of the epiphysis. Type IV is an intraarticular fracture involving the epiphysis, metaphysis, and epiphyseal plate. Type V is a crush injury to the epiphyseal plate. The higher the number, the more likely there will be a growth disturbance due to the injury. Types III, IV, and V often require surgical reduction. *(Barkin, pp. 391–392)*

53. (A) Meckel's diverticulum presents with painless rectal bleeding 40% to 60% of the time. It may cause intestinal obstruction, intussusception, herniation, volvulus, or diverticulitis. Anal fissures are slit-like tears in the anal canal and are usually secondary to passage of large hard stools. Small amounts of bright red blood may be noted on the stool after defecation. Without a history of pain on defecation, other causes of rectal bleeding should be ruled out. Juvenile polyps are always benign, are rare before age 1 and are seen most commonly between 3 to 5 years of age. They present with small amounts of bright blood in the stools, intermittent melena, and painless occult GI bleeding with anemia in previously healthy children. Polyps may act as a lead point for intussusception. Intussusception is marked by sporadic severe abdominal pain, stools with notable blood and mucus, and vomiting. *(Kempe et al, pp. 529–542)*

54. (E) All this information is true. Metabolic abnormalities such as hypoglycemia, hypernatremia, hyponatremia, hypocalcemia, and hypomagnesemia should be considered, as anticonvulsants may be ineffective in the presence of metabolic abnormalities. Respiratory status should be monitored with the use of IV anticonvulsants. *(Barkin, pp. 132–134)*

55. **(C)** The avulsed tooth may be rinsed but not scrubbed because this will remove the cementum that is very important in the success of the tooth reimplantation. Placing the tooth back into the socket or under the tongue is acceptable, gauze will dry out the tooth and decrease success of reimplantation. The dentist should be seen as soon as possible for splinting the tooth in place. *(Barkin, p. 342)*

56. **(E)** Beta hemolytic *Streptococcus* must be considered in the differential, although the finding of a nontender node would tend to "rule-out" this diagnosis. Malignancies are higher on the list of possibilities. The most common site for presentation of Hodgkin's disease is in the cervical glands. The enlargement is firm, nontender, discrete, and may involve one or more nodes. Cat scratch fever usually presents with enlarged, tender nodes within 2 weeks of the primary lesion. The axillary and epitrochlear nodes are most often involved, followed by the cervical nodes. The etiologic agent is believed to be a small gram-negative bacilli. Cat scratch disease is usually self-limiting. Infection with atypical mycobacterium species often presents in 1- to 5-year old children who have no history of exposure to tuberculosis and usually lack systemic symptoms, although fever has been associated with the disease. Excision of the node is curative in 95% of lesions and is the treatment of choice. *(Behrman et al, pp. 640, 710, 1089)*

57. **(D)** The poison control number should be called after determining the amount of the ingested substance. The dose of Syrup of Ipecac is 10 mL, less than 1 year of age; 15 mL; 1 to 12 years; 30 mL, more than 12 years of age. A repeat dose may be given after 20 minutes. Ipecac should not be given to a comatose person or a person with no gag reflex. Serum acetaminophen levels should be drawn at 4 hours postingestion and level of toxicity may be determined by a nomogram. Activated charcoal should not be administered because it inactivates the antidote that is N-acetylcystiene. *(Barkin, p. 279; Handbook/Poisonings, p. 22)*

58. **(A)** Many cases of physical abuse are first suspected because the injury is unexplained, or more commonly an explanation is offered, but is implausible. Often, there are inconsistencies between the history given of a minor accident and the physical findings of a major injury, or between the history and the child's developmental levels, (i.e., a 6-month old baby could not have turned on a hot water faucet that caused burns). In true accidents

parents normally bring their injured children in immediately for examination. Studies have shown that 40% of abused children are not brought to medical attention until the morning after the injury, and another 40% not until 1 to 4 days later. Parents whose children have suffered an accident frequently exhibit a greater degree of emotional turmoil and guilt than do abusive parents. *(Behrman et al, p. 80)*

59. **(A)** The reported rates of adverse reactions are pain at the site, 51%; swelling, 8.9%; fever greater than 38°C, 47%; anorexia, 21%; and vomiting, 6%. Febrile convulsions occur after 0.06% of doses. *(Red Book, p. 321)*

60. **(B)** *H influenzae* is a frequent cause of otitis media, but unencapsulated nontypeable strains are recovered and HIB is very uncommon. Meningitis and epiglottitis are frequent manifestations of systemic HIB infection. Urinary tract infection due to HIB is rare. *(Dajani et al, p. 360)*

61. **(E)** The peak incidence of acute otitis media occurs in the second half of the first year with a second but lower peak between ages 4 and 5. In this study, by age 1, 62.4% of children had more than one episode of acute otitis media and by age 3, 83% of children had experienced acute otitis media at least once. The mean number of incidents of otitis media declined from 1.2 per child during year 1 to 0.4 per child in year 7. *(Teele et al, p. 83)*

62. **(B)** In a girl, puberty is considered delayed if there is no sign of it by age 13. Puberty in a female is considered precocious if it occurs prior to age 8, so breast development prior to age 8 is considered premature thelarche. Puberty in males is *not* delayed until after age 14½. *(Copeland et al, p. 24)*

63. **(B)** Human milk has as two of its many advantages secretory IgA and epidermal growth factor, neither of which is available through commercially prepared formulas. Human milk, however, is lower in vitamin D and has less iron than does formulas. The iron in breast milk is well absorbed by the infant and iron stores are adequate for the first 6 to 9 months in term infants. Premature infants or infants not exposed to sunlight should be supplemented with vitamin D. *(Merenstein et al, pp. 77, 203; Behrman et al, p. 153)*

64. **(B)** The DDST can provide a profile of developmental progress and a means of identifying abnormal delays during infancy and the preschool years. Number 1 is true with the emphasis that the DDST is a screening instrument, not a diagnostic means. Number 3 is true with the emphasis on progressive sequence of developmental tasks that include the

listed areas. Number 2 is incorrect because the DDST is not designed to be an intelligence test; number 4 is incorrect because the DDST in fact is administered easily and quickly without extensive testing material. *(Kempe et al, pp. 33–34)*

65. **(B)** The Apgar method is a practical means for evaluating the status of a newborn infant. Number 1, a score of 0 to 10, is assigned to the newborn at both 1 and 5 minutes. Number 3, there are 5 objective signs evaluated: heartrate, respiratory effort, muscle tone, response to facial irritation, and color. Number 2 is incorrect because it is the 5-minute score that is more predictive of death, neurologic residual, and long-term outcome. However, the 1-minute score is an index of asphyxia and of the need for assisted ventilation. Number 4 is incorrect because each of the five signs receives a possible two points, making a total score of ten the indication of an infant in the best possible condition. *(Behrman et al, pp. 362–363)*

66. **(B)** A Grade I–III, systolic murmur that varies in position, intensity, and activity is present in at least 50% of children. The murmur does not have an associated abnormality of the 2nd heart sound. A click is associated with semilunar valvular lesions. *(Avery et al, pp. 304–305)*

67. **(E)** Pityriasis rosea is a common eruption that is thought to be viral in etiology. It is heralded by a patch that is large (1 to 10 cm in diameter) somewhere on the body, often on the chest or upper extremity. In a few days, multiple raised pink lesions appear, mostly on the trunk, but can involve most of the body. The patient is asymptomatic except for mild pruritus. The lesions last from 2 weeks to 3 months. *(Behrman et al, p. 1412)*

68. **(A)** Lichen sclerosis et atrophicus is a skin disorder characterized by white atrophic, thinning of the skin in a figure-eight pattern around the anus and vagina. Excoriations and secondary infections may occur. *(Behrman et al, p. 1418)*

69. **(D)** Tuberous sclerosis is a dominantly inherited condition that causes mental deficiency and intractable convulsions. There are characteristic cerebral lesions throughout the cortical gray matter. Calcium is often deposited in these lesions and may be visible on x-ray. The most characteristic skin lesion is adenoma sebaceum, which consists of small red or brownish nodules in a butterfly distribution on the nose and cheeks. The lesions appear between 2 and 5 years of age and by late childhood are found in 80% of patients. *(Behrman et al, p. 1309)*

70. **(C)** Chronic eczema is characterized by thickened, dry, and scaly lesions with coarse skin markings, lichenification, and altered pigmentation. *(Behrman et al, p. 1404)*

71. **(E)** The loop of Henle lies between the proximal and distal convoluted tubules. The thick ascending limb rises toward the collecting ducts that later form the ureters. This limb of the loop absorbs sodium chloride quickly, causing a decreased serum osmolality and the tubular fluid concentration of sodium drops to 30 mmol/L. The voltage across the lumen becomes positive because of the addition of Na^+ and flux of H^+. The tubular fluid becomes dilute due to Na loss. However, the concentration of fluid increases in the distal loop when it passes through this region. *(Kelly's Textbook, pp. 733–734)*

72. **(E)** Scleroderma (progressive systemic sclerosis) is associated with 40% to 50% of all death resulting from renal failure. It closely resembles accelerated nephrosclerosis, usually appears in the third to fifth decade, and renal involvement is rarely the presenting symptom. It is a multiorgan disease that also attacks the heart, lungs, colon, jejunum, and ileum. Dysphagia occurs in 90% of patients. There are petechial hemorrhages, wedge-shaped cortical infarcts in the kidney, and diffuse thickening of the skin with telangiectasia and variable pigmentation. *(Harrison's Principles of Internal Medicine, p. 1202)*

73. **(B)** In adult polycystic kidney disease, there are cortical and medullary cysts. There are also hepatic and intracranial ("berry") aneurysms found during work-up. It is an autosomal dominant disease that can also involve the pancreas. Uremia develops slowly and these patients generally live longer than those with other causes of renal insufficiency. *(Harrison's Principles of Internal Medicine, p. 1206)*

74. **(B)** The normal range for serum osmolality is 285 to 295 mOsm/L. It is calculated by

$$2(Na \text{ mmol/L}) + glucose \text{ mmol/L} + BUN \text{ mmol/L}$$
or
$$2(Na + \text{mmol/L}) + \frac{glucose \text{ mg/dL}}{18} + \frac{BUN \text{ mg/dL}}{2.8}$$

Here, 1 mOsm of glucose = 180 mg/L; 1 mOsm of BUN = 28 mg/L. The serum osmolarity is a measure of the concentration of solute in serum concentration of solute, in intracellular and extracellular water.

$$2(140) + \frac{110}{18} + \frac{20}{2.8} = 286$$

Glucose = 110 mg/dL
Sodium = 140 mg/dL
BUN = 20 mg/dL
(Andreoli et al, p. 536)

75. **(A)** Water comprises 50% to 70% of body weight. Distribution of water is chiefly into two areas of the body, namely, the intracellular and extracellular fluid. The percentage attributed to each region is dependent on the amount of adipose (fat) tissue, which has a certain percentage of water. Two thirds of body water is located in intracellular fluid, and one third in extracellular fluid. Extracellular fluid is further divided into plasma and interstitial portions. The total amount of water is regulated by the amount of solvent in each compartment. *(Kelly's Textbook, p. 737)*

76. **(E)** The ability to concentrate the urine is a primary characteristic of the kidney. This is needed to prevent dehydration. This ability is shared by the nephrons, the sodium countercurrent system, the large osmotic gradient between the papilla and cortex, and the loop of Henle. The chief operative ion in water conservation is sodium (Na^+). *(Kelly's Textbook, pp. 734–735)*

77. **(A)** The classic presentation of rheumatoid arthritis is the result of chronic inflammation of synovial membranes. It is the formation of chronic granulation tissue (pannus) resulting from chronic synovitis that produces hydrolytic enzymes. These enzymes are capable of eroding articular cartilage, subchondrial bone, ligaments, and tendons. *(Beeson et al, pp. 1999–2000)*

78. **(D)** The patient presents with a monoarticular arthritis involving the ankle joint. The laboratory investigation reveals an elevated uric acid level and synovial fluid exam shows urate crystals classically seen in gouty arthritis. Bacterial septic arthritis is easily ruled out, as the patient has no fever, and one would expect a synovial white cell count in the range of 50,000 to 200,000. In rheumatoid arthritis, a monoarticular presentation is unlikely. Normal x-ray and urate crystals make the diagnosis of osteoarthritis remote. Pseudogout presents similarly, but crystal exam of the synovial fluid yields the rod-shaped crystals of calcium pyrophosphate. Also, one may find cartilaginous calcification on x-ray in pseudogout. Acute gouty arthritis tends to affect the lower extremities, particularly the metatarsalphalangeal (MTP) joint (75% of patients), but also is seen frequently in the tarsal joints and ankle. The joints of the upper extremities can be affected, particularly the elbow, wrist, and metacarpalphalangeal joints. Shoulder, hips, and sacroiliac joint involvement is rare in pseudogout. *(Beeson et al, pp. 1161–1168; Mercier and Pettid, pp. 169–171)*

79. **(C)** Although pyelonephritis can be asymptomatic during pregnancy, patients are generally fairly sick. They present with fever and chills, nausea, vomiting, and back/flank pain. Often, the typical symptoms of urinary tract infection are not present—such as urinary frequency, urgency, and dysuria. Although premature onset of contractions and, therefore, labor are often the consequence of pyelonephritis in pregnancy, it is not usually the presenting symptom. *(Burrow and Ferris, p. 350)*

80. **(D)** A mother infected with the rubella virus during pregnancy has a very high chance of having a child with congenital rubella syndrome. A generalized viremia, such as described in the question usually precedes the onset of rash by approximately 1 week. In a nonimmune mother who has been infected with the rubella virus, antibody titers will rise 1 to 2 weeks after the onset of rash and 2 to 3 weeks after the onset of viremia. It is, therefore, important to obtain rubella titers immediately after onset of symptoms in order to determine the immune status of the mother. Ideally, these titers should be obtained at the first prenatal visit or prior to conception in order to avoid confusion should the mother be exposed to the virus during pregnancy. All women who do not have immunity to rubella should be vaccinated prior to pregnancy or postpartum. A VDRL would be the most likely other answer, as syphilis acquired during pregnancy is associated with fetal congenital anomalies. Moreover, although secondary syphilis often presents with a rash, the rash typically occurs on palms and soles and is preceded by a history of chancres, usually in the vaginal and cervical areas. Gonorrhea, *Chlamydia*, and group B beta streptococcus will cause infection in the fetus in utero and during delivery, but are not associated with congenital anomalies. *(Cunningham et al, pp. 614–619; pp. 119, 131).*

81. **(E)** Preeclampsia, or more correctly termed *pregnancy-induced hypertension*, classically presents in young nulliparous women. It is characterized by an elevation in blood pressure of 140/90, on two occasions 6 hours apart, proteinuria and generalized edema: edema found in the face and hands. Pregnancy-induced hypertension occurs primarily past 20 weeks' gestation and involves many organ systems including cardiovascular, renal, central nervous system, and hematologic. Although the etiology remains unknown, the basic underlying pathophysiology is that of vasospasm. In most cases, the diagnosis is made if the blood pressure is 140/90, but an elevation of 30 mm Hg above baseline for systolic and 15 mm Hg for diastolic is acceptable. Patients typically have only minimal complaints: headache, spots before eyes, blurred or double vision, and upper abdominal pain. Chronic hypertension would be unlikely in a 16-year old and her first trimester blood pressure was normal. Migraines are not typically associated with hypertension. Although chronic renal disease is a possibility,

the combination of hypertension, proteinuria, and hyperreflexia is more likely preeclampsia. Eclampsia, a major complication of pregnancy-induced hypertension, is the development of generalized tonic–clonic seizure. *(Cunningham et al, pp. 653–654)*

82. **(C)** Treatment of mild preeclampsia prior to term gestation is bed rest; treatment of severe pregnancy-induced hypertension is delivery. To prevent the major and most life-threatening complication of pregnancy-induced hypertension, an eclamptic seizure, magnesium sulfate is administered prior to or concurrent with induction of labor. Although MgSo$_4$ has a slight effect on lowering blood pressure, its primary use is as an anticonvulsant medication. It is used preferentially over other anticonvulsants because of its efficiency in preventing eclamptic seizures and its minimal effect upon the fetus. MgSo$_4$ is usually given in a 4-g bolus, followed by a maintenance dose of 2 g/hour or intramuscular injection of 10 g. Hydrochlorthiazide and furosemide are both diuretics and both previously were used to treat the edema associated with pregnancy-induced hypertension. Subsequently, it has been found that use of diuretics is actually detrimental, because in preeclampsia the intravascular compartment is actually depleted. Lasix (or furosomide) is used in preeclampsia complicated by pulmonary edema. Hydralazine commonly is used in preeclampsia to lower blood pressure, but usually is used only if the diastolic pressure exceeds 110 mm Hg. Diazapan and phenytoin are commonly used antiseizure medications, but their generalized sedative effect on the fetus prevents their routine use. *(Cunningham et al, pp. 627–688; Hacker and Moore, pp. 130–132)*

83. **(B)** Neoplastic changes of the surface epithelium of the cervix are called cervical intraepithelial neoplasm (CIN) or dysplasia. If left untreated, a certain percentage of these neoplastic changes will progress to carcinoma in situ and eventually invasive carcinoma of the cervix. The squamocolumnar junction is the area between the stratified squamous epithelium of the exocervix and the columnar epithelium of the endocervical canal. It is at or very near this junction that the most severe changes of CIN occur. The location of the squamocolumnar junction change with a woman's reproductive stage and age. In women of reproductive age it is located in the external cervical os. In order to best obtain cells from the squamocolumnar junction for a Pap smear, both the endocervix and exocervix are sampled. After the cervix is cleaned of excessive discharge, a cotton tip applicator is inserted into the endocervical canal and then twirled to obtain cells from all sides. This is then applied to a glass slide. A second sample is then obtained from the exocervix with a wooden or plastic spatula or another cotton-tip applicator. This specimen is then placed on the same

glass slide and fixed immediately with 95% ethyl alcohol. The squamocolumnar junction does not typically occur as high as the internal os, nor would dysplastic cells often be found in the posterior vaginal fornix. *(Jones et al, pp. 643–657)*

84. **(E)** The primary means by which oral contraceptives prevent pregnancy is by the deference of ovulation. The effect of estrogen/progesterone in oral contraceptives is to inhibit release of the pituitary gonadotrophins LH and FSH. This in turn prevents the LH surge and, therefore, ovulation. The actual site of action is probably the hypothalamus: the combination of estrogen and progesterone inhibits hypothalamic release of the gonadotrophin-releasing hormone (GnRH) and subsequently the release of the gonadotrophins from the pituitary. Because ovulation does not occur, an embryo does not form. Thus, preventing implantation is not a means by which oral contraceptives prevent pregnancy. Inhibiting the release of prolactin has no effect on preventing ovulation. There is a preovulatory rise of estradiol secretion by the developing follicle, which is a result of FSH stimulation on the ovary. This rise in estrogen may cause the LH surge and, subsequently, ovulation. Because, however, the use of oral contraceptives prevents the release of FSH and LH, the rise in estrogen never takes place. Again, it is the effect of oral contraceptives on the release of gonadotrophins from the pituitary, not any effect of the "pill" directly on the ovary that prevents ovulation. Although oral contraceptives do change the cervical mucus and, therefore, cause the cervix to be impermeable to spermatoza, this is not the primary contraceptive action of the "pill." *(Hacker and Moore, pp. 358–364, 398–400; Jones et al, pp. 210–215)*

85. **(C)** Primary dysmenorrhea is pain that occurs with menstruation without any identifiable pelvic pathology. It typically begins on the first day of menstrual bleeding and occurs for usually only 12 hours. The pain is due to intrinsic uterine factors: exaggerated uterine contractility that is hormonally stimulated. Prostaglandins, found in the musculature of the uterus are synthesized under the influence of progesterone. Therefore, anovulatory cycles, in which there is no development of the corpus luteum, are generally not associated with dysmenorrhea. Because prostaglandins (PG) cause contractions of smooth muscle, it is the excess production of PG that causes more severe dysmenorrhea. The above patient's history is consistent with primary dysmenorrhea: onset usually 2 to 4 years after menarche, no significant previous gynecological history, pain occurring on the first day of the cycle, and no findings on pelvic exam. Primary dysmenorrhea usually responds well to treatment with prostaglandin synthetase inhibitors such as motrin,

anaprox, or indomethocin. Examples of secondary dysmenorrhea would be endometriosis, intrauterine demise, adenomyosis, endometrial polyps, or PID. Prior to the development of PG synthetase inhibitors, tylenol with codeine was used for dysmenorrhea. Because codeine is an addictive narcotic, this medication should not be given, as PG synthetase inhibitors are a better nonaddictive alternative. Because they prevent ovulation, oral contraceptives are acceptable therapy in women with primary dysmenorrhea who are sexually active and require birth control. Nonetheless, the first line of therapy in nonsexually active patients should be PG synthetase inhibitors. Diagnostic laparoscopy would be reserved only for those patients who fail on medication, PG inhibitory and oral contraceptives, and in patients who are strongly suspected of secondary dysmenorrhea. Tocolytic agents should theoretically work, as they are inhibiting uterine contractions, but their side effects and route of administration would mitigate against their usage. *(Gerbie, p. 613)*

86. **(D)** Candida vulvovaginitis is caused by the yeast organism *Candida albicans*. It is characterized by a thick, white "cottage cheese"-like discharge that is pruritic. The hyphae and buds of *C albicans* can be seen on a KOH wet mount. Treatment consists of clotrimazole (Gyne-Lotrimin) or miconazole nitrate (Monistat). Candida vulvovaginitis is more common in diabetics and frequently occurs after systemic antibiotic use and during pregnancy. *(Hacker and Moore, p. 298; Jones et al, pp. 572–573)*

87. **(B)** Atrophic postmenopausal vaginitis occurs when the vaginal mucosa undergoes atrophic changes secondary to absence of estrogen. Because the mucosa is thin and friable, it bleeds easily to the touch and often this is mistaken for postmenopausal bleeding of a more serious origin. In addition to complaints of itching and burning, patients also complain of dyspareunia. Treatment is topical estrogens (suppositories or cream). *(Jones et al, p. 575; Bates, p. 393)*

88. **(A)** *Trichomonas vaginalis* is the protozoan flagellate that causes trichomanas vaginitis. This protozoan is capable of living only in the female vagina and male urethra. It is considered a sexually transmitted disease; the woman's partner should, therefore, be treated. The bubbly greenish-yellow discharge is characteristic of *Trichomonas*. The *Trichomonas* can be seen flagellating on a normal saline wet mount. Treatment is metronidazole (Flagyl) that can be given in a 1-day dose of 2 g or as a 5-to-7 day dose of 250 mg twice daily. It must be remembered that Flagyl has an effect similar to Antabuse. Therefore, when alcohol is ingested while taking Flagyl, violent vomiting will occur. *(Hacker and Moore, p. 298)*

89. **(E)** The gram-negative bacillus *G vaginalis* is responsible for gardnerella vaginitis. The most common presenting complaint is the fishy, musty malodorous discharge. *Gardnerella* can be diagnosed on normal saline wet mount where the bacillus appear as studding on the epithelial cells of the vaginal culture. *(Gerbie, pp. 619–622)*

90. **(C)** A fundal height at the umbilicus roughly corresponds to 20 weeks' gestation. On physical exam, there are several ways of determining fundal height and therefore gestational age. A fundus palpable to the pubic symphysis is 12 weeks; at the umbilicus, 20: those weeks between these two landmarks are approximated. After 20 weeks and before 32 weeks, fundal height is measured with a tape measure in centimeters. Weeks' gestation correspond ($\pm$ 1 cm) to the measured centimeters from the top of the symphysis to the top of the funduu. *(Cunningham, et al, p. 1260)*

91. **(D)** Women who have previously been pregnant will first feel fetal movement between 16 to 18 weeks. With a first pregnancy, a woman will usually feel movement between 18 to 20 weeks. Gestational age can be approximated to when fetal movement is first perceived. *(Cunningham, et al, p. 218)*

92. **(A)** At 6 weeks' gestation, a gestational sac can be seen on abdominal ultrasound. After 8 weeks, the embryo can be seen and measurements of crown–rump length can be made. A fetal heart can be visualized at 7 weeks. *(Cunningham, et al, p. 284; Niswander, p. 29)*

93. **(D)** Maternal serum alpha fetoprotein is a screening test to detect the presence of numerous fetal abnormalities, the most common of which is neural tube defects. The major protein secreted by the early fetus is alpha fetoprotein. This protein is secreted into the amniotic fluid and crosses the fetal membranes into the maternal circulation. The level of alpha fetoprotein is elevated in the amniotic fluid of an abnormal fetus and therefore in the maternal serum. This elevation is best detected between 16 to 20 weeks. In addition to open neural tube defects, other abnormalities detected include congenital nephrosis, esophogeal and duodenal atresia, exophalos, Turner and Potters syndrome, fetal death, or fetal blood or amniotic fluid. *(Cunningham, et al, p. 277)*

94. **(D)** Patients suspected of having a pericardial effusion should have a two-dimensional echocardiogram to confirm the presence and size of a pericardial effusion. Echocardiography provides the most accurate and rapid technique available for evaluating an effusion. A chest x-ray will not show an enlarged cardiac silhouette until at least 250 mL of

fluid have accumulated in the pericardial sac. A CT scan is complementary to the echocardiogram and is effective in diagnosing loculated effusions, hemorrhagic effusions, and pericardial thickening. If an effusion is present and tamponade is suspected, a right heart catheterization can confirm the diagnosis. (*Braunwald, pp. 364, 1491–1492, 1497*)

95.　**(D)** An S_3 gallop is not present with mitral stenosis. An S_3 gallop is associated with rapid ventricular filling and is heard with ventricular dysfunction or with marked left-ventricular volume overload. Mitral stenosis is a low-pitched diastolic murmur heard best at the apex. There may be a loud S_1 and opening snap of the mitral valve. The Graham–Steele murmur of pulmonic regurgitation is due to pulmonary hypertension that can occur with mitral stenosis. The Graham–Steele murmur is a high-pitched, blowing decrescendo murmur best heard along the left sternal border, 2nd to 4th intercostal spaces. (*Braunwald, pp. 1027–1028*)

96.　**(A)** Left ventricular hypertrophy is caused by conditions that lead to pressure or volume overload of the left ventricle. In systemic arterial hypertension, hypertrophic obstructive cardiomyopathy, and aortic stenosis, left ventricular hypertrophy occurs in response to chronic pressure overload. In aortic insufficiency, left ventricular hypertrophy is the result of volume overload. Left ventricular hypertrophy is not seen in mitral stenosis because it does not result in left ventricular volume or pressure overload. (*Clinical Symposia—CIBA pp. 5–7*)

97.　**(B)** The electrocardiogram shows left ventricular hypertrophy. The criteria for LVH include

　　1. Increased QRS voltage in standards leads—R wave in lead I plus S wave in lead III is greater than 25 mm
　　2. Increased precordial voltage S wave in V_1 plus R wave in V_5 or $V_6 > 35$ mm
　　3. ST segment and T wave abnormalities
　　4. Left atrial abnormality
　　(*Clinical Symposia—CIBA p. 5*)

98.　**(C)** The electrocardiogram demonstrates a right bundle branch block (RBBB), hence a delay of right ventricular depolarization. Characteristics of a RBBB include QRS complex greater than 0.12 seconds in duration, terminal broad S wave in lead I and a RSR[1] complex in lead V_1. (*Clinical Symposia-CIBA, p. 6–8*)

99.　**(B)** Diffuse low voltage and electrical alternans may occur in cardiac tamponade. Diffuse low voltage is caused by the attenuation of the electrical signals by the fluid in the pericardial sac. Electrical alternans is caused by the pendulum movement of the heart within the pericardial sac. (*Braunwald, p. 1496*)

100.　**(C)** Tobacco smoking and high blood pressure are major risk factors for the development of coronary artery disease. Nicotine and carbon monoxide affect the heart and coronary arteries by causing an increased myocardial oxygen demand and interfering with the oxygen supply. High blood pressure can result in left ventricular enlargement and dysfunction leading to ischemic heart disease. Caffeine can cause tachycardia and arrhythmias, but there is no proof that it increases the risk of coronary artery disease. Alcohol does not increase the risk of coronary artery disease and some investigations indicate it may increase HDL-cholesterol levels. (*Braunwald, pp. 1153–1184*)

101.　**(B)** Syncope can be due to cardiac arrhythmias. The following arrhythmias are associated with syncope: asystole in the presence of complete heart block, paroxysmal ventricular tachycardia or fibrillation, supraventricular tachycardia or bradycardia, and sick sinus syndrome. (*Braunwald, pp. 890–891*)

102.　**(A)** Patients with acute pericarditis will have ST–T segment elevation that is concave upward and is usually seen in all leads except aV_R and V_1. A pericardial friction rub may be heard. It is a scratching, high-pitched sound and classically has three components. A patient may have dyspnea and breathe shallowly as a result of pleuritic chest pain. The chest pain associated with acute pericarditis is increased when supine and is often relieved by leaning forward. (*Braunwald, pp. 1487–1490*)

103.　**(E)** Secondary causes of hypertension include pheochromocytoma, renal parenchymal disease, use of oral contraceptive pills and primary aldosteronism. A pheochromocytoma is a catecholamine-producing tumor that causes paroxysmal hypertension or persistent hypertension with symptoms of headache, palpitations, sweating, nervousness, weight loss, orthostatic hypotension, and hypermetabolism. Renal parenchymal disease is principally caused by chronic glomerulonephritis. As the renal disease worsens, hypertension develops that can lead to renal insufficiency. Estrogen-containing oral contraceptive pills can cause an elevation in blood pressure. The hypertension is often mild but contributes to the cardiovascular complications from the pill. Primary aldosteronism causes hypertension as a result of volume overload, which then converts to increased peripheral resistance. (*Braunwald, pp. 838–848*)

104.　**(A)** The first heart sound (S_1) is caused by the closure of the mitral and tricuspid valves. It is a high-pitched sound best heard with the diaphragm medial to the apex at the lower sternal border. The S_2 is best heard at the 2nd or 3rd intercostal spaces. The S_1 precedes the palpable upstroke in the carotid pulse, which can help distinguish it from the S_2, which occurs after the peak of the carotid pulse. *(Braunwald, pp. 29–30)*

105. **(A)** Pulmonary rales develop as a result of transudation of fluid into the alveoli and are characteristic of congestive heart failure. Passive congestion of the liver as a result of right heart failure causes hepatomegaly. Congestive hepatomegaly can cause pain, anorexia, and nausea. An S_3 gallop is present with left ventricular failure and is best heard at the apex in the left lateral recumbent position. An S_4 is not a sign of heart failure but is associated with conditions that cause altered compliance of the ventricle (i.e., aortic stenosis, hypertrophic obstructive cardiomyopathy, hypertension). *(Braunwald, pp. 478–482)*

106. **(E)** The most common cause of ST segment elevation is myocardial injury. Injury occurs when there is intense transmural ischemia, which is often caused by narrowing or occlusion of a major coronary artery. Coronary vasospasm can also cause intense transmural ischemia resulting in ST segment elevation. Prinzmetal's angina is caused by coronary vasospasm. In acute pericarditis, the ST segment elevation is usually more generalized and can be seen in many leads. Early repolarization is another cause of ST segment elevation. It is a normal variant and is seen in healthy individuals, particularly blacks, males, and people under 30 years of age. *(Clinical Symposia–CIBA pp. 21–24; Braunwald, pp. 204–205)*

107. **(C)** Manifestations of digitalis intoxication include anorexia and arrhythmias. Arrhythmias can include many different rhythm disturbances, such as ventricular ectopy, ventricular tachycardia, atrioventricular and junctional escape rhythms. Prolonged QT interval is associated with type Ia antiarrhythmic such as quinidine, disopyramide, procainamide. Urinary retention can be a side effect of disopyramide. *(Braunwald, pp. 505–506)*

108. **(E)** Endocarditis prophylaxis is recommended for surgery or instrumentation of the genitourinary or GI tract because of the possibility of bacteremia. Prophylaxis is also recommended for dental procedures and surgery of the upper respiratory tract. *(Schulman, et al, pp. 1124A–1125A)*

109. **(A)** Factors associated with a poor prognosis after an acute myocardial infarction include congestive heart failure, positive stress test after a myocardial infarction, and poor left ventricular systolic function. The most important factor is the state of the left ventricular function. Ventricular arrhythmias in the first 24 hours after a myocardial infarction are often transient and benign. *(Braunwald, pp. 1271, 1291–1293; Rautaharju, pp. 4–52)*

110. **(B)** The Third Joint National Committee on Detection, Evaluation and Treatment of High Blood Pressure have classified mild hypertension as a diastolic blood pressure of 90 to 104 mm Hg. Severe hypertension is a diastolic pressure > 115 mm Hg. Isolated systolic hypertension is commonly seen in the elderly and is classified as a systolic pressure > 160 mm Hg, with diastolic pressure < 90 mm Hg. *(Braunwald, pp. 820–821)*

111. **(D)** Lithium is excreted by the kidneys, and thus blood levels are dependent upon renal function. Lithium can also have long-term effects on renal and thyroid function. Lithium-induced hypothyroidism can be a side effect of lithium administration and is treated with thyroid replacement. Thus, in addition to routine lithium blood levels, renal and thyroid function should be monitored. *(Baldessarini, pp. 96, 115, 119–121)*

112. **(E)** Narcolepsy is a disorder involving more than just excessive daytime sleepiness. Hypersomnolence is more commonly caused by other disorders or poor habits. The diagnosis of true narcolepsy, which is relatively rare, can be made only in the presence of at least one of the other symptoms. Sleep attacks plus cataplexy is considered pathonemonic of narcolepsy. An all-night polysomnograph and daytime sleep latency testing is confirmatory. *(Guilleminault, pp. 338–341)*

113. **(C)** Obstructive sleep apnea is a common cause of excessive daytime somnolence. Snoring is a commonly observable sign of upper airway obstruction. This is not a benign condition. In addition to the debilitating and potentially dangerous nature of sleepiness, lowered PO_2 during sleep and other physiologic changes can lead to hypertension and potentially fatal cardiac arrythmias. *(Lugaresi, et al, p. 498)*

114. **(C)** A statement of suicidal intent by a patient must be taken very seriously. An actively suicidal patient is not a candidate for outpatient treatment because of the potential lethality of an overdose of many psychiatric medications. Initiation of treatment and stabilization is best accomplished in an inpatient setting and can generally be done in a week to 10 days. *(Baldessarini, pp. 195–197)*

115. **(B)** Lyme disease is the leading cause of tick-borne disease in the United States. After the bite of the infected tick, a characteristic expanding annular rash develops, *erythema chronicum migrans*. The

rash may resolve spontaneously and advance to a second stage that includes neurologic and cardiac sequelae. A third stage may develop involving arthritis, which primarily affects the large joints, mostly the knees. The treatment of choice is, in order of preference, tetracycline, penicillin, and erythromycin. *(Harrison's, pp. 658–659; Cecil, pp. 1726–1727; Merck, p. 1251; Mandell, pp. 1346–1347; Krupp, p. 892; Abramowicz, p. 59)*

116. (D) A true converter is one who has 2 consecutive tuberculin skin tests given within 2 years of each other, the first one being read as negative, that is, less than 10 mm induration, and the second one being read as positive, that is, greater than 10 mm induration. The size of the induration must exceed 6 mm between the two readings. The conversion must also not be a result of the "booster" effect. A conversion is an indicator that a new infection has occurred. In any recently infected person, chemoprophylaxis is recommended if the individual is less than 35-years old and has a negative chest x-ray. Household contacts, especially children under 3-years old, are at increased risk for developing the disease, and also should be treated prophylactically. *(Braunwald et al, p. 632; p. 1683; Merck, p. 114; Mandell, p. 1389; Krupp, p. 147)*

117. (B) Hepatitis B surface antigen (HB$_s$Ag) is the first serologic marker of hepatitis B (HBV) infection. It usually occurs during the incubation period and disappears during the recovery phase. The HBV surface antibody (anti-HB$_s$) develops after clinical recovery. It represents past HBV infection. The HBV core antigen (HB$_c$Ag) represents the viral inner core. It is not detectable in serum by conventional lab methods, but only by specialized techniques. The HBV core antibody (anti-HB$_c$) is a marker of acute, persistent, or past infection. The anti-HB$_c$ (IgM) will be positive for 6 to 18 months after infection, and the anti-HB$_c$ (IgG) will remain as the indicator of past infection. There is a "window" period in HBV. This occurs during the transition from the disappearance of HB$_s$Ag and the appearance of anti-HB$_s$. Anti-HB$_c$ (IgM) will be the only indicator of infection during this time. The HBV e antigen (HB$_e$Ag) is only found in HB$_s$Ag positive serum. Its presence in the serum, along with HB$_s$Ag, for more than 10 weeks, correlates with ongoing viral replication and may be a predictor of chronic disease. *(Harrison's pp. 1325–1327; Merck, pp. 859–860; Krupp, pp. 397–398)*

118. (A) Anorexia nervosa is a disorder characterized by a refusal to maintain a normal body weight. The person has a distorted body image and sees herself or himself as fat even when severely undernourished. Such persons are preoccupied with body size

and shape. *(American Psychiatric Association: DSM III, pp. 65–67)*

119. (C) Bulimics have a disorder characterized by binge eating during which they feel a lack of control over their eating behavior. Like anorexics, bulimics, have a preoccupation with their weight and body features. They engage in means to prevent weight gain such as self-induced vomiting, abuse of laxatives, fasting between binges, or overly strenuous exercise. *(American Psychiatric Association, DSM III, pp. 67–69)*

120. (B) Osteoarthritis is the most common disease of axial and peripheral diarthroidal joints. Progressive deterioration and loss of articular cartilage along with reactive changes at joint margins and subchondral bone are characteristic. Heberden's nodes are the formation of spurs at the dorsolateral and medial aspects of the distal interphalangeal (DIP) joints, usually developing slowly over months to years. The DIP joints are usually spared in rheumatoid arthritis (RA). The clinical features of osteoarthritis are usually local and early in the disease pain occurs after joint use, improving with rest. Later in the disease, pain occurs with minimal motion and even at rest. Morning stiffness and swan-neck deformities of the hands are more frequently found in RA. Morning stiffness is thought to be the result of synovial congestion and thickening along with joint effusion. Swan-neck deformity is the hyperextension of the PIP joint and flexion of the DIP joint. *(Rodman et al, pp. 40–41, 104–108)*

121. (B) Septic arthritis is a medical emergency. Failure to rapidly diagnose this condition has the potential to cause permanent damage to the involved joint. Septic arthritis typically affects one joint or a few asymmetrical joints. Patients with septic arthritis usually present with an acute onset of pain, fever, erythema, and swelling of the affected joint; systemic signs of infection are common. Weight-bearing joints (most often the knee) and the wrist most commonly are involved. *(Schwartz, pp. 1983–1984)*

122. (A) The onset of RA is frequently heralded by prodromal symptoms such as fatigue, anorexia, weight loss, weakness, generalized aching, and stiffness. Morning stiffness is frequent (see answer to Question 120) in RA. The DIP joints can be involved in RA, but usually are spared and are involved more consistently in osteoarthritis. *(Rodman et al, pp. 40–41)*

123. (A) Somatiform disorders present in many forms. Symptoms occur in many body systems, commonly GI, cardiovascular, or genitourinary. Often, pain is experienced that cannot be correlated with the anatomic distribution of the nervous system. They occasionally occur concurrent with or subsequent to a genuine physical ailment or trauma. The patient is not conscious of the production of his or her symptoms; they are felt to be "real." *(American Psychiatric Association, DSM III, pp. 255, 263–267)*

124. **(E)** The presence of melancholia (the loss of pleasure in activities) associated with at least three of the following: sleep disturbance, eating disturbance or weight change, reduced energy, inappropriate guilt, loss of libido, reduced concentration, morbid or nihilistic thoughts, or psychomotor changes, fulfill the criteria for diagnosis of major depression. *(Dunner, p. 3)*

125. **(E)** It has been recognized for a long time that schizophrenia occurs in association with many personality types. However, the socially withdrawn type of personality is more strongly represented in schizophrenics and their first-degree relatives. The reason for this is unknown, but it can be a valuable piece of historical information when forming a differential diagnosis. *(Kendell, p. 7)*

126. **(E)** Psychosis is an indication of a brain chemical malfunction. Many different causes must be entertained. The first step in narrowing a differential diagnosis is to take a careful history, including the duration of symptoms and the patient's premorbid level of functioning. One must, of course, rule out nonpsychiatric causes of brain dysfunction. *(Davidson, pp. 1–14)*

127. **(C)** Panic disorder causes discrete episodes of panic that occur spontaneously and often become psychologically linked with the circumstances in which they occur. A phobia is the fear of a single distinct object, such as cats. As opposed to panic disorder, simple phobias are common, result in little debilitation, and do not, in themselves, cause patients to seek treatment. *(American Psychiatric Association, DSM III, pp. 243–245)*

128. **(A)** Imipramine is a tricyclic antidepressant that, in addition to the usual anticholinergic side effects, can produce significant drop in standing blood pressure. This may require discontinuation of the drug and use of another antidepressant. It must be used with care particularly in the elderly because of the hazard of falls. *(Baldessarini, pp. 178–179, 182–183)*

129. **(A)** A borderline personality is distinguished by a great deal of character dysfunction. Such lives are generally marked by one crisis after another, to which the patient responds in impulsive ways. There are periods when reality testing is impaired, but this is generally limited to times of crisis. *(American Psychiatric Association, DSM III, pp. 346–347)*

130. **(D)** Gout has no specific association with sickle cell anemia. Cholelithiasis is commonly associated with sickle cell anemia because of the icterus that occurs secondary to chronic hemolysis, and must always be kept in mind when evaluating the sickle cell patient with abdominal pain (i.e., one cannot automatically assume that such pain is due to sickle cell crisis). Chronic anemia and hypoxemia often lead to a chronic hyperdynamic cardiac state and later to CHF. Skeletal infarction can readily lead to femoral head aseptic necrosis; hepatic infarcts are common and can lead to significant hepatic parenchymal damage. *(Braunwald et al, pp. 1520–1522)*

131. **(E)** This presentation is consistent with a hemolytic anemia. The presence of gallstones in so young a person and the absence of specific symptoms strongly suggests chronic or congenital hemolysis, such as hereditary spherocytosis, rather than an acute acquired hemolytic process, such as autoimmune hemolytic (immunohemolytic) anemia which generally occurs in adults, is often, although not always, acute in presentation, and has a positive direct Coombs test. *(Braunwald et al, pp. 1506–1517)*

132. **(C)** Chronic lymphocytic leukemia (CLL) is a disease usually appearing in the fourth or fifth decade of life or later and is characterized by increased mature appearing lymphocytes in the peripheral blood, associated with spleen, node, and bone marrow, infiltration by a beta-cell neoplasm. It is clinically indistinguishable from diffuse well-differentiated lymphocytic lymphoma. It is a relatively indolent disease that often presents with massive hepatosplenomegaly, peripheral lymphocytosis, and occasionally with lymphadenopathy, with surprisingly few symptoms. Often it is picked up on a routine exam and through CBCs. Stage A, which is lymphocytosis ± mild lymphadenopathy, has a median survival of approximately 7 years. Stage B, lymphocytosis, larger lymphadenopathy, and hepatosplenomegaly, has a median survival of 5 years. Stage C, which is Stage B findings plus anemia and/or thrombocytopenia, has a 2-year median survival. No potentially curative therapy regimen has been found. Single alkylating agents such as low-dose daily or pulse high-dose chlorambucil, or pulse cyclophosphamide, are indicated to palliate hemolytic anemia, symptomatic organomegaly or lymphadenopathy, or systemic symptoms (fever, weight loss, fatigue, night sweats, etc.). Steroid therapy may be of value in instances of hemolytic anemia, which occurs in about 20% of CLL patients, or autoimmune thrombocytopenia (differentiated from thrombocytopenia secondary to neoplastic marrow invasion by presence of antiplatelet antibodies and increased megakaryocytes in the marrow). Splenectomy may be helpful if such problems fail to respond to steroids, but is not otherwise indicated. Radia-

tion therapy may control localized symptomatic disease; interferon is of no value. Hairy cell leukemia, another adult lymphoid leukemia, (seen predominantly in males greater than 40 years of age) must be differentiated from CLL, as interferon *is* very effective in such patients with progressive disease, and alkylating agents are poorly tolerated. As in the other leukemias, infection is a major problem in patients with progressing disease; thus, early diagnosis of infection and initiation of appropriate therapy are essential. *(Braunwald et al, pp. 1548–1550; Eiseman et al, pp. 196–200)*

133. **(D)** A high percentage of patients with PA are of Northern European descent, and are fair haired, and/or prematurely gray. Current thought is that this condition has an immunologic origin, probably an autoimmune response against gastric parietal cells. There is a strong association with other disorders of such origin, including thyroid disorders, Addison's disease, vitiligo, and hypoparathyroidism. Of these, 90% have antiparietal cell antibodies, 50% to 60% have antiintrinsic-factor antibodies. In PA, there is loss of vitamin B_{12} absorption due to the absence of intrinsic factor in the stomach, and gastrin levels are often elevated. Findings may include pallor, slight icterus, smooth (sore) beefy red tongue, mild hepatosplenomegaly, and in more advanced cases, fast pulse, cardiomegaly, CHF, and CNS symptoms (neuropathy, ataxia, weakness, decreased finger coordination, decreased vibratory sense, positive Romberg, Babinski reflexes, and disturbed mentation). CBC and bone marrow demonstrate megaloblastic changes and serum B_{12} levels are low. These patients have a twofold to threefold increased incidence of gastric carcinoma and should be monitored accordingly. *(Braunwald et al, pp. 1499–1501; Hoffbrand and Pettit, pp. 56–57)*

134. **(B)** Thrombocytopenia may be seen in aplastic anemia, leukemias, myelomas, and lymphomas, and may present with petechiae, bruising, purpura, and/or unusual bleeding. All these conditions also cause an increased risk of infection, and an acute pneumonia (or other infection such as cellulitis or perirectal abscess) may well be the presenting complaint. Fever is a nonspecific symptom, and may be due to neoplastic activity or infection. All these conditions often present with anemia, which causes pallor and fatigue. Hepatosplenomegaly and/or lymphomas, and occasionally myelomas, are generally not found in aplastic anemia. Bone pain may occur in leukemias due to increasing activity of neoplastic cells in the marrow, and in myeloma due to skeletal destruction; retroperitoneal lymphadenopathy often causes back pain in lymphoma patients; bone pain is not a specific common finding in aplastic anemia. Weight loss is common in most neoplastic processes, but not in aplastic anemia.

Initial work-up for this patient should include CBC, platelet count, ESR, chemical panel, U/A, protein electrophoresis, and bone marrow aspiration/biopsy, with further work-up to be based on these results (CT scans, lymph node biopsy, lumbar puncture, skeletal survey, etc.). *(Eiseman et al, pp. 193–228)*

135. **(B)** Erythema multiforme is an acute, self-limited eruption of the skin and the mucous membranes. The target or iris lesion, the most characteristic feature of this disease, develops abruptly and symmetrically on extensor surfaces as well as on the palms and soles.

The incorrect answers are A: Erythema marginatum is a specific skin manifestation of rheumatic fever. The lesion may start as an erythematous papule or blotch, spreading peripherally. Lesions may appear on the trunk and the limbs with some pigmentary changes. C: Eruptions with erythema annulare centrifugum begin as erythematous or urticaria-like papules. These spread to form large rings with central clearing. Etiology appears to be related to underlying disease. D: Erythematous, tender nodules usually on the anterior tibia are typical lesions of erythema nodosum. New lesions may be accompanied by fever, chills, and malaise. Numerous etiologies are attributed to this disease. Spontaneous resolution usually occurs. E: The lesions of erythema gyratum repens are rapidly growing scaly, erythematous, concentric bands that may involve the entire body. Underlying malignancy appears to be etiology of this condition. *(Fitzpatrick, pp. 555–556, 1010–1012, 1142–1143, 1859)*

136. **(E)** Basal cell carcinoma (BCC) is the most common malignant skin cancer in light-skinned people. The predominant occurrence is on sun-exposed areas seldom observed before age 40. It rarely metastasizes unless treatment is not initiated promptly once the diagnosis has been made. Treatment modalities include excisional, electro- or cryosurgery or radiation.

The incorrect answers are A: SCC is a skin cancer that develops mostly because of exposure to sunlight and other chemical agents such as arsenic, coal tar, creosote oil. Exposure to x-rays and gamma rays with resulting SCC is experimentally and epidemiologically evident. Treatment of SCC includes electro-, chemo-, and excisional surgery. Radiation therapy may be used where surgical excision may be cosmetically objectionable. B: Primary cutaneous malignant melanoma is the leading fatal illness arising in the skin with an increased incidence expected every year. It is a highly visible tumor and occurs primarily during the productive years except for the lentigo maligna melanoma, which is predominantly seen in the elderly. Sun exposure has been implicated in the etiology of primary melanoma. Recognition of precursor lesions such as lentigo maligna, congenital melanocytic nevi, and the dysplastic nevi, and changes in their variegation is crucial for the improvement of the survival rate. Surgical excision with the margin of these varying according to the depth of the tumor is the definitive therapy. C: Actinic keratosis (AK), a precancerous lesion, presents on sun-exposed areas in almost 100% of the elderly white population. It may also be found on other fair-skinned people from teens on up. AK may progress into a SCC without therapy. Treatment may include topical chemotherapy, cryotherapy, curettage, and electrodesiccation and surgical excision. D: A keratoacanthoma is a fast-growing benign skin tumor believed to arise from the hair follicles. It resembles the SCC during the active growth phase with sunlight, chemical carcinogens, trauma, and genetic predeliction being factors in this. Forms of therapy include topical or intralesional injections of 5-fluorouracil, curettage, surgical excision, and waiting for spontaneous regression. (Fitzpatrick, pp. 733–743, 747–756, 759–771, 766–772, 947–963)

137. **(B)** Macules are flat, nonpalpable lesions marked by pigment alteration, and vary in sizes and shapes. Cafe-au-lait spots and vitiligo are examples of macules.

The incorrect answers are A: Plaques are palpable, raised plateau-like lesions of variable sizes and thickness. The scaly psoriatic plaques are an example of these. C: Wheals are inflamed, flat-topped papules or plaques formed by transient and superficial edema. They may appear as small papules or involve areas as large as the entire back; an example of these would be the wheals in urticaria (hives). D: Pustules are palpable vesicles filled with exudate that contain bacteria as in folliculitis or they may be sterile as in the lesions of pustular psoriasis. E: Scales are palpable results of abnormal shedding or the accumulation of the stratum corneum. An increased rate of cell production appearing as scaly plaques in psoriasis or the scaling with a dermatophyte infection such as tinea versicolor are examples. (Fitzpatrick, pp. 22–37)

138. **(D)** Penicillin is the drug of choice in the treatment of erysipelas, which is usually a group A streptococcal skin infection. Erysipelas, a superficial cellulitis, most often occurs in infants and older adults. The source is commonly the upper respiratory tract.

The incorrect answers are A: As many as 40% of group A streptococci may be resistant to the tetracyclines. B: Cephalothin may be substituted in the very ill patient with a questionable penicillin allergy. C: In the case of an immediate type of reaction, the very ill patient may be treated with vancomycin. E: Nafcillin should be used in the patient with a suspected severe staphylococcal infection. (Fitzpatrick, pp. 2104–2113)

139. **(D)** Acute pyelonephritis is associated with nausea and vomiting, fever, chills, leukocytosis, costovertebral angle tenderness, or pain on deep abdominal palpation. The patient may or may not have cystitis, and can be suffering from headaches or malaise. (Harrison's Principles of Internal Medicine, pp. 1191–1192)

140. **(A)**

141. **(C)**

142. **(D)** Lyme disease begins with the tick bite from Ixodes dammini, which transmits the spirochete Borrelia burgdorferi. The classic rash, erythema chronicum migrans, begins as a macular or maculopapular lesion that expands, leaving centralized clearing. This occurs within 1 month of the tick bite in most patients, and can resolve spontaneously. Within a week to months a second stage of the disease can occur that includes cardiac and neurologic complications. Bilateral Bell's palsy may occur, as well as severe fatigue, peripheral neuropathy, and meningitis. Early manifestations of the disease are treated with tetracycline 250 mg qid for 10 to 21 days, or amoxicillin 250 mg tid for 10 to 21 days. (Harrison's, p. 659, Cecil, pp. 1727–1728; Merck, pp. 1252–1253; Mandell, pp. 1347–1348; Abramowicz, p. 59; Petri, pp. 95–99; Chapel, p. 218)

Rocky Mountain spotted fever (RMSF) is transmitted by the bite of the dog tick, Dermacentor variabilis, or the wood tick, D andersoni. The disease causing organism is Rickettsia rickettsii. The rash of RMSF typically begins as a macular or maculopapular lesion, but progresses to form petechial lesions. The lesions may coalesce to form large hemorrhagic areas. In RMSF, the treatment of choice is either chloramphenicol 50 mg/kg or tetracycline 25 mg/kg divided equally at 6- to 8-hour intervals. (Harrison's, p. 751; Cecil, p. 1743; Merck, p. 151)

143. **(A)** A repeat culture is necessary to document complete eradication of the bacteria. At least 7 to 10 days of antibiotics are needed to completely treat a urinary tract infection (UTI) in pregnancy. A patient who has had one UTI during pregnancy must be constantly monitored for recurrence, as she is now at high risk for subsequent infection. Repeated periodically during the prenatal course, urine cultures will ensure early detection of infection. Chronic suppressive therapy consists of taking a small dose of an antibiotic every day and is indicated only if the patient has subsequent positive cultures with the same infecting organism. It is not indicated for an initial episode of cystitis, although

it may be considered for patients who have had one severe episode of pyelonephritis during pregnancy. *(Burrow and Ferris, p. 348)*

144. (C) There are actually three anatomical changes during pregnancy that predispose the patient to a higher incidence of pyelonephritis. The two above (2 and 4) and decreased bladder tone. Hydronephrosis is found to begin in the first trimester and is predominantly right-sided. Its etiology is controversial, but it is felt to be mechanical, that is, due to obstruction of the ureter by the enlarging uterus and hormonal or changes that occur in the urinary tract as a consequence of the pregnancy hormones. Mechanical and hormonal etiologies probably explain the other two anatomical changes: decreased bladder tone and incomplete bladder emptying. *(Burrow and Ferris, p. 348)*

145. (E) Women who are Rh negative have an absence of the Rho or D antigen on their erythrocytes. If they have an Rh positive baby, this child's positive antigen when crossing the placenta will initiate the production of antibodies (by the mother) against the Rh-positive erythrocytes. These antibodies will either affect a subsequent pregnancy with an Rh-positive baby or affect the current pregnancy if there is a significant feto-maternal hemorrhage. Abortions, whether elective or spontaneous, ectopic and molar pregnancies in Rh-negative mothers have been associated with this isoimmunization process. These mothers should all receive rhogam at the time of abortion. Because of the possibility of feto-maternal hemorrhage following an episode of vaginal bleeding during pregnancy and following amniocentesis, such women should also be treated with rhogam. Finally, because of the possibility of a silent feto-maternal bleed, rhogam is given at 28 weeks in all (except previously isoimmunized) Rh-negative mothers. *(Niswander, pp. 599–604)*

146. (C) Although the percentage of mothers with AIDS who transmit the virus to their offspring is not yet known, it has been estimated at approximately 50%. Because AIDS is a sexually transmitted disease, the mother should be tested for other sexually transmitted diseases. At this time, the effect of pregnancy on the progression of AIDS, particularly those women who are asymptomatic, is unknown. Advising the patient to abort the pregnancy because AIDS will have a definite detrimental effect on the disease process is therefore invalid. Women who develop *P carinii* should definitely be treated, even if the treatment has an adverse affect on the fetus. But there is no reason to treat a woman prophylactically. *(Minkoff, pp. 2714–2717)*

147. (B) Endomyometritis, following cesarean section, is primarily polymicrobial. About 70% of the bacteria recovered are anaerobic: they include anaerobic gram-positive cocci, peptococcus, peptostreptococcus and anaerobic gram-negative species such as bacteroides. Less common are aerobic gram-positive cocci, *S fecalis*, group B beta strep, *S aureus*, *E coli* and enterobacteriaceae. Because these bacteria are usually found in combination, antibiotic therapy is, consequently, in combination. Because anaerobic bacteria are so often involved, there is a need for the addition of clindamycin (or flagyl) to ampicillin and gentamicin. Clindamycin and flagyl are known to be effective against bacteroides species. The combination of gentamicin and clindamycin is usually effective except in infections in which enterobacteriaceae is one of the causative organisms. Neither gentamicin nor clindamycin is effective against this bacteria; therefore, ampicillin must be added. Second- and third-generation cephalosporins such as mefoxin and cefotetan are thought to be as effective as triple antibiotics. *(Cunningham, et al, p. 464; Niswander, p. 406)*

148. (C) CIN II or moderate dysplasia needs to be further evaluated. Colposcopic evaluation allows the examiner to visualize the cervix at 10 to 14 × magnification. This allows for directed biopsy of the squamocolumnar junction and the ability to perform an endocervical curettage. The information obtained from colposcopy and from the Pap smear is then used to form the best plan of treatment for the patient. Prior to the extensive use of colposcopy, cone biopsy was a valid step in the evaluation of a moderate dysplasia. It is currently used diagnostically only if colposcopy is not available. At the present, cone biopsy is more commonly used if the squamocolumnar junction is not adequately visualized on colposcopy; if the Pap smear and colposcopically obtained biopsy do not correlate, and as a presurgical means of staging microinvasive and invasive carcinoma. Simple hysterectomy is not considered a diagnostic procedure, but in women who do not wish for more children it could be a therapeutic procedure. Although cervicitis may occur concurrently with moderate dysplasia, all CIN II/moderate dysplasia requires further evaluation. If the patient does have a cervicitis, treatment prior to colposcopy will aid in a more accurate exam. *(Hacker and Moore, p. 483; Jones, et al, pp. 671–673, pp. 58–64)*

149. (A) A history of previous thromboembolic disease and the history of ischemic heart disease are absolute contraindications to the use of oral contraceptives (OCPs). Use of oral contraception increases the risk of developing venous thrombembolic disease and subsequent pulmonary embolus. The risk is related to the estrogen component and is definitely decreased with lower estrogen doses (less than 50 μg). Development of cardiovascular complications such as myocardial infarction is also increased; the increase is primarily seen in women over the age of 35 and those who smoke. This risk is secondary to the progestational component that increases LDL and lowers HDL. Smoking is not an absolute contraindication to the use of OCPs. Because, however, the risk of developing cardiovascular and thromboembolic complications is increased in women over the age of 30 who smoke, most practitioners would be extremely reluctant to prescribe birth control pills to such a patient. Use of OCPs have been known to increase the severity and frequency of migraine headaches in some patients. Nonetheless, it is not an absolute contraindication and if properly supervised a patient can use the pill if she has a history of migraine. Additional absolute contraindications of OCPs are current pregnancy, cerebral vascular accident, malignant tumor, and abnormal liver function. Patients, especially older women, using OCPs also have a greater risk of developing hypertension. *(Essent, pp. 359–362; Novak, pp. 208–222)*

150. **(B)** It should be explained to a patient contemplating a bilateral tubal ligation that the procedure is permanent. A woman who considers the procedure as reversible has obviously not firmly decided against future childbearing. The success rate of reversal ranges from 30% to 70% and is dependent upon the surgical technique, the original sterilization procedure, and the patient's previous gynecologic history. Laparoscopic ring and clip procedures, and minilap suture and ligation procedures both result in the least amount of tubal damage and greatest amount of remaining tube. These procedures are associated with the best success rate at reversal. Although reversal procedures exist, it must be emphasized to the patient that the original procedure is permanent. The failure rate of tubal ligation is very small, but the major complication of failure is pregnancy. Because the tubes have been damaged, the possibility of the pregnancy developing in the tube is greater. Patients should be informed of this procedural complication as part of the precounseling for tubal ligation. Because all bilateral tubal ligation procedures are performed under sterile technique, there is no increased incidence of PID. There was some suggestion that women who undergo bilateral tubal ligation may later develop dysfunctional uterine bleeding, but the relationship has never been substantiated. *(Hacker and Moore, p. 368)*

151. **(B)** This couple clearly has primary infertility: they have no previous pregnancies and have attempted pregnancy for greater than 1 year without success. A thorough history of both the woman and man together and in separate interviews is essential for the initial work-up of infertility. A woman's past

obstetric, gynecologic, and medical history is important. Because on history this patient has irregular menses, documenting whether ovulation occurs is an important first step. A basal body temperature chart is an easy and accurate means of doing so: the woman takes her temperature each morning before any activity. The basal temperature rises approximately 0.4°F at ovulation and should remain elevated for at least 11 days. Of all infertile couples, 35% have more than one cause; therefore, the male should also undergo an infertility work-up simultaneous to the woman. A semen analysis is an important first step in determining male fertility. A hysterosalpingogram is not a preliminary step in an infertility work-up. Once the preliminary steps have failed to reveal an etiology, however, it is an important means of diagnosing tubal and intrauterine abnormalities. An attempt to measure estrogen levels daily in order to document the pre-LH surge of estrogen and subsequently predict ovulation is time consuming and costly and is, therefore, not done routinely. *(Hacker and Moore, pp. 444–448; Jones, et al, pp. 263–279)*

152. **(E)** Varicella is an acute, highly contagious disease most often occurring in childhood, but can occur at any age, worldwide. The average incubation period is 14 or 15 days with the main route of transmission through the respiratory tract. Presenting signs and symptoms may include a prodrome with a generalized pruritic rash following. Characteristic lesions may present, progressing from erythematous macules to papules, vesicles, and crusts at different stages throughout the disease. Constitutional symptoms are usually mild in normal children. Varicella may be associated with more extensive skin lesions, high fever, severe malaise, pneumonia, and other life-threatening complications in adults and immunologically compromised patients of any age. Treatment is usually symptomatic. *(Fitzpatrick, pp. 2314–2340; Lynch, p. 84)*

153. **(E)** 1. Pemphigus vulgaris may present with flaccid bullae commonly involving the scalp, umbilicus, and other parts of the body, including the mucous membranes. Delay of diagnosis may be life threatening. 2. EBA, a chronic blistering disease, is characterized by blister formation over joint surfaces. Extensor surfaces of the lower legs and the mucous membranes may also be involved. In general, these bullae are tense. 3. Spontaneous bullae may appear in diabetics, usually on the extremities, particularly the feet. In general, the bullae heal without scaring over several weeks. 4. Large tense bullae in bullous pemphigoid are characteristic of this disease. The most common sites include the inner thighs, flexor surfaces of the forearms, axillae, abdomen, and other areas of the body, including the

mucous membranes. This disease occurs predominantly in the sixth, seventh, and eighth decades of life. *(Fitzpatrick, pp. 572–573, 580–581, 589, 2075–2076)*

154. **(A)** 1. Rubella (german measles) is a common viral infection in children and young adults. The rash appears first on the face, then generalizes with discrete erythematous macules and papules clearing within 2 to 4 days, followed by fine desquamation. This is in contrast to rubeola, which persists. 2. Rubeola (measles) is also a highly contagious viral disease in children. Three distinct phases are present in measles: (a) an asymptomatic incubation period of about 10 to 12 days; (b) prodromal period with fever, chills, malaise, coryza, conjunctivitis, and cough; (c) onset of the rash, erythematous macules and papules starting on the face, then spreading downward. Koplik's spots usually appear in the mouth 24 to 48 hours prior to the rash. The average clinical course is about 10 days. Symptomatic therapy is usual unless complications such as encephalitis warrants antibiotic treatment. 3. Kawasaki, a viral illness, has a list of six criteria to establish the diagnosis. (a) The disease begins with a high fever not responding to antipyretics. The fever must last for at least 5 days to be considered compatible with this disease. At the second stage, fever may fluctuate over the next week or two. Often, myringitis and/or diarrhea may follow. A cough may be present as the third manifestation. (b) Conjunctival injection and uveitis may be present in 70% of children. (c) Fissuring red lips and a hypertrophic tongue, as well as small mucosal ulcerations may accompany the illness. (d) Palms and soles that turn bright red and peel as the fever declines are the fourth manifestation of Kawasaki. (e) A skin eruption is the fifth manifestation of which there are several kinds. There is a red, confluent rash with papules or pustules in the diaper area. Another is a scarlatiniform rash. A third type presents with large annular, brownish lesions such as those associated with erythema multiforme. (f) Cervical adenitis is the sixth manifestation. There are many more signs and symptoms than those mentioned, such as abdominal pain and most troublesome of all, cardiovascular disease. No specific form of treatment is available. Scarlet fever is the incorrect answer. It presents with a diffuse erythematous eruption, having a sandpaper quality, a sequela of a group A streptoccal infection in the pharynx. Desquamation usually occurs within 4 to 6 days, lasting several weeks. Other clinical findings include enlarged tonsils, strawberry tongue, and generalized lymphadenopathy. It usually occurs in children; only rarely in adults. Early penicillin therapy prevents development of supporative and nonsupporative sequelae. *(Fitzpatrick, pp. 2108–2111, 2289–2290, 2291–2295, 2376–2382)*

155. **(A)** The risk of HIV transmission to health care workers has been evaluated and demonstrated to be approximately 0.5% (1 in 200) following a single needlestick exposure to HIV-infected blood. Although the incidence of transmission is low, the magnitude of risk emphasizes the need for effective infection control procedures. Universal precautions, treating all blood and body fluids as though infected with HIV, reduces the risk of occupational exposure. Protective measures include handwashing before and after patient contact, proper disposal of sharp objects, no recapping of needles, use of gloves when handling blood or body fluids/tissues, and use of goggles and gowns when splatter of body fluids is anticipated. The use of masks is necessary only with procedures during which there is aerosolization of body fluids or with contagious airborne diseases. No cases of HIV transmission to health care workers from contact with body fluids other than blood have been documented. The potential for hepatitis B virus (HBV) transmission to health care workers after accidental exposure is much greater than HIV transmission. Studies demonstrate that 10% to 30% of health care workers have serologic evidence of past or present HBV exposure. Twelve thousand health care workers become infected with HBV each year, of which 700 to 1200 become chronic carriers. *(MMWR, Vol. 38, No. S-6; Infectious Disease Clinics of North America, Vol. 2. No. 2, Gerberding, pp. 321–328)*

156. **(B)** Kaposi's sarcoma (KS) is the most frequent AIDS-associated malignancy and is seen primarily in homosexual men. Unlike classic KS, which presents as relatively indolent cutaneous lesions, KS in AIDS patients is often aggressive and can be found as cutaneous lesions, visceral lesions, or both. Cutaneous KS can appear on any body surface, but is commonly seen on the face and in the oral cavity. KS may cause pulmonary disease, GI disease leading to gastric outlet obstruction or GI bleeding, and cause lymphatic obliteration leading to severe lymphedema. Pulmonary KS may be seen on chest x-ray as nodular infiltrates, with or without pleural effusions, and patients often present with shortness of breath, hemoptysis, and dyspnea. Definitive diagnosis of Kaposi's sarcoma is readily made by biopsy. Radiotherapy is effective palliative treatment for KS lesions; however, progression and dissemination are not altered with treatment and prognosis is not improved. Multiple cytotoxic chemotherapeutic agents have been used in treatment of visceral KS with varying response rates. Most of these agents, including vincristine, vinblastine, adriamycin, methotrexate, and bleomycin, have been associated with severe toxicities. Alpha-interferon administered parenterally has proven effective against KS, particularly in patients with early disease who do

not yet have marked depletion of CD4 cells. *(Infectious Disease Clinics of North America, Vol. 2, No. 2, Mitsuyasu, pp. 511–523)*

157. **(A)** The first step in evaluating the presence of HIV infection is the HIV antibody status using the enzyme-linked immunosorbent assay (ELISA) technique. HIV antibodies may be detected by this screening method 1 to 2 months after the onset of acute illness. If this test is found to be positive, it is confirmed by the more specific Western Blot (WB) method of HIV antibody detection. HIV serum p24 antigen may be detected by ELISA in the period prior to antibody seroconversion but is less sensitive than antibody status and may be present in the serum for only a brief period of time. Persistent p24 antigenemia or the reappearance of antigenemia is associated with poor clinical outcome and more rapid progression to AIDS. In vitro culture of HIV is used in clinical trials and research, but is rarely indicated in routine practice. T-lymphocyte subset studies are routinely used only in known HIV infected patients. Major subsets include CD4 (T helper) cells and CD8 (T suppressor) cells. A decrease in absolute number of CD4 cells generally correlates with a decline in function of the immune system and an increase in risk of opportunistic infection. *(Tindall, et al, pp. 329–338)*

158. **(C)** The cumulative incidence of reported AIDS cases in the United States is disproportionately higher in blacks and Hispanics. Although 80% of the population in the United States is composed of whites, 59% of all persons with AIDS are white. Conversely, although blacks and Hispanics compose 12% and 6% of the United States population, they make up 27% and 13% of all AIDS cases, respectively. The geographic distribution of AIDS cases throughout the United States has shifted with time. The percent of AIDS cases in New York and San Francisco, although disproportionately larger than other areas in the United States, has gradually decreased since 1983, and these other areas have seen an increase in cases. The proportion of adult AIDS cases in women has increased over time. The highest risk of HIV infection in children occurs in those born to women who are at risk of HIV infection. Women at increased risk should be counseled, tested for HIV antibody status, and advised of the risk of HIV transmission to the fetus should pregnancy arise. As of December 1988, 1.0 to 1.5 million people have been infected with HIV. Using an extrapolation method, projections have been made estimating 365,000 diagnosed AIDS cases in the United States by 1992. *(Centers for Disease Control; pp. 1–38)*

159. **(D)** Lack of clinical improvement after 5 to 7 days of treatment indicates therapeutic failure and the need for replacement with alternate therapy. The addition of high-dose corticosteroid therapy to conventional agents may be successful in improving patients failing to respond to treatment. PCP, which occurs in 80% to 90% of all AIDS patients, is the leading cause of death in these patients. Most patients (approximately 60%) survive their first episode of PCP due to early detection and effective treatment. Clinical presentation is characterized by fever, shortness of breath, and cough. Chest x-ray may reveal diffuse patchy infiltrates; however, it may be normal in up to 30% of patients. A definitive diagnosis of PCP is made only by obtaining pneumocysts on silver stain of sputum, bronchial washings, or lung tissue. *(Hopewell, pp. 409–416; Masur and Kovacs, pp. 421–426; Centers for Disease Control, pp. 1–38)*

160. **(E)** The most reliable indicator of bleeding potential is an accurate history and physical. One must elicit prolonged bleeding or the presence of easy bruising. History of family members with bleeding disorders is important. None of the assays listed completely evaluates the cascade of events associated with the formation of a blood clot. The prothrombin measures only the integrity of Factors II, V, VII, and X, whereas the partial thromboplastin time will evaluate the function of Factors VIII, IX, X, XI, and XII. The measurement of fibrinogen will detect the presence of hypofibrinogenemia, but does not detect abnormalities in fibrinogenolysis. *(Schwartz et al, pp. 87–89)*

161. **(E)** The rectum is the most frequently involved site for idiopathic ulcerative colitis. The disease will often spread proximally and symptoms can often be confused with hemorrhoidal symptoms. *(Schwartz et al, p. 1171)*

162. **(C)** Hypocalcemia results in increased neuromuscular excitability. Chovstek sign involves percussion over the facial nerve in front of the ear with resultant contraction of the facial muscles. The Trousseau sign is a less reliable indication of hypocalcemia in which a carpopedal spasm results from the inflation of a blood pressure cuff on the arm for 3 minutes. *(Schwartz et al, pp. 1620–1621; DeGowin et al, p. 783)*

163. **(D)** Carcinoma is not associated with pancreatitis, which is a painful inflammation of the gland. Carcinoma of the pancreas is almost always a painless entity until late in its course. Alcohol-induced pancreatitis is caused because of precipitation of protein in the pancreas, which acts as a nidus for calcium deposition and ductal obstruction. Similar etiology and ductal obstruction occur with elevated lipids and elevated calcium from hyperlipidemia and hyperparathyroidism, respectively. Gallstone

pancreatitis occurs without obstruction of Wirsung's duct by stones impacted in the distal common bile duct and the resultant edema. *(Schwartz et al, pp. 1350–1351)*

164. (D) An "Apple Core" lesion is the classic finding of carcinoma on barium enema. The abrupt, annular compromise differs from the gradual compression seen in inflammatory processes such as diverticulitis. *(Schwartz et al, pp. 1188–1200; Squire, pp. 208–209)*

165. (C) Homeostatic regulation of thyroid activity begins with thyroid releasing hormone (TRH), which is secreted by the hypothalamus as the result of negative feedback. This in turn causes the pituitary to release thyroid stimulating hormone (TSH), which in turn signals the thyroid gland to release T_4. The T_4 is converted peripherally to T_3, the active form of thyroid hormone. *(Schwartz et al, p. 1550)*

166. (B) Pneumaturia or air in the urine along with fecaluria is diagnostic of a colovesicular fistula (between bladder and colon). This is a consequence of inflammation and perforation along adjacent organs and may result from carcinoma or diverticulitis. *(Schwartz et al, p. 1190)*

167. (A)

Operation	Mortality	Morbidity
Partial gastrectomy	3%	10%
Vagotomy/antrectomy	2%	12%
Vagotomy/pyloroplasty	1%	15%
Vagotomy/drainage	1%	15%
Proximal gastric vagotomy	0.5%	5%

Proximal gastric vagotomy (PGV) leaves vagal innervation to the antral portion of the stomach, and to other intraabdominal organs intact. This, along with low morbidity and mortality rates, has made PGV the procedure of choice for duodenal ulcers when no drainage procedure is required. However, PGV is associated with a 15% recurrence rate. *(Schwartz, pp. 1170–1173)*

168. (C) The chief cells, which are found deep in the glands of the fundus, secrete pepsinogen. Pepsinogen is the inactive precursor of pepsin, which is active in protein breakdown. The G cells secrete gastrin, a hormone. This hormone stimulates the secretion of gastric acid by the parietal cells, and pepsinogen by the chief cells. Glucagon is a hormone secreted by the walls of the stomach and duodenum and also by the alpha cells of the pancreas. Glucagon acts to increase blood glucose levels. *(Schwartz, pp. 1160–1163)*

169. (B) The most common complication of duodenal ulcer is bleeding. This is, however, usually minor, and often presents as melena. If bleeding persists despite adequate medical therapy, endoscopic control is appropriate. The mortality rate is unchanged with endoscopic control. Should an operation become necessary, simple suture ligation would control the bleeding but an antiulcer procedure should be done to prevent recurrence. Total gastrectomy with its associated high rates of morbidity and mortality is reserved for patients with Zollinger–Ellison syndrome or those with multiple recurrences of their ulcers. *(Schwartz, pp. 1168–1170)*

170. (E) Barrett's esophagus is a consequence of the corrosive insult to the lower esophagus as a result of persistent gastroesophageal reflux. A change or destruction of the squamous cell lining of the lower esophagus and a change to columnar epithelial cells is noted. This is also associated with stenosis of the lower esophageal sphincter. These stenotic lesions are readily amenable to esophageal dilation. *(Schwartz et al, p. 1076)*

171. (B) Boerhaave syndrome is a traumatic esophageal rupture following intense straining usually associated with retching. This is an uncommon but life-threatening complication. It is usually associated with severe pain, hematemesis, and, if communicating with the pleural cavity, often associated with respiratory findings of dyspnea or cyanosis. *(Sabiston, pp. 1816–1818)*

172. (C) The Mallory–Weiss syndrome is a result of retching and involves linear tearing of the mucosal lining at the gastroesophageal junction. This is also associated with pain and hematemesis. The pain is not as severe as the pain associated with Booerhave syndrome and is generally a self-limiting condition. *(Schwartz et al, pp. 1103–1104)*

173. (A) The Plummer–Vinson syndrome is also known as sideropenic dysphagia. This is a condition often seen in middle-aged women who have a long-standing history of iron deficiency anemia. They develop dysphagia, which upon endoscopy is noted to be from a fibrous web extending around the esophagus below the cricopharyngus muscles. This syndrome is readily treated with iron supplementation and esophageal dilation. *(Schwartz et al, p. 1103)*

174. (E) Several features of gastric ulcers indicate the need for surgery. Large ulcers, that is, greater than 4 cm may require extensive resection. These usually occur in malnourished, elderly patients. Evidence of deep penetration or association with duodenal ulcers are indications for surgery because of suspicion of malignancy and recurrence, respectively. Finally, failure of medical therapy or recurrence after a period of healing should lead one to consider malignancy and are indications for surgery. *(Schwartz, pp. 1176–1177)*

175. **(A)** Carcinoma is the most common etiology of large bowel obstruction. Volvulus, which involves a torsion of either the cecum or sigmoid represents the second most common cause of large bowel obstruction. Finally, diverticulitis is an infrequent cause of bowel obstruction, generally from a significant abscess formation and resultant inflammation. Ulcerative colitis is not a cause of large bowel obstruction. *(Schwartz et al, pp. 1034–1035; DeGowin et al, pp. 553–555)*

176. **(A)** Parathyroid hormones control the metabolic balances of calcium, phosphorous, and magnesium. Chloride metabolism is regulated via the renal system. The serum levels of calcium are controlled via feedback mechanism involving calcitonin produced from the thyroid gland and parathyroid hormone (PTH), which regulate the release of calcium stores. PTH is secreted from the parathyroid gland in respond to a decrease in serum calcium. *(Schwartz, et al, pp. 1645–1649)*

177. **(C)** Diet and age play prominent roles. Diverticulosis is a disease resulting from highly processed, low-fiber diets of industrialized nations and is rarely seen before the age of 35. The incidence increases with age and by 85, almost 65% of the population will have diverticulosis. *(Schwartz et al, p. 1185)*

178. **(E)** Bilirubin is produced primarily from hemoglobin, but also comes from breakdown products of myoglobin. The liver also synthesizes some bilirubin. From whatever source, once bilirubin is produced, it complexes with albumin to form a stable complex (indirect bilirubin). This complex is not water soluble and therefore is not excreted in the urine. The indirect bilirubin is transported to the hepatic parenchymal cell. Here, the albumin is removed and the bilirubin is conjugated with glucuronic acid to form a diglucuronide that is water soluble (direct bilirubin). Direct bilirubin is excreted into the bile canaliculi, and ultimately makes its way into the intestine where it is acted upon by bacteria forming urobilin and urobilinogen. *(Schwartz, pp. 1091–1094)*

179. **(E)** Distention, tenderness, and tympany, as well as auscultation of rushes and/or tinkling are all associated with bowel obstruction. In addition, the patient may have complaints of nausea and vomiting. Depending upon the level of the bowel obstruction, there may be fecal vomiting and obstipation. *(Schwartz et al, pp. 1034–1038)*

180. **(E)** Shock is usually due to either hemorrhage from the injured arteries or associated injuries. When profound, vasoconstriction may conceal the presence of an arterial injury until blood pressure is restored. The type of trauma—blunt or penetrating—needs to be known. Blunt trauma can cause multiple organ injuries. In the injured extremity, fractures and nerve injuries are commonly present in both types of trauma. Bright red bleeding suggests arterial injury. *(Schwartz, p. 937)*

181. **(C)** Classic stroke from unilateral carotid disease is ipsilateral blindness and contralateral hemiplegia. The presence of aphasia depends on involvement of the dominant cerebral hemisphere. Fleeting neurologic defects, transient monoplegia or hemiplegia, or transient ipsilateral blindness may clear within minutes or hours and are termed *transient ischemic attacks*. *(Schwartz, p. 976)*

182. **(C)** Aneurysm can be defined as the inappropriate dilatation of an artery. There are two types of aneurysms. A fusiform aneurysm is usually due to atherosclerosis and involves the entire circumference of the artery. Saccular aneurysms are focal and usually secondary to traumatic injury, infection, and fibromuscular hyperplasia. Fusiform aneurysms require prosthetic replacement to restore or maintain arterial continuity. Saccular aneurysms may be excised and the artery repaired. *(Schwartz, p. 981)*

183. **(E)** Pacemakers are used when there is an abnormality of cardiac conduction. Arrhythmias and impairment of conduction in the atrioventricular node and the His–Purkinje system are the chief reasons for implantation. Acquired heart block, a fibrosis of the conduction system without other significant cardiac disease, "sick sinus syndrome," an alternating bradycardia and tachycardia, Stokes–Adams attacks, intermittent attacks of syncope, and convulsions with heart block, and complete atrioventricular disassociation, in which there may be periods of transient ventricular syncope, convulsions, and death, all require permanent pacemakers. *(Schwartz, p. 897)*

184. **(B)** The term *restrictive ventilatory disorder* denotes a pattern of abnormalities in lung function. The word restrictive is employed to indicate a restriction of or limitation to the amount of gas within the lungs. Thus, ventilatory disorders are characterized by reduction in lung volume. The hallmark of restriction is a decrease in the vital capacity. Obstructive ventilatory disorder denotes the constellation of abnormalities that resolves from airway obstruction, regardless of its cause. Obstructive disorders are detected mainly by the tests of the behavior of the respiratory system under dynamic conditions. The FeV1/Fvc (Forced expiratory volume in 1 second divided by the forced vital capacity) is the most widely used, although tests of maximal flow volume relationships are being increasingly used. *(Beeson et al, pp. 416–417, 427–428)*

185. **(E)** Patients with pneumonia may present with a variety of clinical manifestations. However, findings disclosed by proper physical examination of the lungs should aid in the formulation of the differential diagnosis. Vocal fremitis is increased in consolidated pneumonias and by inflammation surrounding other pulmonary lesions, by transmitting bronchotracheal air vibration with greater efficiency than do the air-filled pulmonary alveoli. Consolidated pulmonary tissue has increased density as opposed to normal lung tissue, therefore yielding impaired resonance, dullness, and flatness to percussion. This consolidated tissue also transmits whispered syllables distinctly, even when the pathological process is too small to produce bronchial breathing. Rales refer to sounds in the lungs from the movements of fluids or exudates in the airways. Although there are different types of rales, they sound like clicks or small bubbles and occur in bronchiectasis, pneumonia, consolidation, infarction, bronchitis, and TB. *(DeGowin and DeGowin, pp. 296–319)*

186. **(B)** The frequency of different cell types of bronchogenic carcinoma varies in the literature. In general, epidermoid carcinoma occurs with the greatest frequency and constitutes approximately 40% to 50% of pulmonary neoplasms. Adenocarcinoma (bronchogenic and bronchioloalveolar), large cell carcinoma, and small cell anaplastic carcinoma occur at similar rates between 15% to 20%. *(Beeson et al, pp. 458–459)*

187. **(A)** Cheyne–Stokes respiration is the most common form of periodic breathing. Periods of apnea alternate regularly with series of respiratory cycles. In each cycle, the rate and amplitude of successive respirations increase to a maximum, then decrease progressively until the series is terminated with an apneic period. Kussmaul respiration is applied to deep, regular sighing respirations, regardless of rate. This pattern of breathing is seen in diabetic ketoacidosis, uremia, peritonitis, severe hemorrhage, and pneumonia. Biots breathing is an uncommon variant of Cheyne–Stokes respiration, in which periods of apnea alternate irregularly with series of breaths of equal depth. This is most often seen in meningitis. Stridulous breathing is a high-pitched whistling or crowing sound with respirations when the air passes over a partly closed glottis. This occurs with edema of the vocal cords (i.e., infection), neoplasm, abscess of the pharynx, and foreign body in the pharynx. Apnea is simply the absence of respiration. *(DeGowin and DeGowin, pp. 270–281)*

188. **(E)** The clinical manifestations of bronchogenic carcinoma can vary, and many patients are asymptomatic when the pulmonary lesion is discovered. Cough usually productive of scant sputum is a common symptom; hemoptysis occurs frequently secondary to ulceration in the pulmonary lesion. Frequently, because of a significant smoking history, patients with carcinoma also have obstructive pulmonary disease and dyspnea with exertion. Weight loss is another common complaint of bronchogenic carcinoma but generally occurs with more extensive disease beyond the time the neoplasm is limited to the lung. Chest pain may be due to pleural involvement but must also suggest metastatic disease. Pulmonary infections occur distal to the bronchial obstruction and can mask the tumor. Any atypical or recurrent pulmonary infection should suggest carcinoma. Chest x-ray may demonstrate hilar and mediastinal lymph node involvement, pleural effusion, rib metastasis, elevation of a diaphragm, tracheal compression or distortion, and pericardial effusion. Although pulmonary diseases, particularly at end stages, present with similar symptoms, the entire history, physical, laboratory, and roentgenographic findings must be correlated to form the correct diagnosis. Asthma and COPD usually reveal hyperinflation of the lungs and flat diaphragms. Bronchiectasis shows coarse lung markings and even honeycombing due to the abnormal dilatation of the bronchial tree. Chronic bronchitis has been used in various ways, sometimes referring to a simple smoker's cough and at other times to severe COPD. It is usually described as a productive cough that is present on most days for at least 3 months of the year. *(Beeson et al, pp. 457–460)*

189. **(C)** People at risk for pulmonary embolism are those in hypercoagulable states. This may arise from the use of birth control pills, local stasis, immobilization that may be the result of an accident or illness, fractures, obesity, and congestive heart failure. Emboli that cause clinically significant pulmonary insult commonly arise in the ileofemoral and pelvic venous beds. Signs and symptoms often begin abruptly and include dyspnea, cough, anxiety, and chest pain (frequently pleuritic in nature). Hemoptysis may occur; tachycardia and tachypnea are common in this illness. A low-grade fever, hypotension, and cyanosis are also signs of pulmonary embolism. The presence of a deep venous thrombosis aids in the rapid clinical diagnosis. Radiographic evidence of consolidation may be present in cases of pulmonary embolism. *(Mills, p. 535; Beeson et al, pp. 442–444)*

190. **(A)** Therapy for asthma can include all the choices, but inhaled beta-adrenergic agonists provide the most rapid effect and therefore have the best therapeutic index. Use of epinephrine is contraindicated in patients with known cardiac disease and is not recommended in patients older than 50. Aminophyllin, IV and oral, has a slower onset of action

and therapeutic levels must be maintained and monitored. Hydrocortisone also has a delayed onset of action and its use should be limited if possible. *(Beeson et al, pp. 408–410)*

191. **(B)** Vital capacity is the sum of the inspiratory reserve volume, the tidal volume, and the expiratory reserve volume. Any factors that reduce the ability of the lung to expand also reduce the vital capacity. Therefore, fibrotic lung diseases such as tuberculosis, emphysema, chronic asthma, lung cancer, chronic bronchitis, and fibrotic pleurisy can all reduce pulmonary compliance and the vital capacity. For this reason, the vital capacity is the most important of clinical respiratory measurements in assessment of the progression of these diseases. Arterial blood gases are helpful in the objective determination of the oxygenation of the blood, but are not reliable in the assessment of progression in fibrotic diseases. Changes in tidal volume may not become apparent until late in the disease process. *(Krupp et al, p. 126; Guyton, pp. 470–472)*

192. **(B)** Although the location of maximal tenderness may vary with the position of the appendix, in typical acute appendicitis, tenderness will be maximal in the right lower quadrant, near McBurney's point. The psoas sign or other peritoneal signs of irritation such as Rovsing's sign (pressure in LLQ produces pain in the RLQ) or the obturator sign (pain in RLQ with internal rotation of a flexed right thigh in a supine patient) are indicators of local or retroperitoneal irritation. If an inflamed appendix hangs into the pelvis, there may be no abdominal findings and the diagnosis missed unless a rectal examination is done. Cutaneous hyperesthesia is a frequent but inconsistent finding in acute appendicitis. It may be the first positive sign in early appendicitis. *(Schwartz, p. 1317)*

193. **(E)** Venography, the injection of contrast material for direct visualization of the venous system of an extremity is the most accurate method of confirming the diagnosis of venous thrombosis and the extent of involvement. Of the noninvasive studies, duplex scanning, combining ultrasound with real-time B-mode imaging can demonstrate the thrombi within veins only in the extremities, not in the pelvis. Although 95% accurate, impedance plethysmography is unable to detect calf vein thrombosis or differentiate old from new postthrombotic sequelae. Radiolabeled fibrinogen studies cannot detect thrombi in pelvic veins and cannot be used in the presence of a diseased or injured extremity. *(Schwartz, p. 1015)*

194. **(B)** Lymphedema, resulting from an abnormality of the lymphatic system is characteristically firm, rubbery, but nonpitting. It may be unilateral or bilateral. Lymph vesicles may be present containing fluid of high protein concentration. In cardiac and renal disease and cirrhosis, bilateral dependent pitting edema may be present. Venous disease will usually produce unilateral edema and other signs such as brawny discoloration varicose veins; stasis ulcers or dermatitis may also be seen. *(Schwartz, p. 1036)*

195. **(A)** Abdominal aortic aneurysms are the most common of the atherosclerotic aneurysms. Men are affected more frequently than women in a ratio approximating 10:1. Except for traumatic and congenital malformations, almost all peripheral aneurysms result from arteriosclerosis. The majority of peripheral aneurysms are in the popliteal artery. Infrequent sites include the femoral, carotid, and subclavian arteries. *(Schwartz, p. 988)*

196. **(B)** A serum potassium of 5.0 mEq/L is normal. Either deficiency or excess of potassium below 4.0 mEq/L or 6.0 mEq/L can be harmful. Coronary occlusion, anoxia, drugs, and arrhythmias as well as electrolyte abnormalities are the five frequent causes of cardiac arrest or fibrillation. *(Schwartz, p. 852)*

197. **(B)** Patients with cancer of the urinary bladder usually present with painless hematuria. Hematuria, either gross or microhematuria, is present in 95% of the cases at the time of diagnosis and is usually the initial sign. Histologically, 90% of the tumors are transitional cell in type. Adenocarcinoma occurs infrequently. Metastases and local extension usually occur late in the course of the disease. Bladder tumors metastasize via the pelvic lymphatics and by hematogenous routes to bone, liver, and lung, as well as to other sites. The prognosis for bladder cancer is related to the histology of the tumor and its staging. Superficial small tumors may be adequately treated with endoscopic resection and electrodesiccation. The treatment for locally invasive, resectable tumors is preoperative radiation followed by cystectomy, with supravesical diversion of urine. *(Schwartz, pp. 1756–1759)*

198. **(B)** Intermittent claudication is the most common complaint produced by limb ischemia. The pain experienced is felt during exertion, not at rest, and gradually disappears within minutes upon cessation of activity. The symptoms may remain stable for years or improve after exercise programs have been initiated to help develop collateral circulation. Chronic arterial occlusion may progress and intermittent pain involving muscle groups may be supplanted by continuous pain at rest referred to sites most distal to the arterial occlusion. This type of pain worsens with elevation of the extremity and is

relieved by placing the extremity in a dependent position. *(Schwartz, p. 948)*

199. **(B)** Atherosclerosis of the origin of the internal carotid artery is the most common form of extracranial vascular disease. Stenosis involving only the vertebral artery is infrequent and significant only when bilateral or if one vertebral is congenitally absent. Atherosclerotic stenosis or occlusion of the subclavian artery proximal to the site of origin of the vertebral artery produces the subclavian steal syndrome. This phenomenon is not an infrequent finding on angiography, but clinical symptoms are not common because of collateralization. *(Schwartz, pp. 979, 980)*

200. **(B)** In transposition of the great vessels, the two basic handicaps are severe anoxia from the inability to transport oxygen from the lungs to the tissues of the body, and progressive cardiac failure. The severe and rapidly progressive cardiac failure results partly from a high cardiac output and partly from the fact that the coronary arteries are filled with unoxygenated blood resulting in myocardial anoxia. A high percentage of infants are cyanotic at birth and have cardiac failure with dyspnea. Atrial septal defect, ventricular septal defect, and patent ductus arteriosus are not lethal disorders. In patients with tetralogy of Fallot, life expectancy is short; approximately 25% die in the first year, 40% die by 3 years of age, and 70% die by the time they are 10 years old without treatment. *(Schwartz, pp. 772, 775)*

Subspecialty List: Practice Test

Question Numbers and Subspecialty
1. Hypercalcemia
2. Thyroid
3. Adrenal
4. Osteoporosis
5. Diabetes
6. Adrenal
7. Hypocalcemia
8. Hypercalcemia
9. Adrenal
10. Nephrolithiasis
11. Adrenal
12. Lipid metabolism
13. Paget's disease
14. Diabetes
15. Diabetes
16. Pharmacology
17. Pulmonary
18. Seizures
19. Migraine
20. Seizures
21. Spinal cord injury
22. Head injury
23. Hematuria
24. Metabolic acidosis
25. Pyelonephritis
26. Amputation
27. Hemorrhage
28. Fluid resuscitation
29. Small bowel obstruction
30. Acute cholecystitis
31. Mesenteric ischemia
32. Peripheral vascular
33. Soft tissue infection
34. Colorectal surgery
35. Facial fractures
36. Wound care
37. Burns
38. Orthopedics
39. Paracentesis
40. Toxicology
41. Toxicology
42. CPR
43. Trauma
44. Orthopedics
45. Orthopedics
46. Oncology
47. Child abuse
48. Otitis media
49. Pediatric asthma
50. CPR
51. Burns
52. Orthopedics
53. Gastroenterology
54. Seizures
55. Emergency medicine
56. General pediatrics
57. Pediatric poisoning
58. Child abuse
59. Immunizations
60. General pediatrics
61. Otitis media
62. Sexual development
63. Pediatric nutrition
64. Child development
65. Neonatology
66. Pediatric cardiology
67. Dermatology
68. Dermatology
69. Dermatology
70. Dermatology
71. Renal—anatomy and physiology
72. Renal—sclerosis
73. Renal—cysts
74. Renal—osmolality
75. Renal—water metabolism
76. Renal—urine concentration
77. Rheumatology—physiology
78. Rheumatology—gouty arthritis
79. Obstetrics—pyelonephritis
80. Obstetrics—rash
81. Obstetrics—preeclampsia
82. Obstetrics—preeclampsia
83. Gynecology—Pap smear
84. Gynecology—contraception
85. Gynecology—dysmenorrhea
86. Gynecology—vaginal infections
87. Gynecology—vaginal infections

88. Gynecology—vaginal infections
89. Gynecology—vaginal infections
90. Obstetrics—events of pregnancy
91. Obstetrics—events of pregnancy
92. Obstetrics—events of pregnancy
93. Obstetrics—events of pregnancy
94. Cardiology—pericardial effusions
95. Cardiology—physical diagnosis
96. Cardiology—left ventricular hypertrophy
97. Cardiology—EKG
98. Cardiology—EKG
99. Cardiology—EKG findings
100. Cardiology—risk factors
101. Cardiology—syncope
102. Cardiology—pericarditis
103. Cardiology—hypertension
104. Cardiology—anatomy and physiology
105. Cardiology—physical diagnosis
106. Cardiology—EKG findings
107. Cardiology—medications
108. Cardiology—prophylaxis
109. Cardiology—prognosis
110. Cardiology—blood pressure classification
111. Psychiatry—medication
112. Psychiatry—narcolepsy
113. Psychiatry—sleep apnea
114. Psychiatry—management
115. Infectious disease—Lyme disease
116. Infectious disease—TB
117. Infectious disease—hepatitis B
118. Psychiatry—anorexia nervosa
119. Psychiatry—bulimia
120. Rheumatology—osteoarthritis
121. Rheumatology—septic arthritis
122. Rheumatology—rheumatoid arthritis
123. Psychiatry—diagnosis
124. Psychiatry—depression
125. Psychiatry—schizophrenia
126. Psychiatry—psychosis
127. Psychiatry—phobias
128. Psychiatry—medications
129. Psychiatry—borderline personality
130. Hematology/Oncology—Sickle cell anemia
131. Hematology/Oncology—hemolytic anemia
132. Hematology/Oncology—chronic lymphocytic leukemia
133. Hematology/Oncology—pernicious anemia
134. Hematology/Oncology—aplastic anemia
135. Dermatology—erythema multiforme
136. Dermatology—skin cancers
137. Dermatology—skin lesions
138. Dermatology—erysipelas
139. Renal—pyelonephritis
140. Infectious disease—Lyme disease
141. Infectious disease—Rocky Mountain spotted fever
142. Infectious disease—differential diagnosis
143. Obstetrics—infections in pregnancy
144. Obstetrics—infections in pregnancy
145. Obstetrics—rhogam
146. Obstetrics—AIDS
147. Obstetrics—endomyometritis
148. Gynecology—Pap smear
149. Gynecology—contraception
150. Gynecology—sterilization
151. Gynecology—infertility
152. Dermatology—varicella
153. Dermatology—bullae differential diagnosis
154. Dermatology—viral diseases
155. AIDS—transmission
156. AIDS—Karposi sarcoma
157. AIDS—HIV testing
158. AIDS—HIV
159. AIDS—*Pneumocyctis carinii* pneumonia
160. Surgery—bleeding
161. Surgery—ulcerative colitis
162. Surgery—hypocalcemia
163. Surgery—pancreatitis
164. Surgery—radiological findings
165. Surgery—thyroid
166. Surgery—pneumaturia
167. Surgery—morbidity and mortality
168. Surgery—physiology
169. Surgery—duodenal ulcers
170. Surgery—esophageal disorders
171. Surgery—esophageal disorders
172. Surgery—esophageal disorders
173. Surgery—esophageal disorders
174. Surgery—gastric ulcers
175. Surgery—large bowel obstruction
176. Surgery—parathyroid physiology
177. Surgery—diverticulitis
178. Surgery—bilirubin metabolism
179. Surgery—bowel obstruction; physical diagnosis
180. Surgery—vascular trauma
181. Surgery—stroke; signs and symptoms
182. Surgery—aneurysms
183. Surgery—pacemakers; indications
184. Pulmonary—restrictive vs. obstructive disease
185. Pulmonary—pneumonia; physical findings
186. Pulmonary—lung cancer
187. Pulmonary—periodic breathing
188. Pulmonary—lung cancer
189. Pulmonary—pulmonary embolism
190. Pulmonary—asthma treatment
191. Pulmonary—pulmonary function
192. Surgery—appendicitis; physical diagnosis
193. Surgery—venous obstruction; diagnosis
194. Surgery—nonpitting edema; diagnosis
195. Surgery—aneurysms
196. Surgery—causes of atrial fibrillation
197. Surgery—bladder cancer
198. Surgery—claudication
199. Surgery—extracranial vascular disease
200. Surgery—congenital vascular defects

Master Bibliography

Abramowicz M, (ed). Treatment of Lyme disease. *Med Lett*. 1989;31:57-59.

Abramowicz M, (ed). Handbook of antimicrobial therapy. *Med Lett*. 1988, 129-132.

Acker DB, Sachs BP, Friedman EA. Risk factors for shoulder dystocia. *Obset Gynecol*. 1985;66(6):762-767.

Adams JC. Complications of fractures. In: *Outline of Fractures*. Edinburgh: Churchill-Livingston, 1987.

Ahlering T, Weintraub P, Weinburg A, Skinner D. Urologic surgery and trauma. In: Civetta, (ed). *Critical Care*. Philadelphia: JB Lippincott; 1988.

Albarran-Sotelo R, Flint L, Kelley K, (eds). *Instructor's Manual for Basic Life Support*. American Heart Association, 1987.

Aldrich MS. Cardinal manifestations of sleep disorders. In: Kryger, Roth, Dement, (eds). *Principles and Practice of Sleep Medicine*. Philadelphia: WB Saunders; 1989.

American Psychiatric Association. *Diagnostic and Statistical Manual of Mental Disorders*, 3rd ed. Washington, DC: American Psychiatric Association, 1987.

Andreoli T, Carpenter C, Plum F, Smith L, (eds). *Cecil's Essentials of Medicine*, 2nd ed. Philadelphia: WB Saunders, 1990.

Avery ME, First LR, (eds). *Pediatric Medicine*. Baltimore: Williams & Wilkins, 1989.

Avery ME, Tausch HW. *Scaffer's Diseases of the Newborn*, 5th ed. Philadelphia: WB Saunders, 1984.

Baker SP, O'Neil B, Karpf R. *The Injury Fact Book*. Lexington, KY: Lexington Books, 1984.

Baldessarini RJ. *Chemotherapy in Psychiatry*, 2nd ed. Cambridge, MA: Harvard University Press, 1985.

Balfour CN, Balfour HH Jr. Cytomegalovirus is not an occupational risk for nurses in renal transplant and neonatal nurses: Results of a prospective study. *JAMA*. 1986; 256:1909-1914.

Barkin RM. *Emergency Pediatrics*, 2nd ed. St Louis: CV Mosby, 1987.

Barnhart ER. *Physician's Desk Reference*, 44th ed. Oradell, NJ: Medical Economics Co, 1990.

Barrett E, DeFronzo R. Diabetic ketoacidosis: Diagnosis and treatment. *Hosp Pract*. 1984; 19:89-104.

Bates B. *A Guide to Physical Examination and History Taking*, 3rd ed. Philadelphia: JB Lippincott, 1987.

Behrman RE, Vaughn VC. *Nelson's Textbook of Pediatrics*, 13th ed. Philadelphia: WB Saunders, 1987.

Bell DM. Kawasaki update: More answers, fewer questions. *Contemp Pediatr*. 1985;2:20-36.

Benjamin CC. Bacterial pneumonia. In: Tintinalli JE, Krome RL, Ruiz E, (eds). *Emergency Medicine: A Comprehensive Study Guide*. New York: McGraw-Hill, 1988.

Benson H. *The Relaxation Response*. New York: Avon; 1975.

Berger M, Birchtold P. Insulin transport and action at target cells. In: *Joslin's Diabetes Mellitus*, 12th ed. Philadelphia: Lea & Febiger, 1985.

Berkow R, ed. *The Merck Manual of Diagnosis and Therapy*, 15th ed. Rahway, NJ: Merck and Co, 1987.

Bithony WG, Rathbun J. Failure to thrive. In: Levin M, Crocker A, et al, (eds). *Developmental-Behavioral Pediatrics*. Philadelphia: WB Saunders, 1983.

Braunwald E, (ed). *Heart Disease: A Textbook of Cardiovascular Medicine*, 3rd ed. Philadelphia: WB Saunders, 1988.

Braunwald E, Isselbacher KJ, Petersdorf R, et al, (eds). *Harrison's Principles of Internal Medicine*, 11th ed. New York: McGraw-Hill, 1987.

Brent DSA. Suicide and suicidal behavior in children and adolescents. *Pediatr Rev*. 1989; 10:269-275.

Brown SL, Busuttil RW. Portal hypertension. In: Moore W, (ed). *Vascular Surgery, A Comprehensive Review*. New York: Grune & Stratton, 1983.

Burke L. The use of the Friedman curve in labor management. *Cinc J Med*. 1975;56(2):29-36.

Burrow, Ferris. *Medical Complications During Pregnancy*. Philadelphia: WB Saunders, 1988.

Cahill GF, Arky RA, et al. Diabetes mellitus. *Sci Am Med*. VI. January 1987.

Capitulo KL, Maffia A. *The Perinatal Bereavement Team: Development and Function, Women and Loss*. New York: Praeger, 1985.

Carman RA. *Study Skills: A Student's Guide for Survival*, 2nd ed. New York: John Wiley & Sons, 1984.

Center for Disease Control. AIDS and Human Immunodeficiency Virus infection in the United States: 1988 update. *MMWR.* 1989; 38(s-4):1-38, 1989.

Center for Disease Control. Guidelines for prevention of transmission of human immunodeficiency virus and hepatitis B virus to health care workers and public safety workers. *MMWR.* 1989;35(s-6):1-37.

Chapel TA, Riley HD Jr, Russo G, Septimus E. Cutaneous signs of infection. *Patient Care.* 1988;22:185-218.

Clarkin J, Sweeney J. Psychological assessment. *Psychiatry.* 1988;7:5.

Cohn JN. *Drug Treatment of Heart Failure,* 2nd ed. Secaucus, NJ: Advanced Therapeutics Communications International, 1988.

Colloton M. Investigating failure to thrive. *J Am Acad Physic Assist.* 1989;2:10.

Committee on Trauma. *Advanced Trauma Life Support Program of the American College of Surgeons.* Chicago, IL: American College of Surgeons, 1989.

Copeland KC, Brochman RR, Rauk JL. Variations in normal sexual development. *Pediatr Rev.* 1986; 8:18-26.

Cox FL. Principles of the renal regulation of fluids and electrolytes. In: De Vita VT Jr, Dupont HL, Kelley NN, et al (eds). *The Textbook of Internal Medicine.* Philadelphia: JB Lippincott, 1989.

Cox FL, Favus MJ. Nephrolithiasis. In: Braunwald E, Isselbacher KJ, Petersdorf R, et al, (eds). *Harrison's Principles of Internal Medicine,* 11th ed. New York: McGraw-Hill, 1987.

Crapo JD, Hamilton MA, Edgman S, (eds). *Medicine and Pediatrics in One Book.* St. Louis, MO: CV Mosby, 1988.

Cunningham FG, MacDonald PC, Gant NF, (eds). *William's Obstetrics,* 18th ed. Norwalk, CT: Appleton & Lange, 1989.

Dajani AS, Asmar BI, Thirumoorthi MC. Systemic *Haemophilus influenzae* disease: An overview. *J. Pediatr.* 1979;94: 355-364.

Davidson KI. Symptomatic psychoses. *Psychiatry.* 1988;69:1-14.

DeCecco JP, Crawford WR. *The Psychology of Learning and Instruction,* 2nd ed. Englewood Cliffs, NJ: Prentice-Hall, 1974.

DeFronzo RA, Ferrannin E, et al. New concepts in the pathogenesis and treatment of non-insulin dependent diabetes mellitus. *Am J Med.* 1983;74(1a):52-81.

Demling R. Fluid resuscitation. In: Boswick JA, (ed). *The Art and Science of Burn Care.* Rockville, MD: Aspen Publishers, 1987.

Dorsky DI, Crumpacker CS. Drugs five years later: Acyclovir. *Ann Intern Med.* 1987;107(6):859-874.

Dunner DL. Affective disorder: Clinical features. *Psychiatry.* 1988;59:2-3.

Dupont HL, Edelman R, Kimmey M. Infectious diarrhea from A to Z. *Patient Care.* 1987;21:98-137.

Eiseman B, Robinson WA, Steele G Jr. *Follow-up of the Cancer Patient.* New York: Thieme-Stratton, 1982.

Ellinwood E, Woody G, Krichnan R. Treatment for drug abuse. *Psychiatry.* 1988;90:3, 6-12.

Epstein E. *Common Skin Disorders,* 2nd ed. Oradell, NJ: Medical Economics Co, 1983.

Fabrey L, Case SM. Further support for changing multiple-choice answers. *J Med Ed.* June 1985; 488-490.

Fallon J, Eddy J, Weiner L, Pizzo PA. Human Immunodeficiency Virus in children. *J Pediatr.* 1989;114:1-30.

Farer LS, Reichman LB, Stead WW. TB today: Don't count it out. *Patient Care.* 1987;21:141-165.

Federman DD. Thyroid. *Sci Am Med.* May 1989.

Felig P, Baxter JD, et al, (eds). *Endocrinology and Metabolism.* New York: McGraw-Hill, 1987.

Fitzpatrick TB, Eisen AZ, Wolf K, et al. *Dermatology in General Medicine,* 3rd ed. New York: McGraw-Hill, 1987.

Freeman RK, Garite TJ. *Fetal Heart Rate Monitoring.* Baltimore, MD: Williams & Wilkins, 1981.

Galli RL, Spraite DW, Simon RR. *Emergency Orthopedics of the Spine.* Norwalk, CT: Appleton & Lange, 1989.

Georgiade DG, Manstein ME. Maxillofacial trauma. In: Moylan JA, (ed). *Trauma Surgery.* Philadelphia: JB Lippincott, 1988.

Gerber MA, Randolph MD, DeMae K, et al. Failure of once daily penicillin V therapy for streptococcal pharyngitis. *Am J Dis Child.* 1989; 143:153-155.

Gerbie MD. Complications of Menstruation; Abnormal Uterine Bleeding. In: Pernoll ML, Benson RC, (eds). Current *Obstetric & Gynecologic Diagnosis & Treatment,* 6th ed. Norwalk, Conn.: Appleton & Lange, 1987.

Gerkin RD. Cocaine. In: Tintinalli JE, Krome RL, Ruiz E, (eds). *Emergency Medicine, A Comprehensive Study Guide.* New York: McGraw-Hill, 1988.

Goodman LS, Gilman AG. *The Pharmacologic Basis of Therapeutics,* 7th ed. New York: Macmillan, 1985.

Gorman J, Liebowitz M. Panic and anxiety disorders. *Psychiatry.* 1988;32:1-4, 10-11.

Greenberg JS. *Comprehensive Stress Management,* 2nd ed. Dubuque, IA: Wm C Brown, 1987.

Greenfield LJ. Venous and lymphatic disease. In: Schwartz SI, et al (eds). *Principles of Surgery,* 5th ed. New York: McGraw-Hill, 1989.

Grundy SM. Disorders of lipids and lipoproteins. In: Stein JH, (ed). *Internal Medicine,* 2nd ed. Boston: Little, Brown, 1987.

Guilleminault C. Narcolepsy syndrome. In: Kryger, Roth, Dement, (eds). *Principles and Practice of Sleep Medicine.* Philadelphia: WB Saunders, 1989.

Hacker NF, Moore JG. *Essentials of Obstetrics and Gynecology.* Philadelphia: WB Saunders, 1986.

Handbook of Common Poisonings in Children, 2nd ed. Evanston, IL: American Academy of Pediatrics, 1983.

Helzer JE. Schizophrenia: Epidemiology. *Psychiatry.* 1988; 54:4-5.

Herndon DJ, Thompson PB, Brown M, Traber DL. Diagnosis, pathophysiology and treatment of inhalation injury. In: Bostwick JA, (ed). *The Art and Science of Burn Care.* Rockville, MD: Aspen Publishers, 1987.

Hiebert B, Cardinal J, Dumka L, Marx RW. Self-instructed relaxation: A therapeutic alternative. *Biofeedback and Self-Regulation.* December 1983;601-617.

Hoffbrand AV, Pettitt JE. *Clinical Hematology.* London: Gower Medical, 1988.

Hollenberg NK. Vascular injury to the kidney. In: Braunwald E, Isselbacher KJ, Petersdorf R, et al, (eds). *Harrison's Principles of Internal Medicine,* 11th ed. New York: McGraw-Hill, 1987.

Hoppenfeld S. *Physical Examination of the Spine and Extremities.* New York: Appleton-Century-Crofts, 1976.

Hruska KA. Structure and function of the kidneys. In: De Vita VT Jr, Dupont HL, Kelley NN, et al, (eds). *The Textbook of Internal Medicine.* Philadelphia: JB Lippincott, 1989.

Hulse E, Strong W. Participation evaluation for athletes. *Pediatr Rev.* 1987; 9:1-10.

Imparato AM, Riles TS. Peripheral arterial disease. In: Schwartz SI, (ed). *Principles of Surgery,* 5th ed. New York: McGraw-Hill, 1989.

Jenike M. *Handbook of Geriatric Psychopharmacology.* Littleton, MA: PSG Publishing, 1985.

Jones HW, Wentz AC, Burnett LS, (eds). *Novak's Textbook of Gynecology,* 11th ed. Baltimore, MD: Williams & Wilkins, 1988.

Kaplan NM. *Clinical Hypertension,* 4th ed. Baltimore, MD: Williams & Wilkins, 1986.

Kaye R, Oski FA, Barness LA. *Core Textbook of Pediatrics,* 2nd ed. Philadelphia: JB Lippincott, 1982.

Kempe CH, Silver HK, O'Brien D, Fulginiti VA. *Current Pediatric Diagnosis and Treatment,* 9th ed. Norwalk, CT: Appleton & Lange, 1987.

Kendell RE. Schizophrenia: Clinical features. *Psychiatry.* 1988;53:7.

Knobf MK, Lewis KP, Fisher DA, et al. *Cancer Chemotherapy. Treatment and Care.* Boston: HK Hall Medical Publishers, 1981.

Kreisberg RA. Diabetic ketoacidosis: New concepts and trends in pathogenesis and treatment. *Ann Intern Med.* 1978;88:681-695.

Krupp MA. Fluid and electrolyte disorders. In: Krupp MA, Schroeder SA, Tierney LM Jr, (eds). *Current Medical Diagnosis and Treatment.* Norwalk, CT: Appleton & Lange, 1989.

Krupp MA, Schroeder SA, Tierney LM Jr, (eds). *Current Medical Diagnosis and Treatment.* Norwalk, CT: Appleton & Lange, 1987.

Lamers RL. Principles of wound management. In: Roberts JR, Hedges JR, (eds). *Clinical Procedures in Emergency Medicine.* Philadelphia: WB Saunders, 1985.

Lewis M. *Clinical Aspects of Child Development.* Philadelphia: Lea & Febiger, 1982.

Linden CH, Romack BH. Acetaminophen. In: Tintinalli JE, Krome RL, Ruiz E, (eds). *Emergency Medicine, A Comprehensive Study Guide.* New York: McGraw-Hill, 1988.

Lugaresi E, Cirignotta F, Montagna P. Snoring: Pathogenic, clinical, and therapeutic aspects. In: Kryger, Roth, Dement, (eds). *Principles and Practice of Sleep Medicine.* Philadelphia: WB Saunders, 1989.

Luterman A, Curreri P. Chemical burn injury. In: Boswick JA, (ed). *The Art and Science of Burn Care.* Rockville, MD: Aspen Publishers, 1987.

Lynch PJ. *Dermatology for the House Officer,* 2nd ed. Baltimore, MD: Williams & Wilkins, 1987.

Maatsch JL. *The Predictive Value of Medical Subspecialty Examinations: Final Report.* National Center for Health Services Research, Contract N1. HS-02-038-04, 1983.

Management of gestational trophoblastic neoplasia. *Am Coll Obstet Gynecol Tech Bull.* 1980;57:1-7.

Mandell GL, Douglas RG Jr, Bennett JE. *Principles and Practice of Infectious Disease,* 2nd ed. New York: Wiley Medical Publishers, 1985.

Markowitz LE, Preblud SR, Orenstein WA, et al. Patterns of transmission in measles outbreaks in the United States, 1985-1986. *N Engl J Med.* 1989;320:75-81.

Merenstein GB, Gardner SL. *Handbook of Neonatal Intensive Care,* 2nd ed. St. Louis: CV Mosby, 1989.

Minkoff HL. Care of pregnant women infected with Human Immune Deficiency Virus. *JAMA.* 1987;2458: 2714-2717.

Moellering RC Jr, Sande MA, Volverding PA, (eds). *Medical management of AIDS. Infect Dis Clin N Am.* 1988;2(2): 285-555.

Monafo WW, Freeman BM. Electrical and lightning injury. In: Boswick JA, (ed). *The Art and Science of Burn Care.* Rockville, MD: Aspen, 1987.

Molinaro J. A primary care approach to heavy metal poisoning. *J Am Acad Phys Assist.* 1989; 2:260-271.

Moylan JA. Burn injury. In: Moylan JA, (ed). *Trauma Surgery.* Philadelphia: JB Lippincott, 1988.

National Cholesterol Education Program. *Highlights of the report of the expert panel on detection, evaluation, and treatment of high blood cholesterol in adults.* NIH publication 88-2926. Washington, DC: Public Health Service, 1987.

Neinstein L. *Adolescent Health Care. A Practical Guide.* Baltimore, MD: Urban and Schwartzenberg, 1984.

Neshein BI. Induced abortion by the suction method. *Acta Obstet Gynecol Scand.* 1984; 63:591-595.

Niswander KR. *Manual of Obstetrics, Diagnosis and Therapy,* 3rd ed. Boston: Little, Brown, 1987.

O'Shanick G. Closed head injury. *Psychiatry.* 1988;92:4-8.

Pass RF, Huffo C, Ricks R, et al. Increased rate of cytomegalovirus infection among parents of children attending daycare centers. *N Engl J Med.* 1986;314:1414-1418.

Pavikrishnan KP. Viral and mycoplasma pneumonias in adults. In: Tintinalli JE, Krome RL, Ruiz E, (eds). *Emergency Medicine, A Comprehensive Study Guide.* New York: McGraw-Hill, 1988.

Peicher J, Schiff ER. Acute viral hepatitis. *Hosp Med.* June 1988;23-41.

Pelletier KR. *Mind as Healer, Mind as Slayer.* New York: Dell, 1977.

Peyton RB, Wolfe WG. Traumatic thoracic aneurysm. In: Moylan JA, (ed). *Trauma Surgery.* Philadelphia: JB Lippincott, 1988.

Phipps R. *The Successful Student's Handbook: A Step-by-Step Guide to Study, Reading, and Thinking Skills.* Seattle: University of Washington Press, 1983.

Polin RA, Ditmar MF. *Pediatric Secrets.* St. Louis: CV Mosby, 1989.

Ragland G. Diabetic ketoacidosis in adults. In: Tintinalli JE, Krome R1, Ruiz E, (eds). *Emergency Medicine, A Comprehensive Study Guide.* New York:McGraw-Hill, 1988.

Rautaharju PM, Prince RJ, Eifler J, et al. Prognostic value of exercise ECG in men at high risk of future coronary heart disease: Multiple risk factor intervention trial experience. *J Am Coll Cardiol.* 1986;8:1-10.

Reisdoff E, Wiegenstein JG. Carbon monoxide poisoning in adults. In: Tintinalli JE, Krome RL, Ruiz E, (eds). *Emergency Medicine, A Comprehensive Study Guide.* New York: McGraw-Hill, 1988.

Rennenbohm RM. Rheumatic diseases of childhood. *Pediatr Rev.* 1989;6:183-190.

Riley HD Jr, Walker DH. Is it Rocky Mountain spotted fever? *Patient Care.* 1988;22:172-189.

Rosenstein BJ, Fosarelli PD. *Pediatric Pearls: The Handbook of Practical Pediatrics.* Chicago: Year Book Medical Publishers, 1989.

Sacks C. Seizures and status epilepticus in adults. In: Tintinalli JE, Krome RL, Ruiz E, (eds). *Emergency Medicine, A Comprehensive Study Guide.* New York: McGraw-Hill, 1988.

Scheidt S. Basic electrocardiography. Abnormalities of electrocardiographic patterns. *CIBA Clin Symp.* 1984;36:1-32.

Schmitt BD. *Your Child's Health.* Toronto: Bantam Books, 1987.

Schmitt BD. Colic: Excessive crying in newborns. *Clin Perinatol.* 1985;12:441-450.

Schwartz SI, et al (eds). *Principles of Surgery,* 5th ed. New York: McGraw-Hill, 1989.

Shababudin SH. Pattern of answer changes to multiple choice questions in physiology. *Med Ed.* March 1983:316-318.

Sherman S. Acute asthma in adults. In: Tintinalli JE, Krome RL, Ruiz E, (eds). *Emergency Medicine, A Comprehensive Study Guide.* New York: McGraw-Hill, 1988.

Shils ME, Young VR. *Modern Nutrition in Health and Disease,* 7th ed. Philadelphia: Lea & Febiger, 1988.

Shulman ST, Amren DP, Bisro AL, et al. Prevention of bacterial endocarditis. A statement for health professionals by the committee on rheumatic fever and infective endocarditis of the council on cardiovascular disease in the young. *Circulation.* 1984;70:1123-1127.

Simmerman JJ, Fogarty TJ. Acute arterial occlusions. In: Moore W, (ed). *Vascular Surgery, A Comprehensive Review.* New York: Grune & Stratton, 1983.

Simmon RR, Brenner BE. Anesthesia and regional blocks. In: *Emergency Procedures and Techniques.* Baltimore: Williams & Wilkins, 1987.

Simmon RR, Brenner BE. Orthopedic procedures. In: *Emergency Procedures and Techniques.* Baltimore: Williams & Wilkins, 1987.

Simon RR, Koenigsknecht SJ. *Emergency Orthopedics, The Extremities,* 2nd ed. Norwalk, CT: Appleton & Lange, 1987.

Snelbecker GE. *Learning Theory, Instructional Theory and Psychoeducational Design.* Lanham, MD: University Printers of America, 1985.

Spencer FC. Congenital heart disease. In: Schwartz SI, et al (eds). *Principles of Surgery,* 5th ed. New York: McGraw-Hill, 1989.

Spencer FC, Culliford AT. Acquired heart disease. In: Schwartz SI, et al (eds). *Principles of Surgery,* 5th ed. New York: McGraw-Hill, 1989.

Stamm WE, Turck M. Urinary tract infection, pyelonephritis and related conditions. In: Braunwald E, Isselbacher KR, Petersdorf R, et al (eds). *Harrison's Principles of Internal Medicine,* 11th ed. New York: McGraw-Hill, 1987.

Standards and Guidelines for Cardiopulmonary Resuscitation (CPR) and Emergency Cardiac Care (ECC). *JAMA.* 1986;2905-2984.

Stein JH, (ed). *Internal Medicine,* 2nd ed. Boston: Little, Brown, 1987.

Swonger AK, Matejski MP. *Nursing Pharmacology.* Glenview, IL: Scott, Foresman, 1988.

Teele DW, Klein JO, Rosner B, et al. Epidemiology of otitis media during first seven years of life in greater Boston: A prospective, cohort study. *J Inf Dis.* 1989;160:83-94.

Treatment of sexually transmitted diseases. *Med Let Drugs Ther.* 1988;3:15-22.

U.S. Department of Education. *What Works: Research About Teaching and Learning.* Washington, DC: U.S. Department of Education, 1986.

Waller JA. Alcohol and unintentional injury. In: Kissin B, Begleiter H, (eds). *The Biology of Alcoholism*, vol. 4. New York: Plenum.

Warren T. Incision and drainage of cutaneous abscesses and soft tissue infections. In: Roberts JR, (ed). *Clinical Procedures in Emergency Medicine*. Philadelphia: WB Saunders, 1985.

Weiner W Jr, Goetz CG, (eds). *Neurology for the Non-Neurologist*, 2nd ed. Philadelphia: JB Lippincott, 1989.

Welch J, Leichner P. Analysis of changing answers on multiple-choice examination for nationwide sample of Canadian psychiatry residents. *J Med Ed*. February 1988;133-135.

Williams RA. Visceral ischemic syndromes. In: Moore W, (ed). *Vascular Surgery, A Comprehensive Review*. New York: Grune & Stratton, 1983.

Wyngaarden JB, Smith LH, (eds). *Cecil Textbook of Medicine*, 18th ed. Philadelphia: WB Saunders, 1988.

Zarcone VP. Sleep hygiene. In: Kryger, Roth, Dement, (eds). *Principles and Practice of Sleep Medicine*. Philadelphia: WB Saunders, 1989.

Zawacki BE. The local effects of burn injury. In: Boswick JA, (ed). *The Art and Science of Burn Care*. Rockville, MD: Aspen Publishers, 1987.

Zwanger M. Legionnaire's disease. In: Tintinalli JE, Krome RL, Ruiz E., (eds). *Emergency Medicine, A Comprehensive Study Guide*. New York: McGraw-Hill, 1988.